Interpretation of Diagnostic Tests

Interpretation of Diagnostic Tests

A Synopsis of Laboratory Medicine

Fifth Edition

Jacques Wallach, M.D.
Clinical Professor of Pathology,
State University of New York
Health Science Center at Brooklyn;
Attending Pathologist,
Kings County Hospital,
Brooklyn, New York

Little, Brown and Company
Boston/Toronto/London

Fifth Edition

Library of Congress Catalog Card No. 91-75302

ISBN 0-316-92050-9

Printed in the United States of America

INTERPRETATION OF DIAGNOSTIC TESTS: A SYNOPSIS OF LABORATORY MEDICINE is published in the following translations:

First Edition

INTERPRETACIÓN DE LOS DIAGNÓSTICOS DE LABORATORIO: MANUAL SINÓPTICO DE BIOLOGÍA MÉDICA

Ἑρμηνεία τῶν Διαγνωστικῶν Ἐξετάσεων καὶ Δοκιμασιῶν: Συνοητικὸν Ἑγχειρίδιον Ἑργαστηριακῆς Ἰατρικῆς

INTERPRETAÇÃO DOṠ DIAGNÓSTICOS DE LABORATÓRIO

Second Edition

INTERPRETAZIONE DEI TESTS DI LABORATORIO IN MEDICINA

Third Edition

INTERPRETAÇÃO DOṠ DIAGNÓSTICOS DE LABORATÓRIO

INTERPRETAZIONE DEI TESTS DI LABORATORIO IN MEDICINA

INTERPRETACIÓN DE LOS DIAGNÓSTICOS DE LABORATORIO

Fourth Edition

INTERPRETAÇÃO DOṠ DIAGNÓSTICOS DE LABORATÓRIO

RRD-VA

To Doris
and
To Kim, Lisa, and Tracy

Contents

Preface to the Fifth Edition

The role of the laboratory in diagnosis and treatment continues to gain importance as newer tests and analytic methods allow diagnoses that were not possible before. Clinicians increasingly depend on laboratory test data. Now many diagnoses can only be established or etiologies confirmed or appropriate therapy selected by laboratory methods. In the past, laboratory tests were performed only after the history and physical examination had indicated the choice of tests. Currently, laboratory test results are part of most patient-physician encounters and often precede the history and physical examination; they contribute greatly to the selection of additional diagnostic and therapeutic procedures. This edition has been revised to assist in this expanded role of laboratory diagnosis as well as to help with the greater complexity, number, variety, and costs of available tests. With the increased use of reference and distant laboratories, clinicians have less opportunity to receive guidance from local laboratory directors. This book is meant to help clinicians meet these changes.

This fifth edition has been extensively rewritten and reorganized. New tests and recent applications are added, and uses and interpretations of old tests are updated; outmoded tests have been excluded. Technological advances have markedly improved the accuracy and diagnostic value of many tests and thereby altered their utilization and interpretation (e.g., distinguishing parathormone from peptides produced by tumors that simulate the clinical picture of excess hormone production). In some cases, the result has been replacement of older tests by more recent ones (e.g., urine 17-ketosteroids replaced by serum and urine cortisol for the diagnosis of Cushing's syndrome). Examples of new technology include tests based on monoclonal antibodies, DNA probes, polymerase chain reactions, immunochemical and cytochemical staining, and flow cytometry. More sophisticated tests have become more widely available. I have not included tests that are not widely available or established (e.g., cardiac myosin).

Various rare disorders or conditions in which the laboratory minimally contributes to diagnosis have been deleted from this edition in order to make room for newer information and still remain pocket sized. The tables on antibiotics have been removed because of rapid changes in this field and the availability of a number of small, dedicated antibiotic guides.

In Part III, Diseases of Organ Systems, the sequence of test findings has been changed so that the more useful or pathognomic findings are listed first and the incidental or less useful findings appear later. Emphasis is placed on whether findings establish, support, or rule out the diagnosis of that particular disease or are only nonspecific findings that should be noted to avoid confusion. Established diagnostic criteria for many diseases have been included (e.g., systemic lupus erythematosus and diabetes mellitus). Additional tables comparing stages of a disease and comparing similar disorders also appear.

Additional algorithms have been included. They illustrate the diagnostic logic and varying degree of importance of different tests in contrast to simple lists or tables that may lack a sense of direction about how to solve a diagnostic problem. The sequences shown in the flow charts are for illustrative purposes, although many times it is more cost effective or time efficient to perform some tests simultaneously or in a different sequence because they may be part of a test panel. A flow chart, a table of differential diagnosis, a collection of "pearls" (aphorisms), and a list of test findings are all ways of viewing the same disorder; convenience and utility will vary according to the diagnostic problem. They can serve as reminders or guides but none should be substituted for the clinician's judgment and experience. Final steps in the diagnostic workup may not be included because they are obvious or involve nonlaboratory modalities (e.g., imaging). As always in medicine, the reader must remember the complexities of multiple coexisting diseases or sequelae, different stages of disease, varying degree of severity, or the myriad concomitant, sequential, or complicating findings to be considered in the differential diagnosis. Note also that some disorders may appear in more than one category in an algorithm.

Sensitivity, specificity, and predictive values are included for more tests in this edition, but unfortunately there is still a dearth of such data in the literature. Space constraints and the basic nature of this book prevent in-depth explanation of the underlying principles but readers are urged to be familiar with Bayes' theorem and the utility of these concepts, as well as that of receiver-operating characteristic curves, odds, probability, likelihood ratio, and the effect of disease prevalence and level of test results, in order to best request and interpret laboratory data.

This edition has been extensively reorganized to eliminate the time-consuming need to search for information. Tests that refer to one disease are included only in that chapter about the disease. For example, serologic tests for syphilis are now incorporated in the chapter on infectious diseases rather than in a chapter on serologic tests; the same holds true for serologic tests for AIDS and hepatitis. Specific hormone tests are now in the chapter on endocrine diseases rather than in the chapter on normal blood levels. Coagulation tests appear in the chapter on hematologic diseases. Only tests that apply to multiple organ systems or are usually part of a "screening panel" remain in the chapter on core blood analytes. Reference (normal) ranges are included with these tests and a summary of all reference values now appears as a separate chapter so that a reader only needs to look up a value rather than to review a differential diagnosis for a disease. This emphasizes the clinical and diagnostic orientation and lessens the focus on laboratory tests per se, although the information about each test remains as complete as before.

I have not incorporated Système International (SI) units in the text because most physicians are not sufficiently accustomed to them and my goal remains to provide a simple, quick reference source. However, a table for converting SI and conventional units is included at the back.

In response to suggestions from some readers, more current references are included. There is also a new chapter on therapeutic drug monitoring, toxic substances, and drugs of abuse, reflecting the increased clinical importance of these topics.

The purposes of previous editions for the last two decades still hold true today. The value of this book is even greater now because of the larger number of tests available, their higher costs, and the determination of government and other third-party payers to restrain health costs. The utility of this book has been confirmed by the hundreds of thousands of copies in use in many languages, the many favorable comments received from all over the world, and the number of authors who have tried to emulate it. It is particularly gratifying that previous editions have been found so useful by a wide range of students (in medicine, dentistry, nursing, medical technology, and veterinary medicine) and colleagues in all of the clinical specialties as well as in pathology.

Making current medical information in its most useful form available to students and colleagues continues to be a most rewarding professional experience and a most important facet of my teaching and practice of laboratory medicine. For this reason, the fifth edition will have a companion electronic version for use on personal computers to allow more frequent updating at shorter intervals than is practical for a book. Electronic retrieval will also permit faster, simpler, easier cross-checking, and integrating data from various sections of the book (e.g., normal values, drug interferences, and alterations in various diseases) as an "electronic index."

These changes have been made without losing the organization, format, style, pocket-size portability, ease of use, nominal cost, thoroughness, and practicality of current information, which were the goals of previous editions.

I continue to welcome suggestions, ideas, and criticisms from all readers.

J. W.

Preface to the Previous Editions

Results of laboratory tests may aid in
- Discovering occult disease
- Preventing irreparable damage (e.g., phenylketonuria)
- Early diagnosis after onset of signs or symptoms
- Differential diagnosis of various possible diseases
- Determining the stage of the disease
- Estimating the activity of the disease
- Detecting the recurrence of disease
- Monitoring the effect of therapy
- Genetic counseling in familial conditions
- Medicolegal problems, such as paternity suits

This book is written to help the physician achieve these purposes with the least amount of
- Duplication of tests
- Waste of patient's money
- Overtaxing of laboratory facilities and personnel
- Loss of physician's time
- Confusion caused by the increasing number, variety, and complexity of tests currently available. Some of these tests may be unrequested but performed as part of routine surveys or hospital admission multitest screening.

In order to provide quick reference and maximum availability and usefulness, this handy-sized book features
- Tabular and graphic style of concise presentation
- Emphasis on serial time changes in laboratory findings in various stages of disease
- Omission of rarely performed, irrelevant, esoteric, and outmoded laboratory tests
- Exclusion of discussion of physiologic mechanisms, metabolic pathways, clinical features, and nonlaboratory aspects of disease
- Discussion of only the more important diseases that the physician encounters and should be able to diagnose

This book is not
- An encyclopedic compendium of clinical pathology
- A technical manual
- A substitute for good clinical judgment and basic knowledge of medicine

Deliberately omitted are
- Technical procedures and directions
- Photographs and illustrations of anatomic changes (e.g., blood cells, karyotypes, isotope scans)
- Discussions of quality control
- Selection of a referral laboratory
- Performance of laboratory tests in the clinician's own office
- Bibliographic references, except for the most general reference texts in medicine, hematology, and clinical pathology and for some recent references to specific conditions

The usefulness and need for a book of this style, organization, and contents have been increased by such current trends as
- The frequent lack of personal assistance, advice, and consultation in large commercial laboratories and hospital departments of clinical pathology, which are often specialized and fragmented as well as impersonal
- Greater demand for the physician's time

The development of many new tests

The lack of adequate teaching of laboratory medicine in most medical schools. Faculty and administrators still assume that this essential area of medicine can be learned "intuitively" as it was 20 years ago and that it therefore requires little formal training. This attitude ignores changes in the number and variety of tests now available as well as their increased sophistication and basic value in establishing a diagnosis

The contents of this book are organized to answer the questions most often posed by physicians when they require assistance from the pathologist. There is no other single adequate source of information presented in this fashion. It appears from numerous comments I have received that this book has succeeded in meeting the needs not only of practicing physicians and medical students but also of pathologists, technologists, and other medical personnel. It has been adopted by many schools of nursing and of medical technology, physicians assistant training programs, and medical schools. Such widespread acceptance confirms my original premise in writing this book and is most gratifying.

A perusal of the table of contents and index will quickly show the general organization of the material by type of laboratory test or organ system or certain other categories. In order to maintain a concise format, separate chapters have not been organized for such categories as newborn, pediatric, and geriatric periods or for primary psychiatric or dermatologic diseases. A complete index provides maximum access to this information.

Obviously these data are not original but have been adapted from many sources over the years. Only the selection, organization, manner of presentation, and emphasis are original. I have formulated this point of view during 40 years as a clinician and pathologist, viewing with pride the important and growing role of the laboratory but deeply regretting its inappropriate utilization.

This book was written to improve laboratory utilization by making it simpler for the physician to select and interpret the most useful laboratory tests for his clinical problems.

J. W.

Acknowledgments

I thank my colleagues in various parts of the world who have shared their clinical and laboratory problems with me. The universal need to convert an ever-expanding mass of raw laboratory data into accessible, clinically usable information has become a matter of increasing significance throughout the medical community and a chief concern of mine in producing this book and in other teaching and research efforts. The need for expeditious, unencumbered information has been repeatedly confirmed during the teaching of medical students and house officers, in the daily practice of clinical pathology, by discussions with physicians in many countries that I have visited or in which I have worked or taught, and by the translation of these volumes into various languages. I am rewarded by numerous instances of friendship, criticism, kindness, and help, and by learning far more than I could include in this small volume. I continue to be gratified and stimulated beyond expectation.

My thanks to the staff of Little, Brown and Company, especially to Jon Sarner, Editorial Assistant Marie Salter, and Editorial Intern Terri Blow, who performed meticulous, difficult, day-to-day work on the raw manuscript; Susan Pioli and Lynne Herndon for their outstanding help and cooperation; and Betty Herr Hallinger who again prepared an outstanding index that greatly facilitates the use of this book.

The friendship, love, care, and generosity of my wife Doris can never be sufficiently acknowledged.

I
Normal Values

Notice

The indications and dosages of all drugs in this book have been recommended in the medical literature and conform to the practices of the general medical community. The medications described do not necessarily have specific approval by the Food and Drug Administration for use in the diseases and dosages for which they are recommended. The package insert for each drug should be consulted for use and dosage as approved by the FDA. Because standards for usage change, it is advisable to keep abreast of revised recommendations, particularly those concerning new drugs.

1

Normal Blood Levels (Reference Values)

INTRODUCTION TO NORMAL VALUES (REFERENCE RANGES)

In the majority of laboratory measurements, the combination of short-term physiologic variation and analytic error is sufficient to render the interpretation of single determinations difficult when the concentrations are in the borderline range.

The reader must always keep in mind that all values given in this book are to be used as general guidelines rather than rigid separations of normal from abnormal or diseased from healthy. Considerable variation in test results is due not only to instrumentation, methodology, and other laboratory techniques but also to more subtle preanalytic factors such as position or condition of patient (e.g., supine or upright, fasting or postprandial), time of day, age, sex, climate, effect of diet or drugs, characteristics of test population. It is therefore essential that the clinician use the reference ranges from the laboratory that is performing those particular tests and which it has determined for its own procedures, patient population, etc. Too many misunderstandings result from attempts to apply normal ranges of one laboratory to test results from another laboratory. Misinterpretation of laboratory data due to this error, as well as from overemphasizing the significance of borderline values, has caused immeasurable emotional pain and economic waste for innumerable patients. The clinician is referred elsewhere for more detailed discussions of this topic.

Special notation should be made on the laboratory test request form when it is particularly germane to a test, e.g., time when blood is drawn is important when the tested component is subject to marked diurnal variation (cortisol, iron), relation to meals (glucose) or IV infusions (electrolytes), source of specimen (arterial or capillary rather than venous blood). Many tests can be properly interpreted only when such information is known.

Some tests are performed too infrequently to be included in this list; other tests have such wide reference ranges that interlaboratory utility is limited.

A review of the texts, reference books, and current literature in clinical pathology often reveals surprising and considerable discrepancy between well-known sources. The following pages of normal laboratory values were summarized from my own experience as well as what seemed to be the best and most current sources of data available.

I have used my own experience and clinical judgment in selecting the most useful data to be included.

Some analytes are very specialized, and these values appear with the disorder in question rather than in the section on normal values (e.g., hormone levels, microbiologic data in chapter on infectious diseases).

GENERAL PRINCIPLES

Many clinicians are still largely unaware of the reasoning process that they pursue in seeking a diagnosis and tend to follow an empirical path that was previously successful or was learned during early training periods by observing their mentors during clinical rounds without appreciating the rationale for selecting, ordering, and interpreting laboratory tests; this is often absorbed in a subliminal, informal, or rote fashion. The need to control health care costs and many recent studies on laboratory test utilization have emphasized the need for a selective approach.

Table 1-1. Normal Leukocyte Differential Count in Peripheral Blood

	Segmented Neutrophils		Band* Neutrophils		Eosinophils		Basophils		Lymphocytes		Monocytes	
Age	%	No./ cu mm	%	No./ cu mm	%	No./ cu mm	%	No./ cu mm	%	No./ cu mm	%	No./ cu mm
At birth	47 ± 15	8400	14.1 ± 4	2540	2.2	400	0.6	100	31 ± 5	5500	5.8	1050
12 hr	53	12,100	15.2	3460	2.0	450	0.4	100	24	5500	5.3	1200
24 hr	47	8870	14.2	2680	2.4	450	0.5	100	31	5800	5.8	1100
1 wk	34	4100	11.8	1420	4.1	500	0.4	50	41	5000	9.1	1100
2 wk	29	3320	10.5	1200	3.1	350	0.4	50	48	5500	8.8	1000
4 wk	25 ± 10	2750	9.5 ± 3	1150	2.8	300	0.5	50	56 ± 15	6000	6.5	700
2 mo	25	2750	8.4	1100	2.7	300	0.5	50	57	6300	5.9	650
4 mo	24	2730	8.9	1000	2.6	300	0.4	50	59	6800	5.2	600
6 mo	23	2710	8.8	1000	2.5	300	0.4	50	61	7300	4.8	580
8 mo	22	2680	8.3	1000	2.5	300	0.4	50	62	7600	4.7	580

10 mo	22	2600	8.3	1000	2.5	300	0.4	50	63	7500	4.6	550
12 mo	23	2680	8.1	990	2.6	300	0.4	50	61	7000	4.8	550
2 yr	25	2660	8.0	850	2.6	280	0.5	50	59	6300	5.0	530
4 yr	34 ± 11	3040	8.0 ± 3	710	2.8	250	0.6	50	50 ± 15	4500	5.0	450
6 yr	43	3600	8.0	670	2.7	230	0.6	50	42	3500	4.7	400
8 yr	45	3700	8.0	660	2.4	200	0.6	50	39	3300	4.2	350
10 yr	46 ± 15	3700	8.0 ± 3	645	2.4	200	0.5	40	38 ± 10	3100	4.3	350
12 yr	47	3700	8.0	640	2.5	200	0.5	40	38	3000	4.4	350
14 yr	48	3700	8.0	640	2.5	200	0.5	40	37	2900	4.7	380
16 yr	49 ± 15	3800	8.0 ± 3	620	2.6	200	0.5	40	35 ± 10	2800	5.1	400
18 yr	49	3800	8.0	620	2.6	200	0.5	40	35	2700	5.2	400
20 yr	51	3800	8.0	620	2.7	200	0.5	40	33	2500	5.0	380
21 yr	51 ± 15	3800	8.0 ± 3	620	2.7	200	0.5	40	34 ± 10	2500	4.0	300

*Note that these values are higher than those found in other references. They have been obtained by using strict criteria in differentiating segmented from band forms. I do not classify a neutrophil as a segmented form unless a typical threadlike filament is visible.

Source: Data from JB Miale, *Laboratory Medicine—Hematology* (6th ed.). St. Louis: Mosby, 1982; average values based on the average leukocyte counts taken from EC Albritton, *Standard Values in Blood*. Philadelphia: Saunders, 1952.

Table 1-2. Normal Values for Red Corpuscles at Various Ages

Age	Red Cell Count (millions/cu mm)	Hemoglobin (gm/dl)	Vol. Packed RBC (ml/dl)	Corpuscular Values			
				MCV (cu μ)	MCH (γγ)	MCHC (%)	MCD (μ)
First day	5.1 ± 1.0	19.5 ± 5.0	54.0 ± 10.0	106	38	36	8.6
2–3 days	5.1	19.0	53.5	105	37	35	
4–8 days	5.1	18.3 ± 4.0	52.5	103	36	35	
9–13 days	5.0	16.5	49.0	98	33	34	
14–60 days	4.7 ± 0.9	14.0 ± 3.3	42.0 ± 7.0	90	30	33	8.1
3–5 mo	4.5 ± 0.7	12.2 ± 2.3	36.0	80	27	34	7.7
6–11 mo	4.6	11.8	35.5 ± 5.0	77	26	33	7.4
1 yr	4.5	11.2	35.0	78	25	32	7.3
2 yr	4.6	11.5	35.5	77	25	32	
3 yr	4.5	12.5	36.0	80	27	35	7.4
4 yr	4.6 ± 0.6	12.6	37.0	80	27	34	
5 yr	4.6	12.6	37.0	80	27	34	
6–10 yr	4.7	12.9	37.5	80	27	34	7.4
11–15 yr	4.8	13.4	39.0	82	28	34	
Adults							
Females	4.8 ± 0.6	14.0 ± 2.0	42.0 ± 5.0	87 ± 5	29 ± 2	34 ± 2	7.5 ± 0.3
Males	5.4 ± 0.8	16.0 ± 2.0	47.0 ± 5.0	87 ± 5	29 ± 2	34 ± 2	7.5 ± 0.3

MCV = mean corpuscular volume; MCH = mean corpuscular hemoglobin; MCHC = mean corpuscular hemoglobin concentration; MCD = mean corpuscular diameter.

Source: Data from MM Wintrobe et al., *Clinical Hematology* (8th ed.). Philadelphia: Lea & Febiger, 1981. P. 1891.

Some important principles in utilizing laboratory (and all other) tests are as follows:

1. Under the best of circumstances, no test is perfect (e.g., 100% sensitivity, specificity, predictive value). In any specific case, the results may be misleading.
2. Choosing tests should be based on the prior probability of the diagnosis being sought, which affects the predictive value of the test. This prior probability is determined by the history, physical examination, and prevalence of the disorder being sought, which is why history and physical examination should precede ordering tests.
3. Any particular laboratory result may be incorrect for a large variety of reasons regardless of the high quality of the laboratory; all such results should be rechecked. If indicated, a new specimen sample should be submitted, with careful confirmation of patient identification, prompt delivery to the laboratory, and immediate processing; in some circumstances, confirmation of test results at another laboratory may be indicated.
4. The greater the degree of abnormality of the test result, the more likely that a confirmed abnormality is significant or represents a real disorder.
5. Tables of reference values represent statistical data for 95% of the population; values outside of these ranges do not necessarily represent disease. Results may still be within the reference range but be elevated above the patient's baseline, which is why serial testing is important in a number of conditions. For example, in acute myocardial infarction, the rise in serum total creatine kinase (CK) may be abnormal for that patient although the value may be within "normal" range.
6. An individual's test values, when performed in a good laboratory, tend to remain fairly constant over a period of years when performed with comparable technology; comparison of results with previous values obtained when the patient was not ill (if available) is often a better reference value than "normal" ranges.
7. Multiple test abnormalities are more likely to be significant than single test abnormalities. When two or more tests for the same disorder are positive, the results reinforce the diagnosis, but when only one test is positive and the other is not positive, the strength of the interpretation is diluted.
8. Characteristic laboratory test profiles that are described in the literature and in this book represent the full-blown picture of the well-developed or far-advanced case, but all abnormal tests may be present simultaneously in only a small fraction (e.g., one-third) of patients with that condition.
9. Excessive repetition of tests is wasteful, and the excess burden increases the possibility of laboratory errors. Appropriate intervals between tests should be dictated by the patient's clinical condition.
10. Tests should only be performed if they will alter the patient's diagnosis, prognosis, treatment, or management. Incorrect test values or isolated individual variation in results may cause "Ulysses syndrome" and result in loss of time, money, and peace of mind.
11. Clerical errors are far more likely than technical errors to cause incorrect results. Greatest care should be taken to completely and properly label and identify every specimen, which should *always* be accompanied by a test requisition form. Busy hospital laboratories receive inordinate numbers of unlabelled, unidentified specimens each day, which are useless, burdensome, and sometimes dangerous.
12. Reference ranges vary from one laboratory to another; the user should know what these ranges are for each laboratory used and should also be aware of variations due to age, sex, race, size, and physiologic status (e.g., pregnancy, lactation) that apply to the particular patient. These "normal" ranges represent collected statistical data rather than classification of patients as having disease or being healthy. This is best illustrated in the use of *multitest* chemical profiles for screening persons known to be free of disease. The

probability of any given test being abnormal is about 2–5%, and the probability of disease if a screening test is abnormal is generally low (0–15%). The frequency of abnormal single tests is 1.5% (albumin) to 5.9% (glucose) and up to 16.6% for sodium. Based on statistical expectations, when a panel of 8 tests is performed in a multiphasic health program, 25% of the patients have one or more abnormal results, and when the panel includes 20 tests, 55% have one or more test abnormalities.*

13. The effect of drugs on laboratory test values must never be overlooked. The clinician should always be aware of what the patient has been taking, including over-the-counter medications, vitamins, iron, etc. These effects may produce false negative as well as false positive results; for example, vitamin C may produce a false negative test for occult blood in the stool.

HEMATOLOGY REFERENCE VALUES

Complete blood count (CBC)	
Leukocyte (WBC) count	4300–10,800/cu mm (see Tables 1-1 and 1-2, pp. 4–6)
Methemoglobin	< 3% of total
Carboxyhemoglobin	< 5% of total
Haptoglobins	Genetic absence in 1% of population
Newborns	Absent in 90%; 10 mg/dl in 10%
1–6 months	Gradual increase to 30 mg/dl
6 months–17 years	40–180 mg/dl
Adults	40–270 mg/dl
Osmotic fragility of RBC	Increased if hemolysis occurs in > 0.5% NaCl Decreased if incomplete in 0.3% NaCl
Erythrocyte sedimentation rate (ESR)	
Wintrobe	
Males	0–10 mm in 1 hour
Females	0–15 mm in 1 hour
Westergren	
Males	0–13 mm in 1 hour
Females	0–20 mm in 1 hour
Blood volume	
Males	75 ml/kg body weight
Females	67 ml/kg body weight (8.5–9.0% body weight in kg)
Plasma volume	
Males	44 ml/kg body weight
Females	43 ml/kg body weight
RBC volume	
Males	30 ml/kg body weight
Females	24 ml/kg body weight
RBC survival time (^{51}Cr)	Half-life: 25–35 days
Reticulocyte count	0.5–2.5% of erythrocytes
Plasma iron turnover rate	38 mg/24 hours (0.47 mg/kg)
Delta-aminolevulinic acid	1.5–7.5 mg/24-hour urine

*Data from GD Friedman et al., Biochemical screening tests: Effect of panel size on medical care. *Arch Intern Med* 129:91, 1972.

Ferritin	
Newborns	25–200 ng/ml
1 month	200–600 ng/ml
2–5 months	50–200 ng/ml
6 months–15 years	7–142 ng/ml
Adult males	20–300 ng/ml
Adult females	20–120 ng/ml
Borderline (males or females)	10–20 ng/ml
Iron excess	> 400 ng/ml
Hemoglobin electrophoresis	
Hgb A	
0–30 days	10–40%
6 months–adult	> 95%
Hgb A2	
0–30 days	< 1%
1 year–adult	1.5–3.0%
Borderline	3.0–3.5%
HgbF	< 2%
No abnormal Hgb variants	
Hemoglobin F, RBC	Hgb F remaining in < 1% of RBC
Hemoglobin, plasma	
≥ 18 years old	< 15 mg/dl
Infants and neonates	May be higher
Hemosiderin, urine	Negative
Iron, liver tissue	530–900 μg/gm dry weight
Iron, urine	100–300 ng/24 hours
Iron, serum	
0–30 days	95–225 μg/dl
1–48 months	60–116 μg/dl
5–17 years	50–200 μg/dl
Adult males	75–175 μg/dl
Adult females	65–165 μg/dl
Iron-binding capacity	250–450 μg/dl
% saturation	20–50%
Transferrin	240–480 mg/dl
Ceruloplasmin	23–43 mg/dl
Copper	75–145 μg/dl
Leukocyte alkaline phosphatase (LAP) score	Score of 40–100
Lysozyme (muramidase), plasma	0.2–15.8 μg/ml
Lysozyme (muramidase), urine	< 3 mg/24 hours
Myoglobin, serum	90 ng/ml
Myoglobin, urine	0–2 mg/ml
Glucose 6-phosphate dehydrogenase (G-6-PD) erythrocyte	
2–17 years	6.4–15.6 units/gm hemoglobin
≥ 18 years	8.6–18.6 units/gm hemoglobin
Pyruvate kinase, erythrocyte	2.0–8.8 units/gm hemoglobin
Folate	Low: < 2.0 ng/ml Normal: 2.0–20.0 ng/ml Elevated: > 20.0 ng/ml
Vitamin B_{12} assay	Low: < 100 pg/ml Indeterminate: 100–200 pg/ml Normal: 200–1100 pg/ml Elevated: > 1100 pg/ml
Unsaturated vitamin B_{12}–binding capacity	870–1800 pg/ml
Urobilinogen, urine	< 4 mg/24 hours
Urobilinogen, stool	50–300 mg/24 hours

BLOOD COAGULATION TESTS—REFERENCE VALUES

Platelet count	140,000–340,000/cu mm (Rees-Ecker) 150,000–350,000/cu mm (Coulter counter)
Bleeding time (Simplate)	3.0–9.5 minutes
Clot retraction, qualitative	Begins in 30–60 minutes; complete within 24 hours, usually within 6 hours
Coagulation time (Lee-White)	6–17 minutes (glass tubes) 19–60 minutes (siliconized tubes)
Euglobulin lysis	No lysis in 2 hours
Fibrinogen split products	Negative at > 1 : 4 dilution Positive at > 1 : 8 dilution
Fibrinolysins	No clot lysis in 24 hours
Partial thromboplastin time, activated (aPTT)	25–38 seconds
Prothrombin time (PT), one stage	±2 seconds of control (control should be 11–16 seconds)
Thrombin time (TT)	±5 seconds of control
Coagulation factor assay	
I (fibrinogen)	150–350 mg/dl
II (prothrombin)	60–140%
V (accelerator globulin)	60–140%
VII (proconvertin-Stuart)	70–130%
VIII (antihemophilic globulin)	50–200%
IX	60–140%
X (Stuart factor)	70–130%
XI	60–140%
XII (Hageman factor)	60–140%
XIII	50–200%
Factor VIII related antigen	45–185%
Coagulator factor VIII inhibitor	Negative
Platelet aggregation	Full response to adenosine diphosphate (ADP), epinephrine and collagen
Platelet antibody	Negative
Ristocetin-Willebrand factor	45–140%
Antithrombin III, plasma	
Immunologic	17–30 mg/dl
Functional	80–120%
Protein S	
Total, plasma	60–140%
Free, plasma	60–140%
Whole blood clot lysis	No clot lysis in 24 hours

BLOOD CHEMISTRIES—REFERENCE VALUES

(alphabetic)

These values will vary, depending on the individual laboratory as well as the methods used. Each clinician should compare the transferability of these data to their own situation.

Acetone	0.3–2.0 mg/dl
Aldolase	
0–3 years	< 16.3 units/L
4–16 years	< 8.3 units/L
Adults (≥ 17 years)	< 7.4 units/L

Ammonia			12–55 μg/dl
Amylase (total)			
< 18 years			0–260 units/L
adults (≥ 18 years)			35–115 units/L
Base, excess			
Newborns			−10 to −2 mEq/L
Infants			−7 to −1 mEq/L
Children			−4 to +2 mEq/L
Adults			−2 to +3 mEq/L
Bicarbonate			
	Age (years)		
	Males	**Females**	
	1–2	1–3	17–25 mEq/L
	3–4	4–5	18–26 mEq/L
	4–5	6–7	19–27 mEq/L
	6–7	8–9	20–28 mEq/L
	≥ 8*	≥ 10*	21–29 mEq/L
Bilirubin			
Total			< 1.6 mg/dl
Direct			
1 month–adult			< 0.5 mg/dl
Calcium			
	Age (years)		
	Males	**Females**	
Total			
	1–14	1–11	9.6–10.6 mg/dl
	15–16		9.5–10.5 mg/dl
	17–18	12–14	9.5–10.5 mg/dl
	19–21		9.3–10.3 mg/dl
	> 21*	> 18*	8.9–10.1 mg/dl
Ionized			
	1–19	1–17	4.9–5.5 mg/dl
	≥ 20*	> 18*	4.75–5.3 mg/dl
Carbon dioxide			
Total (content)			
Arterial			19–24 mEq/L
Venous			22–26 mEq/L
PCO_2 arterial or capillary			
Infants			27–40 mm Hg
Male adults			35–48 mm Hg
Female adults			32–45 mm Hg
PCO_2 venous			6–7 mm Hg > arterial blood
Ceruloplasmin			23–43 mg/dl
Chloride			
1–17 years			102–112 mEq/L
≥ 18 years			100–108 mEq/L
Cholesterol (see Lipid Fractionation, p. 14)			
Cholinesterase			
Plasma			7–25 units/ml
RBC			0.65–1.3 pH units
Copper			70–150 μg/dl

*Adult values.

Creatine kinase (CK) (Ektachem)	
1–3 years	60–305 units/L
4–6 years	75–230 units/L
7–9 years	60–365 units/L
Males	
10–11 years	55–215 units/L
12–13 years	60–330 units/L
14–15 years	60–335 units/L
16–19 years	55–370 units/L
Females	
10–11 years	80–230 units/L
12–13 years	50–295 units/L
14–15 years	50–240 units/L
16–19 years	45–230 units/L
Creatine kinase isoenzymes	MB < 5%
Creatinine	

Age (years) Males	Females	
1–2	1–3	0.2–0.6 mg/dl
3–4	4–5	0.3–0.7 mg/dl
5–9	6–8	0.5–0.8 mg/dl
10–11	≥ 9*	0.6–0.9 mg/dl
12–13		0.6–1.0 mg/dl
14–15		0.7–1.1 mg/dl
≥ 16*		0.8–1.2 mg/dl

Cryoglobulins	0
Fibrinogen	150–350 mg/dl
Gamma-glutamyl transpeptidase (GGT) (Ektachem)	
1–3 years	6–19 units/L
4–6 years	10–22 units/L
7–9 years	13–25 units/L
Males	
10–11 years	17–30 units/L
12–13 years	17–44 units/L
14–15 years	12–33 units/L
16–19 years	11–34 units/L
Females	
10–11 years	17–28 units/L
12–13 years	14–25 units/L
14–15 years	14–26 units/L
16–19 years	11–28 units/L
Glucose (fasting)	60–100 mg/dl (depends on method)
Iron, serum	
0–30 days	95–225 μg/dl
1–48 months	60–116 μg/dl
5–17 years	50–200 μg/dl
Adult males	75–175 μg/dl
Adult females	65–165 μg/dl
Iron-binding capacity	250–450 μg/dl
% saturation	20–50%
Isocitric dehydrogenase (ICD)	3–85 units/L

*Adult values.

Lactic acid	
Venous	4.5–23 mg/dl
Arterial	4.5–14 mg/dl
Lactic dehydrogenase (LDH) (Ektachem)	
1–3 years	500–920 units/L
4–6 years	470–900 units/L
7–9 years	420–750 units/L
Males	
10–11 years	432–700 units/L
12–13 years	470–750 units/L
14–15 years	360–730 units/L
16–19 years	340–670 units/L
Females	
10–11 years	380–770 units/L
12–13 years	380–640 units/L
14–15 years	390–580 units/L
16–19 years	340–670 units/L
Lactic dehydrogenase isoenzymes	
I	17–28%
II	30–36%
III	19–25%
IV	10–16%
V	6–13%
Lead	< 20 μg/dl
Leucine aminopeptidase (LAP)	Depends on method
Lipase	< 1.5 units/ml
Lipid fractionation (see Tables 1-3 and 1-4, pp. 14 and 15)	
Cholesterol esters	60–75% of total
Phospholipids	180–320 mg/dl
Magnesium	1.7–2.1 mg/dl
Myoglobin, serum	≤ 90 ng/ml
Osmolality	275–295 mOsm/kg
Oxygen	
Saturation, arterial	96–100% of capacity
Tension, PO_2 arterial	
While breathing room air	
Newborns	60–75 mm Hg
< 60 years	> 85 mm Hg
60 years	> 80 mm Hg
70 years	> 70 mm Hg
80 years	> 60 mm Hg
90 years	> 50 mm Hg
While breathing 100% oxygen	> 500 mm Hg
pH, arterial	7.35–7.45
Phenylalanine	
≤ 1 week	0.69–2.05 mg/dl
< 1 month	0–2 mg/dl
< 16 years	0.43–1.42 mg/dl
≥ 16 years	0.68–1.12 mg/dl
Tyrosine	
≤ 1 week	0.60–2.20 mg/dl
< 16 years	0.47–1.34 mg/dl
≥ 16 years	0.82–1.99 mg/dl
Prostate specific antigen	
> 40 years	≤ 4.0 ng/ml
≤ 40 years	≤ 2.7 ng/ml
Prostatic acid phosphatase (PAP), serum	< 3.7 ng/ml

Table 1-3. Lipid Fractionation—Desirable Levels*

	Cholesterol (mg/dl)						Triglycerides (mg/dl)				
	Males		Females		Males	Females
Age (years)	5p 95p	75p†	5p 95p	75p†	5p 95p	5p 95p
5–9	126–191	172	122–209	173	27–102	34–76
10–14	130–204	179	124–217	174	30–103	33–121
15–19	114–198	167	125–212	175	31–124	32–122
20–24	128–216	185	128–209	181	34–137	32–97
25–29	140–236	202	134–218	190	40–157	33–100
30–34	150–250	216	141–229	199	43–171	35–106
35–39	156–264	226	147–240	209	45–182	38–110
40–44	162–274	235	155–253	219	48–189	40–117
45–49	166–280	242	162–265	229	50–193	41–122
50–54	170–286	246	171–278	241	50–195	43–128
55–59	173–291	250	179–291	253	51–197	45–134
60–64	175–295	253	188–306	265	51–198	47–140
65–69	176–298	255	197–320	278	51–199	50–147
70–74	177–299	256	207–336	291	51–199	52–154
> 74	178–300	257	217–352	306	51–199	54–162

p = percentile (e.g., 5p = 5th percentile).
*Data are presented as "desirable levels" rather than "reference ranges" or "normal values."
†75th percentile has been recommended as upper limit for serum cholesterol and LDL cholesterol.

Phosphatase, acid, serum
- Adult males: 2.5–11.7 units/L
- Adult females: 0.3–9.2 units/L

Phosphatase, alkaline (Ektachem)
- 1–3 years: 145–320 units/L
- 4–6 years: 150–380 units/L
- 7–9 years: 175–420 units/L
- Males
  - 10–11 years: 135–530 units/L
  - 12–13 years: 200–495 units/L
  - 14–15 years: 130–525 units/L
  - 16–19 years: 65–260 units/L
- Females
  - 10–11 years: 130–560 units/L
  - 12–13 years: 105–420 units/L
  - 14–15 years: 70–230 units/L
  - 16–19 years: 50–130 units/L

Phosphorus

Age (years)		
Male	Female	
1–4	1–7	4.3–5.4 mg/dl
5–13		3.7–5.4 mg/dl
	8–13	4.0–5.2 mg/dl
14–15		3.5–5.3 mg/dl
	14–15	3.5–4.9 mg/dl
16–17	16–17	3.1–4.7 mg/dl
≥ 18*	≥ 18*	2.5–4.5 mg/dl

*Adult values.

Table 1-4. Lipid Fractionation—Desirable Levels*

	HDL Cholesterol				LDL Cholesterol			
	Males		Females		Males		Females	
Age (years)	5p 95p	70p	5p 95p	70p	5p 95p	75p†	5p 95p	75p†
6–11	30–70	55	34–65	59	60–140	114	60–150	114
12–14	30–65	50	30–65	49	60–140	111	60–150	114
15–19	30–60	53	33–65	47	60–140	113	60–150	118
20–29	30–65	55	34–75	47	60–175	131	60–160	128
30–39	30–70	60	35–80	47	70–190	147	70–170	140
40–49	30–70	63	35–80	47	70–205	160	80–190	150
> 50	30–70	65	35–80	47	80–220	170	80–200	164

p = percentile (e.g., 5p = 5th percentile).
*Data are presented as "desirable levels" rather than "reference ranges" or "normal values."
†75th percentile has been recommended as upper limit for serum cholesterol and LDL cholesterol.

Potassium	
1–16 years	3.7–5.0 mEq/L
≥ 16 years	3.6–4.8 mEq/L

Proteins, serum (Behring LN Nephelometer)	Total (gm/dl)	Albumin (gm/dl)
< 5 days	5.4–7.0	2.6–3.6
1–3 years	5.9–7.0	3.4–4.2
4–6 years	5.9–7.8	3.5–5.2
7–9 years	6.2–8.1	3.7–5.6
10–19 years	6.3–8.6	3.7–5.6

Globulin	2.3–3.5 gm/dl
Prealbumin	18–36 mg/dl
Electrophoresis	
Albumin	52–68% of total
Globulin	
$Alpha_1$	4.2–7.2% of total
$Alpha_2$	6.8–12.0% of total
Beta	9.3–15.0% of total
Gamma	13–23% of total
$Alpha_1$ antitrypsin	> 180 mg/dl
Z heterozygotes	79–171 mg/dl
Z homozygotes	19–31 mg/dl
Haptoglobins	Genetic absence in 1% of population
Newborns	Absent in 90%; 10 mg/dl in 10%
1–6 months	Gradual increase to 30 mg/dl
6 months–17 years	40–180 mg/dl
Adults	40–270 mg/dl
Transferrin	240–480 mg/dl
Total complement	25–110 units
C1 esterase inhibitor	8–24 mg/dl
C1q complement component	7–15 mg/dl
C2 (second component of complement)	50–250% of normal
C3 (third component of complement)	70–150 mg/dl

C4 (fourth component of complement) 10–30 mg/dl
C5 (fifth component of complement) 9–18 mg/dl
Fibrinogen 150–400 mg/dl
Cryoglobulins 0

Immunoglobulins

	IgG (mg/dl)	IgA (mg/dl)	IgM (mg/dl)
0–4 months	141–930	5–64	14–142
5–8 months	250–1190	10–87	24–167
9–11 months	320–1250	17–94	
1–3 years	400–1250		
1–2 years			35–242 F†
			35–200 M†
2–3 years		24–192	41–242 F
			41–200 M
4–6 years	560–1307	26–232	
7–9 years	598–1379	26–232	
10–12 years	638–1453	45–285	
13–15 years	680–1531	47–317	
16–17 years	724–1511	55–377	
≥ 18 years*	700–1500	60–400	60–300
4–17 years			56–242 F
			47–200 M

IgE

	Mean (units/ml)	+2SD (units/ml)
Cord serum	< 12	< 12
1–11 months	< 12	56
1 year	< 12	83
2–4 years	< 12	130
5–80 years	20	367

IgD 0–14 mg/dl

Sodium 135–145 mEq/L

Transaminase (Ektachem)

SGOT (AST)

1–3 years	20–60 units/L
4–6 years	15–50 units/L
7–9 years	15–40 units/L
Males	
10–11 years	10–60 units/L
12–15 years	15–40 units/L
16–19 years	10–45 units/L
Females	
10–11 years	10–40 units/L
12–15 years	10–30 units/L
16–19 years	5–30 units/L

SGPT (ALT) (Ektachem)

1–3 years	5–45 units/L
4–6 years	10–25 units/L
7–9 years	10–35 units/L
Males	
10–11 years	10–35 units/L
12–13 years	10–55 units/L

*Adult values.
†F = females; M = males.

14–15 years	10–45 units/L
16–19 years	10–40 units/L
Females	
10–13 years	10–30 units/L
14–15 years	5–30 units/L
16–19 years	5–35 units/L
Urea nitrogen (BUN)	
1–3 years	10–36 mg/dl
4–13 years	15–36 mg/dl
14–19 years	17–45 mg/dl
Uric acid	
Females	
1–4 years	2.2–5.1 mg/dl
5–6 years	2.3–5.3 mg/dl
7–8 years	2.3–5.5 mg/dl
9–12 years	2.3–5.8 mg/dl
≥ 13 years*	2.3–6.0 mg/dl
Males	
1–10 years	2.4–5.4 mg/dl
11–12 years	2.8–6.0 mg/dl
13–14 years	3.5–7.0 mg/dl
15–16 years	4.1–7.9 mg/dl
≥ 17 years*	4.3–8.0 mg/dl

NORMAL BLOOD AND URINE HORMONE LEVELS

Adrenocorticotropic hormone (ACTH), plasma	≤ 60 pg/ml
Aldosterone, serum	
0–3 weeks	16.5–154.0 ng/dl
1–11 months	6.5–86.0 ng/dl
1–10 years	
Supine	3.0–39.5 ng/dl
Upright	3.5–124.0 ng/dl
≥ 11 years	1–21 ng/dl
Aldosterone, urine	
0–30 days	7–11 μg/24 hrs
1–11 months	0.7–22.0 μg/24 hrs
≥ 1 year	2–16 μg/24 hours

Androstenedione, serum	**Males**	**Females**
0–7 years	0.1–0.2 ng/ml	0.1–0.3 ng/ml
8–9 years	0.1–0.3 ng/ml	0.2–0.5 ng/ml
10–11 years	0.3–0.7 ng/ml	0.4–1.0 ng/ml
12–13 years	0.4–1.0 ng/ml	0.8–1.9 ng/ml
14–17 years	0.5–1.4 ng/ml	0.7–2.2 ng/ml
≥ 18 years	0.3–3.1 ng/ml	0.2–3.1 ng/ml

Angiotensin converting enzyme, serum (SACE)	
≤ 1 year	10.9–42.1 μ/L
1–2 years	9.4–36.0 μ/L
3–4 years	7.9–29.8 μ/L
5–9 years	9.6–35.4 μ/L
10–12 years	10.0–37.0 μ/L

*Adult values.

13–16 years	9.0–33.4 μ/L	
17–19 years	7.2–26.6 μ/L	
≥ 20 years	6.1–21.1 μ/L	
Calcitonin, plasma	**Males**	**Females**
Basal	≤ 19 pg/ml	< 14 pg/ml
Calcium infusion (2.4 mg calcium/kg)	≤ 190 pg/ml	≤ 130 pg/ml
Pentagastrin infusion (0.5 μg/kg)	≤ 110 pg/ml	≤ 30 pg/ml
Catecholamine fractionation, free, plasma	**Supine**	**Standing**
Norepinephrine	70–750 pg/ml	200–1700 pg/ml
Epinephrine	≤ 110 pg/ml	≤ 140 pg/ml
Dopamine	< 30 pg/ml (any posture)	
Catecholamine fractionation, urine		
Epinephrine		
< 1 year	< 2.5 μg/24 hours	
1–2 years	< 3.5 μg/24 hours	
2–3 years	< 6.0 μg/24 hours	
4–9 years	0.2–10.0 μg/24 hours	
10–15 years	0.5–20.0 μg/24 hours	
≥ 16 years	0–20 μg/24 hours	
Norepinephrine		
< 1 year	0–10 μg/24 hours	
1 year	1–17 μg/24 hours	
2–3 years	4–29 μg/24 hours	
4–6 years	8–45 μg/24 hours	
7–9 years	13–65 μg/24 hours	
≥ 10 years	15–80 μg/24 hours	
Dopamine		
< 1 year	< 85 μg/24 hours	
1 year	10–140 μg/24 hours	
2–3 years	40–260 μg/24 hours	
≥ 4 years	65–400 μg/24 hours	
Metanephrines, urine	< 1.3 mg/24 hours	
Chorionic gonadotropins		
Beta-subunit, serum		
Females	< 5 IU/L	
Postmenopausal females	< 9 IU/L	
Males	< 2.5 IU/L	
CSF	≤ 1.5 IU/L	
Corticoids (includes cortisol, corticosterone, 11-deoxycortisol), plasma (for general screening)	A.M.: 7–25 μg/dl P.M.: 2–14 μg/dl	
Cortisol, free, urine	24–108 μg/24 hours	
Cortisol, plasma (not for general screening)	**Males**	**Females**
0–5 years	8–17 μg/dl	5–11 μg/dl
6–8 years	5–11 μg/dl	7–13 μg/dl
9 years	4–9 μg/dl	9–14 μg/dl
10–11 years	4–8 μg/dl	6–11 μg/dl
12–13 years	8–14 μg/dl	7–14 μg/dl
14–17 years	4–16 μg/dl	4–19 μg/dl
≥ 18 years (A.M.)	7–25 μg/dl	7–25 μg/dl
(P.M.)	2–14 μg/dl	2–14 μg/dl

Deoxycorticosteroids, plasma (for metyrapone test)		
A.M.	0–5 μg/dl	
P.M.	0–3 μg/dl	
Dehydroepiandrosterone sulfate (DHEA-S), serum		
0–30 days	**Males**	**Females**
Premature	0.25–10.0 μg/ml	0.25–10.0 μg/ml
Full-term	0.25–2.0 μg/ml	0.25–2.0 μg/ml
1–16 years	< 0.5 μg/ml	< 0.5 μg/ml
≥ 17 years	< 6.0 μg/ml	< 3.0 μg/ml
Estradiol, serum		
Children	< 1 ng/dl	
Adult males	1–5 ng/dl	
Premenopausal adult females	3–40 ng/dl	
Postmenopausal females	< 3 ng/dl	
Estrogen receptor assay (ERA), tissue		
Negative	< 3 fmol/mg cytosol protein	
Borderline	3–9 fmol/mg cytosol protein	
Positive	≥ 10 fmol/mg cytosol protein	
Follicle-stimulating hormone (FSH), serum		
Children ≤ 8 years old	< 5 IU/L	
Males ≥ 9 years old	< 22 IU/L	
Females 9–15 years	< 22 IU/L	
Females > 15 years	< 30 IU/L	
Postmenopausal females	2–3 × cycling level	
Gastrin, serum	< 300 pg/ml	
	Males	**Females**
Growth hormone, serum	≤ 5 ng/ml	≤ 10 ng/ml
Homovanillic acid (HVA), urine		
< 1 year	< 35 μg/mg creatinine	
> 1 year	< 23 μg/mg creatinine	
2–4 years	< 13.5 μg/mg creatinine	
5–9 years	< 9 μg/mg creatinine	
10–14 years	< 12 μg/mg creatinine	
15–18 years	< 2 μg/mg creatinine	
Adults	< 8 mg/24 hours	
5-Hydroxyindoleacetic acid (5-HIAA), urine	≤ 6 mg/24 hours	
17-Hydroxyprogesterone, serum		
Males	< 220 ng/dl	
Prepubertal	< 110 ng/dl	
Females		
Follicular phase	< 80 ng/dl	
Luteal phase	< 285 ng/dl	
Postmenopausal	< 51 ng/dl	
Prepubertal	< 100 ng/dl	
Newborns	< 630 ng/dl	
Insulin, serum	< 20 μU/ml	
Borderline	21–25 μU/ml	
17-Ketogenic steroids, urine		
Adults		
Males	4–14 mg/24 hours	
Females	2–12 mg/24 hours	
Children		
0–10 years	0.1–4 mg/24 hours	
11–14 years	2–9 mg/24 hours	

17-Ketosteroids, urine	
Adults	
Males	6–21 mg/24 hours
Females	4–17 mg/24 hours
Children	
0–10 years	0.1–3 mg/24 hours
11–14 years	2–7 mg/24 hours
17-Ketosteroids, fractionation, urine	See Table 1-5, p. 21.
Luteinizing hormone (LH), serum	
Children	< 15 IU/L
Adult males	4–24 IU/L
Adult females, non-midcycle	< 30 IU/L
Adult females, midcycle	30–150 IU/L
Postmenopausal females	30–120 IU/L
Parathyroid hormone (PTH), serum	1.0–5.0 pmol/L
N-terminal	< 6.1 pmol/L
C-terminal	≤ 50 μLeq/ml
Pregnanetriol, urine	
0–6 years	0–0.2 mg/24 hours
7–16 years	0.3–1.1 mg/24 hours
Adults	< 2.0 mg/24 hours
Progesterone, serum	
Males	
0–1 year	87–337 ng/dl
2–9 years	12–14 ng/dl
Postpuberty	< 100 ng/dl
Females, premenopausal	
0–1 year	87–337 ng/dl
2–9 years	20–24 ng/dl
Puberty through adolescence	Increasing values
Follicular phase	< 70 ng/dl
Luteal phase	200–2000 ng/dl
Prolactin, serum	
Males	0–20 ng/ml
Females	0–23 ng/ml
Renin activity (peripheral vein specimen), plasma	
Na-depleted, upright	
18–39 years	2.9–24.0 ng/ml/hour
> 40 years	2.9–10.8 ng/ml/hour
Na-replete, upright	
18–39 years	≤ 0.6–4.3 ng/ml/hour
≥ 40 years	≤ 0.6–3.0 ng/ml/hour
Sex hormone binding globulin (SHBG), serum	
Adult males	10–80 nmol/L
Adult nonpregnant females	20–130 nmol/L

Somatomedin-C, plasma

	Percentiles of S-C in ng/ml	
	Males	**Females**
0–5 years	0–103	0–112
6–8 years	2–118	5–128
9–10 years	15–148	24–158
11–13 years	55–216	65–226
14–15 years	114–232	124–242
16–17 years	84–221	94–231
18–19 years	56–177	66–186

Table 1-5. 17-Ketosteroids (Fractionation), Urine (mg/24 hours)

	Adult Females	Adult Males	Males 10–15 yr	Females 10–15 yr	6–9 yr	3–5 yr	1–2 yr	0–1 yr
Pregnanediol	0–4.5	0–1.9	0.1–1.2	0.1–0.7	<0.5	<0.3	<0.1	<0.1
Androsterone	0–3.1	0.9–6.1	0.2–2.0	0.5–2.5	0.1–1.0	<0.3	<0.3	<0.1
Etiocholanolone	0.1–3.5	0.9–5.2	0.1–1.6	0.7–3.1	0.3–1.0	<0.7	<0.4	<0.1
Dehydroepiandrosterone	0–1.5	0–3.1	<0.4	<0.4	<0.2	<0.1	<0.1	<0.1
Pregnanetriol	0–1.4	0.2–2.0	0.2–0.6	0.1–0.6	<0.3	<0.1	<0.1	<0.1
Δ5-Pregnanetriol	0–0.4	0–0.4	<0.3	<0.3	<0.2	<0.2	<0.1	<0.1
11-Ketoandrosterone	0–0.3	0–0.5	<0.1	<0.1	<0.1	<0.1	<0.1	<0.1
11-Ketoetiocholanolone	0–1.0	0–1.6	<0.3	0.1–0.5	0.1–0.5	<0.4	<0.1	<0.1
11-Hydroxyandrosterone	0–1.1	0.2–1.6	0.1–1.1	0.2–1.0	0.4–1.0	<0.4	<0.3	<0.3
11-Hydroxyetiocholanolone	0.1–0.8	0.1–0.9	<0.3	0.1–0.5	0.1–0.5	<0.4	<0.1	<0.1
11-Ketopregnanetriol	0–0.5	0–0.5	<0.3	<0.2	<0.2	<0.2	<0.2	<0.2

Source: De Leavelle (Ed), *Mayo Medical Laboratories Handbook*. Rochester, MN: Mayo Medical Laboratories, 1990.

20–24 years	75–142	64–131
25–29 years	65–131	55–121
30–34 years	58–122	47–112
35–39 years	51–115	40–104
40–44 years	46–109	35–98
45–49 years	43–104	32–93
≥ 50 years	40–100	29–90
Testosterone, serum	**Total**	**Free**
Children	Values increase through puberty and adolescence	
Males	300–1200 ng/dl	9–30 ng/dl
Females	20–80 ng/dl	0.3–1.9 ng/dl
Thyroxine (T4), serum		
Free	0.7–2.0 ng/dl	
Total		
1–9 years	6.0–12.5 ng/dl	
10–17 years	5.0–11 ng/dl	
Females ≥ 18, males ≥ 24 years	5.0–12.5 ng/dl	
Triiodothyronine (T3), serum		
Free	2.2–7.2 pmol/L	
Total		
1–14 years	125–250 ng/dl	
15–23 years	100–220 ng/dl	
≥ 24 years	80–180 ng/dl	
Borderline increase	181–230 ng/dl	
Triiodothyronine, reverse (rT3) serum	0.18–0.51 nmol/L	
T3 resin uptake, serum	25–35%	
Thyroid-stimulating hormone, sensitive (S-TSH), serum		
1–19 years	0.4–7.0 mIU/L	
20–29 years	0.4–5.0 mIU/L	
30–39 years	0.4–5.5 mIU/L	
40–49 years	0.4–6.0 mIU/L	
50–59 years	0.4–7.0 mIU/L	
60–69 years	0.4–8.0 mIU/L	
70–79 years	0.4–9.0 mIU/L	
≥ 80 years	0.4–10.0 mIU/L	
Thyroglobulin, serum	3–42 ng/ml	
Thyroxine-binding globulin (TBG), serum		
1–6 years	17–26 μg/dl	
7–23 years (females)	15–26 μg/dl	
7–13 years (males)	15–24 μg/dl	
14–18 years (males)	13–22 μg/dl	
19–23 years (males)	11–20 μg/dl	
≥ 24 years	16–24 μg/dl	
Thyroid antibodies (antimicrosomal and antithyroglobulin)	< 1 : 100	
Vanillylmandelic acid (VMA), urine		
< 1 year	< 27 μg/mg creatinine	
1 year	< 18 μg/mg creatinine	
2–4 years	< 13 μg/mg creatinine	
5–9 years	< 8.5 μg/mg creatinine	
10–14 years	< 7 μg/mg creatinine	
15–18 years	< 5 μg/mg creatinine	
Adults	< 9 mg/24 hours	
Vasoactive intestinal polypeptide (VIP), plasma	< 75 pg/ml	

NORMAL BLOOD ANTIBODY LEVELS FOR SEROLOGIC TESTS FOR INFECTIOUS AGENTS

Amebiasis (*Entamoeba histolytica*)	
No invasive disease	< 1 : 32
Borderline	< 1 : 32–1 : 64
Active or recent infection	≥ 128
Current infection	> 1 : 256
Aspergillosis	Negative
Blastomycosis	Negative (test is positive in < 50% of cases)
Brucellosis	< 1 : 80
Candidosis	Negative (test positive in 25% of normal population)
Chlamydia IgG (lymphogranuloma venereum, psittacosis)	≤ 1 : 640
Cold agglutinin titer	< 1 : 16
Cryptococcosis antigen, serum or CSF	Negative
Cytomegalovirus*	
IgG	< 1 : 5
IgM	< 1 : 10
Echinococcosis	Negative
Epstein-Barr virus IgG early antigen	< 1 : 10
Hepatitis	See pp. 666–667.
Herpes simplex	
IgG	< 1 : 5
IgM	< 1 : 10
Heterophil	Titer < 1 : 56 or absorption pattern showing no 2 × titer reduction
Histoplasmosis, serum or CSF	Negative
Influenza A or B*	
IgG or IgM	< 1 : 10
Lyme disease (*Borrelia burgdorferi*)	
Nonreactive	< 249 antibody response units (ABR)
Weakly reactive	250–999 ABR
Reactive	> 1000 ABR
Monospot screen	Negative
Mumps*	
IgG	< 1 : 5
IgM	< 1 : 10
Murine typhus IgG	< 1 : 32
Mycoplasma pneumoniae IgG or IgM	< 1 : 10
Q fever*	< 1 : 2
Respiratory syncytial virus	
IgG	< 1 : 5
IgM	< 1 : 10
Rocky Mountain spotted fever IgG*	≤ 1 : 32
Rubella	
IgG	≤ 1 : 8 indicates little or no immunity
IgM	Negative

*Presence of IgM antibodies or ≥ fourfold rise in IgG titer between acute and convalescent phase sera drawn within 30 days of each other indicates recent infection. Generally, presence of IgG indicates past exposure and possible immunity. Congenital infections require serial sera from both mother and infant. Passively acquired antibodies in infant will decay in 2–3 months. Antibody levels that are unchanged or increased in 2–3 months indicate active infection. Absence of antibody in mother rules out congenital infection in infant.

Rubeola serum or CSF	
IgG	< 1 : 5
IgM	< 1 : 10
Scrub typhus	≤ 1 : 40
St. Louis encephalitis*	< 1 : 10
Sporotrichosis	< 1 : 80
Streptococcal	

	ASO	Anti-DNase-B
Preschool	< 85 units	< 60 units
School age	< 170 units	< 170 units
Adults	< 85 units	< 85 units

Syphilis	Negative
Syphilis serology	See pp. 638–640.
Toxoplasmosis	
IgG	
No previous infection (except eye)	< 1 : 16
Prevalent in general population	1 : 16–1 : 256
Suggests recent infection	> 1 : 256
Indicates active infection	≥ 1 : 1024
IgM	
Indicates active infection (adults)	≥ 1 : 64
Children—any titer is significant	
Trichinosis*	< 1 : 5
Tularemia	< 1 : 40
Varicella-zoster IgG or IgM	< 1 : 10

NORMAL BLOOD ANTIBODY LEVELS

Acetylcholine	
Receptor binding antibodies	≤ 0.03 nmol/L
Receptor blocking antibodies	< 25% blockade of ACh receptors
Receptor modulating antibodies	<20% loss of ACh receptors
Anti-ds-DNA antibodies	< 70 units
Borderline	70–200 units
Positive	> 200 units
Antiextractable nuclear antigens (anti-RNP, anti-Sm, anti-SSB, anti-SSA)	Negative
Antiglomerular basement membrane antibody	Negative
Antimitochondrial antibodies	Negative
Antinuclear antibodies (ANA)	Negative
C1 esterase inhibitor	8–24 mg/dl
C1q	7–15 mg/dl
C2	50–250% of normal
C3	70–150 mg/dl
C4	10–30 mg/dl
C5	9–18 mg/dl
Complement, total	41–90 hemolytic units
Granulocyte antibodies	Negative
HLA-B27, present in:	Whites: 6–8% Blacks: 3–4% Orientals: 1%

*Presence of IgM antibodies or ≥ fourfold rise in IgG titer between acute and convalescent phase sera drawn within 30 days of each other indicates recent infection. Generally, presence of IgG indicates past exposure and possible immunity. Congenital infections require serial sera from both mother and infant. Passively acquired antibodies in infant will decay in 2–3 months. Antibody levels that are unchanged or increased in 2–3 months indicate active infection. Absence of antibody in mother rules out congenital infection in infant.

Intrinsic factor blocking antibody	Negative
Parietal cell antibodies	Negative
Prostate-specific antigen (PSA), serum	
Males ≤ age 40	≤ 2.7 ng/ml
Males > age 40	≤ 4.0 ng/ml
Prostatic acid phosphatase (PAP), serum	< 3.7 ng/ml
Rheumatoid factor	
Latex agglutination	Negative
Rate nephelometry	
Nonreactive	0–39 IU/ml
Weakly reactive	40–79 IU/ml
Reactive	≥ 80 IU/ml
Smooth muscle antibody	Negative
Striated muscle antibodies	< 1 : 60
Thyroid (thyroglobulin, microsomal)	< 1 : 100

NORMAL BLOOD LEVELS FOR METABOLIC DISEASES

(U = urine; S = serum; P = plasma; B = whole blood; F = skin fibroblasts; L = leukocytes; RBC = erythrocytes; St = stool)

Acid mucopolysaccharides (U)	Age dependent
Alpha$_1$ antitrypsin (S)	126–226 mg/dl
Alpha-fucosidase (F)	1.3–3.6 units/gm cellular protein
(L)	0.49–1.76 units/gm cellular protein
Alpha-galactosidase (Fabry's disease) (S)	0.016–0.2 units/L
(F)	0.24–1.10 units/gm cellular protein
(L)	0.60–3.63 units/10^{10} cells
Alpha-L-iduronidase (Hurler's, Scheie's syndrome) (F)	0.44–1.04 units/gm cellular protein
(L)	0.17–0.54 units/10^{10} cells
Alpha-mannosidase (mannosidosis) (F)	0.71–5.92 units/gm cellular protein
(L)	1.50–3.33 units/10^{10} cells
Alpha-*N*-acetylglucosaminidase (Sanfilippo Type B) (S)	0.09–0.58 units/L
(F)	0.076–0.291 units/gm cellular protein
Arylsulfatase A (mucolipidosis, Type II and III) (F)	2.28–15.74 units/gm cellular protein
(L)	> 2.5 units/10^{10} cells
(U)	> 1 unit/L
Arylsulfatase B (F)	1.6–14.9 units/gm cellular protein
Beta-galactosidase (Gm$_1$, gangliosidosis, Morquio's syndrome) (F)	4.7–19.1 units/gm cellular protein
(L)	1.01–6.52 units/10^{10} cells
Beta-glucosidase (Gaucher's disease) (F)	3.80–8.70 units/gm cellular protein
(L)	0.08–0.35 units/10^{10} cells
Beta-glucuronidase (MPS VII) (F)	0.34–1.24 units/gm cellular protein
Carbohydrate (U)	Negative
Cystine (U)	
< 1 month	15–108 mg/gm creatinine
1–5 months	16–90 mg/gm creatinine

6–11 months	17–76 mg/gm creatinine
1–2 years	13–59 mg/gm creatinine
3–15 years	2.6–13 mg/24 hours
> 16 years and adults	7–28 mg/24 hours
Fatty acid profile of serum lipids	
Linoleate	≥ 25% of fatty acids in serum lipids
Arachidonate	≥ 6% of fatty acids in serum lipids
Palmitate	18–26% of fatty acids in serum lipids
Phytanate	≤ 0.3% of fatty acids in serum lipids (> 0.5% suggests Refsum's disease)
Free fatty acids (S)	239–843 μEq/L
Galactokinase	
< 2 years old	20–80 mU/gm hemoglobin
≥ 2 years old	12–40 mU/gm hemoglobin
Galactose (U)	Not detectable
Galactose 1-phosphate uridyltransferase (galactosemia) (B)	18.5–28.5 units/gm hemoglobin
Galactosylceramide-beta-galactosidase (Krabbe's disease, globoid cell leukodystrophy (F)	10.3–89.7 mU/gm cellular protein
(L)	21.5–59.2 mU/gm cellular protein
Glucose 6-phosphate (G-6-PD) dehydrogenase (B)	
2–17 years old	6.4–15.6 units/gm hemoglobin
≥17 years old	8.6–18.6 units/gm hemoglobin
Glucose phosphate isomerase (B)	10.6–38.2 units/gm hemoglobin
Hexosaminidase, total (S)	10.4–23.8 units/L
Hexosaminidase A, ≥ 5 years old (Tay-Sachs, GM_2, gangliosidosis)	Normal: 56–80% of total Indeterminate: 50–55% Abnormal: < 50%
Homogentisic acid (U)	Negative
Hydroxyproline, total (24-hour U)	
< 5 years old	100–400 μg/mg creatinine
5–12 years	100–150 μg/mg creatinine
≥ 19 years	15–45 mg/24 hours
Females ≥ 19 years	0.4–2.9 mg/2-hour specimen
Males ≥ 18 years	0.4–5.0 mg/2-hour specimen
35S Mucopolysaccharide turnover (MPS I, II, III, VI, VII) (F)	Normal or abnormal turnover
Phenylalanine (P)	
≤ 1 week of age	0.69–2.0 mg/dl (42–124 μmol/L)
< 16 years old	0.43–1.4 mg/dl (26–86 μmol/L)
> 16 years old	0.68–1.1 mg/dl (41–68 μmol/L)
Porphyrins, total (RBC)	16–60 μg/dl packed cells
Porphyrins	
Total (P)	≤ 1 μg/dl
Fractionation	≤ 1 μg/dl for any fraction
Porphyrins (St)	
Coproporphyrin	≤ 200 μg/24 hours
Protoporphyrin	≤ 1500 μg/24 hours
Uroporphyrin	≤ 1000 μg/24 hours
Porphyrins (U)	
Uro (octacarboxylic)	
Males	≤ 46 μg/24 hours

Females	≤ 22 μg/24 hours	
Hepatocarboxylic		
Males	≤ 13 μg/24 hours	
Females	≤ 9 μg/24 hours	
Hexacarboxylic		
Males	≤ 5 μg/24 hours	
Females	≤ 4 μg/24 hours	
Pentacarboxylic		
Males	≤ 4 μg/24 hours	
Females	≤ 3 μg/24 hours	
Copro (tetracarboxylic)		
Males	≤ 96 μg/24 hours	
Females	≤ 60 μg/24 hours	
Porphobilinogen	Normal: ≤ 1.5 mg/24 hours Marginal: 1.5–2.0 mg/24 hours Excess: > 2.0 mg/24 hours	
Protoporphyrins (RBC)		
Free	1–10 μg/dl packed RBCs	
Zinc-protoporphyrin	10–38 μg/dl packed RBCs	
Phytanic acid (Refsum's disease) (S)	Negative: ≤ 0.3% Borderline: 0.3–0.5% > 0.5% suggests Refsum's disease.	
Sphingomyelinase (Niemann-Pick disease) (F)	1.53–7.18 units/gm cellular protein	
Tyrosine (P)		
≤ 1 week	0.6–2.2 mg/dl	(33–122 μmol/L)
< 16 years	0.47–2.0 mg/dl	(26–110 μmol/L)
> 16 years	0.8–1.3 mg/dl	(45–74 μmol/L)
Uroporphyrinogen synthase (RBC)		
Males	7.9–14.7 nM/sec/L	
Females	8.0–16.8 nM/sec/L Marginal values 6.0–8.0 nM/sec/L are suggestive but indeterminate. Values < 6.0 nM/sec/L are definite for acute, intermittent porphyria.	
Vitamin D		
25-Hydroxyvitamin D (S)	14–42 ng/ml (winter) 15–80 ng/ml (summer) < 15 ng/ml may be vitamin D deficiency.	
1,25-Dihydroxyvitamin D	15–60 pg/ml	

BIBLIOGRAPHY

Lockitch G, et al. Age- and sex-specific pediatric reference intervals: various analytes. *Clin Chem* 34/8:1618, 1988.

Burritt ME, et al. Pediatric reference intervals for 19 biologic variables in healthy children. *Mayo Clin Proc* 65:329, 1990.

Leavelle DE (Ed). *Mayo Medical Laboratories Interpretive Handbook*. Rochester, MN: Mayo Medical Laboratories, 1990.

Case Records of the Massachusetts General Hospital. *N Engl J Med* 314:39, 1986; 315:1606, 1986.

Tietz NW. *Clinical Guide to Laboratory Tests*. Philadelphia: Saunders, 1990.

Critical Values*

These levels may indicate the need for prompt clinical intervention. Any *sudden change* in values may also be critical.

Exact levels should be determined in conjunction with the laboratory performing the tests.

HEMATOLOGY

	Low	**High**
WBC	<1500/cu mm	>15,000/cu mm
WBC in CSF	None	Increased
CSF containing blasts or malignant cells		
Packed cell volume (hematocrit)	<15 vol%	>55 vol%
Hemoglobin	<5 gm/dl	>18 gm/dl
Platelet count	<30,000/cu mm	>1,000,000/cu mm
Platelet count (pediatric)	<20,000/cu mm	>1,000,000/cu mm
Prothrombin time	None	>40 seconds or 3 × control level
Activated partial thromboplastin time	None	>90 seconds
Positive test for fibrin split products, protamine sulfate, high heparin level		
Presence of blast cells, sickle cells		
New diagnosis of leukemia, sickle cell anemia, aplastic crisis		

BLOOD CHEMISTRY

	Low	**High**
Total serum bilirubin (newborns)	None	>18 mg/dl
Serum calcium	<6 mg/dl	>14 mg/dl
Serum glucose	<40 mg/dl	>700 mg/dl
Serum glucose (newborns)	<30 mg/dl	>300 mg/dl
Serum phosphorus	<1 mg/dl	None
Serum potassium	<2.5 mEq/L	>6.5 mEq/L
Serum potassium (newborns)	<2.5 mEq/L	>8.0 mEq/L
Serum sodium	<120 mEq/L	>160 mEq/L
Serum bicarbonate	<10 mEq/L	>40 mEq/L
Blood PCO_2	<20 mmHg	>70 mmHg
Blood pH	<7.2 units	>7.6 units
Blood PO_2	<40 mmHg	None
Creatinine kinase	None	>3–5 × ULN
CK-MB	None	>5%
CSF total protein	None	>45 mg/dl
CSF glucose	<80% of blood level	

*Source: Data from GJ Kost, Critical limits for urgent clinician notification at US medical centers. *JAMA* 263: 704, 1990.

MICROBIOLOGY

Positive blood culture
Positive CSF Gram's stain, culture, or India ink preparation
Positive culture from body fluid (e.g., pleural, peritoneal, joint)
Positive acid-fast stain or culture
Presence of malarial or other blood parasites
Positive rapid antigen detection for *Cryptococcus,* group B streptococci, *Haemophilus influenzae* b, or *Neisseria meningitidis*
Stool culture positive for *Salmonella, Shigella,* or *Campylobacter*

URINALYSIS

Strongly positive test for glucose and ketone
Presence of pathological crystals (urate, cysteine, leucine, tyrosine)

SEROLOGY

Incompatible cross match
Positive test for hepatitis, syphilis, AIDS

THERAPEUTIC DRUGS

	Blood Levels
Tobramycin	>12 μg/ml (peak)
Carbamazepine	>20 μg/ml
Ethosuximide	>200 μg/ml
Phenobarbital	>60 μg/ml
Phenytoin	>40 μg/ml
Primidone	>24 μg/ml
Lithium	>2 mEq/L
Lidocaine	>9 μg/ml
Quinidine	>10 μg/ml
Theophylline	>25 μg/ml
Digoxin	>2.5 ng/ml
Digitoxin	>35 ng/ml
Salicylate	>700 μg/ml

II
Specific Laboratory Examinations

3

Core Blood Analytes—Alterations by Diseases

SERUM GLUCOSE

May Be Increased In

Diabetes mellitus, including
- Hemochromatosis
- Cushing's syndrome (with insulin-resistant diabetes)
- Acromegaly and gigantism (with insulin-resistant diabetes in early stages; hypopituitarism later)

Increased circulating epinephrine
- Adrenalin injection
- Pheochromocytoma
- Stress (e.g., emotion, burns, shock, anesthesia)

Acute pancreatitis

Chronic pancreatitis (some patients)

Wernicke's encephalopathy (vitamin B_1 deficiency)

Some CNS lesions (subarachnoid hemorrhage, convulsive states)

Effect of drugs (e.g., corticosteroids, estrogens, alcohol, phenytoin, thiazides, propranolol, chronic hypervitaminosis A)

WHO defines unequivocal increase of fasting serum (or plasma) glucose as ≥ 140 mg/dl on more than one occasion or any glucose ≥ 200 mg/dl.

May Be Decreased In

Pancreatic disorders
- Islet cell tumor, hyperplasia
- Pancreatitis
- Glucagon deficiency

Extrapancreatic tumors
- Carcinoma of adrenal gland
- Carcinoma of stomach
- Fibrosarcoma
- Other

Hepatic disease
- Diffuse severe disease (e.g., poisoning, hepatitis, cirrhosis, primary or metastatic tumor)

Endocrine disorders
- Hypopituitarism and Addison's disease
- Hypothyroidism
- Adrenal medulla unresponsiveness
- Early diabetes mellitus

Functional disturbances
- Postgastrectomy
- Gastroenterostomy
- Autonomic nervous system disorders

Pediatric anomalies
- Prematurity
- Infant of diabetic mother
- Ketotic hypoglycemia
- Zetterstrom's syndrome
- Idiopathic leucine sensitivity
- Spontaneous hypoglycemia in infants

Enzyme diseases
- von Gierke's disease
- Galactosemia
- Maple syrup urine disease
- Fructose intolerance

Other
- Exogenous insulin (factitious)
- Oral hypoglycemic medications (factitious)
- Leucine sensitivity
- Malnutrition
- Hypothalamic lesions
- Alcoholism

Blood samples in which serum is not separated from blood cells will show glucose values decreasing at rate of 7 mg/dl/hour at room temperature.

SERUM UREA NITROGEN (BUN)

Increased In

Impaired kidney function (see Serum Creatinine, p. 35)

Prerenal azotemia—any cause of reduced renal blood flow
- Congestive heart failure
- Salt and water depletion (vomiting, diarrhea, diuresis, sweating)
- Shock

Postrenal azotemia—any obstruction of urinary tract (increased BUN/creatinine ratio)
- Increased protein catabolism (serum creatinine remains normal)
- Hemorrhage into gastrointestinal tract
- Acute myocardial infarction
- Stress

Decreased In

Severe liver damage (liver failure)
- Drugs
- Poisoning
- Hepatitis
- Other

Increased utilization of protein for synthesis
- Late pregnancy
- Infancy
- Acromegaly
- Malnutrition
- Anabolic hormones

Diet
- Low-protein and high-carbohydrate
- IV feedings only
- Impaired absorption (celiac disease)
- Malnutrition

Nephrotic syndrome (some patients)

Syndrome of inappropriate secretion of antidiuretic hormone (SIADH)

A low BUN of 6–8 mg/dl is frequently associated with states of overhydration.

A BUN of 10–20 mg/dl almost always indicates normal glomerular function.

A BUN of 50–150 mg/dl implies serious impairment of renal function.

Markedly increased BUN (150–250 mg/dl) is virtually conclusive evidence of severely impaired glomerular function.

In chronic renal disease, BUN correlates better with symptoms of uremia than does the serum creatinine.

SERUM CREATININE

Increased In

Diet
- Ingestion of creatinine (roast meat)

Muscle disease
- Gigantism
- Acromegaly

Prerenal azotemia (see Serum Urea Nitrogen [BUN], p. 34)

Postrenal azotemia (see Serum Urea Nitrogen [BUN], p. 34)

Impaired kidney function; 50% loss of renal function is needed to increase serum creatinine from 1.0 to 2.0 mg/dl; therefore not sensitive to mild to moderate renal injury.

Serum creatinine is a more specific and sensitive indicator of renal disease than BUN. Use of simultaneous BUN and creatinine determinations provides more information in conditions listed in the next section.

Decreased In

Not clinically significant

Artifactual (e.g., marked increase of serum bilirubin)

BUN/CREATININE RATIO

(see also Table 15-3, p. 564)

Normal range for healthy person on normal diet = 12–20; most individuals are 12–16. Because of considerable variability, this should be used only as a rough guide.

Increased Ratio with Normal Creatinine In

Prerenal azotemia (BUN rises without increase in creatinine) (e.g., heart failure, salt depletion, dehydration, blood loss) due to decreased glomerular filtration rate

Catabolic states with increased tissue breakdown

GI hemorrhage

High protein intake, especially in uremia

Impaired renal function plus
- Excess protein intake or production or tissue breakdown (e.g., GI bleeding, thyrotoxicosis, infection, Cushing's syndrome, high-protein diet, surgery, burns, cachexia, high fever)
- Urine reabsorption (e.g., ureterocolostomy)
- Patients with reduced muscle mass (subnormal creatinine production)

Certain drugs (e.g., tetracycline, glucocorticoids)

Increased Ratio with Elevated Creatinine In

Postrenal azotemia (BUN rises disproportionately more than creatinine) (e.g., obstructive uropathy)

Prerenal azotemia superimposed on renal disease

Decreased Ratio with Decreased BUN In

Acute tubular necrosis

Low-protein diet, starvation, severe liver disease and other causes of decreased urea synthesis

Repeated dialysis (urea rather than creatinine diffuses out of extracellular fluid)

Inherited hyperammonemias (urea is virtually absent in blood)

SIADH (due to tubular secretion of urea)

Pregnancy

Decreased Ratio with Increased Creatinine In

Phenacemide therapy (accelerates conversion of creatine to creatinine)
Rhabdomyolysis (releases muscle creatinine)
Muscular patients who develop renal failure

Inappropriate Ratio

Diabetic ketoacidosis (acetoacetate causes false increase in creatinine with certain methodologies, resulting in normal ratio when dehydration should produce an increased BUN/creatinine ratio)
Cephalosporin therapy (interferes with creatinine measurement)

SERUM CREATINE

Increased In

High dietary intake (meat)
Destruction of muscle
Hyperthyroidism (this diagnosis almost excluded by normal serum creatine)
Active rheumatoid arthritis
Testosterone therapy

Decreased In

Not clinically significant
Drugs (e.g., trimethoprim/sulfamethoxazole [TMP/SMX], cimetidine, cefoxitin)
Artifactual (e.g., diabetic ketoacidosis)

SERUM URIC ACID

Levels are very labile and show day-to-day and seasonal variation in same person; also increased by emotional stress, total fasting.

Increased In

Renal failure (does not correlate with severity of kidney damage; urea and creatinine should be used)
Gout (see pp. 257–259)
25% of relatives of patients with gout
Asymptomatic hyperuricemia (e.g., incidental finding with no evidence of gout; clinical significance not known, but people so afflicted should be rechecked periodically for gout). The higher the level of serum uric acid, the greater the likelihood of an attack of acute gouty arthritis.
Increased destruction of nucleoproteins
- Leukemia, multiple myeloma
- Polycythemia
- Lymphoma, especially postirradiation
- Other disseminated neoplasms
- Cancer chemotherapy (e.g., nitrogen mustards, vincristine, mercaptopurine)
- Hemolytic anemia
- Sickle cell anemia
- Resolving pneumonia
- Toxemia of pregnancy (serial determinations to follow therapeutic response and estimate prognosis)
- Psoriasis (one-third of patients)

Diet
- High-protein weight reduction diet
- Excess nucleoprotein (e.g., sweetbreads, liver)

Miscellaneous
- von Gierke's disease
- Lead poisoning
- Lesch-Nyhan syndrome

- Maple syrup urine disease
- Down's syndrome
- Polycystic kidneys
- Calcinosis universalis and circumscripta
- Some drugs (e.g., thiazides, furosemide, ethacrynic acid, and all diuretics except spironolactone, mercurials, and ticrynafen; small doses of salicylates [<4 gm/day])
- Hypoparathyroidism
- Primary hyperparathyroidism
- Hypothyroidism
- Sarcoidosis
- Chronic berylliosis
- Some patients with alcoholism
- Patients with arteriosclerosis and hypertension *(Serum uric acid is increased in 80% of patients with elevated serum triglycerides.)*
- Certain population groups (e.g., Blackfoot and Pima Indians, Filipinos, New Zealand Maoris)
- Metabolic acidosis

Most common causes in hospitalized men are azotemia, metabolic acidosis, diuretics, gout, myelolymphoproliferative disorders, other drugs, unknown causes.

*"It is difficult to justify therapy in asymptomatic persons with hyperuricemia to prevent gouty arthritis, uric acid stones, urate nephropathy or risk of cardiovascular disease."**

Decreased In

Administration of adrenocorticotropic hormone (ACTH)
Administration of uricosuric drugs (e.g., high doses of salicylates, probenecid, cortisone, allopurinol, coumarins)
Wilson's disease
Fanconi's syndrome
Acromegaly (some patients)
Celiac disease (slightly)
Pernicious anemia in relapse (some patients)
Xanthinuria
Administration of various other drugs (x-ray contrast agents, glyceryl guaiacolate)
Neoplasms (occasional cases) (e.g., carcinomas, Hodgkin's disease)
Healthy adults with isolated defect in tubular transport of uric acid (Dalmatian dog mutation)

Unchanged In

Colchicine administration

SERUM SODIUM

(see Fig. 3-1, p. 38; Fig. 3-2, p. 39; Table 3-1, pp. 40–41; Causes of Hyponatremias, pp. 546–547; "Essential" Hypernatremia, p. 547]

Changes in serum sodium most often reflect changes in water balance rather than sodium balance. If patient has not received a large load of sodium, hypernatremia suggests need for water, and values < 130 mEq/L suggest overhydration.

*Source: WB Duffy et al., *JAMA* 246:2215, 1981.

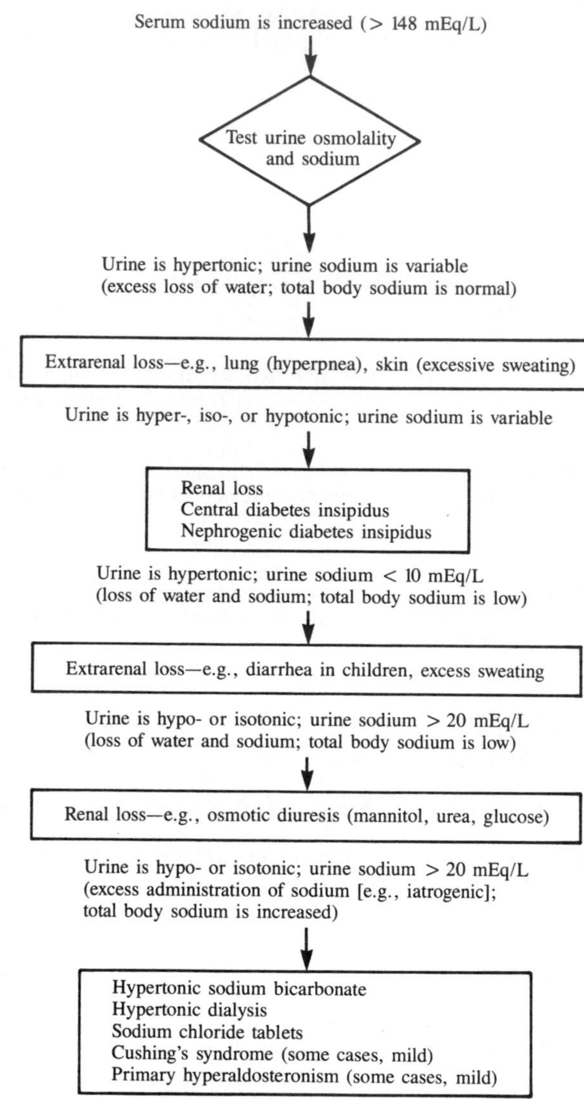
Serum sodium is increased (> 148 mEq/L)
Test urine osmolality and sodium
Urine is hypertonic; urine sodium is variable (excess loss of water; total body sodium is normal)
Extrarenal loss—e.g., lung (hyperpnea), skin (excessive sweating)
Urine is hyper-, iso-, or hypotonic; urine sodium is variable
Renal loss
Central diabetes insipidus
Nephrogenic diabetes insipidus
Urine is hypertonic; urine sodium < 10 mEq/L
(loss of water and sodium; total body sodium is low)
Extrarenal loss—e.g., diarrhea in children, excess sweating
Urine is hypo- or isotonic; urine sodium > 20 mEq/L
(loss of water and sodium; total body sodium is low)
Renal loss—e.g., osmotic diuresis (mannitol, urea, glucose)
Urine is hypo- or isotonic; urine sodium > 20 mEq/L
(excess administration of sodium [e.g., iatrogenic];
total body sodium is increased)
Hypertonic sodium bicarbonate
Hypertonic dialysis
Sodium chloride tablets
Cushing's syndrome (some cases, mild)
Primary hyperaldosteronism (some cases, mild)
Hypotonic urine = urine osmolality < 800 mOsm/L
Isotonic urine = urine osmolality is between 800 mOsm/L and plasma osmolality
Hypertonic urine = urine osmolality > 800 mOsm/L

Fig. 3-1. Flow chart for hypernatremia.

Serum sodium decreased (< 135 mEq/L)
(dilutional or depletional)

↓

Test serum osmolality and urine sodium

↓

(1) Urine sodium > 20 mEq/L (e.g., **acute and chronic renal failure**)
Urine sodium < 10 mEq/L (e.g., **congestive heart failure, nephrotic syndrome, cirrhosis**)
(Dilutional—i.e., extracellular fluid volume increased > increased total body sodium and patient has edema)

(2) Urine sodium > 20 mEq/L
(Dilutional—i.e., increased extracellular fluid volume without edema)
Stress, pain
Glucocorticoid deficiency
SIADH (see p. 551; is now chief cause of hyponatremia in hospitalized patients; diagnosis principally by exclusion but should be considered when there is low BUN and uric acid)
Hypothyroidism (only in presence of gross myxedema)
Drugs that stimulate antidiuretic hormone release (e.g., chlorpropamide, tolbutamide, clofibrate, morphine, barbiturates, carbamazepine, acetaminophen, isoproterenol, indomethacin)

(3) Urine sodium < 10 mEq/L
(Dilutional—i.e., decreased extracellullar fluid volume < decreased total body sodium)
Extrarenal loss (e.g., **vomiting, diarrhea, burns, pancreatitis, peritonitis)**

(4) Urine sodium > 20 mEq/L
(Dilutional—i.e., decreased extracellular fluid volume < decreased total body sodium)
Renal loss (e.g., diuresis [diuretics, mannitol, glucose, urea], ketonuria, metabolic alkalosis, salt-losing nephritis [renal cystic disease, chronic interstitial nephritis, incomplete urinary tract obstruction, analgesic nephropathy], renal tubular acidosis)

(5) Spurious
Serum osmolality is normal
Hyperlipidemia (also causes spurious hyperchloremia)
Hyperproteinemia (e.g., multiple myeloma)
(Hyperlipidemia and hyperproteinemia cause spurious results only with flame photometric but not with specific ion electrode techniques for measuring sodium)
Serum osmolality is increased
Hyperglycemia (serum sodium decreases 1.7 mEq/L for every increase of serum glucose of 100 mg/dl)
Administration of mannitol

Fig. 3-2. Flow chart for hyponatremia.

Table 3-1. Urine and Blood Changes in Electrolytes, pH, and Volume in Various Conditions

Measurement	Pulmonary Emphysema	Congestive Heart Failure	Excessive Sweating	Diarrhea	Pyloric Obstruction	Dehydration	Starvation	Malabsorption	Salicylate Intoxication	Primary Aldosteronism
Blood										
Sodium	N	N or D	D	D	D	I	N	D	N	I
Potassium	N	N	N	D	D	N	D	D	N or D	D
Bicarbonate	I	N	N	D	I	N or D	D	N or D	D	I
Chloride	D	D	D	D	D	I	N	N	I	D
Volume	N or I	I	N	D	D	D	N or D	D	N	N
Urine										
Sodium	D	D	D	D	D	I	N or I	D	I	D
Potassium	N	N	N	N or D	N	I	I or N	D	N or I	I
pH	D	N	N	D	I	D	D	N or D	I	N or D
Volume	N	D	N	D	D	D	I	N	N	I

N = normal; D = decreased; I = increased; V = variable.

Measurement	Adrenal Cortical Insufficiency	Diabetes Insipidus	Diabetic Acidosis	Mercurial Diuretic Administration	Thiazide Diuretic Administration	Ammonium Chloride Administration	Diamox Administration	Renal Tubular Acidosis	Chronic Renal Failure	Acute Renal Failure
Blood										
Sodium	D	N or I	D	D	D	D	D	D	D	D
Potassium	I	N	N or I	D	D	D	D	D	N or D	I
Bicarbonate	N or D	N	D	I	D	D	D	D	D	D
Chloride	D	I	D	D	D	I	I	I	D or N	I
Volume	D	D	D	D	D	D	D	D	V	I
Urine										
Sodium	I	N	I	I	I	I	I	I	I	D
Potassium	N or D	N	I	I	I	I	I	I	I	D
pH	N or I	N	D	D	N or I	I	I	I	I	N or I
Volume	N or D	I	I	I	I	I	I	I	V*	D

*Usually increased.

SERUM OSMOLALITY

Hyperosmolality

Due To

Hyperglycemia
- Diabetic ketoacidosis
- Nonketotic hyperglycemia coma (see p. 487)
  - Clinical picture: A middle-aged or older person with diabetes of recent onset or unrecognized diabetes, who shows neurologic symptoms (e.g., convulsions or hemiplegia) and then becomes stuporous or comatose.
  - Serum glucose is very high but, contrary to expectation in diabetic coma, ketosis is minimal and plasma acetone is not found.
  - Increased serum osmolality (normal = 280–300 mOsm/L). In mildly drowsy patients, mean is 320 mOsm/L. At level of 350 mOsm/L, there will be some confusion or some stupor. At 400 mOsm/L, most patients are obtunded. State of consciousness does not correlate with height of acidemia.

    Osmolality should be determined routinely in grossly unbalanced diabetic patients.

  - Determinations of blood sodium and potassium levels are not useful in diagnosis or in estimating net ion losses but are performed to monitor changes in sodium and potassium during therapy.
  - Laboratory findings are those due to complications or precipitating factors (e.g., pneumonia, pancreatitis, stroke).
  - Some precipitating factors
    - Drugs (e.g., thiazides, steroids, phenytoin, propranolol)
    - Glucose overloading (e.g., hyperalimentation, dialysis, IV infusions in treatment of burns)
    - Dehydration
    - Pancreatitis with major shift of fluids
    - Cerebral or cardiovascular accident

Hypernatremia with dehydration
- Diarrhea, vomiting, fever, hyperventilation, inadequate water intake
- Diabetes insipidus—central
- Nephrogenic diabetes insipidus—congenital or acquired (e.g., hypercalcemia, hypokalemia, chronic renal disease, sickle cell disease, effect of some drugs)
- Osmotic diuresis—hyperglycemia, administration of urea or mannitol

Hypernatremia with normal hydration—due to hypothalamic disorders
- Insensitivity of osmoreceptors (essential hypernatremia)—water loading does not return serum osmolality to normal; chlorpropamide may lower serum sodium toward normal.
- Defect in thirst (hypodipsia)—forced water intake returns serum osmolality to normal.

Hypernatremia with overhydration—iatrogenic or accidental (e.g., infants given feedings with high sodium concentrations or given $NaHCO_3$ for respiratory distress or cardiopulmonary arrest)

Alcohol ingestion is the commonest cause of hyperosmolar state and of coexisting coma and hyperosmolar state.

HYPOSMOLALITY (equivalent to hyponatremia)

Due To

Hyponatremia with hypovolemia
- Adrenal insufficiency (e.g., salt-losing form of congenital adrenal hyperplasia, congenital adrenal hypoplasia, hemorrhage into adrenals, inadequate replacement of corticosteroids, inappropriate tapering of steroids)

Renal losses
GI tract loss (e.g., vomiting, diarrhea)
Other losses (e.g., burns, peritonitis, pancreatitis)
Hyponatremia with normal volume or hypervolemia (dilutional syndromes)
Congestive heart failure, cirrhosis, nephrotic syndrome
SIADH

Urine and plasma osmolality are more useful to diagnose state of hydration than changes in hematocrit, serum proteins, and BUN, which are more dependent on other factors than hydration.

Changes in serum sodium most often reflect changes in water balance rather than sodium balance. If patient has not received a large load of sodium, hypernatremia suggests need for water, and hyponatremia suggests overhydration.

Formulas for *calculation* or *prediction* of serum osmolality:

$$\text{mOsm/L} = (2 \times \text{serum Na}) + \frac{\text{serum glucose}}{18} + \frac{\text{BUN}}{2.8} \text{ (in mg/dl)} \quad \text{or}$$

$$= (2 \times \text{serum Na}) + \frac{\text{serum glucose}}{20} + \frac{\text{BUN}}{3.0} + 9 \text{ (in mg/dl)} \quad \text{or}$$

$$= (2 \times \text{serum Na}) + \text{serum glucose (mmol/L)} + \text{BUN (mmol/L)}$$

Difference between measured and calculated values is <10 in healthy persons.
If measured − calculated osmolality > 10 (osmotic gap), one of the following is present:
Laboratory analytic error
Decreased serum water content
Hyperlipidemia (serum will appear lipemic)
Hyperproteinemia (total protein > 10 gm/dl)
Additional low-molecular-weight substances are in serum (measured osmolality will be >300 mOsm/kg water):
Ethanol
Methanol
Isopropyl alcohol
Ethylene glycol (when large amounts are ingested)
Acetone
Ethyl ether
Paraldehyde
Mannitol
Severely ill patients, especially those in hemorrhagic shock

Difference between measured and calculated values can be used to estimate the blood alcohol. Since serum osmolality increases 22 mOsm/kg for every 100 mg/dl of ethanol:

$$\text{Estimated blood alcohol (mg/dl)} = \text{osmotic gap} \times \frac{100}{22}$$

Osmotic gap can also be used to detect accumulation of infused mannitol in serum.

Serum osmolality is also used to determine serum water deviation from normal for evaluation of hyponatremia (see Causes of Hyponatremias, pp. 546–547; Table 14-24, p. 550)

SERUM POTASSIUM

(see also Table 3-1, pp. 40–41)

Increased In

Potassium retention
- Glomerular filtration rate <3–5 ml/min
  - Oliguria due to any condition (e.g., renal failure)
  - Chronic nonoliguric renal failure associated with dehydration, obstruction, trauma, or excess potassium
  - Excess dietary intake or rapid potassium infusion
- Glomerular filtration rate >20 ml/min
  - Decreased (aldosterone) mineralocorticoid activity
    - Addison's disease
    - Hypofunction of renin-angiotensin-aldosterone system (see p. 514)
    - Pseudohypoaldosteronism
    - Aldosterone antagonist drugs (e.g., spironolactone, captopril, heparin)
  - Increased or normal aldosterone
    - Drugs (e.g., spironolactone, triamterene, amiloride)
  - Mineralocorticoid-resistant syndromes
    - Primary tubular disorders
      - Hereditary
      - Acquired (e.g., systemic lupus erythematosus [SLE], amyloidosis, sickle cell nephropathy*, obstructive uropathy*, interstitial nephritis*, renal allograft transplant, chloride shift)

Potassium redistribution
- Familial hyperkalemic periodic paralysis (Gamstorp's disease, adynamia episodica hereditaria)
- Acute acidosis (especially hyperchloremic metabolic acidosis; less with respiratory; little with metabolic acidosis due to organic acids) (e.g., diabetic ketoacidosis, lactic acidosis, acute renal failure, acute respiratory acidosis)
- Decreased insulin
- Beta-adrenergic blockade
- Drugs (e.g., succinylcholine, great excess of digitalis, arginine infusion)
- Intravascular hemolysis (e.g., transfusion reaction, hemolytic anemia), rhabdomyolysis

Increased supply of potassium
- Laboratory artifacts (e.g., hemolysis during venipuncture, conditions associated with thrombocytosis [>1,000,000/cu mm] or leukocytosis [>100,000/cu mm], incomplete separation of serum and clot)
- Prolonged tourniquet use and hand exercise when drawing blood
- Potassium value can be elevated ~15% in slight hemolysis (Hgb ≤ 50 mg/dl); elevated ~30–50% in moderate hemolysis (Hgb > 100 mg/dl). Thus potassium status can be assessed with slight hemolysis but not with moderate hemolysis.

Decreased In

(see Table 13-2, p. 395)

Excess renal excretion
- Osmotic diuresis of hyperglycemia (e.g., uncontrolled diabetes)
- Nephropathies
  - Renal tubular acidosis (proximal or distal) (see pp. 560–562)
  - Bartter's syndrome (see pp. 510, 511)
  - Liddle's syndrome (see pp. 511, 514)
  - Magnesium depletion
- Drugs
  - Diuretics
  - Mineralocorticoids (e.g., aldosterone, desoxycorticosterone, fludrocor-

*Increased renin and aldosterone may be low.

tisone acetate, high doses of cortisone; some cases of Cushing's syndrome, especially due to ectopic ACTH production; renal vascular disease, malignant hypertension, renin-producing tumors) by excess administration or production by tumor
Antibiotics (e.g., amphotericin B, gentamicin, carbenicillin, ticarcillin)
Glycyrrhizic acid (licorice)

Nonrenal causes of excess potassium loss
- Gastrointestinal
  - Vomiting
  - Diarrhea
  - Neoplasms (e.g., villous adenoma of colon, pancreatic islet cell tumor that produces vasoactive intestinal polypeptide > 200 pg/ml)
  - Excessive spitting (sustained expectoration of all saliva in neurotic persons and to induce weight loss in professional wrestlers)
- Skin
  - Excessive sweating
  - Cystic fibrosis
  - Extensive burns
  - Draining wounds
- Cellular shifts
  - Respiratory alkalosis
  - Insulin
  - Adrenergic activity (e.g., epinephrine, albuterol)
  - Barium chloride poisoning
  - Treatment of megaloblastic anemia with vitamin B_{12} or folic acid
  - Classic periodic paralysis
  - Physiologic (e.g., highly trained athletes)

Diet
- Severe eating disorders (e.g., anorexia nervosa, bulimia)
- Dietary deficiency

SERUM CHLORIDE

Used with sodium, potassium, and carbon dioxide to assess electrolyte, acid-base, and water balance. Usually changes in same direction as sodium, except in metabolic acidosis with bicarbonate depletion and metabolic alkalosis with bicarbonate excess when serum sodium levels may be normal.

Increased In

Metabolic acidosis associated with prolonged diarrhea with loss of $NaHCO_3$
Renal tubular diseases with decreased excretion of H^+ and decreased reabsorption of HCO_3^- ("hyperchloremic metabolic acidosis")
Respiratory alkalosis (e.g., hyperventilation, severe CNS damage)
Excessive administration of certain drugs (e.g., NH_4Cl, IV saline, steroids, salicylate intoxication; acetazolamide therapy)
Some cases of hyperparathyroidism
Diabetes insipidus, dehydration
Sodium loss > chloride loss (e.g., diarrhea, intestinal fistulas)
Bromism
Ureterosigmoidostomy

Decreased In

Prolonged vomiting or suction (loss of HCl)
Metabolic acidoses with accumulation of organic anions (see Anion Gap Classification, pp. 393–394)
Chronic respiratory acidosis
Salt-losing renal diseases
Adrenocortical insufficiency
Primary aldosteronism

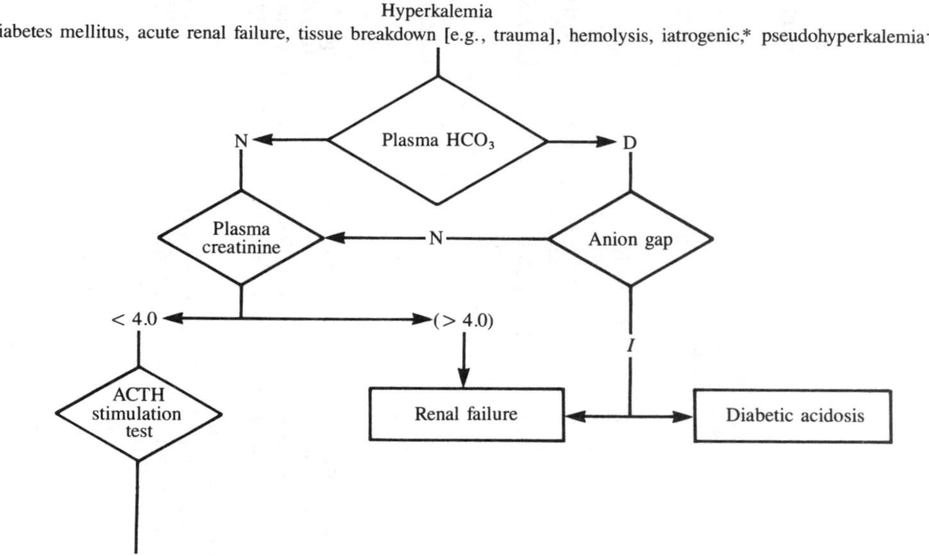
Hyperkalemia
(exclude diabetes mellitus, acute renal failure, tissue breakdown [e.g., trauma], hemolysis, iatrogenic,* pseudohyperkalemia†)
Plasma HCO3
N
D
Plasma creatinine
N
Anion gap
< 4.0
(> 4.0)
I
ACTH stimulation test
Renal failure
Diabetic acidosis

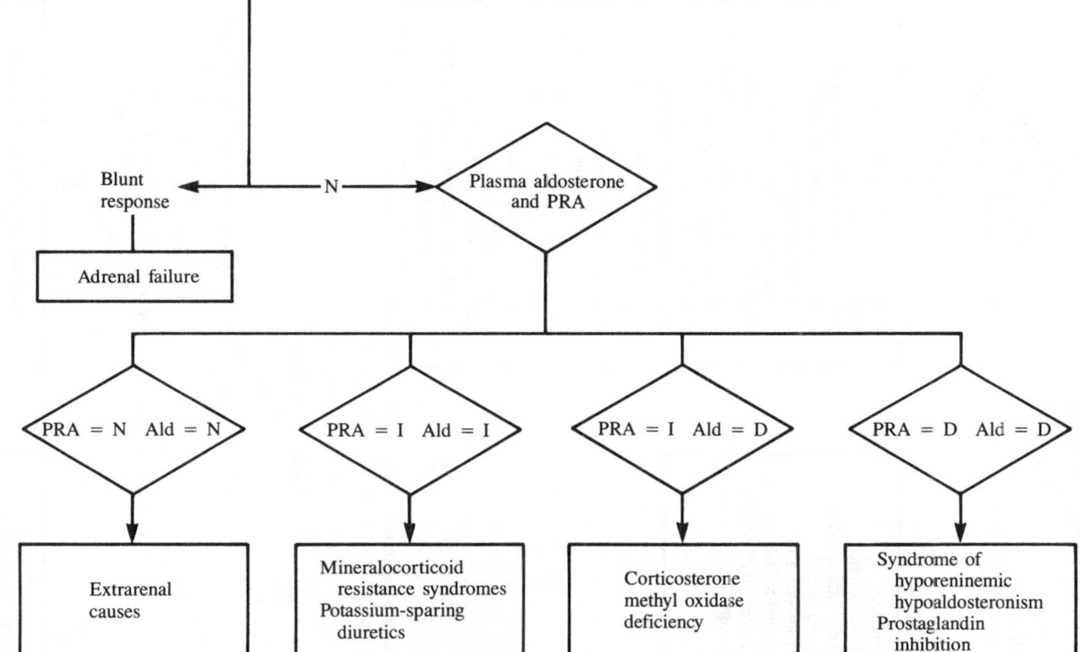

*Potassium-sparing diuretics, administration of potassium (e.g., blood transfusions, salt substitutes, potassium penicillin)

†Pseudohyperkalemia = WBC > 100,000/cu mm or platelet count > 1,000,000/cu mm (serum potassium > plasma potassium)

Fig. 3-3. Flow chart for hyperkalemia. (PRA = plasma renin activity; N = normal; D = decreased; I = increased; Ald = aldosterone.)

CO_2 > 30 mmol/L

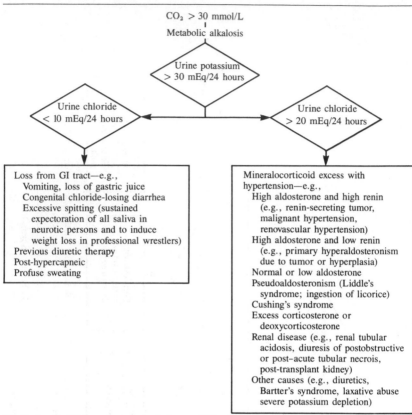

Metabolic alkalosis

Urine potassium > 30 mEq/24 hours

Urine chloride < 10 mEq/24 hours

Urine chloride > 20 mEq/24 hours

Loss from GI tract—e.g.,
- Vomiting, loss of gastric juice
- Congenital chloride-losing diarrhea
- Excessive spitting (sustained expectoration of all saliva in neurotic persons and to induce weight loss in professional wrestlers)

Previous diuretic therapy

Post-hypercapneic

Profuse sweating

Mineralocorticoid excess with hypertension—e.g.,
- High aldosterone and high renin (e.g., renin-secreting tumor, malignant hypertension, renovascular hypertension)
- High aldosterone and low renin (e.g., primary hyperaldosteronism due to tumor or hyperplasia)
- Normal or low aldosterone
- Pseudoaldosteronism (Liddle's syndrome; ingestion of licorice)
- Cushing's syndrome
- Excess corticosterone or deoxycorticosterone
- Renal disease (e.g., renal tubular acidosis, diuresis of postobstructive or post–acute tubular necrois, post-transplant kidney)
- Other causes (e.g., diuretics, Bartter's syndrome, laxative abuse severe potassium depletion)

Change in pH of 0.1 causes reciprocal change of 0.6 mEq/L in serum potassium in hyperchloremic acidosis, but < 0.4 mEq/L in other acid-base disturbances.

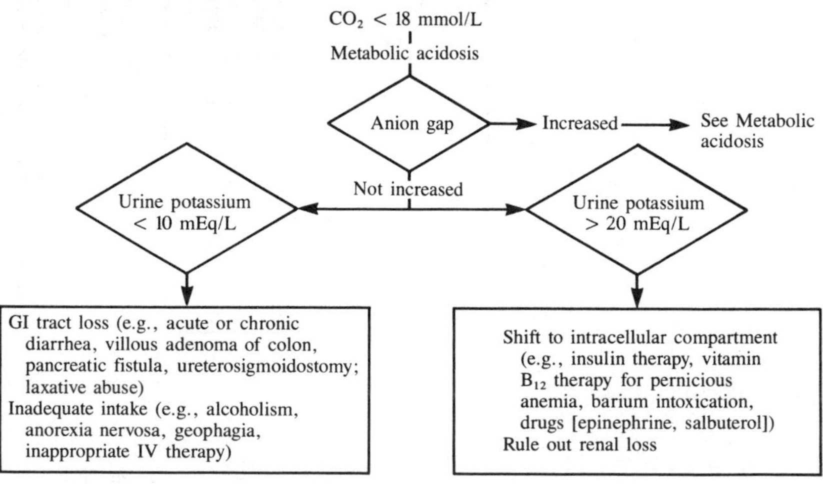

Fig. 3-4. Flow chart for hypokalemia.

Expansion of extracellular fluid (e.g., SIADH, hyponatremia, water intoxication, congestive heart failure)
Burns

SERUM MAGNESIUM

Increased In

Iatrogenic (is usual cause; most often with acute or chronic renal failure)
- Antacids containing magnesium
- Enemas containing magnesium
- Parenteral nutrition
- Magnesium for eclampsia or premature labor
- Lithium carbonate intoxication

Renal failure; in chronic renal failure, hypermagnesemia is inversely related to residual renal function.
Diabetic coma before treatment
Hypothyroidism
Addison's disease and after adrenalectomy
Controlled diabetes mellitus in older patients
Accidental ingestion of large amount of seawater

Signs	*Serum Levels in Adults*
Neuromuscular depression, hypotension	>4–6 mg/dl
Difficulty in urination	>5 mg/dl
CNS depression	6–8 mg/dl
Coma	12–17 mg/dl

Decreased In
(almost always due to GI or renal disturbance)

GI disease
- Malabsorption (e.g., sprue, small-bowel resection, biliary and intestinal fistulas, abdominal irradiation, celiac disease, and other causes of steatorrhea)
- Abnormal loss of GI fluids (e.g., chronic ulcerative colitis, Crohn's disease, villous adenoma, carcinoma of colon, laxative abuse, prolonged aspiration of intestinal contents)

Renal disease
- Chronic glomerulonephritis
- Chronic pyelonephritis
- Renal tubular acidosis
- Diuretic phase of acute tubular necrosis
- Postobstructive diuresis
- Drug injury
  - Diuretics (e.g., furosemide, thiazides, ethacrynic acid)
  - Antibiotics (e.g., gentamicin, tobramycin, carbenicillin, ticarcillin, amphotericin B, aminoglycosides)
  - Antineoplastic (e.g., cisplatin)
  - Cyclosporine
- Tubular losses due to ions or nutrients
  - Hypercalcemia
  - Diuresis due to glucose, urea, or mannitol
  - Phosphate depletion
  - Extracellular fluid volume expansion

Nutritional
- Prolonged parenteral fluid administration without magnesium (usually >3 weeks)
- Acute alcoholism and alcoholic cirrhosis
- Starvation with metabolic acidosis
- Kwashiorkor, protein-calorie malnutrition

Endocrine
- Hyperthyroidism
- Aldosteronism (primary and secondary)
- Hyperparathyroidism and other causes of hypercalcemia
- Hypoparathyroidism
- Diabetes mellitus (in 25–75% of patients)

Metabolic
- Excessive lactation
- Third trimester of pregnancy
- Insulin treatment of diabetic coma

Other
- Lytic tumors of bone
- Active Paget's disease of bone due to increased uptake by bone
- Acute pancreatitis
- Transfusion of citrated blood
- Severe burns
- Sweating
- Sepsis
- Hypothermia

Magnesium deficiency may cause apparently unexplained hypocalcemia and hypokalemia; the patients may have neurologic and GI symptoms (see Serum Calcium, next sections).

Approximately ninety percent of patients with high or low serum magnesium levels are not clinically recognized; therefore routine inclusion of magnesium with electrolyte measurements has been suggested.

SERUM TOTAL CALCIUM

(see Fig. 3-5)

Ninety percent of cases of hypercalcemia are due to hyperparathyroidism, neoplasms, or granulomatous diseases.

Hypercalcemia of sarcoidosis, adrenal insufficiency, and hyperthyroidism tends to be found in clinically evident disease.

Concomitant hypokalemia is not infrequent in hypercalcemia.

Concomitant dehydration is almost always present because hypercalcemia causes nephrogenic diabetes insipidus.

Increased In

Hyperparathyroidism
- Primary
- Secondary
  - Acute and chronic renal failure
  - Postrenal transplant
  - Osteomalacia with malabsorption
  - Aluminum-associated osteomalacia

Malignant tumors (especially breast, lung, kidney; 2% of patients with Hodgkin's or non-Hodgkin's lymphoma)
- Direct bone metastases (up to 30% of these patients) (e.g., breast cancer, Hodgkin's and non-Hodgkin's lymphoma, leukemia, pancreatic cancer, lung cancer)
- Osteoclast activating factor (e.g., multiple myeloma, adult T-cell lymphoma, Burkitt's lymphoma)
- Humoral hypercalcemia of malignancy
- Increased 1,25-dihydroxyvitamin D_3 (e.g., Hodgkin's and non-Hodgkin's lymphoma)

Effect of drugs
- Vitamin D intoxication
- Milk-alkali (Burnett's) syndrome

- Acute osteoporosis (e.g., immobilization of young patients or in Paget's disease)
- Diuretics (thiazide and chlorthalidone rarely increase serum calcium >1.0 mg/dl)
- Therapeutic agents (estrogens, androgens, progestins, tamoxifen, lithium)
- Others (e.g., vitamin A, thyroid hormone)

Other endocrine conditions
- Hyperthyroidism (in 20–40% of patients; usually <14 mg/dl)
- Some patients with hypothyroidism, Cushing's syndrome, adrenal insufficiency acromegaly)
- Multiple endocrine neoplasia

Granulomatous disease (e.g., sarcoidosis, tuberculosis, mycoses, berylliosis)
Artifactual (e.g., venous stasis during blood collection by prolonged application of tourniquet, use of cork-stoppered test tubes; elevated serum protein; dehydration)
Renal transplantation
Polyuric phase of acute renal failure
Miscellaneous
- Familial hypocalciuric hypercalcemia
- Rhabdomyolysis causing acute renal failure
- Porphyria
- Dehydration with hyperproteinemia
- Hypophosphatasia
- Idiopathic hypercalcemia of infancy

Decreased In

Hypoparathyroidism
- Surgical
- Idiopathic
- Pseudohypoparathyroidism

Chronic therapeutic use of anticonvulsant drugs (e.g., phenobarbital, phenytoin)
Malabsorption of calcium and vitamin D
Obstructive jaundice
Hypoalbuminemia
- Cachexia
- Nephrotic syndrome
- Sprue
- Celiac disease
- Cystic fibrosis of pancreas

Chronic renal disease with uremia and phosphate retention; Fanconi's syndrome; renal tubular acidosis
Acute pancreatitis with extensive fat necrosis
Insufficient calcium, phosphorus, and vitamin D ingestion
- Bone disease (osteomalacia, rickets)
- Starvation
- Late pregnancy

Certain drugs
- Mithramycin (for cancer chemotherapy)
- Citrated banked blood in recipient
- Fluoride intoxication
- Gentamicin
- Anticonvulsants
- Hypomagnesemia (e.g., due to cisplatin cancer chemotherapy)
- Hyperphosphatemia (e.g., laxatives, phosphate enemas, chemotherapy of leukemia or lymphoma, rhabdomyolysis)
- Loop-active diuretics
- Calcitonin

Neonates born of complicated pregnancies
- Hyperbilirubinemia
- Respiratory distress, asphyxia
- Cerebral injuries

Artifactual
- Hypoalbuminemia
- Hemodilution

Total serum protein and albumin should always be measured simultaneously for proper interpretation of serum calcium levels, since 0.8 mg of calcium is bound to 1.0 gm of albumin in serum; binding to globulin only affects total calcium if globulin > 6 gm/dl.

Hyponatremia (<120 mEq/L) increases protein-bound fraction of calcium, thereby slightly increasing the total calcium (opposite effect in hypernatremia).

SERUM IONIZED CALCIUM

45–50% of calcium is ionized; 40% is bound to albumin; 15% is bound to other anions (e.g., sulfate, phosphate, lactate, citrate); only ionized fraction is physiologically active. Total calcium levels may be deceiving since they may be unchanged even if ionized calcium level is changed; e.g., increased blood pH increases protein-bound calcium and decreases ionized calcium, and parathyroid hormone has the opposite effect (blood pH should always be performed with ionized calcium). However, in critically ill patients, elevated total serum calcium usually indicates ionized hypercalcemia, and a normal total serum calcium is evidence against ionized hypocalcemia.

Ionized calcium is the preferred measurement rather than total calcium because it is physiologically active and can be rapidly measured, which may be essential in certain situations (e.g., liver transplantation, rapid or large transfusion of citrated blood make interpretation of total calcium nearly impossible).

Reference ranges for ionized calcium vary with method and type of sample preparation (e.g., brand of heparin used) and should be determined by each laboratory. Sample ranges are

Age	Values
1 day	1.11–1.31 mmol/L
3 days	1.16–1.36 mmol/L
5 days	1.24–1.44 mmol/L
1 year–adult	1.29–1.31 mmol/L
Adults	1.15–1.35 mmol/L

Life-threatening complications are frequent when serum ionized calcium < 2 mg/dl (<0.50 mmol/L).

With multiple blood transfusions, ionized calcium < 3 mg/dl (<0.95 mmol/L) may be an indication to administer calcium.

Increased In

Normal total serum calcium associated with hypoalbuminemia may indicate ionized hypercalcemia.

~25% of patients with hyperparathyroidism have normal total but increased ionized calcium levels.

Decreased In

Hyperventilation (e.g., to control increased intracranial pressure) (total serum calcium may be normal)

Administration of bicarbonate to control metabolic acidosis

Increased serum free fatty acids (increase calcium binding to albumin) due to

- Certain drugs (e.g., heparin, intravenous lipids, epinephrine, norepinephrine, isoproterenol, alcohol)
- Severe stress (e.g., acute pancreatitis, diabetic ketoacidosis, sepsis, acute myocardial infarction)
- Hemodialysis

Increase of ions to which calcium is bound
- Phosphate (e.g., phosphorus administration in treatment of diabetic ketoacidosis, chemotherapy causing tumor lysis syndrome, rhabdomyolysis)
- Bicarbonate
- Citrate (e.g., during blood transfusion)
- Radiographic contrast media containing calcium chelators (edetate, citrate)

Hypoparathyroidism (primary, secondary)
Vitamin D deficiency
Hypo- or hypermagnesemia (see pp. 49–50); patients respond to serum magnesium that becomes normal but not to calcium therapy.
Toxic shock syndrome
Fat embolism

Hypokalemia protects the patient from hypocalcemic tetany; correction of hypokalemia without correction of hypocalcemia may provoke tetany.

SERUM PHOSPHORUS

Increased In

- Acute or chronic renal failure (most common cause) with decreased glomerular filtration rate (GFR)
- Increased tubular reabsorption
  - Hypoparathyroidism
    - Idiopathic
    - Surgical
    - Irradiation
    - Surgical
  - Secondary hyperparathyroidism (renal rickets)
  - Pseudohypoparathyroidism
  - Other endocrine disorders
    - Addison's disease
    - Acromegaly
  - Sickle cell anemia
- Increased phosphate load
  - Exogenous
    - Phosphate enemas, laxatives, or infusions
    - Excess vitamin D intake
    - Massive blood transfusions
    - IV therapy for hypophosphatemia or hypercalcemia
    - Milk-alkali (Burnett's) syndrome (some patients)
  - Endogenous (high tissue turnover)
    - Neoplasms (e.g., myelogenous leukemia)
    - Excessive breakdown of tissue (e.g., chemotherapy for neoplasms, rhabdomyolysis, lactic acidosis, acute yellow atrophy)
    - Bone disease
      - Healing fractures
      - Multiple myeloma (some patients)
      - Paget's disease (some patients)
      - Osteolytic metastatic tumor in bone (some patients)
    - Childhood
- Miscellaneous
  - High intestinal obstruction
  - Sarcoidosis (some patients)
  - Magnesium deficiency

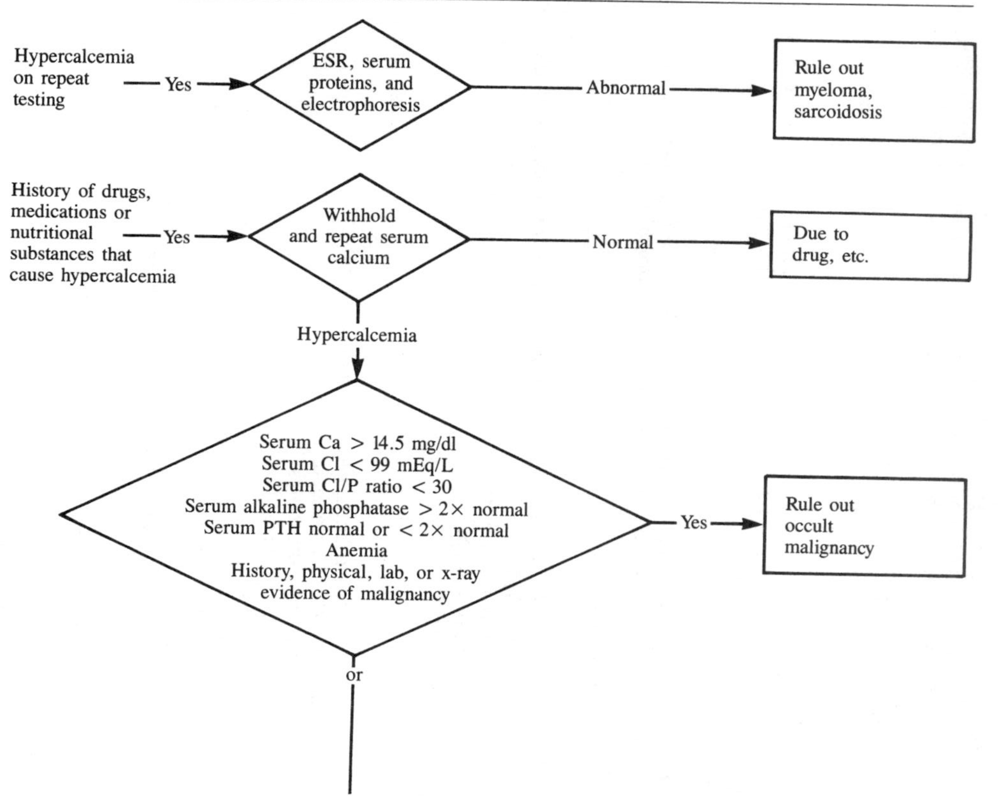
Hypercalcemia on repeat testing
Yes
ESR, serum proteins, and electrophoresis
Abnormal
Rule out myeloma, sarcoidosis
History of drugs, medications or nutritional substances that cause hypercalcemia
Yes
Withhold and repeat serum calcium
Normal
Due to drug, etc.
Hypercalcemia
Serum Ca > 14.5 mg/dl
Serum Cl < 99 mEq/L
Serum Cl/P ratio < 30
Serum alkaline phosphatase > 2× normal
Serum PTH normal or < 2× normal
Anemia
History, physical, lab, or x-ray evidence of malignancy
Yes
Rule out occult malignancy
or

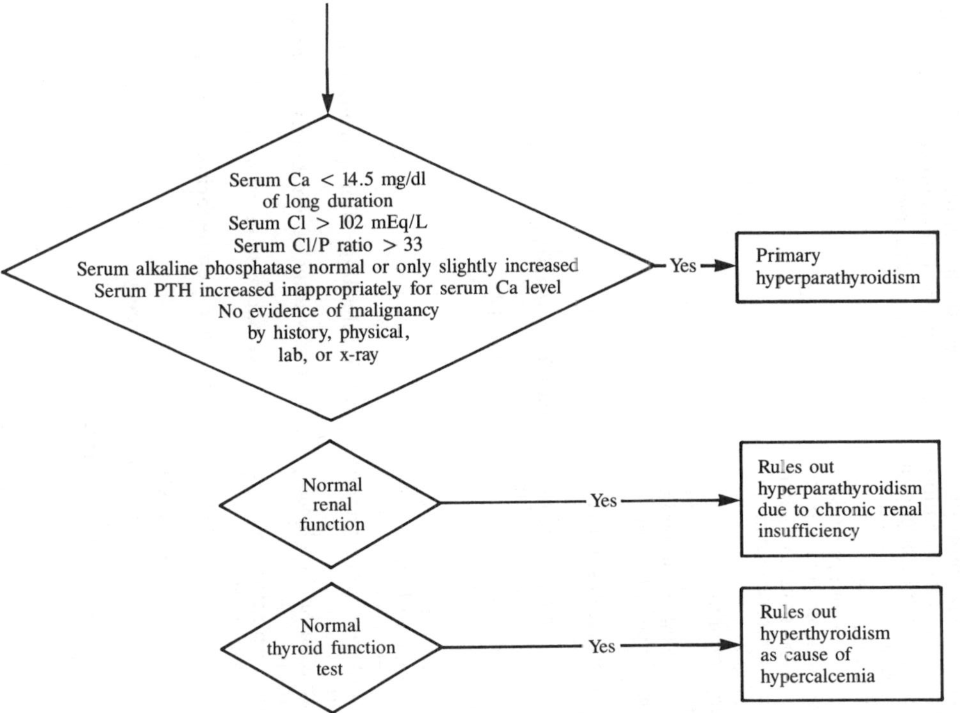

Fig. 3-5. Flow chart for diagnosis of hypercalcemia. (Data from ET Wong and EF Freier, The differential diagnosis of hypercalcemia: An algorithm for more effective use of laboratory tests. *JAMA* 247:75, 1982; KR Johnson and AT Howarth, Differential laboratory diagnosis of hypercalcemia. *CRC Crit Rev Clin Lab Sci* 21:51, 1984.)

Serum magnesium should always be measured in any patient with hypocalcemia.

Artifactual increase by hemolysis of blood.

Decreased In

(Mechanisms of hypophosphatemia are intracellular shift of phosphate, increased loss [via kidney or intestine], or decreased intestinal absorption, usually associated with prior phosphorus depletion. Often, more than one mechanism is operative.)

Renal or intestinal loss
- Administration of diuretics
- Renal tubular defects (e.g., Fanconi's syndrome)
- Primary hyperparathyroidism
- Idiopathic hypercalciuria
- Hypokalemia
- Hypomagnesemia
- Dialysis
- Primary hypophosphatemia
- Idiopathic hypercalciuria
- Acute gout

Decreased intestinal absorption
- Malabsorption
- Vitamin D deficiency and/or resistance, osteomalacia
- Malnutrition, vomiting, diarrhea
- Administration of phosphate-binding antacids*

Intracellular shift of phosphate
- Alcoholism*
- Diabetes mellitus*
- Acidosis (especially ketoacidosis)
- Hyperalimentation*
- Nutritional recovery syndrome* (rapid refeeding after prolonged starvation)
- Administration of IV glucose (e.g., recovery after severe burns, hyperalimentation)
- Alkalosis, respiratory (e.g., gram-negative bacteremia) or metabolic
- Salicylate poisoning
- Administration of anabolic steroids, androgens, epinephrine, glucagon, insulin
- Cushing's syndrome (some patients)
- Prolonged hypothermia (e.g., open heart surgery)

SERUM ALKALINE PHOSPHATASE

(see also Table 14-6, pp. 472–473)

Increased In

Increased deposition of calcium in bone
- Osteitis fibrosa cystica (hyperparathyroidism)
- Paget's disease (osteitis deformans)
- Healing fractures (slightly)
- Osteoblastic bone tumors (osteogenic sarcoma, metastatic carcinoma)
- Osteogenesis imperfecta (due to healing fractures)
- Familial osteoectasia
- Osteomalacia
- Rickets
- Polyostotic fibrous dysplasia
- Late pregnancy; reverts to normal level by 20th day postpartum

*Conditions associated with severe hypophosphatemia.

Children
Administration of ergosterol
Liver disease—any obstruction of biliary system
Nodules in liver (metastatic tumor, abscess, cyst, parasite, amyloid, tuberculosis, sarcoid, or leukemia)
Biliary duct obstruction (e.g., stone, carcinoma)
Cholangiolar obstruction in hepatitis
Adverse reaction to therapeutic drug (e.g., chlorpropamide)
(progressive elevation of serum alkaline phosphatase may be first indication that drug therapy should be halted)
Chronic therapeutic use of anticonvulsant drugs (e.g., phenobarbital, phenytoin)
Placental origin—appears 16–20th week of normal pregnancy, increases progressively up to onset of labor, disappears 3–6 days after delivery of placenta. May be increased during complications of pregnancy (e.g., hypertension, preeclampsia, eclampsia, threatened abortion) but difficult to interpret without serial determinations.
Intestinal origin—is a component in ~25% of normal sera; increases after eating in these persons. Has been reported to be increased in cirrhosis, various diseases of GI tract, chronic hemodialysis. Benign familial hyperphosphatasemia (see p. 478).
Ectopic production by neoplasm without involvement of liver or bone (e.g., Hodgkin's disease, cancer of lung or pancreas)
Marked hyperthyroidism in some patients (bone origin)
Some patients with myocardial, pulmonary, renal (one-third of cases), or splenic infarction, usually during phase of organization
Intravenous injection of albumin; sometimes marked increase (e.g., 10 times normal level) lasting for several days (placental origin)
Hyperphosphatasia (liver and bone isoenzymes)
Primary hypophosphatemia (often increased)
Alkaline phosphatase isoenzyme determinations are not clinically useful; heat inactivation may be more useful to distinguish bone from liver source of increased alkaline phosphatase. Or use serum gamma-glutamyl transpeptidase (GGT) or leucine aminopeptidase (LAP).

Increase in cases of metastases to bone is marked only in prostate carcinoma. Increase > 2 times upper limit of normal in patients with primary breast or lung tumor with osteolytic metastases is more likely due to liver than bone metastases.

Whenever the alkaline phosphatase is elevated, a simultaneous elevation of 5′-nucleotidase (5′-N) establishes biliary disease as the cause of the elevated alkaline phosphatase. If the 5′-N is not increased, the cause of the elevated alkaline phosphatase must be found elsewhere, e.g., bone disease.

Marked elevation in absence of liver disease is most suggestive of Paget's disease of bone or metastatic carcinoma from prostate.

Normal In

Inherited metabolic diseases (Dubin-Johnson, Rotor's, Gilbert's, Crigler-Najjar syndromes; types I–V glycogenoses, mucopolysaccharidoses; increase in Wilson's disease and hemochromatosis related to hepatic fibrosis)
Consumption of alcohol by healthy persons (in contrast to GGT); may be normal even in alcoholic hepatitis.
In acute icteric viral hepatitis, increase is <2 times normal in 90% of cases, but when alkaline phosphatase is high and serum bilirubin is normal, rule out infectious mononucleosis as cause of hepatitis.

Decreased In

Excess vitamin D ingestion
Milk-alkali (Burnett's) syndrome

Scurvy
Hypophosphatasia
Hypothyroidism
Pernicious anemia in one-third of patients
Celiac disease
Malnutrition
Collection of blood in EDTA, fluoride, or oxalate anticoagulant

SERUM LEUCINE AMINOPEPTIDASE (LAP)

Parallels serum alkaline phosphatase except that

LAP is usually normal in the presence of bone disease or malabsorption syndrome.

LAP is a more sensitive indicator of choledocholithiasis and of liver metastases in anicteric patients.

When serum LAP is increased, urine LAP is almost always increased; but when urine LAP is increased, serum LAP may have already returned to normal.

5′-NUCLEOTIDASE (5′-N)

Increased Only In

Obstructive type of hepatobiliary disease

May be an early indication of liver metastases in the cancer patient, especially if jaundice is absent.

Normal In

Pregnancy and postpartum period (in contrast to serum LAP and alkaline phosphatase); therefore may aid in differential diagnosis of hepatobiliary disease occurring during pregnancy.

SERUM GAMMA-GLUTAMYL TRANSPEPTIDASE (GGT)

Increased In

Liver disease. Generally parallels changes in serum alkaline phosphatase, LAP, and 5′-N but is more sensitive.

Acute hepatitis. Elevation is less marked than that of other liver enzymes, but it is the last to return to normal and therefore is useful to indicate recovery.

Chronic hepatitis. Increased more than in acute hepatitis. More elevated than SGOT and SGPT. In dormant stage, may be the only enzyme elevated.

Cirrhosis. In inactive cases, average values are lower than in chronic hepatitis. Increases greater than 10–20 times in cirrhotic patients suggest superimposed primary carcinoma of the liver.

Primary biliary cirrhosis. Elevation is marked.

Fatty liver. Elevation parallels that of SGOT and SGPT but is greater.

Obstructive jaundice. Increase is faster and greater than that of serum alkaline phosphatase and LAP.

Liver metastases. Parallels alkaline phosphatase; elevation precedes positive liver scans.

Cholestasis. In mechanical and viral cholestasis, GGT and LAP are about equally increased, but in drug-induced cholestasis, GGT is much more increased than LAP.

Children. Much more increased in biliary atresia than in neonatal hepatitis (300 units/L is useful differentiating level). Children with $alpha_1$ antitrypsin deficiency have higher levels than other patients with biliary atresia.

Pancreatitis. Always elevated in acute pancreatitis. In chronic pancreatitis, is increased when there is involvement of the biliary tract or active inflammation.

Acute myocardial infarction. Increased in 50% of the patients. Elevation begins on fourth to fifth day, reaches maximum at 8–12 days. With shock or acute right heart failure, may have early peak within 48 hours, with rapid decline followed by later rise.

Heavy use of alcohol, barbiturates, or phenytoin (Dilantin). Is the most sensitive indicator of alcoholism, since elevation exceeds that of other commonly assayed liver enzymes.

Some cases of carcinoma of prostate.

Neoplasms, even in absence of liver metastases; especially malignant melanoma, carcinoma of breast and lung; highest levels in hypernephroma.

Gross obesity (slight increase)

Normal In

Women during pregnancy (in contrast to serum alkaline phosphatase and LAP) and children over 3 months of age; therefore may aid in differential diagnosis of hepatobiliary disease occurring during pregnancy and childhood.

Bone disease or patients with increased bone growth (children and adolescents); therefore useful in distinguishing bone disease from liver disease as a cause of increased serum alkaline phosphatase.

Renal failure

Strenuous exercise

Principal uses are as sensitive indicator of alcoholism and for differential diagnosis of liver disease in children and pregnant women that alters other serum enzymes (e.g., alkaline phosphatase and LAP).

SERUM BILIRUBIN

Increased In

(see also Chap. 9, Hepatobiliary Diseases and Diseases of Pancreas)

Hepatic cellular damage

Biliary duct obstructions

Hemolytic diseases

Prolonged fasting

Direct (conjugated) bilirubin

- <20% of total: due to hemolysis or constitutional hyperbilirubinemia (e.g., Gilbert's disease, Crigler-Najjar syndrome)
- 20–40% of total: more suggestive of hepatic than posthepatic jaundice
- 40–60% of total: occurs in either hepatic or posthepatic jaundice
- >50% of total: more suggestive of posthepatic than hepatic jaundice

Increased conjugated bilirubin may be associated with normal total bilirubin in up to one-third of patients with liver diseases.

Total serum bilirubin >40 mg/dl indicates hepatocellular rather than extrahepatic obstruction.

A 48-hour fast produces a mean increase of 240% in normal patients and 194% in those with hepatic dysfunction.

Decreased In

Ingestion of certain drugs (e.g., barbiturates)

SERUM GLUTAMIC-OXALOACETIC TRANSAMINASE (SGOT) (ASPARTATE AMINOTRANSFERASE [AST])

Increased In

Acute myocardial infarction (see also Chap. 6, Cardiovascular Diseases); especially useful in patients tested >48 hours after onset of symptoms. Level reflects size of infarct.

Liver diseases (see also Chap. 9, Hepatobiliary Diseases and Diseases of Pancreas)
- Active necrosis of parenchymal cells is suggested by extremely high levels
  - Acute viral hepatitis shows greatest increases; may be 20–100 times normal.
- Is often used as surrogate test for screening blood donors.

Hepatotoxic drugs (e.g., salicylates)

Musculoskeletal diseases, including trauma, surgery, and IM injections

Acute pancreatitis

Other
- Myoglobinuria
- Intestinal injury (e.g., surgery, infarction)
- Local irradiation injury
- Pulmonary infarction (relatively slight increase)
- Cerebral infarction (increased in following week in 50% of patients)
- Cerebral neoplasms (occasionally)
- Renal infarction (occasionally)
- "Pseudomyocardial infarction" pattern. Administration of opiates to patients with diseased biliary tract or previous cholecystectomy causes increase in lactic dehydrogenase (LDH) and especially SGOT. SGOT increases by 2–4 hours, peaks in 5–8 hours; increase may persist for 24 hours; elevation may be 2½–65 times normal.
- Drugs (e.g., heparin therapy)
- Rapid rise and decline suggest extrahepatic biliary disease
- Burns
- Heat exhaustion
- Mushroom poisoning
- Lead poisoning (not useful for screening)

Decreased In

Azotemia

Chronic renal dialysis

Falsely Increased In

(because enzymes are activated during test)

Therapy with Prostaphlin, Polycillin, opiates, erythromycin

Calcium dust in air (e.g., due to construction in laboratory)

Falsely Decreased In

(because of increased serum lactate–consuming enzyme during test)

Diabetic ketoacidosis

Beriberi

Severe liver disease

Chronic hemodialysis (reason unknown)

Uremia—proportional to BUN level (reason unknown)

Normal In

Angina pectoris

Coronary insufficiency

Pericarditis

Congestive heart failure without liver damage

SGOT varies <10 units/day in the same person.

SERUM GLUTAMIC-PYRUVIC TRANSAMINASE (SGPT)

(alanine aminotransferase [ALT])

Generally parallels SGOT, but the differences (SGOT/SGPT ratio) may be useful in differential diagnosis.

Also Increased In

Obesity (not SGOT)
Severe preeclampsia (both)
Rapidly progressing acute lymphoblastic leukemia (both)
Levels in females ~75% of those in males

SGOT/SGPT RATIO*

(normal = 0.7–1.4 depending on methodology)

Increased In

Drug hepatotoxicity (>2.0)
Alcoholic hepatitis (>1.5 is highly suggestive; may be 2.0–6.0)
Cirrhosis (1.4–2.0)
Intrahepatic cholestasis (>1.5)
Hepatocellular carcinoma
Chronic hepatitis (slightly increased; 1.3)

Decreased In

Acute viral hepatitis (usually ≤0.65; ratio 0.3–0.6 is a good prognostic sign, but higher ratio of 1.2–1.6 is a poor prognostic sign)
Extrahepatic cholestasis (normal or slightly decreased; 0.8)

SERUM LACTIC DEHYDROGENASE (LDH)

Increased In

Acute myocardial infarction (AMI). Serum LDH is almost always increased, beginning in 10–12 hours and reaching a peak (of about 3 times normal), in 48–72 hours. The prolonged elevation of 10–14 days is particularly useful for late diagnosis when the patient is first seen after sufficient time has elapsed for creatine kinase (CK) and SGOT to become normal. Levels > 2000 units suggest a poorer prognosis. Because many other diseases may increase the LDH, isoenzyme studies should be performed. Increased serum LDH, with a ratio of LDH_1/LDH_2 > 1 ("flipped" LDH), occurs in acute renal infarction, pernicious anemia, and hemolysis associated with hemolytic anemia or prosthetic heart valves as well as in AMI. In AMI, flipped LDH usually appears between 12 and 24 hours and is present within 48 hours in 80% of patients; after 1 week it is still present in <50% of patients, even though total serum LDH may still be elevated; flipped LDH never appears before CK-MB isoenzyme. LDH_1 may remain elevated after total LDH has returned to normal; with small infarcts, LDH_1 may be increased when total LDH remains normal. (See Serum Creatine Kinase [CK] Isoenzymes, p. 62.)
AMI with congestive heart failure. May show increase of LDH_1 and LDH_5.
Congestive heart failure alone. LDH isoenzymes are normal.
Insertion of intracardiac prosthetic valves consistently causes chronic hemolysis with increase of total LDH and of LDH_1 and LDH_2. This is also often present before surgery in patients with severe hemodynamic abnormalities of cardiac valves.
Cardiovascular surgery. LDH is increased up to 2 times normal without cardiopulmonary bypass and returns to normal in 3–4 days; with extracorporeal

*Data from R Reg, Aminotransferases in disease. *Clin Lab Med* 9:667, 1989.

circulation, it may increase up to 4–6 times normal; increase is more marked when transfused blood is older.

Hepatitis. Most marked increase is of LDH_5, which occurs during prodromal stage and is greatest at time of onset of jaundice; total LDH is also increased in 50% of the cases. LDH_5 is also increased with other causes of liver damage (e.g., chlorpromazine hepatitis, carbon tetrachloride poisoning, exacerbation of cirrhosis, biliary obstruction) even when total LDH is normal. Liver disease, per se, does not produce marked increase of total LDH or LDH_5. *If liver disease is suspect but total LDH is very high and isoenzyme pattern is nonspecific, rule out cancer.*

Untreated pernicious anemia. Total LDH (chiefly LDH_1) is markedly increased, especially with hemoglobin <8 gm/dl. Hemolytic anemia can probably be ruled out if LDH_1 and LDH_2 are not increased in an anemic patient. Normal in iron deficiency anemia, even when very severe.

Malignant tumors. Increased in ~50% of patients with carcinoma, especially in advanced stages. In patients with cancer, a higher LDH level generally indicates a poorer prognosis. Whenever the total LDH is increased and the isoenzyme pattern is nonspecific or cannot be explained by obvious clinical findings (e.g., myocardial infarction, hemolytic anemia), cancer should always be ruled out. Increased in ~60% of patients with lymphomas and lymphocytic leukemias. Increased in ~90% of patients with acute leukemia; degree of increase is not correlated with level of WBC; relatively low levels in lymphatic type of leukemia.

Increased in 95% of patients with myelogenous leukemia. (See also Chap. 12, Hematologic Diseases.)

Disease of muscle (see pp. 240, 242). Marked increase of LDH_5 is likely due to anoxic injury of striated muscle.

Electrical and thermal burns and trauma. Marked increase of total LDH (about the same as in myocardial infarction) and LDH_5.

Pulmonary embolus and infarction—*pattern of increased LDH with increased LDH_3 and normal SGOT 24–48 hours after onset of chest pain* (see Serum Lactic Dehydrogenase [LDH] Isoenzymes).

Renal diseases. LDH_4 and LDH_5 may be increased in nephrotic syndrome. LDH_1 and LDH_2 may be increased in nephritis. In renal cortical infarction, total LDH may be increased with $LDH_1 > LDH_2$. *Rule out renal infarction if LDH_1 is increased in the absence of myocardial infarction or anemia; increased LDH is out of proportion to SGOT and alkaline phosphatase levels.* Generally not clinically useful but may mimic pattern of AMI.

Other causes of hemolysis

- Artifactual (e.g., poor venipuncture, failure to separate clot from serum, heating of blood)
- Various hemolytic conditions in vivo (e.g., hemolytic anemias)

Miscellaneous conditions (may be related to hemolysis, involvement of liver, striated muscle, heart)

- Various infectious and parasitic diseases
- Hypothyroidism, subacute thyroiditis
- Collagen vascular diseases
- Acute pancreatitis
- Intestinal obstruction
- Sarcoidosis

Decreased In

X-ray irradiation

SERUM LACTIC DEHYDROGENASE (LDH) ISOENZYMES

Interpretation of this test must be correlated with clinical status of the patient. Do serial determinations to obtain maximum information.

Condition	LDH Isoenzyme Increased
AMI	I and II
Acute renal cortical infarction	I and II
Pernicious anemia	I
Sickle cell crisis	I and II
Electrical and thermal burn, trauma	V
Mother carrying erythroblastotic child	IV and V
AMI with acute congestion of liver	I and V
Early hepatitis	V (may become normal even when SGPT is still rising)
Malignant lymphoma	III and IV (may even increase II) (reflects effect of chemotherapy)
SLE	III and IV
Dermatomyositis	V
Carcinoma of prostate	V
Pulmonary embolus and infarction	II and III
Pulmonary embolus with acute cor pulmonale causing acute congestion of liver	III and V

Increased total LDH with normal distribution of isoenzymes may be seen in myocardial infarction, arteriosclerotic heart disease with chronic heart failure, various combinations of acute and chronic diseases (this may represent a general stress reaction).

About 50% of patients with malignant tumors have altered LDH patterns. This change often is nonspecific and of no diagnostic value. Solid tumors, especially of germ cell origin, may increase LDH_1.

In megaloblastic anemia, hemolysis, and renal cortical infarction, the isoenzyme pattern may mimic myocardial infarction, but the time to peak value and the increase help to differentiate.

SERUM ALPHA-HYDROXYBUTYRIC DEHYDROGENASE (α-HBD)

Increased In

Acute myocardial infarction. Is more specific than SGOT and LDH but less specific than CK and LDH isoenzymes.

Other conditions that cause elevation of fast-moving LDH in serum (e.g., muscular dystrophy, megaloblastic anemia)

Increase is always accompanied by increased LDH activity.

May Be Slightly Increased In

Heart failure

Nephrosis

Normal In

Angina pectoris

SERUM CREATINE KINASE (CK)

Increased In

Necrosis or acute atrophy of cardiac muscle (see also Chap. 6, Cardiovascular Diseases)
- AMI
- Severe myocarditis

Necrosis or acute atrophy of striated muscle (see also Chap. 11, Musculoskeletal System and Joint Diseases)
- Progressive muscular dystrophy
- Amyotrophic lateral sclerosis (>40% of cases)

Polymyositis (70% of cases; average 20 times upper limit of normal [ULN])
Thermal and electrical burns (values usually higher than in AMI)
Rhabdomyolysis (especially with trauma and severe exertion; also after alcohol or other drug abuse); associated with myoglobinemia and myoglobinuria; marked increase may be 1000 times ULN
Severe or prolonged exercise (begins 3 hours after start of exercise; peaks after 8–16 hours; usually normal by 48 hours)
Status epilepticus
Postoperative state. Increase may last up to 5 days. Greater increase with use of electrocautery in surgery
Chemical toxicity (benzene ring compounds [e.g., xylene] depolarize surface membrane and leach out low-molecular-weight enzymes, producing very high levels of total CK (100% MM) with increased LDH of 3–5 times normal.

Half of patients with extensive brain infarction. Maximum levels in 3 days; increase may not appear before 2 days; levels usually less than in AMI and remain increased for longer time; return to normal within 14 days; high mortality associated with levels >300 IU. Elevated serum CK in brain infarction may obscure diagnosis of concomitant AMI.
Parturition and frequently the last few weeks of pregnancy
Malignant hyperthermia (see pp. 115–121)
Endocrine myopathy
Hypothyroidism—increased 4–8 times ULN in 60–80% of cases; becomes normal within 6 weeks of replacement therapy.
Acromegaly—increased 2 times ULN.

Slight Increase Occasionally In

IM injections. Variable increase after IM injection to 2–6 times normal level. Returns to normal 48 hours after cessation of injections.
Muscle spasms or convulsions in children
Electrical cardiac defibrillation or countershock in 50% of patients; returns to normal in 48–72 hours.

Normal In

Angina pectoris
Pericarditis
Pulmonary infarction
Renal infarction
Liver disease
Biliary obstruction
Some muscle disorders
Neurogenic muscle atrophy
Thyrotoxicosis
Steroid myopathy
Pernicious anemia
Most malignancies
Following cardiac catheterization and coronary arteriography unless myocardium has been injured by catheter

SERUM CREATINE KINASE (CK) ISOENZYMES

MB Isoenzyme May Be Increased In

Necrosis of cardiac muscle
AMI (see pp. 115–119)
Cardiac contusion
Cardiac surgical procedures
Cardioversion (>400 joules)
Percutaneous transluminal coronary angioplasty

Pericarditis
Prolonged supraventricular tachycardia
Noncardiac causes
Skeletal muscle trauma
Skeletal muscle diseases (e.g., myositis, muscular dystrophies)
Reye's syndrome
Hypothyroidism
Alcoholism
Peripartum period
Acute cholecystitis
Carcinomas (e.g., prostate, breast)
Drugs (e.g., aspirin, tranquilizers)

BB Isoenzyme May Be Increased In

Malignant hyperthermia, uremia, brain infarction (see Serum Creatine Kinase, p. 62) or anoxia, necrosis of intestine, various neoplasms, biliary atresia. It is rarely encountered clinically.

SERUM ISOCITRATE DEHYDROGENASE (ICD)

Increased In

Liver disease
Early viral hepatitis, hepatitis of infectious mononucleosis and of liver poisons—ICD > 25 IU, becomes normal in 2–3 weeks
Metastatic carcinoma—ICD < 20 IU
Cirrhosis—normal or slightly increased
Extrahepatic biliary obstruction—normal
Neonatal biliary atresia—may be increased
With protein malnutrition—may be increased
Active placental degeneration
Placental infarction
Preeclampsia
Some cases of carcinoma without liver metastases

Normal In

AMI
Pregnancy

SERUM ALDOLASE (ALD)

Increased In

Cell destruction
AMI
Burns
Acute hepatitis
Muscular dystrophies (especially Duchenne type), myopathies, polymyositis
Carcinoma of prostate
20% of cancer patients—more frequent with liver involvement

Normal In

Neurogenic muscle atrophy
Cirrhosis (or may be slightly increased)
Obstructive jaundice (or may be slightly increased)

SERUM ORNITHINE CARBAMYL TRANSFERASE (OCT)

Increased In

Liver cell damage (e.g., hepatitis, metastatic carcinoma, cirrhosis, acute cholecystitis)
Intestinal mucosa damage (e.g., enteritis, infarction)

Alcohol consumption
Prolonged exercise (some patients)

BLOOD AMMONIA

(normal <40 μmol/L; infants at term <100 μmol/L [venous] or <150 μmol/L [capillary]; premature infants <300 μmol/L)

Increased In

Transient hyperammonemia in newborn; unknown etiology; may be life-threatening in first 48 hours.

Moribund children. Moderate increases (≤300 μmol/L) without being diagnostic of a specific disease.

May occur in any patient with severe liver disease (e.g., acute hepatic necrosis, terminal cirrhosis, hepatectomy). Not useful to assess degree of dysfunction; e.g., in Reye's syndrome, hepatic function improves and ammonia level falls even in patients who finally die of this.

Increased in most casees of hepatic coma but correlates poorly with degree of encephalopathy. *In cirrhosis, blood ammonia may be increased after portacaval anastomosis.*

Some inherited metabolic disorders, especially ornithine carbamoyltransferase, citrullinemia, argininosuccinic aciduria

GU tract infection with distention and stasis

Sodium valproate therapy

Should be measured in cases of unexplained lethargy and vomiting, encephalopathy or any neonate with unexplained neurological deterioration.

Decreased In

Hyperornithinemia (deficiency of ornithine aminotransaminase activity) with gyrate atrophy of choroid and retina

SERUM TOTAL PROTEIN

Increased In

Hypergammaglobulinemias (mono- or polyclonal)
Hypovolemic states

Decreased In

Nutritional deficiency
- Malabsorption
- Kwashiorkor
- Marasmus

Decreased or ineffective protein synthesis
- Severe liver disease
- Agammaglobulinemia

Increased loss
- Renal (e.g., nephrotic syndrome)
- GI disease (e.g., protein-losing enteropathies, surgical resection)
- Severe skin disease (e.g., burns, pemphigus vulgaris, eczema)

Increased catabolism
- Fever
- Inflammation
- Hyperthyroidism
- Malignancy
- Chronic diseases

Dilutional
- IV fluids
- SIADH
- Water intoxication

SERUM ALBUMIN

(generally parallels total protein except when total protein changes are due to gamma globulins)

Increased In

Dehydration (relative increase)
IV albumin infusions

Decreased In

Inadequate intake (e.g., malnutrition)
Decreased absorption (e.g., malabsorption syndromes)
Increased need (e.g., hyperthyroidism, pregnancy)
Impaired synthesis (e.g., liver diseases, chronic infection, hereditary analbuminemia)
Increased breakdown (e.g., neoplasms, infection, trauma)
Increased loss (e.g., edema, ascites, burns, hemorrhage, nephrotic syndrome, protein-losing enteropathy)
Dilutional (e.g., IV fluids, SIADH, psychogenic diabetes/water intoxication)

SEPARATION OF SERUM PROTEINS (IMMUNODIFFUSION, ELECTROPHORESIS)

Diagnosis of Specific Diseases

Multiple myeloma
Waldenström's macroglobulinemia
Hypogammaglobulinemia
- Agammaglobulinemia
- Agamma-A-globulinemia
- Analbuminemia

Bisalbuminemia
Afibrinogenemia
Atransferrinemia
Wilson's disease

Other Changes

Nonspecific changes in serum proteins
Protein pattern changes in urine, cerebrospinal fluid, peritoneal fluid, etc.

SERUM PROTEIN GAMMOPATHIES

(localized or general increase in immunoglobulins demonstrated by serum immunoelectrophoresis)

Monoclonal

(hyperproteinemia very frequent)
IgG gammopathy with or without Bence Jones protein (60% of patients)
IgA gammopathy (16% of patients)
IgM gammopathy (15% of patients)
Bence Jones gammopathy (light-chain disease) (9% of patients)
IgE gammopathy (heavy-chain disease), very rare
IgD gammopathy, very rare

Only two-thirds of patients with monoclonal gammopathy are symptomatic (IgG, IgA, IgD, and Bence Jones gammopathies are associated with classic picture of multiple myeloma—see pp. 345–347).
IgM gammopathy is associated with classic picture of macroglobulinemia—see pp. 350–351).

Classic (associated with increased serum M protein > 3 gm/dl and increased number of plasma cells in marrow > 25%)
- Multiple myeloma

Waldenström's macroglobulinemia
Certain malignant lymphomas

Idiopathic (not associated with diseases in classic group) (serum M protein usually < 2 gm/dl; plasma marrow cells usually 5–25% of total marrow white cells)

In apparently healthy persons

Associated with various diseases (e.g., diabetes mellitus, cirrhosis, abnormalities of lipid metabolism, chronic infections, collagen diseases, myeloproliferative diseases, and neoplasms not of lymphocyte or plasma cell origin)

Either type may be familial.

Polyclonal Gammopathy with Hyperproteinemia

Collagen diseases (e.g., SLE, rheumatoid arthritis, scleroderma)
Liver disease (e.g., chronic hepatitis, cirrhosis)
Chronic infection (e.g., chronic bronchitis and bronchiectasis, lung abscess, tuberculosis, osteomyelitis, subacute bacterial endocarditis, infectious mononucleosis, malaria)
Miscellaneous (e.g., sarcoidosis, malignant lymphoma, acute myeloid and monocytic leukemia, diabetes mellitus)
Idiopathic (family of patients with SLE)

IMMUNOGLOBULIN G (IgG)

Increased In

IgG myeloma
Sarcoidosis
Chronic liver disease (e.g., cirrhosis)
Sarcoidosis
Autoimmune diseases
Parasitic diseases
Chronic infection

Decreased In

Acquired immunodeficiency
Hereditary deficiencies
Protein-losing syndromes
Pregnancy
Non-IgG myeloma
Waldenström's macroglobulinemia

IMMUNOGLOBULIN M (IgM)

Increased In

Liver disease
Chronic infections
Waldenström's macroglobulinemia

Decreased In

Hereditary deficiency
Acquired immunodeficiency
Protein-losing syndromes
Non-IgM myeloma
Infancy, early childhood

IMMUNOGLOBULIN A (IgA)

Increased In
(in relation to other immunoglobulins)

Gamma-A myeloma (M component)
Cirrhosis of liver
Chronic infections
Rheumatoid arthritis with high titers of rheumatoid factor
SLE (some patients)
Sarcoidosis (some patients)
Wiskott-Aldrich syndrome
Other

Decreased In
(alone)

Normal persons (1 : 700)
Hereditary telangiectasia (80% of patients)
Type III dysgammaglobulinemia
Malabsorption (some patients)
SLE (occasionally)
Cirrhosis of liver (occasionally)
Still's disease (occasionally)
Recurrent otitis media (occasionally)
Non-IgA myeloma
Waldenström's macroglobulinemia
Acquired immunodeficiency

Table 3-2. Serum Immunoglobulin Changes in Various Diseases

Disease	IgG	IgA	IgM
Immunoglobulin disorders (see Table 12-22, pp. 354–355)			
Lymphoid aplasia	D	D	D
Agammaglobulinemia	D	D	D
Type I dysgammaglobulinemia (selective IgG and IgA deficiency)	D	D	N or I
Type II dysgammaglobulinemia (absent IgA and IgM)	N	D	D
IgA globulinemia	N	D	N
Ataxia-telangiectasia	N	D	N
Multiple myeloma, macroglobulinemia, lymphomas (see pp. 350, 340)			
Heavy-chain disease	D	D	D
IgG myeloma	I	D	D
IgA myeloma	D	I	D
Macroglobulinemia	D	D	I
Acute lymphocytic leukemia	N	D	N
Chronic lymphocytic leukemia	D	D	D
Acute myelogenous leukemia	N	N	N
Chronic myelogenous leukemia	N	D	N
Hodgkin's disease	N	N	N
Liver diseases			
Hepatitis	I	I	I
Laennec's cirrhosis	I	I	N
Biliary cirrhosis	N	N	I
Hepatoma	N	N	D
Miscellaneous			
Rheumatoid arthritis	I	I	I
Systemic lupus erythematosus	I	I	I
Nephrotic syndrome	D	D	N
Trypanosomiasis	N	N	I
Pulmonary tuberculosis	I	N	N

N = normal; I = increased; D = decreased.

Decreased In
(combined with other immunoglobulin decreases)

Agammaglobulinemia
- Acquired
  - Primary
  - Secondary (e.g., multiple myeloma, leukemia, nephrotic syndrome, protein-losing enteropathy)
- Congenital

Hereditary thymic aplasia
Type I dysgammaglobulinemia (decreased IgG and IgA and increased IgM)
Type II dysgammaglobulinemia (absent IgA and IgM and normal levels of IgG)
Infancy, early childhood

IMMUNOGLOBULIN E (IgE)

Increased In

Atopic diseases
- Exogenous asthma in ~60% of patients

Table 3-3. Changes in Serum Immunoproteins in Various Conditions

Condition	Albumin	$Alpha_1$ Antitrypsin	Haptoglobin	Transferrin	C3
Acute inflammation	D	I	I	D	Slight I
Chronic inflammation	D	V–I	V–I	D	Slight I
Chronic liver disease	D	V–I	V	D	V–D
Obstructive jaundice	N	N	V–I	N	I
Hemolytic anemia	N	N	D	N	N
Iron deficiency	N	N	N	I	N
Acute glomerulonephritis	N	N	N	N	D
Systemic lupus erythematosus	D	I	D[a]	D	V–D[b]
$Alpha_1$ antitrypsin deficiency	N	D	N	N	N
Analbuminemia	D	N	N	N	N
Agammaglobulinemia	N	N	N	N	N
IgG myeloma	D	N	N	N	N
IgA myeloma	D	N	N	N	N
Waldenström's macroglobulinemia	D	N	N	N	N

N = normal; D = decreased; I = increased; V = variable.
[a]D with associated hemolytic anemia.
[b]N if immunosuppressive treatment is effective.

Hay fever in ~30% of patients
Atopic eczema
Influenced by type of allergen, duration of stimulation, presence of symptoms, hyposensitization treatment
Parasitic diseases (e.g., ascariasis, visceral larva migrans, hookworm disease, schistosomiasis, *Echinococcus* infestation)
E-myeloma

Normal or Low In
Asthma

A normal serum IgE level excludes the diagnosis of bronchopulmonary aspergillosis.

Decreased In
Hereditary deficiencies
Acquired immunodeficiency
Ataxia-telangiectasia
Non-IgE myeloma

IMMUNOGLOBULIN D (IgD)

Increased In
Chronic infection (moderately)
IgD myelomas (greatly)
Autoimmune disease

Decreased In
Hereditary deficiencies
Acquired immunodeficiency
Non-IgD myeloma
Infancy, early childhood

APOLIPOPROTEINS

Apolipoprotein A-I

(Decreased level is associated with increased risk of CHD.)
Reference values
Males: 1.15–1.9 gm/L
Females: 1.15–2.2 gm/L

Increased In
Familial hyperalphalipoproteinemia
Pregnancy
Estrogen therapy
Alcohol consumption
Exercise

Decreased In
Tangier disease
"Fish-eye" disease
Familial hypoalphalipoproteinemia
Type I and V hyperlipoproteinemia
Diabetes mellitus
Cholestasis
Hemodialysis
Infection
Drugs (e.g., diuretics, beta-blockers, androgenic steroids, glucocorticoids, cyclosporine)

Apolipoprotein A-II

Reference values: 0.21–0.53 gm/L

Increased In
Alcohol consumption

Decreased In
Tangier disease
Cholestasis
Cigarette smoking

Apolipoprotein A-IV
Reference values (fasting): 0.13–0.16 gm/L

Increased In
Postprandial lipemia

Decreased In
Abetalipoproteinemia
Chronic pancreatitis
Malabsorption
Obstructive jaundice
Acute hepatitis
Total parenteral nutrition

Apolipoprotein (a)
(increased risk of CHD with serum levels > 0.30 gm/L)
Reference values
Whites: 0.0–0.60 gm/L
Blacks: 0.0–0.70 gm/L

Increased In
Pregnancy
Patients who have had AMI

Decreased In
Drugs (e.g., nicotinic acid, neomycin, anabolic steroids)

Apolipoprotein B-48
Normally absent during fasting.

Increased In
Hyperlipoproteinemia (Types I, V)
Apo E deficiency

Decreased In
Liver disease
Hypo- and abetalipoproteinemia
Malabsorption

Apolipoprotein B-100
(Increased levels are associated with increased risk of CHD.)
Reference values
Males: 0.17–1.6 gm/L
Females: 0.6–1.5 gm/L

Increased In
Hyperlipoproteinemia (Types IIa, IIb, IV, V)
Familial hyperapobetalipoproteinemia
Nephrotic syndrome
Pregnancy
Biliary obstruction
Hemodialysis
Cigarette smoking
Drugs (e.g., diuretics, beta-blockers, cyclosporine, glucocorticoids)

Decreased In
Hypo- and abetalipoproteinemia
Type I hyperlipoproteinemia (hyperchylomicronemia)
Liver disease
Exercise
Infections
Drugs (e.g., cholesterol-lowering drugs, estrogens)

Apolipoprotein C-1
Reference values: 0.05–0.11 gm/L

Increased In
Hyperlipoproteinemia (Types I, III, IV, V)

Decreased In
Tangier disease

Apolipoprotein C-II
Reference values
Males: 0.02–0.08 gm/L
Females: 0.01–0.06 gm/L

Increased In
Hyperlipoproteinemia (Types I, III, IV, V)

Decreased In
Tangier disease
Hypoalphalipoproteinemia
Apo C-II deficiency
Nephrotic syndrome

Apolipoprotein C-III
(with combined hereditary apo A-I and apo C-III deficiency, increased risk of premature CHD)
Reference values
Males: 0.05–0.18 gm/L
Females: 0.04–0.16 gm/L

Increased In
Hyperlipoproteinemia (Types III, IV, V)

Decreased In
Tangier disease
Combined with hereditary deficiency apo A-1

Apolipoprotein E
Reference values
Males: 0.01–0.06 gm/L
Females: 0.01–0.05 gm/L

Increased In
Hyperlipoproteinemia (Types I, III, IV, V)
Pregnancy
Cholestasis
Multiple sclerosis in remission
Drugs (e.g., dexamethasone)

Decreased In
Drugs (e.g., ACTH)

SERUM CHOLESTEROL, HDL-CHOLESTEROL, LDL-CHOLESTEROL, TRIGLYCERIDES

See Disorders of Lipid Metabolism, pp. 406–418.

SERUM VITAMIN D

Increased In
1,25-Dihydroxyvitamin D
- Hyperparathyroidism
- Sarcoidosis
- Idiopathic calcium nephrolithiasis

25-Hydroxyvitamin D
- Vitamin D toxicity

Decreased In
1,25-Dihydroxyvitamin D
- Hypoparathyroidism
- Chronic renal failure

25-Hydroxyvitamin D
- Vitamin D deficiency
- Inadequate exposure to ultraviolet light
- Malabsorption syndromes
- Hepatocellular disease
- Nephrotic syndrome (some patients)
- Drugs (e.g., high-dosage glucocorticoid or anticonvulsant therapy)

ACUTE INFLAMMATORY REACTANTS

Erythrocyte sedimentation rate (ESR) (see next section)
Serum C-reactive protein (CRP) (see p. 76)

Total WBC, neutrophils and bands
Acute phase reactants in serum are not used for this purpose (except CRP), but it is important to recognize this cause of increase when they are used in testing for other conditions (e.g., ceruloplasmin).
- CRP
- Fibrinogen
- Ferritin
- Haptoglobin
- Ceruloplasmin
- $Alpha_1$ antitrypsin
- $Alpha_1$ acid glycoprotein

Serum complement (see pp. 78–81)

ERYTHROCYTE SEDIMENTATION RATE (ESR)

(see Table 3-4, p. 75)

Indicates presence and intensity of an inflammatory process; never diagnostic of a specific disease.

May Be Useful To

Detect occult disease (e.g., screening program), but a normal ESR does not exclude malignancy or other serious disease.
Monitor the course or response to treatment of certain diseases (e.g., temporal arteritis, polymyalgia rheumatica, acute rheumatic fever, rheumatoid arthritis, SLE, Hodgkin's disease, tuberculosis).

ESR is normal in 5% of patients with rheumatoid arthritis and with SLE.

Assist in differential diagnosis (e.g., acute myocardial infarction as opposed to angina pectoris; early acute appendicitis versus ruptured ectopic pregnancy or acute pelvic inflammatory disease; rheumatoid arthritis as opposed to osteoarthritis, acute versus quiescent gout).
Confirm or exclude a diagnosis (a normal ESR virtually excludes diagnosis of temporal arteritis or polymyalgia rheumatica; >50 mm/hour in 90% of these patients).
In patients with cancer, ESR > 100 mm/hour indicates metastases.
Is said rarely (6 in 10,000) to be useful for screening of asymptomatic persons after history and physical examination.
Unexplained increase with no detectable disease occurs in <3% of cases.

Increased In

Anemia: ESR is said to be useful to differentiate iron deficiency anemia (ESR normal) from anemia of acute or chronic disease alone or combined with iron deficiency in which ESR is almost always increased.
Macrocytosis
Hypercholesterolemia
Chronic inflammatory diseases, especially collagen and vascular diseases
Increased fibrinogen, gamma or beta globulins

Decreased In

Polycythemia, vera or secondary
Abnormal RBCs especially sickle cells; hereditary spherocytosis; acanthocytosis
Microcytosis (e.g., hemoglobin disease)
Hypofibrinogenemia (e.g., disseminated intravascular coagulation [DIC], massive hepatic necrosis)
Cachexia
Overanticoagulation
High WBC Count

Formula for normal-range Westergren ESR:

Table 3-4. Changes in Erythrocyte Sedimentation Rate*

Disease	Increased In	Not Increased In
Infectious	Tuberculosis (especially) Acute hepatitis Many bacterial infections	Typhoid fever Undulant fever Malarial paroxysm Infectious mononucleosis Uncomplicated viral diseases
Cardiac	Acute myocardial infarction Active rheumatic fever After open-heart surgery	Angina pectoris Active renal failure with heart failure
Abdominal	Acute pelvic inflammatory disease Ruptured ectopic pregnancy Pregnancy—third month to about 3 weeks postpartum Menstruation	Acute appendicitis (first 24 hours) Unruptured ectopic pregnancy Early pregnancy
Joint	Rheumatoid arthritis Pyogenic arthritis	Degenerative arthritis
Miscellaneous	Significant tissue necrosis especially neoplasms (most frequently malignant lymphoma, cancer of colon and breast) Increased serum globulins (e.g., myeloma, cryoglobulinemia, macroglobulinuria) Decreased serum albumin Hypothyroidism Hyperthyroidism Acute hemorrhage Nephrosis, renal disease with azotemia Arsenic and lead intoxication Dextran and polyvinyl compounds in blood Temporal arteritis Polymyalgia rheumatica	Peptic ulcer Acute allergy

*Extreme elevation of ESR is found particularly in association with malignancy (most frequently malignant lymphoma, carcinomas of colon and breast), hematologic diseases (most frequently myeloma), collagen diseases (e.g., rheumatoid arthritis, SLE), renal diseases (especially with azotemia), infections, drug fever, and other conditions (e.g., cirrhosis). Westergren method is more accurate; Wintrobe method is more convenient.

$$\text{Men: ESR} = \frac{\text{age (years)}}{2}$$

$$\text{Women: ESR} = \frac{[\text{age(years)} + 10]}{2}$$

Hyperviscosity syndrome should be suspected in patients with hyperproteinemia (e.g., multiple myeloma, Waldenström's macroglobulinemia) with rouleaux formation but no increase of ESR.

SERUM C-REACTIVE PROTEIN (CRP)

(an acute-phase reactant; quantitative test is superior; normal < 8 mg/L)

Increased In

In general parallels ESR but is not influenced by anemia, polycythemia, congestive heart failure, hypergammaglobulinemia. Most useful as indicator of activity in a rheumatic disease (e.g., rheumatoid arthritis, rheumatic fever).

Inflammatory disorders:

- In any acute inflammatory change, CRP shows an earlier (begins in 4–6 hours), more intense increase than ESR; with recovery, disappearance of CRP precedes the return to normal of ESR. CRP disappears when the inflammatory process is suppressed by steroids or salicylates.
- Rheumatoid arthritis, rheumatic fever, seronegative arthritides (e.g., Reiter's syndrome), vasculitis syndromes (e.g., hypersensitivity vasculitis).
- In inflammatory bowel disease, CRP is significantly higher in Crohn's disease than in ulcerative colitis and corresponds to relapse, remission, and response to therapy in Crohn's disease.

Tissue injury or necrosis:

- AMI: CRP appears within 24–48 hours, begins to fall by the third day, and becomes negative after 1–2 weeks; correlates with peak CK-MB levels, but CRP peak occurs 1–3 days later. Failure of CRP to return to normal indicates tissue damage in the heart or elsewhere. Not increased by angina in absence of tissue necrosis.
- Infarction of other tissues
- Increased by rejection of kidney or marrow transplant but not by heart transplant.
- Malignant diseases, especially breast, lung, GI tract. May be a useful tumor marker since a high CRP is often present when carcinoembryonic antigen (CEA) and other tumor markers are not increased.
- Following surgery: CRP increases within 4–6 hours to peak at 48–72 hours (usually at 25–35 mg/dl). Begins to decrease after third postoperative day; failure to fall is more sensitive indicator of complications (e.g., infection, pulmonary infarction) than WBC, ESR, temperature, pulse rate.
- Burns

Infections:

- Highest levels are found in bacterial infections (>100 μg/ml).
- May be useful to monitor disease activity in bacterial and viral infections.
- Useful for diagnosis of postoperative and intercurrent infection:
  - Active severe SLE produces almost no increase of CRP unless infection is present.
  - Leukemia: Fever, blast crisis, or cytotoxic drugs cause only modest elevation of CRP, but intercurrent infection stimulates significantly higher CRP levels and is particularly useful to monitor response to antibiotic therapy.
- Lower in viral compared to bacterial infection but may be very high in both. CSF CRP has been reported specific to differentiate bacterial from viral meningitis.
- Other infections (e.g., neonatal, GU, GI and biliary tracts, pelvic inflammatory disease, CNS)

"PREGNANCY" TEST

(immunoassay detection of human chorionic gonadotropin [hCG] in urine, blood)

Positive In

Pregnancy. Test becomes positive as early as 4 days after expected date of menstruation; it is >95% reliable by 10th–14th day. hCG increases to peak at 60th–70th day, then drops progressively.

Hydatidiform mole, choriocarcinoma. Test negative 1 or more times in >60% and negative at all times in >20% of these patients, for whom more sensitive methods (e.g., radioimmunoassay) should be used. Quantitative titers should be performed for diagnosis and for following the clinical course of patients with these conditions.

False negative results may occur with dilute urine or in cases of missed abortion, dead fetus syndrome, ectopic pregnancy. False positive results may occur with bacterial contamination, with protein or blood in urine, or in patients on methadone therapy.

With the latex agglutination type of test, only urine should be used if patient has rheumatoid arthritis.

Older methods injecting specimens into animals are no longer in use.

Leukocyte alkaline phosphatase scoring may also be used as a test for pregnancy (see pp. 265–266).

See also Urinary Chorionic Gonadotropins, pp. 107, 539.

ANTISTREPTOCOCCAL ANTIBODY TITERS (ASOT)

A high or rising titer is indicative only of current or recent streptococcal infection.

- Direct diagnostic value in
  - Scarlet fever
  - Erysipelas
  - Streptococcal pharyngitis and tonsillitis
- Indirect diagnostic value in
  - Rheumatic fever
  - Glomerulonephritis

Antibody appears as early as 1 week after infection; titer rises rapidly by 3–4 weeks and then declines quickly; may remain elevated for months.

Even in severe streptococcal infection, there will be an elevated ASO titer in only 70–80% of patients.

Individual determinations depend on various factors (e.g., duration and severity of infection, antigenicity) and are of limited clinical value. Serial determinations are most desirable; a 4 times increase in ASO titer confirms immunologic response to streptococcal organisms.

Conditions	Usual ASO Titer (Todd Units)
Normal persons	12–166
Active rheumatic fever	500–5000
Inactive rheumatic fever	12–250
Rheumatoid arthritis	12–250
Acute glomerulonephritis	500–5000
Streptococcal upper respiratory tract infection	100–333
Collagen diseases	12–250

False positives are associated with tuberculosis, liver disease (e.g., active viral hepatitis), bacterial contamination.

Latex agglutination method may give a false positive in markedly lipemic or contaminated specimens.

Other streptococcal antigens may be tested:

- Antistreptococcal hyaluronidase (ASH) (significant titer >128)
- Antideoxyribonuclease (DNase B) (significant titer >10)

Useful In

Detecting subclinical streptococcal infection
Differential diagnosis of joint pains of rheumatic fever and rheumatoid arthritis

ASOT is increased in only 30–40% of patients with streptococcal pyoderma and 50% of patients with poststreptococcal glomerulonephritis; DNase antibodies are the most sensitive indicators of these conditions. DNase B titers may also be helpful in diagnosis of delayed sequelae of Sydenham's chorea, since they are detectable for several months.

SERUM COMPLEMENT

Normal In

Renal diseases
- IgG-IgA nephropathy (Berger's disease)
- Idiopathic rapidly progressive glomerulonephritis
- Antiglomerular basement membrane disease
- Immune-complex disease
- Negative immunofluorescence findings

Systemic diseases
- Polyarteritis nodosa
- Hypersensitivity vasculitis
- Wegener's granulomatosis
- Schönlein-Henoch purpura
- Goodpasture's syndrome
- Visceral abscess

Decreased In (Acquired)

Common diseases associated with arthritis
- SLE
- Prodromal HBV hepatitis
- Essential mixed cryoglobulinemia
- Sjögren's syndrome
- Serum sickness
- Short-bowel syndrome

Common diseases associated with vasculitis
- SLE
- Rheumatoid vasculitis
- Essential mixed cryoglobulinemia
- Sjögren's syndrome
- Hypocomplementemic vasculitis

Common diseases associated with nephritis

	% of Cases in Which Occurs
Acute poststreptococcal glomerulonephritis	Transient (3–8 week) decline in C3
Membranoproliferative glomerulonephritis	
Type I ("classic")	50–80%
Type II ("dense deposit disease")	80–90%; C3 often remains depressed
SLE	
Focal	75%
Diffuse	90%
Subacute bacterial endocarditis	90%
Cryoglobulinemia	85%
"Shunt" nephritis	90%

Table 3-5. Immunologic Tests

Antibody Test	Interpretation
Acetylcholine receptor	Result < 1 unit makes the diagnosis of myasthenia gravis unlikely; result > 5 units confirms diagnosis of myasthenia gravis. Test may be negative in ocular myasthenia, Eaton-Lambert syndrome, and treated or inactive generalized myasthenia gravis.
Antiadrenal	High titers are characteristic of autoimmune hypoadrenalism (70%); not found in Addison's disease due to tuberculosis.
Antiglomerular basement membrane	High titer strongly suggests, but negative results do not rule out, Goodpasture's syndrome.
Anti-intrinsic factor	Antibodies indicate overt or latent pernicious anemia; present in ~75% of cases.
Antimitochondrial	Absence is strong evidence against primary biliary cirrhosis (PBC). High titer strongly suggests PBC. Low titers are seen frequently in other liver diseases.
Antirheumatoid arthritis nuclear antigen	Found in 87% of patients with rheumatoid arthritis and in 15% of SLE cases.
Antireticulin	Presence supports the diagnosis of gluten-sensitive enteropathy. Especially useful in childhood where positive in 80% of cases.
Antiskin, interepithelial	Positive test confirms diagnosis of pemphigus and is helpful in evaluating bullous diseases. Positive in >90% of pemphigus cases; absence largely excludes that diagnosis. Rise and fall of titer may indicate impending relapse or effective control of disease. High sensitivity; lower specificity.
Antiskin, dermal-epidermal	Positive in >80% of bullous pemphigus cases. Absence does not exclude that diagnosis. Some correlation of titer and severity. Low sensitivity; high specificity.
Antistriational	Absence is strong evidence against the presence of thymoma in myasthenia gravis. May be positive in some patients with myasthenia gravis alone, thymoma alone, and in drug reactions, e.g., penicillamine.
Antithyroglobulin and antithyroid microsome antibodies	Absence of both antibodies is strong evidence against autoimmune thyroiditis. Persistent thyroid microsome may be predictive of elevated TSH (72%). Positive thyroid antibody titers and elevated TSH are associated with risk of hypothyroidism of 5% per year, even with initially normal T-4.
Thyroid-stimulating immunoglobulin (TSI)	Elevated TSI occurs in >90% of Graves' disease. Failure of TSI to fall after antithyroid therapy predicts relapse. Elevated TSI in a patient who is HLA-DR3 positive predicts poor response to antithyroid therapy and suggests need for alternate mode of treatment.

Source: Data from JB Peter, *Use and Interpretation of Tests in Clinical Immunology* (7th ed). Omaha: Interstate Press, 1990.

Serum sickness
Atheromatous emboli

Decreased In (Inherited)

	Deficient Complement
SLE	C1qINH, C1q, C1r, C1s, C2, C4, C5, C8
Hereditary angioedema	C1qINH
Familial Mediterranean fever	C5aINH
Urticarial vasculitis	C3
Glomerulonephritis	C1r, C2
Severe combined immunodeficiency	C1q
X-linked hypogammaglobulinemia	C1q
Recurrent infections	C3, C3bINH
Recurrent neisserial infections	C5, C6, C7, C8

Increased In
Inflammatory conditions that increase acute-phase reactants

Individual Complement Levels

CH50 is useful for screening, since a normal result indicates classic complement pathway is functionally intact. Decrease indicates 50–80% of normal amounts have been depleted. Detects all inborn and most acquired complement deficiencies.

C3 is useful for screening for classic and activation of alternate complement pathway. May be increased in subacute inflammation, biliary obstruction, nephrotic syndrome, corticosteroid therapy. May be decreased in immune complex disease (especially lupus nephritis), acute poststreptococcal glomerulonephritis, hypercatabolism (especially C3b inactivator deficiency), massive necrosis and tissue injury, sepsis, viremia, hereditary deficiency, infancy.

C3 or CH50 may be useful for monitoring disease activity in SLE but usefulness may vary from case to case.

C2 may be decreased in immune complex disease (especially lupus nephritis), hereditary angioedema, hereditary deficiency, infancy.

C4 may be decreased in immune complex disease (especially lupus nephritis), hereditary angioneurotic edema, hereditary deficiency, acute glomerulonephritis, infancy, or when classic pathway is activated.

C1 esterase inhibitor deficiency is characteristic of hereditary angioedema. In heterozygote, C1 inhibitor is substantially decreased. Patients have low CH100, C4, and C2 during attacks.

C1q can be very low in acquired angioedema, severe combined immunodeficiency, and X-linked hypogammaglobulinemia. May be decreased in SLE, infancy.

Absence of or marked decrease in any of the components of complement will cause absence of or marked decrease in the total hemolytic complement assay, but mild to moderate decrease of an individual component of complement may not alter this total.

Deficiency of early classic pathway components (C1q, r, s, C2, C4)
- Serum shows absence of hemolytic complement activity.
- The affected component is absent or decreased on immunochemical testing.
- Opsonic activity and generation of chemotactic activity are defective.
- Infections are not a problem (due to alternative pathway being intact).
- Symptoms due to collagen vascular disorders (e.g., nephritis, arthritis)

Deficiency of C3 and C5
- Serum shows absence of hemolytic complement activity.
- C3 or C5 is absent or decreased in serum.
- Defective opsonic capacity and chemotactic activity

Severe recurrent infections (e.g., pneumonia, sepsis, otitis media, chronic diarrhea)
Often respond to fresh plasma

Deficiency of late classic pathway components (C6, C7, C8)
Serum shows absence of hemolytic complement activity.
Normal opsonization and generation of chemotactic factor
Total absence of individual component
Recurrent systemic infection due to *Neisseria gonorrhoeae* or *Neisseria meningitidis*

FLUORESCENT ANTIBODY TESTS

Antimitochondrial antibodies are found in ~85% of patients with primary biliary cirrhosis but almost never in diffuse extrahepatic biliary obstruction; therefore, antibodies are useful in differentiating these two conditions.

May also be found in two other liver disorders associated with autoimmune disease: active chronic hepatitis and cryptogenic cirrhosis.

Smooth-muscle antibodies may be found in ~80% of patients with chronic active hepatitis (lupoid hepatitis) and in patients with biliary cirrhosis.

Antibodies against the cross-striations of skeletal muscle are present in 30–40% of patients with myasthenia gravis; a changing titer may indicate response to treatment or thymectomy.

COLD AUTOHEMAGGLUTINATION

Increased In

Primary atypical (virus) pneumonia (30–90% of patients): titer ≥ 1:14–1:224. Negative titer does not rule out primary atypical pneumonia (see p. 648).
Atypical hemolytic anemia
Paroxysmal hemoglobinuria
Raynaud's disease
Cirrhosis of the liver
Trypanosomiasis
Malaria
Infectious mononucleosis
Adenovirus infections
Influenza
Psittacosis
Mumps
Measles
Scarlet fever
Rheumatic fever

4

Urine

NORMAL VALUES

Specific gravity	1.003–1.030
pH	4.6–8.0 (average = 6.0), depending on diet
Total solids	30–70 gm/L (average = 50). To estimate, multiply last two figures of specific gravity by 2.66 (Long's coefficient).
Osmolality	500–1200 mOsm/L
Volume	
Adults	600–2500 ml/24 hours (average = 1200) Night volume usually < 700 ml with specific gravity < 1.018 or osmolality > 825 mOsm/kg of body weight in children Ratio of night to day volume 1 : 2–1 : 4
Infants	
Premature	1–3 ml/kg/hour
Full-term	15–60 ml/24 hours
2 weeks	250–400 ml/24 hours
8 weeks	250–400 ml/24 hours
1 year	500–600 ml/24 hours
Protein	Qualitative = 0 0–0.1 gm/24 hours
Glucose	Qualitative = 0 ≤ 0.3 gm/24 hours
Ketones	Qualitative = 0
Chloride	140–250 mEq/L
Calcium	< 150 mg/24 hours on low-calcium (Bauer-Aub) diet
Phosphorus	1 gm/24 hours (average), depending on diet
Urobilinogen	0–4 mg/24 hours
Porphobilinogen	0–2 mg/24 hours
Uroporphyrin	0
Coproporphyrin	50–300 μg/24 hours 0–75 μg/24 hours in children weighing < 80 pounds
Amylase	260–950 Somogyi units/24 hours
Lead	< 0.08 μg/ml or 120 μg/24 hours
Delta-aminolevulinic acid	1.5–7.5 mg/24 hours
Homogentisic acid	0
Hemoglobin and myoglobin	0
Creatinine	1.0–1.6 gm/24 hours (15–25 mg/kg of body weight/24 hours)
Creatine	< 100 mg/24 hours (< 6% of creatinine) Higher in children (< 1 year: may = creatinine; older children: ≤ 30% of creatine) and during pregnancy (≤ 12% of creatinine)

Cystine or cysteine	0
Oxalate	
Males	≤ 55 mg/24 hours
Females	≤ 50 mg/24 hours
Uric acid	
Males	≤ 800 mg/24 hours
Females	≤ 750 mg/24 hours
Phenylpyruvic acid	0
Microscopic examination	≤ 1–2 RBC, WBC, epithelial cells/hpf; occasional hyaline cast/lpf
Addis count (no longer performed)	
RBC	≤ 1,000,000/24 hours
Casts	≤ 100,000/24 hours
WBC + epithelial cells	≤ 2,000,000/24 hours

DIPSTICK URINALYSIS

For detection of proteinuria, sensitivity and specificity = 95–99%; positive predictive value for renal disease = 0–1.4% (in young populations).

For detection of hematuria, specificity = 65–99% compared to microscopy; positive predictive value for significant disease = 0–2% and for possibly significant disease = 6–58%.

Therefore screening of asymptomatic young adults is not recommended.*

For detection of WBC, sensitivity = 100% for > 50 WBCs/hpf, 90% for 21–50 WBCs, 60% for 12–20 WBCs, 44% for 6–12 WBCs.

For detection of bacteria, sensitivity = 73% for "large" numbers, 46% for "moderate" numbers.†

Combined positive esterase and nitrate strips is sufficient indication for colony count to identify bacteriuria.

Dipstick (leukocyte esterase) of first-catch urine is a cost-effective way to detect asymptomatic urethritis (*Chlamydia, Neisseria*) in males.

DETECTION OF BACTERIURIA

A colony count is significant (> 85% sensitivity) if there are > 100,000 bacteria/cu mm under the following conditions: Periurethral area has first been thoroughly cleaned with soap; a midstream, clean-catch, first morning specimen is submitted in a sterilized container; and the specimen is refrigerated until the colony count is performed. Transport tubes have an inhibitory effect and should be used. When urine is allowed to remain at room temperature, the number of bacteria doubles every 3–45 minutes. Suprapubic sterile needle aspiration is the most reliable sampling technique, and the presence of any organisms on culture is virtually diagnostic of urinary tract infection (97% sensitivity); it is the only acceptable method in infants, as urine collection bags have a very high false positive rate; compared to urethral catheterization of adults, it is more accurate, simpler, and less traumatic. Colony counts < 10,000/cu mm in the absence of therapy largely rule out bacteriuria. Colony counts > 10,000/cu mm of a single or predominant organism should be considered positive in symptomatic patients. Three or more species with none being predominant (i.e., > 80% of the growth) almost always represents specimen contamination. False low colony counts may occur with a high rate of urinary flow, low urine specific gravity, low urine pH, presence of antibacterial drugs, or inappropriate cultural techniques (e.g., tubercle bacilli, *Mycoplasma, Ureaplasma urealyticum, Chlamydia trachomatis,* anaerobes). Positive significant single culture is 95% reliable, and repeat is unnecessary. Prostatic localization for diagnosis of chronic bacterial prostatitis: three glass-voided bladder

*Data from S Woolhandler et al., *JAMA* 262:1214, 1989.
†Data from DA Propp et al., *Ann Emerg Med* 18:560, 1989.

urine specimens and then one of prostatic secretions (by prostatic massage) will show a greater (usually 10 times) colony count in the third and prostatic specimens compared to the first urine specimen, but reverse finding in urethritis. Nonbacterial prostatitis is much commoner than chronic bacterial prostatitis: ≥ 10 polymorphonuclear leukocytes (PMNs)/hpf in prostatic secretions with negative cultures of urine and prostatic fluid.

Direct microscopic examination of uncentrifuged urine, unstained or gram-stained, that shows 1 PMN or 1 organism/hpf has sensitivity of 85% and specificity of 60%. It may show > 10% false positive results. With pyuria and bacteriuria, a Gram's stain to differentiate gram-positive cocci (e.g., enterococci or staphylococci) from gram-negative bacilli will indicate appropriate immediate initial therapy. Microscopic detection of pus cells is less sensitive and produces more false positive results than detection of bacteria. On urine microscopic examination, ≤ 50% of patients with bacteriuria may not show significant numbers of WBCs; however, ≥ 10 WBCs/hpf is associated with bacteriuria in ~90% of cases. "Sterile" pyuria (i.e., pyogenic infection is absent) or absence of bacilli (< 1 bacillus in multiple oil-immersion fields or 20–40 bacteria/hpf in centrifuged sediments) should cast doubt on diagnosis of untreated bacterial urinary tract infection (UTI) and may occur in renal tuberculosis, chemical inflammation, mechanical inflammation (e.g., calculi, instrumentation), early acute glomerulonephritis prior to appearance of hematuria or proteinuria, extreme dehydration, hyperchloremic renal acidosis, nonbacterial gastroenteritis and respiratory tract infections, and after administration of oral polio vaccine. Presence of both bacteria and WBCs has a higher predictive value than either alone. Large numbers of squamous epithelial cells may indicate a specimen that contains greater numbers of bacteria from the vagina or perineum rather than the urinary tract.

Dye tests (bacterial reduction of nitrate to nitrite; tetrazolium reduction) do not detect 10–50% of infections. Bacteria show great variability in rate of dye reduction; some important bacteria do not reduce dye at all; e.g., coliforms are more likely to be detected than enterococci. If overnight urine specimen is impossible to obtain, then urine should incubate in patient's bladder for ≥ 4 hours. High doses of vitamin C may cause false negative test for nitrite and also for glucose.

Decreased glucose in urine (< 2 mg/dl) in properly collected first morning urine (no food or fluid intake after 10 P.M., no urination during night) correlates well with colony count.

A culture should be performed for identification of the organism and determination of sensitivity when these screening tests are positive. If culture shows a common gram-positive saprophyte, it should be repeated because the second culture is often negative. Causative bacteria are usually enteric organisms; < 10% are gram-positive cocci (see Table 16-1, p. 608). If culture shows mixed flora, contamination should be suspected and culture should be repeated; but true mixed infections may occur after instrumentation or with chronic infection. *If* Pseudomonas *or* Proteus *is found, the patient may have an anatomic abnormality. If an organism other than* Escherichia coli *is found, the patient probably has chronic pyelonephritis even if this is the first clinical episode of infection.* In women, > 80% of UTI are due to *E. coli* and a smaller percent are due to *Staphylococcus saprophyticus,* and less often to other aerobic gram-negative bacilli. In men, gram-negative bacilli cause ~75% of UTI, but *E. coli* causes only ~25% of infections in men and < 50% of infections in boys. Other common gram-negative bacilli are *Proteus* and *Providencia* species. Gram-positive organisms (especially enterococci and coagulase-negative staphylococci) cause about 20% of infections in men and boys, but *S. saprophyticus* is rare. *Gardnerella vaginalis* is found in < 3% of bacteriuric men.

Antibody coating of bacteria (immunofluorescence assay) is positive in bacteria originating from kidney but negative in bacteria from lower tract infection. False positives may occur with heavy proteinuria, prostatitis, and contamina-

Table 4-1. Sensitivity, Specificity, and Predictive Values of Tests in Predicting Bacteriuria (10^5 colonies/ml)

Test	Sensitivity (%)	Specificity (%)	Predictive Value (%) of Positive Test	Predictive Value (%) of Negative Test
>5 WBC/hpf	80	83	46	96
>10 WBC/hpf	63	90	53	93
Nitrite	69	90	57	94
Leukocyte esterase	71	85	47	94
Nitrite + leukocyte esterase (either positive)	86	86	54	97

tion with vaginal or rectal bacteria. False negatives may occur in early infection. Test is less reliable in children and adults with neurogenic bladder. Test is not generally available and is not recommended for routine use.

With pyuria and bacteriuria, alkaline pH may indicate infection with urea-splitting organism (e.g., *Proteus;* less often *Pseudomonas* or *Klebsiella*) or an infected stone.

WBC casts are pathognomonic of renal infection but are absent in most cases; therefore are only useful if present.

Decreased concentrating ability occurs in renal but not bladder infections; persistent dilute urine (low specific gravity or osmolarity) suggests renal rather than bladder infection if patient is not forcing fluid. This is not a sensitive or specific test because of overlapping values, even though it is more marked in bilateral than unilateral infection and concentrating ability increases with cure.

Bacteriuria may be found in

- 10% of patients who are pregnant
- 15% of patients with diabetes mellitus
- 20% of patients with cystocele
- ~50% of patients with dysuria
- 70% of patients with prostatic obstruction
- Up to 5% of patients during catheterization
- 95% of patients (untreated) with an indwelling catheter for > 4 days
- Should be searched for in elderly patients with altered mental status and infants with failure to thrive, persistent fever, or lethargy.

EOSINOPHILURIA*

(should be performed using Hansel's rather than Wright's stain; refers to > 1% of urinary leukocytes as eosinophils)

May Be Found In

Acute interstitial nephritis (drug-induced); sensitivity = 60–90%, specificity > 85%, positive predictive value ~50%, negative predictive value 98%. May be useful to distinguish this syndrome from acute tubular necrosis, in which it is absent.

*Data from HL Corwin, BA Bray, and MH Haber, The detection and interpretation of urinary eosinophils. *Arch Pathol Lab Med* 113:1256, 1989.

Acute glomerulonephritis (rapidly progressive; acute, including poststreptococcal)
IgA nephropathy (Schönlein-Henoch purpura)
Chronic pyelonephritis
Acute rejection of renal allograft
Obstructive uropathy
Prostatitis
Eosinophilic cystitis due to *Schistosoma haematobium*
Bladder cancer

URINE VOLUME

Anuria (excretion < 100 ml/24 hours)

May Be Due To

Bilateral complete urinary tract obstruction
Acute cortical necrosis
Necrotizing glomerulonephritis
Certain causes of acute tubular necrosis

Oliguria (excretion usually < 400 ml/24 hours; < 15–20ml/kg/24 hours in children)

May Be Due To

Prerenal, renal, or postrenal causes.

Polyuria (normal or increased urine excretion in presence of increasing serum creatinine and BUN)

May Be Due To

Diabetic ketoacidosis
Partial obstruction of urinary tract with impaired urinary concentration function
Some types of acute tubular necrosis (e.g., due to aminoglycosides)

URINE SPECIFIC GRAVITY

Increased in

Temperature
Proteinuria
Glucosuria
Sucrosuria (see p. 164)
Radiographic contrast medium (frequently 1.040–1.050)
Mannitol
Dextran
Diuretics
Antibiotics
Detergent
(Urinometer readings should be corrected by adding [or subtracting] 0.001 to specific gravity reading for each 3°C above [or below] calibration temperature [respectively]. Subtract 0.003 for each 1 gm/dl of protein and 0.004 for each 1 gm/dl of glucose from temperature-compensated specific gravity.)

Specific gravity compares mass of a solution to an equal volume of water (i.e., related to but not an exact measure of number of solute particles; osmolality measures the exact number of solute particles and is a constant weight-weight relationship. Osmolarity is 1 osmol of nonelectrolyte in 1 L of water and varies with the volume-expanding effect of the dissolved substance and the proportional effect of temperature on the fluid volume. Osmolality is the preferred unit of measure.).

Decreased volume of concentrated urine (specific gravity > 1.030 and osmolality > 500 mOsm/kg) is diagnostic of prerenal azotemia.

Urine-plasma osmolality ratio is more accurate than urine osmolality or specific gravity to distinguish prerenal azotemia (with increased ratio) from acute tubular necrosis (with decreased ratio that is rarely > 1.5).

See also urine concentration and dilution tests, p. 555.

URINARY DIAGNOSTIC INDICES

See pp. 563, 565–567 and Table 15-3, p. 564.

PROTEINURIA

(see Table 15-11, pp. 604–607)

Found in 1–9% of cases on routine screening.

Refers to protein excretion > 150 mg/day in adults and > 100 mg/day in children < age 10 or > 140 mg/m^2/day. Significant proteinuria is > 300 mg/day in adults. > 1000 mg/day makes a diagnosis of renal parenchymal disease very likely. > 2000 mg/day in adults or > 40 mg/m^2 in children usually indicates glomerular etiology. ≥ 3500 mg/day or protein-creatinine ratio > 3.5 points to a nephrotic syndrome.

When a 24-hour urine cannot be reliably collected, a spot urine for urine protein-creatinine ratio (especially after first morning specimen and before bedtime and if renal function is not severely impaired) often correlates well. Normal < 0.2; > 3.5 in nephrosis.

Dipstick is sensitive to ~30 mg/dl of protein; 1+ = 100 mg/dl; 2+ = 300 mg/dl; 4+ = 1000 mg/dl; may be falsely negative with predominantly low molecular weights or nonalbumin proteins. Positive dipstick should always be followed by a sulfosalicylic acid test, which is sensitive to 5–10 mg/dl of protein; may be falsely negative with very alkaline urine; may be falsely positive due to certain drugs (e.g., x-ray contrast media, high doses of penicillin, chlorpromazine, tolbutamide, sulfa drugs). When the sulfosalicylic acid test shows a significantly higher concentration than the dipstick in an adult, immunoelectrophoresis should be performed to rule out Bence-Jones proteinuria. Association with hematuria indicates high likelihood of disease.

Due To

Orthostatic (postural)

- First morning urine before arising shows high specific gravity but no protein.
- Protein only appears after person is upright; usually < 1.5 gm/day.
- Urine microscopy is normal.
- Is usually considered benign and slowly disappears with time but is still present in 50% of persons 10 years later.
- Progressive renal insufficiency does not occur.
- Occurs in 15% of apparently healthy young men and 3% of otherwise healthy persons and some patients with resolving acute pyelonephritis or glomerulonephritis
- Renal biopsy, electron microscopy, and immunofluorescent stains show pathologic changes in some patients.

Transient

- Commonly found in routine urinalysis of asymptomatic healthy children and young adults initially but not subsequently
- Progressive renal disease is not present.
- Functional occurs in 10% of hospital medical patients; associated with high fever, congestive heart failure, hypertension, stress, exposure to cold, strenuous exercise, seizures. Usually < 2 gm/day; disappears with recovery from precipitating cause. Progressive renal disease is not present.

Persistent
- Glomerular
  - Idiopathic (e.g., membranoproliferative glomerulonephritis, membranous glomerulopathy, minimal change disease, focal segmental glomerulosclerosis)
  - Secondary
    - Infection (e.g., poststreptococcal, hepatitis B)
    - Drugs (e.g., nonsteroidal anti-inflammatory drugs, heroin, gold, captopril, penicillamine)
    - Autoimmune (e.g., SLE, rheumatoid arthritis, dermatomyositis, polyarteritis, Goodpasture's syndrome, Schönlein-Henoch purpura, ulcerative colitis)
    - Hereditary and metabolic (e.g., diabetes mellitus, Fabry's disease, Alport's syndrome)
- Decreased tubular reabsorption
  - Acquired
    - Drugs (e.g., phenacetin, aminoglycoside, lithium, methicillin, etc.)
    - Heavy metal (e.g., lead, mercury, cadmium)
    - Sarcoidosis
    - Acute tubular necrosis
    - Interstitial nephritis
    - Renal graft rejection
    - Balkan nephropathy
  - Congenital (e.g., Fanconi's syndrome, oculocerebrorenal syndrome)
  - Hereditary (e.g., Wilson's disease, medullary cystic disease, oxalosis, cystinosis)
- Increased plasma levels of normal or abnormal proteins (e.g., Bence Jones proteins, myoglobin, lysozyme in monocytic or myelocytic leukemias)

Some common causes of low-grade proteinuria (< 1 gm/24 hours)
- Idiopathic low-grade proteinuria—normal history and physical examination, renal function, and urine sediment with no hematuria
- Nephrosclerosis
- Polycystic kidney disease
- Medullary cystic disease
- Chronic obstruction of urinary tract
- Chronic interstitial nephritis (e.g., analgesic abuse, uric acid, oxalate, hypercalcemia, hyopokalemia, lead, cadmium)

RENAL DISEASES THAT MAY BE FOUND WITHOUT PROTEINURIA

Congenital abnormalities
Renal artery stenosis
Obstruction of GU tract
Pyelonephritis
Stone
Tumor
Polycystic kidneys
Hypercalcemic nephropathy
Hypokalemic nephropathy
Prerenal azotemia

SOME GLOMERULAR CAUSES OF PROTEINURIA

Immune complexes (e.g., nephritis of systemic lupus erythematosus (SLE), poststreptococcal glomerulonephritis, membranous glomerulonephritis)
Antiglomerular basement membrane antibodies (e.g., Goodpasture's syndrome)
Deposition of abnormal material (e.g., amyloidosis, diabetes mellitus)
Pyelonephritis
Vascular disease (e.g., hypertension, congestive heart failure)
Congenital (e.g., Alport's syndrome of progressive interstitial nephritis and progressive nerve deafness)

Unknown etiology (e.g., lipoid nephrosis)
Physiologic (e.g., orthostatic, exercise, fever)

SOME TUBULAR CAUSES OF PROTEINURIA

Fanconi's syndrome
Renal tubular acidosis
Medullary cystic disease
Pyelonephritis
Cystinosis
Wilson's disease
Oculocerebral renal syndrome
Renal transplantation
Sarcoidosis
Cadmium toxicity
Balkan nephropathy

POSTRENAL PROTEINURIA

Primarily associated with epithelial tumors of bladder or renal pelvis
Degree of proteinuria related to size and invasiveness; generally < 1 gm/day (similar to pyelonephritis) and includes IgM

DIFFERENTIATION OF URINARY PROTEINS

Precipitated by 5% Sulfosalicylic Acid

On boiling, precipitate remains
- Albumin
- Globulin
- Pseudo-Bence-Jones protein

On boiling, precipitate disappears
- Bence-Jones protein
- A "proteose"

Precipitated at 40–60°C

Resuspend precipitate in normal urine and equal volume of 5% sulfosalicylic acid and boil.

Precipitate dissolves
- Bence-Jones protein

Precipitate does not dissolve
- Pseudo-Bence-Jones protein

CAUSES OF FALSE POSITIVE TESTS FOR PROTEINURIA

(see also pp. 738–739)

	Dipstick	Sulfosalicylic Acid
Gross hematuria	+	+
Highly concentrated urine	+	+
Highly alkaline urine (pH > 8) (e.g., GU tract infection with urea-splitting bacteria)	+	−
Antiseptic contamination (e.g., banzalkonium, chlorhexidine)	+	−
Phenazopyridine	+	−
Radiopaque contrast media	−	+
Tolbutamide metabolities	−	+
High levels of cephalosporin or penicillin analogs	−	+
Sulfonamide metabolites	−	+

Dipstick for positive protein

Sulfosalicylic acid test

Negative

Confirm with repeat testing
Rule out false positive causes

Disproportionately positive

No further testing

Negative

Repeat tests

Rule out Bence Jones (BJ) protein (in adults)

Positive

< 150 mg/day

Quantitative measurement*

< 2 gm/day

> 2 gm/day ($> 40\ mg/m^2/hour$ in children)

Urinalysis

Isolated proteinuria†	Not isolated proteinuria†	Sediment "nephritic"	Not "nephritic" sediment

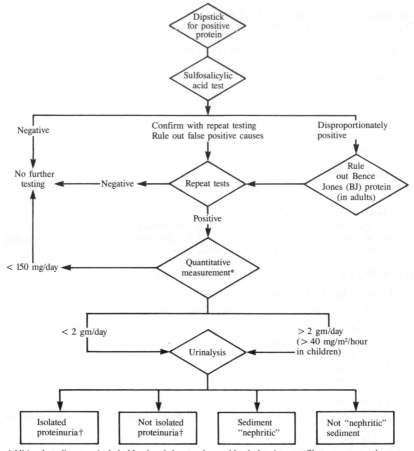

Additional studies may include blood and throat cultures, blood chemistry profiles, serum complement, ASOT, ANA, cryoglobulins, BJ protein, renal biopsy, nephrologist consultation

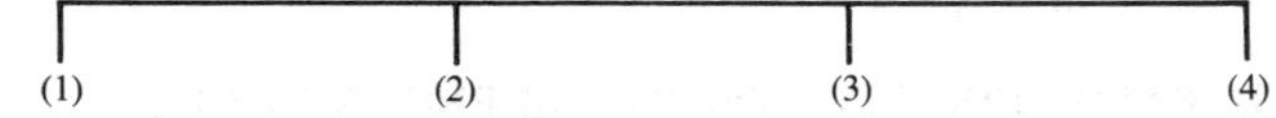

(1) Isolated proteinuria: follow for orthostatic, nonorthostatic, functional proteinuria, or possible early renal disease. IVP, periodic renal function tests, and urinalysis.
(2) Not isolated proteinuria < 2 gm/day may occur in some glomerular diseases where there is marked hypoalbuminemia or marked impairment of glomerular filtration or overflow proteinuria (e.g., BJ proteinuria) or tubular proteinuria (e.g., hereditary, metabolic, inflammatory conditions). Also acute tubular necrosis.
(3) "Nephritic" sediment may occur in various types of glomerulonephritis, SLE, SBE, mixed cryoglobulinemia, hereditary nephritis, IgA nephropathy.
(4) Proteinuria > 2 gm/day without "nephritic" sediment may occur in glomerular proteinura (e.g., diabetes mellitus, focal glomerulosclerosis, amyloidosis, preeclampsia, minimal-change nephrotic syndrome, membranous nephropathy, some infections [HBV, syphilis, malaria], drugs).

*Check creatinine to assure 24-hour sample collection.
†Isolated proteinuria = no findings of GU tract abnormalities, renal manifestations of systemic disease, hypertension, decreased renal function, or abnormal renal sediment.

"Nephritic" sediment = RBCs or RBC casts; other casts and WBCs may or may not be present.

Fig. 4-1. Flow chart for diagnosis of proteinuria.

PROTEINURIA PREDOMINANTLY GLOBULIN RATHER THAN ALBUMIN

Multiple myeloma
Macroglobulinemia
Primary amyloidosis
Adult Fanconi's syndrome (some patients)

BENCE JONES PROTEINURIA

About 20% of tests will be false positive (i.e., urine electrophoresis does not show a spike, and immunoelectrophoresis does not show a monoclonal light chain) due to

- Connective tissue disease (e.g., rheumatoid arthritis, SLE, scleroderma, polymyositis, Wegener's granulomatosis)
- Chronic renal insufficiency
- Lymphoma and leukemia
- Metastic carcinoma of lung, GI or GU tracts
- High doses of penicillin and aminosalicylic acid
- Presence of x-ray contrast media

80% of tests are true positive due to

- Myeloma (70% of all positive tests)
- Cryoglobulinemia
- Waldenström's macroglobulinemia
- Primary amyloidosis
- Adult Fanconi's syndrome
- Hyperparathyroidism
- Benign monoclonal gammopathy

Positive test for Bence Jones proteinuria by heat test should always be confirmed by electrophoresis and immunoelectrophoresis of concentrated urine. Heat test is not reliable and should not be used for diagnosis.
"Dipstick" test for albumin does not detect Bence Jones protein.

BETA$_2$ MICROGLOBULIN

Normal < 1 mg/day by ELISA or RIA

Increased In

Tubular disease (> 50 mg/day)

- Heavy-metal poisoning (e.g., mercury, cadmium, cis-platinum)
- Drug toxicity (e.g., aminoglycosides, cyclosporine)
- Hereditary (e.g., Fanconi's syndrome, Wilson's disease, cystinosis)
- Pyelonephritis
- Renal allograft rejection
- Others (e.g., nephrocalcinosis)

Difficulty due to need for 24-hour timed collection, instability at room temperature, acid urine, and presence of pyuria.

(Serum levels may also be increased due to increased production in hepatitis, sarcoiditis, Crohn's disease, vasculitis, certain malignancies prevents diagnostic utility.)

RETINOL BINDING PROTEIN

Increased in proximal tubular dysfunction. Correlates with beta$_2$ microglobulin excretion but not affected by acid urine. More sensitive than *N*-acetyl-beta-D-glucosaminidase excretion. May show false negative due to low serum level in vitamin A deficiency.

POSITIVE REDUCING SUBSTANCES (BENEDICT REACTIONS) IN URINE

Glycosuria
- Hyperglycemia
  - Endocrine (e.g., diabetes mellitus, pituitary, adrenal, thyroid disease)
  - Nonendocrine (e.g., liver, CNS diseases)
  - Due to administration of hormones (e.g., adrenocorticotropic hormone [ACTH], corticosteroids, thyroid, epinephrine) or drugs (e.g., morphine, anesthetic drugs, tranquilizers)
- Renal
  - Tubular origin (serum glucose < 180 mg/dl; oral and IV glucose tolerance tests [GTT] are normal; ketosis is absent)
  - Fanconi's syndrome
  - Toxic renal tubular disease (e.g., due to lead, mercury, degraded tetracycline)
  - Inflammatory renal disease (e.g., acute glomerulonephritis, nephrosis)
- Glomerular due to increased glomerular filtration rate (GFR) without tubular damage
- Idiopathic

Melituria (5% of cases of melituria in the general population are due to renal glycosuria [incidence = 1:100,000], pentosuria [incidence = 1:50,000], essential fructosuria [incidence = 1:120,000])
- Hereditary (e.g., galactose, fructose, pentose, lactose)
  - Galactose (classic and variant forms of galactosemia)
  - Fructose (fructosemia, essential fructosuria, hereditary fructose intolerance)
  - Lactose (lactase deficiency, lactose intolerance)
  - Phenolic compounds (phenylketonuria, tyrosinosis)
  - Xylulose (pentosuria)
- Neonatal (e.g., physiologic lactosuria, sepsis, gastroenteritis, hepatitis)
- Lactosuria during lactation
- Xylose (excessive ingestion of fruit)

Non-sugar-reducing substances (e.g., ascorbic acid, glucuronic acid, homogentisic acid, salicylates)

Galactosuria (in galactosemia) shows a positive urine reaction with Clinitest but negative with Clinistix and Tes-Tape.

False negative tests for glucose may occur in presence of ascorbic acid using glucose oxidase paper test (Labstix); found in > 1% of routine urine analyses in hospital.

KETONURIA

(ketone bodies [acetone, beta-hydroxybutyric acid, acetoacetic acid] appear in urine)

Occurs In

Metabolic conditions
- Diabetes mellitus
- Renal glycosuria
- Glycogen storage disease

Dietary conditions
- Starvation
- High-fat diets

Increased metabolic requirements
- Hyperthyroidism
- Fever
- Pregnancy and lactation
- Other

False positive results may occur after injection of bromsulphalein (BSP test).

DISEASES ASSOCIATED WITH SPECIFIC ODORS OF URINE

(and other body fluids)

Condition	Odor
Maple syrup urine disease	Maple syrup, burned sugar
Oasthouse urine disease, methionine malabsorption	Brewery, oasthouse
Methylmalonic, propionic, isovaleric, and butyric/hexanoic acidemia	Sweaty feet
Tyrosinemia	Cabbage-like, fishy
Trimethylaminuria	Stale fish
Hypermethioninemia	Rancid butter, rotten cabbage
Phenylketonuria	Musty, mousy
Ketosis	Sweet
Cystinuria, homocystinuria	Sulfurous

SUBSTANCES AND CONDITIONS THAT MAY CAUSE ABNORMAL COLOR OF URINE*

(see also pp. 737–738)

Red
- No specific test (chlorzoxazone, ethoxazene, oxamniquine, phenothiazines, rifampin)
- Acid urine only (phenolphthalein)

Red or pink
- No specific test (chloroquine, ethoxazene, ibuprofen, iron sorbitex, pamaquine, phenacetin, phenothiazines, phensuximide, phenytoin)
- Acid urine only (beets, blackberries)
- Alkaline urine only (anthraquinone laxatives, rhubarb, santonin; eosin produces green fluorescence)
- Darkens on standing (porphyrins)
- On contact with hypochlorite bleach (toilet bowl cleaner) (aminosalicylic acid)

Purple
- No specific test (chlorzoxazone)
- Alkaline urine only (phenolphthalein)
- Darkens on standing (porphyrins; fluoresces with ultraviolet light)

Red-brown
- No specific test (aminopyrine, aniline dyes, antipyrine, doxorubicin, ibuprofen, phenacetin, phenothiazines, phensuximide, phenytoin)
- Acid urine only (methemoglobin, metronidazole)
- Alkaline urine only (anthraquinone laxatives, levodopa, methyldopa, parahydroxyphenylpyruvic acid, phenazopyridine)
- Positive *o*-toluidine test for blood
  - Centrifuged specimen shows RBC in base if blood, pink supernatant plasma if hemoglobin, but clear plasma if myoglobin
- Green in reflected light (antipyrine)

Brown-black
- Ferric chloride test (blue-green with homogentisic acid) (black with melanin or melanogen; nitroprusside test is red with melanin, black with melanogen)
- Darkens on standing (homogentisic acid, melanin, melanogen, nitrobenzene, parahydroxyphenylpyruvic acid [alkaline urine only], phenol, cresol)

*Data from R Raymond and WE Yarger, Abnormal urine color: Differential diagnosis. *South Med J* 81:837, 1988.

Yellow-brown
- No specific test (niridazole, nitrofurantoin, pamaquine, primaquine, sulfamethoxasole)
- Darkens on standing in acid urine (anthraquinone laxatives, rhubarb)
- Positive test for bile (bilirubin, urobilin)

Yellow
- No specific test (fluorescein dye, phenacetin, riboflavin, trinitrophenol)
- Acid urine only (quinacrine, santonin)
- Alkaline urine only (beets)
- Positive test for bile (bilirubin, urobilin)

Yellow-orange
- No specific test (aminopyrine, warfarin)
- Alkaline urine only (anisindione, sulfasalazine)
- Positive test for bile (bilirubin, urobilin)
- Color increases with HCl (phenazopyridine)
- Ether soluble (carrots, vitamin A)

Yellow-green or brown-green
- Darkens on standing (cresol, phenol [chloraseptic], methocarbamol, resorcinol)
- Positive test for bile (biliverdin)

Blue-green
- No specific test (chlorophyll breath mints [Clorets], Evans blue dye, guaiacol, magnesium salicylate [Doan's Pills], methylene blue, thymol)
- Darkens on standing (methocarbamol, resorcinol)
- Blue fluorescence in acid urine (triamterene)
- *Pseudomonas* infection (rare)

Milky
- Lipuria
- Chyluria
- Many PMNs

Colorless
- Specific gravity
  - High (diabetes mellitus with glycosuria; positive test for glucose)
  - Low (diabetes insipidus, recent fluid intake)
  - Variable (diuretics, ethyl alcohol, hypercalcemia)

Clear to deep yellow
- Normal (due to urochrome pigment)

Sickle cell crises produce a characteristic dark-brown color independent of volume or specific gravity that becomes darker on standing or on exposure to sunlight. Increase in total porphyrins, coproporphyrins, and uroporphyrins is routinely shown; increase in the porphyrin precursors (delta-aminolevulinic acid and porphobilinogen) occasionally occurs.

Red urine may be caused by ingestion of beets, blackberries, certain cold-drink and food dyes, certain drugs (e.g., phenolphthalein in laxatives); presence of urates and bile may also cause red urine.

Darkening of urine on standing, alkalinization, or oxygenation is nonspecific and may be due to melanogen, hemoglobin, indican, urobilinogen, porphyrins, phenols, salicylate metabolites (e.g., gentisic acid), homogentisic acid (due to alkaptonuria; if acid pH, may not darken for hours) and may appear in tyrosinosis. Darkened urine may follow administration of metronidazole (Flagyl).

Biliverdin: Blue or green color is due to oxidation of bilirubin in poorly preserved specimens. Gives negative diazo tests for bilirubin (Ictotest), but oxidative tests (Harrison spot test) may still be positive.

Methylene blue ingestion may cause a similar urine color. Blue urine occurs very rarely in *Pseudomonas* infection.

Blue diaper syndrome results from indigo blue in urine due to familial metabolic

defect in tryptophan absorption associated with idiopathic hypercalcemia and nephrocalcinosis.
Red diaper syndrome is due to a nonpathogenic chromobacterium (*Serratia marcescens*) that produces a red pigment when grown aerobically at 25–30°C.
White cloud is due to excessive oxalic acid and glycolic acid in urine; occurs in oxalosis (primary hyperoxaluria).
Hemoglobin
Myoglobin
Melanin
Porphyrins
Chyluria
Lipuria

URINE UROBILINOGEN

Increased In

Increased hemolysis (e.g., hemolytic anemias)
Hemorrhage into tissues (e.g., pulmonary infarction, severe bruises)
Hepatic parenchymal cell damage (e.g., cirrhosis, acute hepatitis in early and recovery stages)
Cholangitis

Decreased In

Complete biliary obstruction

PORPHYRINURIA

(due mainly to coproporphyrin)

Lead poisoning
Cirrhosis
Infectious hepatitis
Passive in newborn of mother with porphyria; lasts for several days
Porphyria

HEMATURIA

< 3% of normal persons have ≥ 3 RBCs/hpf or > 1000 RBCs/cu ml (no easy conversion formula between these two methods). Abnormal range is > 5 RBCs/hpf. Centrifuged fresh urine sediment should be examined under high dry magnification. Routine screening of all adults is not recommended.
Dipsticks (orthotolidine or peroxidase) detect heme peroxidase activity in RBCs, hemoglobin, or myoglobin with reported sensitivity of 91–100% and specificity of 65–99%; may miss 10% of patients with microscopic hematuria. Orthotolidine test strips are sensitive to about 3–10 RBCs/hpf. Is more reliable in hypotonic urine (lyses RBCs) than hypertonic urine. False positives may be due to oxidizing contaminants (e.g., bacterial peroxidases, povidone, hypochlorite) and false negatives due to reducing agents (e.g., ascorbic acid) or pH < 5.1.
Hematuria found in 18% of persons after very strenuous exercise.
In microscopic hematuria, number of RBCs is not related to the significance of the causative lesion.
Presence of blood clots virtually rules out glomerular origin of blood. Large thick clots suggest bladder origin; small stringy clots suggest upper tract.
Wright's stain or phase microscopy in urine sediment is said to show distortion with crenation and uneven hemoglobin distribution of < 80% of RBCs of glomerular origin; if > 80% are similar to RBCs in peripheral blood, the source is likely to be distal to glomeruli. With an automated RBC counter that produces size distribution curves, urine RBC size distribution has been reported less than venous RBCs in glomerulonephritis and greater than either venous RBCs (nonglomerular) or both (mixed) types in lower GU tract lesions.

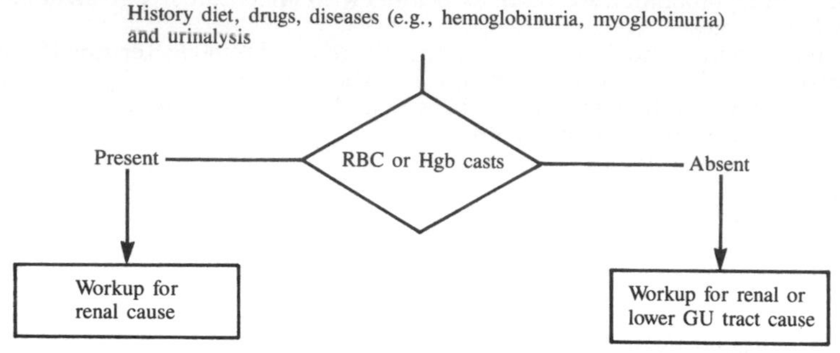

Fig. 4-2. Flow chart for red or brown urine.

RBC casts or hemoglobin casts indicate blood is of glomerular origin, but their absence does not rule out glomerular disease.

Gross hematuria that is initial suggests origin in urethra distal to urogenital diaphragm; terminal suggests origin in bladder neck or prostatic urethra; total suggests origin in bladder proper or upper urinary tract.

Proteinuria may occur with gross hematuria. In nonglomerular hematuria, sufficient proteinuria to produce 2+ dipstick requires equivalent of 25 ml of blood/L of urine (if Hct is normal), which would cause gross hematuria; in glomerular hematuria, proteins filter through glomerulus out of proportion to RBCs. Therefore microscopic hematuria with 2+ protein on dipstick favors glomerular origin; one exception is papillary necrosis, which may show 2+ proteinuria with nonglomerular type of RBCs.

Pyuria or WBC casts suggest inflammation or infection of GU tract.

False causes of hematuria include vaginal bleeding, factitious, red diaper syndrome, drugs, foods (e.g., beets, blackberries, rhubarb), pigmenturia (porphyria, hemoglobinuria, myoglobinuria).

Persistent or intermittent hematuria should always be evaluated; one episode of microscopic hematuria usually does not require full evaluation (e.g., may be due to viral infection, mild trauma, exercise).

Some causes of hematuria in adults*

	Gross (%)	**Microscopic** (%)
GU tract cancer	22.5	5.1
Kidney	3.6	0.5
Prostate	2.4	0.5
Ureter	0.8	0.2
Bladder	15	4
Other lesions		
GU tract infection	33	4.3
Calculi	11	5
Benign prostatic hypertrophy	13	13
Renal		2.2
Systemic (e.g., hemophilia, thrombocytopenia, dicumarol overdose)	1	
No source found	8.4	43

*Data from JM Sutton, Evaluation of hematuria in adults. *JAMA* 263:2475, 1990.

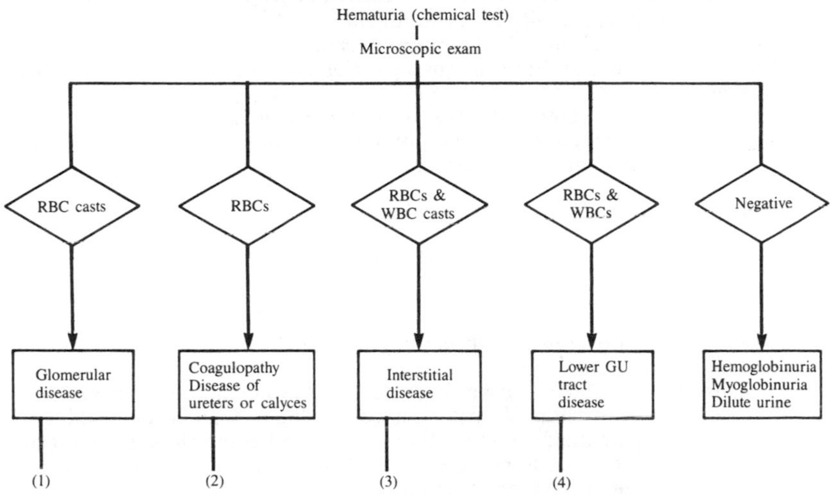

(1) Hypertension, diabetes mellitus, glomerulonephritis, immune-complex or postinfectious glomerular disease, drug reaction, endocarditis, embolic diseases. Tests: ASOT, ANA, C3, HB_SAb, renal biopsy.
(2) Calculi, papillary necrosis, polycystic disease, sickle cell disease; GU tract trauma, neoplasm, or parasites. Tests: Cytology, CAT scan, ultrasound, IVP.
(3) Pyelonephritis, tuberculosis, sarcoidosis, drug reaction. Tests: Urine cultures, lymph node biopsy.
(4) GU tract infection (e.g., prostatitis, urethritis, vaginitis), reflux, GU tract carcinoma. Tests: Urine cultures, cytology, cystoscopy, ultrasound.

Fig. 4-3. Flow chart for diagnosis of microhematuria.

PRINCIPAL CAUSES OF ASYMPTOMATIC HEMATURIA IN CHILDREN

Glomerular

Acute postinfectious glomerulonephritis
Membranoproliferative glomerulonephritis
IgG-IgA nephropathy (Berger's disease)
Hereditary nephritis
SLE
Schönlein-Henoch purpura
Benign familial hematuria
Benign recurrent hematuria

Nonglomerular

Polycystic kidneys
Renal tumors
Renal tuberculosis
Vascular abnormalities (e.g., renal hemangioma, essential hematuria)
Hematologic conditions (e.g., sickle cell trait, coagulation disorders)
Hydronephrosis
GU tract infection, foreign body, calculi, etc. (usually symptomatic)

BENIGN FAMILIAL OR RECURRENT HEMATURIA

Asymptomatic hematuria without proteinuria
Other laboratory and clinical findings are normal.
Renal biopsy is normal on light microscopy, electron microscopy, and immunofluorescence.
Other family members may also have asymptomatic hematuria.
Should gradually clear spontaneously; annual screening for other abnormalities should be performed until condition clears.

HEMOGLOBINURIA

Renal threshold is 100–140 mg/dl plasma.

Due To

Infarction of kidney
Hematuria (due to any cause) with hemolysis in urine
Intravascular hemolysis due to
- Parasites (e.g., malaria, Oroya fever due to *Bartonella bacilliformis*)
- Infection (e.g., clostridial, *E. coli* bacteremia due to transfused blood)
- Antibodies (e.g., transfusion reactions, acquired hemolytic anemia, paroxysmal cold hemoglobinuria, paroxysmal nocturnal hemoglobinuria)
- Disseminated intravascular coagulation
- Inherited hemolytic disorders (e.g., sickle cell disease, thalassemias, glucose-6-PD deficiency, pyruvate kinase deficiency, hereditary spherocytosis)
- Fava bean sensitivity
- Mechanical (e.g., prosthetic heart valve)
- Hypotonicity (e.g., transurethral prostatectomy with irrigation of bladder with water, hemodialysis accidents)
- Chemicals (e.g., naphthalene, sulfonamides)
- Thermal burns injuring RBCs
- Strenuous exercise and march hemoglobinuria

False positive (Occultest) results may occur in the presence of pus, iodides, bromides.

Serum is pink due to free hemoglobin but clear due to myoglobin.

HEMOSIDERIN IN URINE

Centrifuged specimen of random urine incubated for 10 minutes with Prussian blue stain shows blue granules. Granules are located in cells but if these have disintegrated, free granules may be predominant.
Normal—absent
Present in intravascular hemolysis even when hemoglobinuria is absent (e.g., paroxysmal nocturnal hemoglobinuria).

MYOGLOBINURIA

(due to rhadomyolysis)

Renal threshold is 20 mg/dl plasma.
Diagnosis based on
- Positive benzidine or *o*-toluidine test of urine that contains few or no RBCs when urine is red or brown. This is the simplest and most practical initial test. Tests may be positive even when urine is normal in color.
- Serum is clear (not pink) unless renal failure is present in contrast to hemoglobinemia.
- Serum haptoglobin is normal (in contrast to hemoglobinemia).
- Serum enzymes of muscle origin (e.g., creatine kinase [CK]) are increased.

Identification of myoglobin in urine by various means
Immunodiffusion is most sensitive and specific.
Ultracentrifugation and electrophoresis lack specificity.
Spectrophotometry shows similar peaks for myoglobin and hemoglobin.
Precipitation by ammonium sulfate may give false negative results.

Hereditary
Phosphorylase deficiency (McArdle syndrome)
Metabolic defects (e.g., associated with muscular dystrophy)

Sporadic
Ischemic (e.g., arterial occlusion) (in acute myocardial infarction, levels > 5 mg/ml occur within 1–2 hours and precede ECG and serum CK and CK-MB changes). Has 100% sensitivity but is less specific than CK-MB elevation.
Crush syndrome
Exertional (e.g., exercise, some cases of march hemoglobinuria, electric shock, convulsions, and seizures)
Metabolic myoglobinuria (e.g., Haff disease, alcoholism, seasnake bite, carbon monoxide poisoning, diabetic acidosis, hypokalemia, malignant hyperpyrexia, systemic infection, barbiturate poisoning)
In up to 50% of patients with progressive muscle disease (e.g., dermatomyositis, polymyositis, SLE, others) in active stage
Various drugs and chemicals, especially illicit (e.g., cocaine, heroin, methadone, amphetamines, diazepam)

MELANOGENURIA

In some patients with malignant melanoma, when the urine is exposed to air for several hours, colorless melanogens are oxidized to melanin, and urine becomes deep brown and later black.

Is also said to occur in some patients with Addison's disease or hemochromatosis and in intestinal obstruction in blacks.

Confirmatory tests
Ferric chloride test
Thormählen's test
Ehrlich's test

None of these is consistently more reliable or sensitive than observation of urine for darkening.

Melanogenuria occurs in 25% of patients with malignant melanoma; it is said to be more frequent with extensive liver metastasis. It is not useful for judging completeness of removal or early recurrence.

Beware of false positive red-brown or purple suspension due to salicylates.

CHYLURIA

Due To

Obstruction of the lymphochylous system, usually filariasis. Microfilariae appear in the urine for 6 weeks after acute infection, then disappear unless endemic.

Trauma to chest or abdomen

Abdominal tumors or lymph node enlargement

Milky urine is due to chylomicrons recognized as fat globules by microscopy (this is almost entirely neutral fat). Protein is normal or low. Hematuria is common. Specific gravity is low, and reaction is acid.

A test meal of milk and cream may cause chyluria in 1–4 hours.

Laboratory findings due to pyelonephritis that is often present.

LIPURIA

Lipids in the urine include all fractions. Double refractile (cholesterol) bodies can be seen. There is a high protein content.

May Occur In

Hyperlipidemia due to
- Nephrotic syndrome
- Severe diabetes mellitus
- Severe eclampsia

Extensive trauma with bone fractures
Phosphorus poisoning
Carbon monoxide poisoning

URINE ELECTROLYTES

Value may be limited due to failure to obtain 24-hour excretion levels rather than random samples or administration of diuretics.

See Table 15-3, p. 564.

Table 4-2. Urine Electrolytes in Various Metabolic Conditions

Metabolic Problem	Cause	Urine Electrolytes*
Volume depletion	Extrarenal sodium loss	Sodium < 10 mEq/L
	Adrenal insufficiency or renal salt wasting	Sodium > 10 mEq/L
Acute oliguria	Prerenal azotemia	Sodium < 10 mEq/L
	Acute tubular necrosis	Sodium > 30 mEq/L
Hyponatremia	Severe volume depletion: edematous states	Sodium < 10 mEq/L
	Inappropriate antidiuretic hormone secretion; adrenal insufficiency; salt-wasting nephropathies	Sodium ≥ dietary intake
Hypokalemia	Extrarenal potassium loss	Potassium < 10 mEq/L
	Renal potassium loss (often associated with diuretic therapy)	Potassium > 10 mEq/L
Metabolic alkalosis	Chloride-responsive alkalosis	Chloride < 10 mEq/L
	Chloride-resistant alkalosis	Chloride parallels dietary intake

*Values based on patient not receiving diuretics.

URINE CALCIUM

Increased In

Hyperparathyroidism
Idiopathic hypercalciuria
High-calcium diet
Excess milk intake
Immobilization (especially in children)
Lytic bone lesions
  Metastatic tumor
  Multiple myeloma
  Osteoporosis (primary or secondary to hyperthyroidism, Cushing's syndrome, acromegaly)
Excess vitamin D ingestion
Drug therapy
  Mercurial diuretics
  Ammonium chloride
Fanconi's syndrome
Renal tubular acidosis
Sarcoidosis
Glucocorticoid excess due to any cause
Rapidly progressive osteoporosis
Paget's disease

Decreased In

Hypoparathyroidism
Rickets, osteomalacia
Familial hypocalciuric (benign) hypercalcemia
Steatorrhea
Renal failure
Metastatic carcinoma of prostate

SOME CAUSES OF HYPERCALCIURIA WITHOUT HYPERCALCEMIA

Idiopathic hypercalciuria
Sarcoidosis
Glucocorticoid excess due to any cause
Hyperthyroidism
Rapidly progressive bone diseases, Paget's disease, immobilization, malignant tumors
Renal tubular acidosis
Medullary sponge kidney
Furosemide administration

URINE CREATINE

Increased In

Physiologic states
  Growing children
  Pregnancy
  Puerperium (2 weeks)
  Starvation
  Raw meat diet
Increased formation
  Myopathy
    Amyotonia congenita
    Muscular dystrophy
    Poliomyelitis
    Myasthenia gravis
    Crush injury
    Acute paroxysmal myoglobinuria

- Endocrine diseases
    - Hyperthyroidism
    - Addison's disease
    - Cushing's syndrome
    - Acromegaly
    - Diabetes mellitus
    - Eunuchoidism
    - Therapy with ACTH, cortisone, or desoxycorticosterone acetate.
- Increased breakdown
    - Infections
    - Burns
    - Fractures
    - Leukemia
    - SLE

Decreased In

Hypothyroidism

URIC ACID–CREATININE RATIO

Ratio > 1.0 in most patients with acute renal failure due to hyperuricemia, but lower in other causes of acute renal failure.

FERRIC CHLORIDE TEST OF URINE

(primarily used as screening test for phenylketonuria)

Positive In	Phenistix Color
Phenylketonuria (unreliable for diagnosis)	Gray-green
Tyrosinuria (transient elevation in newborns)	Green
Maple syrup urine disease	Negative
Alkaptonuria	Negative
Histidinemia	Blue-gray to green
Tyrosinosis	Green (fades quickly)
Oasthouse urine disease	—
Bilirubin	—
Lactic acidosis	Gray
Melanin	—
Methionine malabsorption	—
Pyruvic acid	Yellow
Xanthurenic acid	Negative
Acetoacetic acid	Negative
Drugs	
Para-aminosalicylic acid	Purple
Phenothiazines	Purple
Salicylates	Purple

A positive test should always be followed by other tests (e.g., chromatography of blood and urine) to rule out genetic metabolic disorders.

DISORDERS FREQUENTLY ASSOCIATED WITH URINARY CRYSTALS

Disorder	Substance
Massive hepatic necrosis (acute yellow atrophy) tyrosinemia, tyrosinosis	Tyrosine
Cystinuria, cystinosis	Cystine
Fanconi's syndrome	Leucine
Hyperoxaluria, oxalosis	Calcium oxalate

Lesch-Nyhan syndrome	Uric acid
Orotic aciduria	Orotic acid
Xanthinuria	Xanthine

URINARY EXCRETION OF SOME RENAL ENZYMES

Lactic Dehydrogenase (LDH) Activity

Increased In

Carcinoma of kidney, bladder, and prostate in a high proportion of cases; may be useful for detection of asymptomatic lesions or screening of susceptible population groups and differential diagnosis of renal cysts

Other renal diseases

- Active glomerulonephritis, SLE with nephritis, nephrotic syndrome, acute tubular necrosis, diabetic nephrosclerosis, malignant nephrosclerosis, renal infarction
- Active pyelonephritis (25% of patients), cystitis, and other inflammations

Instrumentation of the GU tract (especially cystoscopy with retrograde pyelography); transient increase is < 1 week.

Myocardial infarction and other conditions with considerably increased serum levels

Normal In

Benign nephrosclerosis
Pyelonephritis (most patients)
Obstructive uropathy
Renal stones
Polycystic kidneys
Renal cysts

The test is not useful in routine screening for malignancy of kidney, renal pelvis, and bladder, since increased levels suggest GU tract disease but do not indicate its nature. Increased values usually precede clinical symptoms.

Precautions: 8-hour overnight urine collection, clean-voided to prevent bacterial and menstrual contamination. Refrigerate until analysis is begun. Specimen must be dialyzed to remove inhibitors in urine. Urinalysis should be performed first, since false positive LDH may occur if there are > 10 bacteria/hpf or if RBCs or hemolyzed blood is present.

L-Alanine Aminopeptidase (LAP)
(derived from proximal tubule brush borders)

Normal is 1500–3700 mU/24 hours in women and 2000–6000 mU/24 hours in men. Affected by diuresis and circadian rhythm but not by proteinuria or bacteriuria.

Increased by all types of proximal tubular injury and other renal diseases (e.g., glomerular disease, tumors), which makes test too sensitive and nonspecific.

N-Acetyl-beta-D-glucosaminidase (NAG)
(derived from proximal tubule lysozymes)

Increased in many types of renal disease, causing low specificity; therefore not clinically useful. Correlates with degree of albuminuria.

Lysozyme

Increased in acute monocytic and myelomonocytic leukemias.

URINARY EXCRETION OF RENAL ANTIGENS
(derived from proximal tubule brush borders)

Low levels in normal persons

May Be Useful To

Distinguish cases of prerenal azotemia and glomerular disease (with low levels) from increased levels in acute renal failure due to proximal tubular disease.
Follow course of renal transplant patients.
Distinguish pyelonephritis from cystitis.

URINARY EXCRETION OF FORMIMINOGLUTAMIC ACID (FIGLU)

Histidine loading is followed after 3 hours by a 5-hour urine collection. Normal is < 2 mg/hour or 3 mg/dl.

Increased In

Folic acid deficiency; is no longer used in this diagnosis.

URINARY 5-HYDROXYINDOLEACETIC ACID (5-HIAA)

Increased In

Carcinoid syndrome
Ingestion of bananas, tomatoes, avocados, red plums, walnuts, eggplant, reserpine (Serpasil), mephenesin carbamate, phenothiazine derivatives, Lugol's solution

Normal is 2–9 mg/day; in carcinoid syndrome, 5-HIAA is > 40 mg/day, often 300–1000 mg/day.

URINARY ALDOSTERONE

Increased In

Primary and secondary aldosteronism (see pp. 503, 508–511)

Decreased In

Hypoadrenalism
Panhypopituitarism

URINARY CATECHOLAMINES (NOREPINEPHRINE, NORMETANEPHRINE)*

Increased In

Pheochromocytoma
Neural crest tumors (neuroblastoma, ganglioneuroma, ganglioblastoma)
Progressive muscular dystrophy and myasthenia gravis (some patients)
May also be increased by vigorous exercise prior to urine collection (≤ 7 times)
False increase may be due to drugs that produce fluorescent urinary products (e.g., tetracyclines, Aldomet, epinephrine and epinephrine-like drugs, large doses of vitamin B complex; see pp. 742–743). *Avoid such medications for 1 week before urine collection.*
Has also been reported in
- Guillain-Barré syndrome
- Acute intermittent porphyria
- Brain tumor
- Carcinoid syndrome
- Acute psychosis
- Clonidine withdrawal

URINE VANILLYLMANDELIC ACID (VMA)

(VMA is the urinary metabolite of both epinephrine and norepinephrine.)

Increased In

Pheochromocytoma
Neuroblastoma, ganglioneuroma, ganglioblastoma

*Not all methods include dopamine in determination of total catecholamines.

Beware of false positive results due to certain foods (e.g., coffee, tea, chocolate, vanilla, some fruits and vegetables, especially bananas); certain drugs (e.g., vasopressor drugs); some antihypertensive drugs (e.g., methyldopa). Monoamine oxidase inhibitors may increase metanephrine and decrease VMA. *(See p. 743.)*

URINARY 17-KETOSTEROIDS (17-KS)

Increased In

Adrenocortical hyperplasia (causing Cushing's syndrome, adrenogenital syndrome)
Adrenocortical adenoma or carcinoma
Arrhenoblastoma and lutein cell tumor of ovary (if androgenic)
Interstitial cell tumor of testicle
Pituitary tumor or hyperplasia
ACTH administration
Severe stress
Third trimester of pregnancy
Testosterone administration
Nonspecific chromagens in urine

Decreased In

Addison's disease
Panhypopituitarism
Hypothyroidism (myxedema)
Generalized wasting diseases
Nephrosis
Hypogonadism in men (castration)
Primary ovarian agenesis

Urinary 17-KS may have a daily variation of 100% in the same individual.

URINARY 17-KETOSTEROIDS BETA FRACTION

Increased In

Adrenal carcinoma

URINARY 17-KETOSTEROIDS BETA-ALPHA RATIO

Beta fraction is largely dehydroepiandrosterone; alpha fraction is mostly androsterone and etiocholanolone.

Normal: Beta-alpha ratio is usually < 0.2.

Adrenocortical hyperplasia: Ratio is usually normal; even when it is increased, it is rarely > 0.3.

Adrenal carcinoma: Ratio is usually 0.28–0.4. In adults, some patients may have a ratio > 0.2, but the ratio is increased in most cases in children. The ratio is most helpful if it is > 0.4, when it is most indicative of carcinoma. Unless the total 17-KS is increased, the beta-alpha ratio is not likely to be abnormal.

BLOOD AND URINARY CORTICOSTEROIDS (17-KETOGENIC STEROIDS)

Increased In

Adrenal hyperplasia
Adrenal adenoma
Adrenal carcinoma
ACTH therapy
Stress

Decreased In
Addison's disease
Panhypopituitarism
Cessation of corticosteroid therapy
General wasting disease

URINARY PORTER-SILBER REACTION

This reaction measures only OH at C-17 and C-21 and O= at C-20; does not measure pregnanetriol and other C-20 OH compounds.

Increased In
Cushing's syndrome (sometimes markedly)
Severe stress (e.g., eclampsia, pancreatitis [may be marked], infection, burns, surgery)
Third trimester of pregnancy (moderately)
Early pregnancy (slightly)
Severe hypertension (slightly)
Virilism (slightly)

Decreased or Normal In
Addison's disease
Hypopituitarism

Certain drugs (e.g., paraldehyde) interfere with determination.

URINARY DEHYDROISOANDROSTERONE (ALLEN BLUE TEST)

Increased In
Adrenal carcinoma

URINARY PREGNANEDIOL

Increased In
Luteal cysts of ovary
Arrhenoblastoma
Hyperadrenocorticism

Decreased In
Toxemia of pregnancy
Fetal death
Threatened abortion (some patients)
Amenorrhea

URINARY PREGNANETRIOL

Increased In
Adrenogenital syndrome (congenital adrenal hyperplasia)

URINARY ESTROGENS

Increased In
Granulosa cell tumor of ovary
Theca cell tumor of ovary
Luteoma of ovary
Interstitial cell tumor of testis
Pregnancy
Hyperadrenalism
Liver disease

Decreased In

Primary hypofunction of ovary
Secondary hypofunction of ovary

URINARY CHORIONIC GONADOTROPINS

(see also "Pregnancy" Test, p. 77)

Increased In

Normal pregnancy
Hydatidiform mole (sometimes markedly; after 12 weeks of pregnancy, > 500,000 IU/24 hours usually is associated with moles; > 1,000,000 is almost always associated with moles).
Chorionepithelioma (sometimes markedly)
- Of uterus
- Of testicle

Normal In

Nonpregnant state
Fetal death

URINARY PITUITARY GONADOTROPINS

This is a practical assay only for combined follicle-stimulating hormone and interstitial cell-stimulating hormone.

Increased In

Menopause
Male climacteric
Primary hypogonadism
Early hyperpituitarism

Decreased In

Secondary hypogonadism
Simmonds' disease
Late hyperpituitarism

OTHER PROCEDURES

Urine findings in various diseases (see Table 15-11, pp. 604–607)
See also specific tests on urine in various chapters (e.g., Chap. 8, Gastrointestinal Diseases; Chap. 12, Hematologic Diseases; Chap. 13, Metabolic and Hereditary Diseases; Chap. 14, Endocrine Diseases).

5

Nuclear Sex Chromatin and Karyotyping

NUCLEAR SEXING

Epithelial cells from buccal smear (or vaginal smear, etc.) are stained with cresyl violet and examined microscopically.

A dense body (Barr body) on the nuclear membrane represents one of the X chromosomes and occurs in 30–60% of female somatic cells. The maximum number of Barr bodies is 1 less than the number of X chromosomes.

If there are $< 10\%$ of the cells containing Barr bodies in a patient with female genitalia, karyotyping should be done to delineate probable chromosomal abnormalities.

A normal count does not rule out chromosomal abnormalities.

- 2 Barr bodies may be found in
  - 47 XXX female
  - 48 XXXY male (Klinefelter's syndrome)
  - 49 XXXYY male (Klinefelter's syndrome)
- 3 Barr bodies may be found in
  - 49 XXXXY male (Klinefelter's syndrome)

EVALUATION OF SEX CHROMOSOME IN LEUKOCYTES

Presence of a "drumstick" nuclear appendage in ~3% of leukocytes in normal females indicates the presence of 2 X chromosomes in the karyotype. It is not found in males.

It is absent in the XO type of Turner's syndrome.

There is a lower incidence of drumsticks in Klinefelter's syndrome (XXY) as opposed to the extra Barr body. (*Mean lobe counts of neutrophils are also decreased.*)

Incidence of drumsticks is decreased and mean lobe counts are lower also in mongolism.

Double drumsticks are exceedingly rare and diagnostically impractical.

SOME INDICATIONS FOR CHROMOSOME ANALYSIS (KARYOTYPING)

Suspected Autosomal Syndromes

Down's (mongolism)

E^{18} trisomy

D^{13} trisomy

Cri du chat syndrome

Suspected Sex-Chromosome Syndromes

Klinefelter's XXY, XXXY

Turner's XO

"Superfemale" XXX, XXXX

"Supermale" XYY

"Funny-looking kid" syndromes, especially with multiple anomalies including mental retardation and low birth weight

Possible myelogenous leukemia to demonstrate Philadelphia chromosome (22)

Ambiguous genitalia

Infertility (some patients)

Repeated miscarriages

Primary amenorrhea or oligomenorrhea

Mental retardation with sex anomalies

Hypogonadism

Delayed puberty

Abnormal development at puberty

Disturbances of somatic growth

ASSAY (cDNA probe) FOR REARRANGEMENT OF *bcr* GENE

Recently, special procedures using Southern blot techniques following gel electrophoresis for DNA fragment size fractionation can demonstrate reciprocal translocation of DNA from chromosome 9 (including the *abl* locus) to 22 (breakpoint cluster [*bcr*]) giving rise to shorter chromosome 22 (Philadelphia chromosome [Ph1]). This is found in 95% of patients with chronic granulocytic leukemia (CML), 5–10% of acute lymphoblastic leukemia (ALL), and 1–2% of patients with acute myelogenous leukemia. Presence of Ph1 affects response to therapy and survival. This rearrangement of *bcr* is typical of Ph1-positive CML patients and is found in ~30% of Ph1-positive AML patients. This assay can be done on peripheral blood as well as marrow, does not require dividing cells, and is more sensitive than routine cytogenetic analysis.

Table 5-1. Chromosome Number and Karyotype in Various Clinical Conditions

Clinical Condition	Chromosome Number and Karyotype	Incidence
Normal	46 XY	
Normal female	46 XX	
Suspected autosomal syndromes		
Down's (mongolism; trisomy 21)	47 XX, G+ or 47 XY, G+	1 in 700 live births (2% are 46 count due to translocation and have 10% risk of Down's syndrome in subsequent pregnancies; 2% are 46/47 mosaics)
D_1 trisomy	47 XX, D+ or 47 XY, D+	1 in 5000 live births
	Translocations	Rare
	Mosaics	Rare
E_{18} trisomy	47 XX, E+ or 47 XY, E+	1 in 3000 live births
	Translocations	Rare
	Mosaics	Rare
D_{13} trisomy		
Cri du chat syndrome	46 with partial B deletion	1 in 30,000 births
Suspected sex-chromosome syndromes		
Klinefelter's syndrome	47 XXY	1 in 600 live male births
	48 XXXY	Rare
	48 XXYY	Rare
	49 XXXXY	Rare
	49 XXXYY	Rare
	Mosaics	Infrequent
Turner's syndrome	45 XO	1 in 3000 live female births
	46 XX	Rare
	Mosaics	Infrequent
"Superfemale"	47 XXX	1 in 1000–2000 live female births
	48 XXXX	Rare
	49 XXXXX	Rare
	Mosaics	Rare
"Supermale"	47 XXY	1 in 1000 live male births

ASSAY FOR REARRANGEMENT OF GENES FOR IMMUNOGLOBULIN HEAVY (IgH) AND LIGHT (IgL-kappa) CHAINS AND FOR REARRANGEMENT OF BETA AND GAMMA T CELL RECEPTOR GENES (beta-TCR, gamma-TCR)*

Allows classification of almost all cases of ALL as T, B, or pre-B types. Confirms pathologic-immunologic diagnoses of T and B cell lymphomas that are difficult to classify. Virtually all cases of non-T, non-B leukemias are recognized as pre-B types. Up to 90% of cases of non-Hodgkin's lymphoma are derived from B cells. Their immunophenotypic abnormalities can be used to distinguish them from benign reactions in lymph nodes.

CHROMOSOME ABNORMALITIES IN MALIGNANT HEMATOLOGIC DISORDERS†

At initial diagnosis, routine cytogenetic studies show chromosomal abnormality in > 50% of cases.

Acute nonlymphocytic leukemia	54%
Acute lymphocytic leukemia	41%
Chronic granulocytic leukemia	94%
Myelodysplastic syndrome	39%
Lymphoma	71%

Structural abnormalities include translocations, deletions, isochromosomes, inversions, duplications and numeric anomalies (e.g., trisomies, monosomies). If an abnormal chromosome clone is not observed, the analysis should be considered not diagnostic.

*Data from Specialty Laboratories, Inc., San Diego, CA.

†Data from GW Dewald et al., Chromosome abnormalities in malignant hematologic disorders. *Mayo Clin Proc* 60:675, 1985.

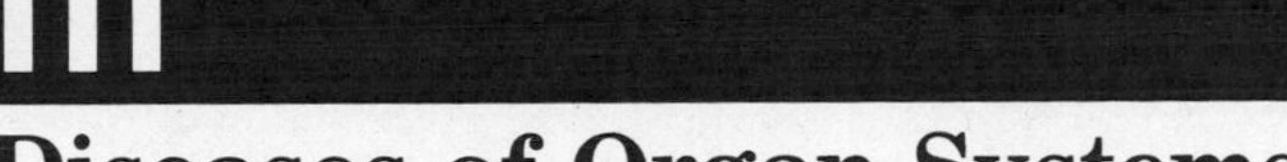

III
Diseases of Organ Systems

6

Cardiovascular Diseases

HYPERTENSION

(present in 18% of adults in the United States)

Laboratory findings due to the primary disease. These conditions are often occult or unsuspected and should always be carefully ruled out, since many of them represent curable causes of hypertension.

- Systolic hypertension
  - Hyperthyroidism
  - Chronic anemia with hemoglobin < 7 gm/dl
  - Arteriovenous fistulas—advanced Paget's disease of bone; pulmonary arteriovenous varix
  - Beriberi
- Systolic and diastolic hypertension
  - Essential (primary) hypertension (causes > 90% of cases of hypertension)
  - Secondary hypertension (causes < 10% of cases of hypertension)
    - Endocrine diseases
      - Adrenal
        - Pheochromocytoma (< 0.64% of cases of hypertension)
        - Aldosteronism (< 1% of cases of hypertension)
        - Cushing's syndrome
      - Pituitary disease
        - Signs of hyperadrenal function
        - Acromegaly
      - Hyperthyroidism
      - Hyperparathyroidism
    - Renal diseases
      - Vascular (4% of cases of hypertension)
        - Renal artery stenosis (usually due to atheromatous plaque in elderly patients and fibromuscular hyperplasia in younger patients) (0.18% of cases of hypertension)
        - Nephrosclerosis
        - Embolism
        - Arteriovenous fistula
        - Aneurysm
      - Parenchymal
        - Glomerulonephritis
        - Pyelonephritis
        - Polycystic kidneys
        - Kimmelstiel-Wilson syndrome
        - Amyloidosis
        - Collagen diseases
        - Renin-producing renal tumor (Wilms' tumor; renal hemangiopericytoma)
        - Miscellaneous
        - Urinary tract obstructions
    - Central nervous system diseases
      - Cerebrovascular accident
      - Brain tumors
      - Poliomyelitis
    - Other
      - Toxemia of pregnancy
      - Polycythemia

In children < 18 years of age, causes of hypertension are

Renal disease	61–78%
Cardiovascular disease	13–15%
Endocrine	6–9%
Miscellaneous	2–7%
Essential	1–16%

Laboratory findings indicating the functional renal status (e.g., urinalysis, serum urea nitrogen [BUN], creatinine, uric acid, serum electrolytes, phenolsulfonphthalein [PSP], creatinine clearance, radioisotope scan of kidneys, renal biopsy). The higher the uric acid in uncomplicated essential hypertension, the less the renal blood flow and the higher the renal vascular resistance.

Laboratory findings due to complications of hypertension (e.g., congestive heart failure, uremia, cerebral hemorrhage, myocardial infarction)

Laboratory findings due to administration of some antihypertensive drugs

- Oral diuretics (e.g., benzothiadiazines)
  - Increased incidence of hyperuricemia (to 65–75% of hypertensive patients from incidence of 25–35% in untreated hypertensive patients)
  - Hypokalemia
  - Hyperglycemia or aggravation of preexisting diabetes mellitus
  - Less commonly, bone marrow depression, aggravation of renal or hepatic insufficiency by electrolyte imbalance, cholestatic hepatitis, toxic pancreatitis
- Hydralazine
  - Long-term dosage of > 200 mg/day may produce syndrome not distinguishable from SLE. Usually regresses after drug is discontinued. Antinuclear antibody may be found in ≤ 50% of asymptomatic patients.
- Methyldopa
  - ≤ 20% of patients may have positive direct Coombs' test, but relatively few have hemolytic anemia. When drug is discontinued, Coombs' test may remain positive for months but anemia usually reverses promptly.
- Abnormal liver function tests indicate hepatocellular damage without jaundice associated with febrile influenza-like syndrome.
  - Rheumatoid arthritis and lupus erythematosus (LE) tests may occasionally be positive.
  - Rarely, granulocytopenia or thrombocytopenia may occur.
- Monoamine oxidase inhibitors (e.g., pargyline hydrochloride)
  - Wide range of toxic reactions, most serious of which are
    - Blood dyscrasias
    - Hepatocellular necrosis
- Diazoxide
  - Sodium and fluid retention
  - Hyperglycemia (usually mild and manageable by insulin or oral hypoglycemic agents)

When hypertension is associated with decreased serum potassium, rule out

- Primary aldosteronism
- Pseudoaldosteronism (due to excessive ingestion of licorice)
- Secondary aldosteronism (e.g., malignant hypertension)
- Hypokalemia due to diuretic administration
- Potassium loss due to renal disease
- Cushing's syndrome

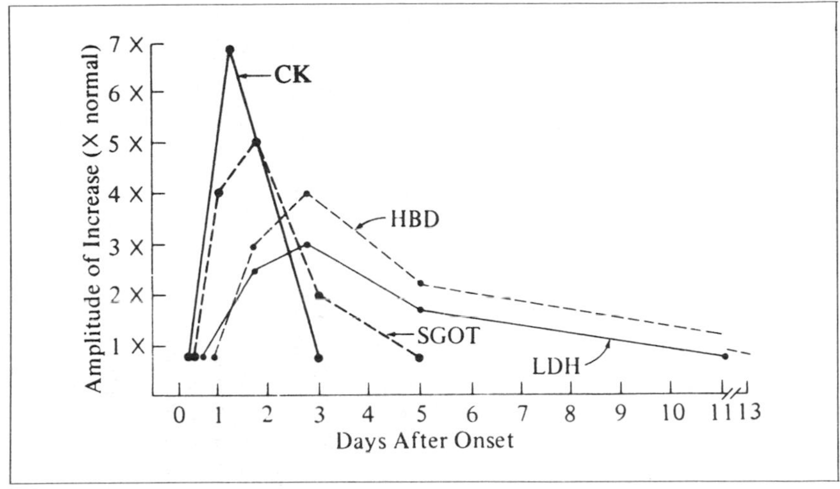

Fig. 6-1. Sequential changes in serum enzymes after acute myocardial infarction.

ACUTE MYOCARDIAL INFARCTION (AMI)*

(see Fig. 6-1 and Tables 6-1 through 6-3)

Laboratory Determinations Required

Because ECG changes may be inconclusive (e.g., masked by bundle branch block or Wolff-Parkinson-White syndrome or may not reveal intramural or diaphragmatic infarcts)

For differential diagnosis (e.g., angina pectoris, pulmonary infarction)

Normal serum enzyme levels during 48 hours after onset of clinical symptoms indicate no MI.

To follow the course of the patient with acute MI

To estimate prognosis (e.g., marked elevation of serum enzyme [4–5 times normal] correlates with increased incidence of ventricular arrhythmia, shock, heart failure, and with higher mortality)

Blood should be drawn promptly after onset of symptoms. Repeat determinations should be performed at appropriate intervals (see Fig. 6-1) and also if symptoms recur or new signs or symptoms develop. Changes may indicate extension or additional MI or other complications (e.g., pulmonary infarction).

Specific Findings

Serum creatine kinase (CK) is particularly valuable for the following reasons:

- Serial total CK has sensitivity of 98% early in course of MI but false positive rate of 15% due to many causes of increased CK (see pp. 62–64).
- It allows early diagnosis because increased levels appear within 3–6 hours after onset and peak levels in 24–36 hours.
- It is a more sensitive indicator than other enzymes because an increased CK level shows a larger amplitude of change (6–12 times normal).

*Data from NJ Pappas, Enhanced cardiac enzyme profile. *Clin Lab Med* 9:689, 1989; JA Lott and JM Stang, Differential diagnosis of patients with abnormal creatine kinase isoenzymes. *Clin Lab Med* 9:627, 1989.

Table 6-1. Summary of Increased Serum Enzyme Levels After Acute Myocardial Infarction[a]

Serum Enzymes	Earliest Increase (hours)	Maximum Level (hours)	Return to Normal by (days)	Amplitude of Increase × Normal	Comment[b]
CK	3–6	24–36	3	7	Recommended for early diagnosis
MDH	4–6	24–48	5	4	Early use parallels CK; no advantage over other enzymes; technically difficult to do
SGOT	6–8	24–48	4–6	5	
LDH	10–12	48–72	11	3	See α-HBD; isoenzyme determination to differentiate pulmonary infarction, congestive heart failure, etc.
α-HBD	10–12	48–72	13	3–4	Particularly useful for later diagnosis (in 2nd week) when other enzymes have returned to normal, because of longer duration of increased activity; more specific than LDH
ALD	6–8	24–48	4	4	
SGPT	Usually normal unless liver damage due to congestive heart failure, shock, drug therapy (e.g., Coumadin)				
ICD	Usually normal				

[a]The time periods all represent average values.

[b]Least number of false positive results occur with tests of CK, α-HBD, heat-stable LDH.

Table 6-2. Comparison of Sensitivity and Specificity of Various Tests for Myocardial Infarction*

Test	Sensitivity (%)	Specificity (%)
ECG	63–84	100
SGOT increased	89–97	48–88
CK increased	93–100	57–88
CK-MB increased	94–100	93–100
LDH increased	87	88
$LDH_1 > LDH_2$ (on third day after chest pain)	61–90	94–99

*Range of values because different studies used various methods, time periods after onset of symptoms, benchmarks for establishing the diagnosis, etc. Refers to levels in serum.

High sensitivity of CK-MB is combined with the high specificity of LDH isoenzymes by ordering both performed on same specimen where the diagnosis is uncertain.

Table 6-3. Triad of Laboratory Tests Suggested for Differential Diagnosis of Acute Myocardial Infarction[a]

	Serial Tests Done Within 2 Days of Onset		
	SGOT	LDH	Serum Bilirubin
Acute myocardial infarction	I	I	N
Angina pectoris	N	N	N
Pulmonary embolism or infarction[b]	Usually N	I	I ≅ 20% of patients
Pneumonia or atelectasis	N	N	N
Congestive heart failure	N	N	May be slightly I
Pulmonary embolism and myocardial infarction	I	I	I

I = increased; N = normal.

[a] Not useful in presence of severe liver disease.

[b] "Triad" of increased LDH and serum bilirubin associated with normal SGOT is found in only ≅ 15% of patients.

Less diagnostic confusion occurs because CK is not increased by diseases often associated with MI (e.g., liver damage due to congestion, drug therapy, may increase serum glutamic-oxaloacetic transaminase [SGOT]) or that may be difficult to distinguish from MI (e.g., pulmonary infarction may increase lactic dehydrogenase [LDH]).

It returns to normal by third day; a poorer prognosis is suggested if the increase lasts more than 3–4 days. Reinfarction is indicated by an elevated level after the fifth day that had previously returned to normal.

It is useful in differential diagnosis of diseases with normal enzyme level (e.g., angina pectoris) or from those with increased levels of other enzymes (e.g., increased LDH in pulmonary infarction).

Serial CK-MB levels provide the best laboratory discrimination between the presence or absence of myocardial necrosis and has become the "gold standard" for diagnosis within 24 hours of onset of symptoms. In AMI, CK-MB usually is evident at 4–8 hours, peaks at 15–24 hours (mean peak = 16 times normal), with sensitivity and specificity each > 97% within the first 48 hours. By 72 hours, two-thirds of patients still show some increase in CK-MB. More frequent sampling (every 6 hours) is more likely to identify a peak value; in elderly patients, a peak may be the only abnormality. False negative results may be due to incorrect sampling (e.g., only once in 24 hours) or sampling too late after MI.

~5% of AMI patients (especially in older age groups) have abnormal CK-MB but normal CK due to lower CK reference values. (Normal serum CK values decline with age and sedentary or bedridden status.)

CK-MB should be reported in units as well as percentage, since if there is injury of both cardiac and skeletal muscle (e.g., perioperative AMI), CK-MB percentage may not appear increased.

MB isoenzyme may also be increased in

- Cardiac trauma
- Myocarditis (some cases)
- Congestive heart failure (moderate)
- Coronary angiography (transient)
- Cardiac surgery (transient) and heart valve replacement
- Muscular dystrophy, polymyositis, collagen vascular diseases (especially SLE), massive myoglobinuria, or rhabdomyolysis
- Electrical and thermal burns and trauma (~50% of patients; but not supported by $LDH_1 > LDH_2$)
- Rocky Mountain spotted fever
- Reye's syndrome
- Hyperthermia, hypothermia
- Hypothyroidism (some cases)
- Hypo- and hyperthyroidism and chronic renal failure may cause persistent increase, although the proportion of CK-MB remains low.

MB isoenzyme is **not increased** in

- Angina
- Cardiac arrest or cardioversion not due to AMI
- Cardiac hypertrophy or cardiomyopathy unless there is myocarditis or heart failure
- Cardiac pacemaker or catheterization (including Swan-Ganz)
- Cardiopulmonary bypass
- IM injections (total CK may be increased)
- Seizures (total CK may be markedly increased)
- Brain infarction or injury (total CK may be increased)
- Pulmonary embolism

In one protocol the criteria for AMI are an increasing (above reference range) and then decreasing CK-total and CK-MB in serial specimens drawn on admission and at 8- or 12-hour intervals; this is considered almost pathognomonic in patients in whom AMI is strongly suspected; no blood need be collected after 48 hours in patients with uneventful course. LDH studies are done only if patient's symptoms occurred > 12–24 hours before admission or if history or ECG is still suggestive of AMI.

In another ("classic") protocol, patients with suspected acute MI have blood samples taken on admission and at 24 and 48 hours; isoenzyme determinations should be performed if total CK or LDH is increased. If increased CK-MB and flipped LDH both occur in any of the blood specimens (not necessarily at the same time), it is virtually certain that the patient has AMI, and there is no need for further diagnostic testing; if these criteria are not met within 48 hours, acute myocardial necrosis is considered ruled out and enzyme measurement can be terminated. CK isoenzyme determinations are generally not performed unless total CK is > 75% upper limit of normal. An elevated CK-MB in the presence of normal total CK should be questioned (although total CK may be very low in small or sedentary or older persons).

Single CK-MB values in emergency room patients have a sensitivity of only 18% within 4 hours of chest pain and 50% at 4–12 hours; specificity is 88%; thus single tests are usually not recommended for screening in the ER.

In patients with delayed admission, serial blood samples for LDH total and isoenzymes and SGOT are occasionally useful when CK and CK-MB are no longer diagnostic; when CK and CK-MB are positive, LDH and SGOT studies are not cost-effective and usually add little useful information.

CK and CK-MB isoenzyme are also increased after cardiac surgery so a diagnosis of AMI cannot be made until 12–24 hours after surgery; typically AMI patients have higher peak values of CK, CK-MB, and myoglobin; patients without AMI have earlier peaks that return to basal values more rapidly; diagnostic value of enzymes are diminished after cardiac surgery. CK-MB is probably the only useful laboratory test for diagnosis of perioperative AMI because hemolysis and skeletal muscle injury increase other enzyme levels. Significant increases in CK, CK-MB, and myoglobin are also common after percutaneous transluminal angioplasty of coronary arteries. Balloon angioplasty may also cause increased CK-MB and myoglobin. Cardiac trauma and contusions, electrical injury, and inflammatory myocarditis may produce enzyme changes that cannot be distinguished from AMI. Other causes of CK-MB changes are given on pp. 63–64.

Recent innovations are CK-MM and CK-MB isoform measurements. Reagent manufacturers claim much higher proportions of MI patterns appear earlier in serum, before CK-MB or total CK, but methodology is not yet widely available.

Serum LDH is almost always increased, beginning in 10–12 hours and reaching a peak in 48–72 hours (of about 3 times normal). The prolonged elevation of 10–14 days is particularly useful for late diagnosis if the patient is first seen after sufficient time has elapsed for CK to become normal. Levels > 2000 units suggest a poorer prognosis. Because many other diseases may increase the LDH, isoenzyme studies should be performed. Increased serum LDH with an LDH_1/LDH_2 ratio > 1 ("flipped" LDH) may occur in acute renal infarction and hemolysis associated with hemolytic anemia, pernicious anemia, prosthetic heart valves, or pregnancy, as well as in AMI. In AMI, flipped LDH usually appears in 12–24 hours, peaks at 55–60 hours, and is present within 48 hours in 80% of patients; after 1 week, it is still present in < 50% of patients even though total serum LDH may still be elevated. Flipped LDH never appears before CK-MB. LDH_1 may remain elevated after total LDH has returned to normal; with small infarcts, LDH_1 may be increased while total LDH remains normal. Flipped LDH may reverse several times within 2–3 days. LDH_1/total LDH > 0.4 or LDH_1 > 90 units/L has also been used instead of flipped LDH_1/LDH_2 ratio.

SGOT has been replaced by CK and LDH determinations (see above) but may be useful when CK determinations are no longer elevated (i.e., first blood sample is collected > 24 hours after onset) for the following reasons:

SGOT is increased in > 95% of the patients when blood is drawn at the appropriate time.

It allows early diagnosis because increased levels appear within 6–8 hours and peak levels in 24 hours. Usually returns to normal in 4–6 days.

Peak level is usually ~200 units (5 times normal). A higher level (> 300 units), along with a more prolonged increase, suggests a poorer prognosis.

Reinfarction is indicated by a rise following a return to normal.

SGPT is usually not increased unless there is liver damage due to congestive heart failure, drug therapy, etc.

SGOT/SGPT ratio > 3 : 1 or that rises more than 2 times supports diagnosis of AMI if the following are excluded: certain hepatocellular injuries (e.g., acetaminophen overdose, severe ethanol toxicity), hepatic carcinoma, severe hepatic congestion, cirrhosis, severe skeletal muscle injury. May be helpful in evaluating LDH results and when blood is drawn late after onset of symptoms and CK-MB has declined to normal or borderline levels.

Serum alpha-hydroxybutyric dehydrogenase (α-HBD) parallels increase of fast-moving LDH with peak (3–4 times normal) in 48 hours and persistent elevation for up to 2 weeks. Serum malic dehydrogenase (MDH) may be useful on rare occasions; an early increase (4–6 hours) parallels changes in CK.

Serum ICD is normal.

Leukocytosis is almost invariable; commonly detected by second day but may occur as early as 2 hours. Usually the WBC is 12,000–15,000; up to 20,000 is not rare; sometimes it is very high. Usually there are 75–90% neutrophilic leukocytes with only a slight shift to the left. Leukocytosis is likely to develop before fever.

Erythrocyte sedimentation rate (ESR) is increased, usually by second or third day (may begin within a few hours); peak rate is in 4–5 days, persists for 2–6 months. Increased ESR is sometimes more sensitive than WBC, as it may occur before fever and it persists after temperature and WBC have returned to normal. Degree of increase of ESR does not correlate with severity or prognosis.

Glycosuria and hyperglycemia occur in ≤ 50% of patients.

Glucose tolerance is decreased.

Increased serum myoglobin peaks and returns to normal earlier than CK; useful for diagnosis within 6 hours of onset of symptoms. Myoglobinuria often occurs (see pp. 98–99).

Thrombolytic agents (e.g., streptokinase, urokinase, tissue plasminogen activator) alter the enzyme patterns. After successful reperfusion, enzymes show an earlier rise (3–4 hours after AMI), earlier peak (6–14 hours after AMI), and higher levels of CK-total and CK-MB compared to nonperfused patients. Peak CK-MB after reperfusion occurs in ~6–10 hours. Isoforms have also been recommended for this study with MB_2 peak parallel to CK-MB but occurring about 2 hours earlier. One protocol to determine if thrombolytic therapy is successful measures total CK and CK-MB every half hour for the first 3 hours, then every 1–3 hours up to 24 hours. The CK-total and CK-MB increase simultaneously (by 13–57%) if reperfusion has occurred.

Differential Diagnosis

Serum enzymes not elevated in angina pectoris; increased levels mean MI or another condition.

Serum enzymes usually show little or no increase in inflammatory myocardial lesions (e.g., rheumatic fever) unless disease is severe. (Salicylates may cause some increase of SGOT and SGPT due to liver damage.)

Little or no change occurs in chronic heart failure.

Some increase of SGOT and serum glutamic-pyruvic transaminase (SGPT) may occur in acute heart failure due to liver congestion; it is quickly reversed with appropriate therapy. There may be marked increase in cardiac tamponade due to pericardial effusion.

SGPT is higher than SGOT (which is only slightly increased) in pulmonary infarction and upper abdominal disease (e.g., liver injury) (see SGOT/SGPT ratio (p. 60).

Findings due to underlying coronary heart disease

CORONARY HEART DISEASE (CHD)

Increased risk factors

- Increased serum total and LDL cholesterol, decreased HDL cholesterol, and various ratios (see pp. 70–75)
- Increased serum triglycerides is not considered an independent risk factor.
- Recent reports suggest that apolipoprotein A-I and apolipoprotein B may be better discriminators of CHD than cholesterol levels, and low ratio of apolipoprotein A-I to apolipoprotein B may be best predictor. (Variation in methodology and lack of interlaboratory standardization make this difficult to evaluate presently.)
- Clinical evidence of CHD or atherosclerosis in patient $<$ age 40, family history of premature CHD, hypertension, males, smokers

Lipoprotein electrophoresis (see Table 13-6, pp. 410–413) shows a specific abnormal pattern in $< 2\%$ of Americans (usually Types II, IV). The chief purpose of the test is to identify rare familial disorders (I, III, V) to anticipate problems in children.

Lipoprotein electrophoresis may be indicated if serum triglycerides $>$ 300 mg/dl, fasting serum is lipemic, or there is hyperglycemia, significant glycosuria, impaired glucose tolerance, increased serum uric acid ($>$ 8.5 mg/dl).

Perform laboratory tests to rule out diabetes mellitus, liver disease, nephrotic syndrome, dysproteinemias, hypothyroidism.

CONGESTIVE HEART FAILURE

Renal changes: Urine—slight albuminuria ($<$ 1 gm/day) is common. There are isolated RBCs and WBCs, hyaline, and (sometimes) granular casts. Urine is concentrated, with specific gravity $>$ 1.020. Oliguria is a characteristic feature of right-sided failure. PSP excretion and urea clearance are usually depressed. Moderate azotemia (BUN usually $<$ 60 mg/dl) is evident with severe oliguria; may increase with vigorous diuresis. (*Primary renal disease is indicated by proportionate increase in serum creatinine and low specific gravity of urine despite oliguria.*)

ESR may be decreased because of decreased serum fibrinogen.

Plasma volume is increased. Serum albumin and total protein are decreased, with increased gamma globulin. Hematocrit reading is slightly decreased, but red cell mass may be increased.

Urine sodium is decreased. Plasma sodium and chloride tend to fall but may be normal before treatment. Total body sodium is markedly increased. Plasma potassium is usually normal or slightly increased (because of shift from intracellular location); may be somewhat reduced with hypochloremic alkalosis due to some diuretics. Total body potassium is decreased. Saliva sodium and chloride are decreased and potassium is increased.

Liver function changes (see pp. 204–205).

Laboratory findings due to underlying disease (e.g., rheumatic fever, viral myocarditis, bacterial endocarditis, chronic severe anemia, hypertension, hyperthyroidism, Hurler's syndrome)

- Acidosis (reduced blood pH) occurs when renal insufficiency is associated or there is CO_2 retention due to pulmonary insufficiency, low plasma sodium, or ammonium chloride toxicity.
- Alkalosis (increased blood pH) occurs in uncomplicated heart failure itself, in hyperventilation, in alveolar-capillary block due to associated pulmo-

nary fibrosis, after mercurial diuresis that causes hypochloremic alkalosis, because of potassium depletion.

Alkalosis (with normal or increased blood pH) showing increased plasma bicarbonate and moderately increased PCO_2 after acute correction of respiratory acidosis is due to CO_2 retention when there is chloride deficit and usually decreased potassium.

ACUTE RHEUMATIC FEVER

Serologic titers: one of these three is elevated in 95% of patients with acute rheumatic fever; if all are normal, a diagnosis of rheumatic fever is less likely.

Antistreptolysin O (ASO) titer increase indicates recent hemolytic streptococcus infection and indirectly corroborates clinical findings of rheumatic fever. Increased titer develops only after the second week and reaches a peak in 4–6 weeks. Increasing titer is more significant than a single determination. Titer is usually > 250 units; more significant if > 400–500 units. A normal titer helps to rule out clinically doubtful rheumatic fever. Sometimes ASO is not increased even when other titers (antifibrinolysin, antihyaluronidase) are increased. Increased titer is found in 80% of patients within the first 2 months. Height of titer is not related to severity; rate of fall is not related to course of disease.

Antihyaluronidase titer of 1000–1500 follows recent streptococcus A disease and ≤ 4000 with rheumatic fever. Average titer is higher in early rheumatic activity than in subsiding or inactive rheumatic fever or nonrheumatic streptococcal disease or nonstreptococcal infections. Antihyaluronidase titer is increased as often as ASO and antifibrinolysin titers.

Antifibrinolysin (antistreptokinase) titer is increased in rheumatic fever and in recent hemolytic streptococcus infections.

ESR increase is a sensitive test of rheumatic activity; returns to normal with adequate treatment with adrenocorticotropic hormone (ACTH) or salicylates. It may remain increased after WBC becomes normal. It is said to become normal with onset of congestive heart failure even in the presence of rheumatic activity. It is normal in uncomplicated chorea alone.

C-reactive protein (CRP) parallels ESR.

Serum proteins are altered, with decreased serum albumin and increased $alpha_2$ and gamma globulins. (*Streptococcus A infections do not increase $alpha_2$ globulin.*) Fibrinogen is increased.

WBC may be normal but usually is increased (10,000–16,000/cu mm) with shift to the left; increase may persist for weeks after fever subsides. Count may decrease with salicylate and ACTH therapy.

Anemia (hemoglobin usually 8–12 gm/dl) is common; gradually improves as activity subsides; microcytic type. Anemia may be related to increased plasma volume that occurs in early phase of acute rheumatic fever.

Urine: There is a slight febrile albuminuria. Often mild abnormality of Addis count (protein, casts, RBCs, WBCs) indicates mild focal nephritis. Concomitant glomerulonephritis appears in ≤ 2.5% of cases.

Blood cultures are usually negative. Occasional positive culture is found in 5% of patients (bacteria usually grow only in fluid media, not on solid media), in contrast to bacterial endocarditis.

Throat culture is often negative for group A streptococci.

Serum glutamic-oxaloacetic transaminase (SGOT) may be increased, but is normal unless the patient has cardiac failure with liver damage.

Determine clinical activity–follow ESR, CRP, and WBC. Return to normal should be seen in 6–12 weeks in 80–90% of patients; it may take ≤ 6 months. Normal findings do not prove inactivity if patient is receiving hormone therapy. When therapy is stopped after findings have been suppressed for 6–8 weeks, there may be a mild rebound for 2–3 days and then a return to normal. Relapse after cessation of therapy occurs within 1–8 weeks.

VALVULAR HEART DISEASE

Laboratory findings due to associated or underlying or predisposing disease (e.g., syphilis, rheumatic fever, carcinoid syndrome, genetic disease of mucopolysaccharide metabolism, congenital defects)

Laboratory findings due to complications (e.g., heart failure, bacterial endocarditis, embolic phenomena)

VIRAL MYOCARDITIS

(routine autopsy incidence of 1.2–3.5%)

May be due to Coxsackie A and B, echovirus, poliomyelitis, influenza A and B, cytomegalovirus (CMV), Epstein-Barr, adenovirus, rubeola, mumps, rubella, variola, vaccinia, varicella zoster, rabies, lymphocytic choriomeningitis, chikungunya, dengue, yellow fever

Increased ESR

Mild to moderate leukocytosis

Increased serum CK, SGOT, LDH is common only in early stages

Serologic tests for viral antigen, IgM antibody, or changed titer using acute and convalescent paired sera

Radionuclide scintigraphic sequential imaging using technetium 99m pyrophosphate and gallium 67

Biopsy of right ventricular muscle showing > 5 lymphocytes/hpf and degeneration of muscle fibers

BACTERIAL ENDOCARDITIS

Blood culture is positive in 80–90% of patients. *Streptococcus viridans* causes 40–50% of cases, *Staphylococcus aureus* 15–20%, *Streptococcus pneumoniae* 5%, and enterococcus 5–10%. Other causes may be gram-negative bacteria (about 10% of cases—e.g., *Escherichia coli, Pseudomonas aeruginosa, Klebsiella, Proteus*) and fungi (e.g., *Candida, Histoplasma, Cryptococcus*).

Proper blood cultures require adequate volume of blood, at least 5 cultures taken during a period of several days with temperature 101°F or more (preferably when highest), anaerobic as well as aerobic growth, variety of enriched media, prompt incubation, prolonged observation (growth is usual in 1–4 days but may require 2–3 weeks). Beware of negative culture due to recent antibiotic therapy. Beware of transient bacteremia following dental procedures, tonsillectomy, etc., which does not represent bacterial endocarditis (in these cases, streptococci usually grow only in fluid media; in bacterial endocarditis, many colonies also occur on solid media). Blood culture is also negative in bacterial endocarditis due to *Rickettsia burnetii,* but Phase 1 complement fixation test is positive.

Positive blood cultures may be more difficult to obtain in prosthetic valve endocarditis (due to unusual and fastidious organisms), right-sided endocarditis, uremia, and long-standing endocarditis. A single positive culture must be interpreted with extreme caution. Aside from the exceptions noted in this paragraph, the diagnosis should be based on 2 or more cultures positive for the same organism.

Serum bactericidal test measures ability of serial dilutions of patient's serum to sterilize a standardized inoculum of his infecting organisms; it is sometimes useful to demonstrate inadequate antibiotic levels or to avoid unnecessary drug toxicity.

Progressive normochromic normocytic anemia is a characteristic feature; in 10% of patients, hemoglobin is < 7 gm/dl. Rarely there is a hemolytic anemia with a positive Coombs' test. Serum iron is decreased. Bone marrow contains abundant hemosiderin. WBC is normal in ~50% of patients and elevated ≤ 15,000/cu mm in the rest, with 65–86% neutrophils. Higher WBC indicates presence of a complication (e.g., cerebral, pulmonary). Occasionally there is leukopenia. Monocytosis may be pronounced. Large macrophages may occur in peripheral blood.

Platelet count is usually normal, but occasionally it is decreased; rarely purpura occurs.

Serum proteins are altered, with an increase in gamma globulin; therefore positive ESR, cryoglobulins, rheumatoid factor, etc., are found.

Hematuria (usually microscopic) occurs at some stage in many patients due to glomerulitis, renal infarct, or focal embolic glomerulonephritis. Albuminuria is almost invariable even without these complications. Renal insufficiency with azotemia and fixed specific gravity is infrequent now. Nephrotic syndrome is rare.

CSF findings in various complications, meningitis, brain abscess

Laboratory findings due to underlying or predisposing diseases
- Rheumatic heart disease
- Congenital heart disease
- Infection of genitourinary system
- Other

MYXOMA OF LEFT ATRIUM OF HEART

Anemia that is hemolytic in type and mechanical in origin (due to local turbulence of blood) is to be looked for and may be severe. Bizarre poikilocytes may be seen in blood smear. Reticulocyte count may be increased. Other findings may reflect effects of hemolysis or compensatory erythroid hyperplasia. The anemia is recognized in ~50% of patients with this tumor. Increased serum LDH reflects hemolysis.

Serum gamma globulin is increased in ~50% of patients. IgG may be increased.

Increased ESR is a reflection of abnormal serum proteins.

Platelet count may be decreased (possibly the cause here also is mechanical) with resultant findings due to thrombocytopenia.

Negative blood cultures differentiate this tumor from bacterial endocarditis.

Occasionally WBC is increased, and CRP may be positive.

Laboratory findings due to complications
- Emboli to various organs (increased SGOT may reflect many small emboli to striated muscle)
- Congestive heart failure

These findings are reported much less frequently in myxoma of the right atrium, which is more likely to be accompanied by secondary polycythemia than anemia.

POSTCOMMISSUROTOMY SYNDROME

This condition occurs after cardiac surgery (e.g., commissurotomy, correction of pulmonary stenosis with atrial septal defect); it is the same as the postcardiac injury syndrome.

Increased WBC, ESR, CRP (present by the second day).

SGOT is increased to 4–7 times normal by the second day.

COR PULMONALE

Secondary polycythemia

Increased blood CO_2 when cor pulmonale is secondary to chest deformities or pulmonary emphysema

Laboratory findings of the primary lung disease (e.g., chronic bronchitis and emphysema, multiple small pulmonary emboli, pulmonary schistosomiasis)

ACUTE PERICARDITIS

Due To

Active rheumatic fever (40% of patients)

Bacterial infection (20% of patients)

Other infections (e.g., viral, rickettsial, parasites)
Uremia (11% of patients)
Benign nonspecific pericarditis (10% of patients)
Neoplasms (3.5% of patients)
Collagen disease (e.g., SLE, polyarteritis nodosa) (2% of patients)
Acute myocardial infarction, postcardiac injury syndrome
Trauma
Myxedema
Others (e.g., hypersensitivity, unknown origin or in association with various syndromes)

Findings

See appropriate sections for laboratory findings of primary disease.
Radioisotope scan of cardiac pool
WBC: usually increased in proportion to fever; normal or low in viral disease and tuberculous pericarditis; markedly increased in suppurative bacterial pericarditis
Examination of aspirated pericardial fluid (see Table 7-2, p. 135)
- Smears and cultures for pyogenic bacteria and tubercle bacilli
- Cytologic examination for LE cells and neoplastic cells

CHRONIC PERICARDIAL EFFUSION

See appropriate sections for primary diseases and sections (Table 7-2, p. 135) on body fluids.

Due To

Tuberculosis
Metastatic tumor
Myxedema
SLE

Rarely Due To

Severe anemia
Polyarteritis nodosa
Irradiation therapy
Endomyocardial fibrosis of Africa
Scleroderma
Rheumatoid arthritis
Mycotic infections
Idiopathic causes

AORTIC ARCH SYNDROME (TAKAYASU'S SYNDROME; PULSELESS DISEASE)

WBC usually normal
Serum proteins abnormal with increased gamma globulins (mostly composed of IgM)
Increased ESR

Women patients have a continuous high level of urinary total estrogens (rather than the usual rise during luteal phase after a low excretion during follicular phase).

LOEFFLER'S PARIETAL FIBROPLASTIC ENDOCARDITIS

Eosinophilia ≤ 70%; may be absent at first but appears sooner or later
WBC frequently increased
Laboratory findings due to frequently occurring
- Mural thrombi in heart and embolization of spleen and lung
- Mitral and tricuspid regurgitation

SHOCK

Leukocytosis is common, especially with hemorrhage. There may be leukopenia when shock is severe, as in gram-negative bacteremia. Circulating eosinophils are decreased.

Hemoconcentration (e.g., dehydration, burns) or hemodilution (e.g., hemorrhage, crush injuries, and skeletal trauma) takes place.

Hyperglycemia occurs early.

Acidosis appears when shock is well-developed, with increased blood lactate, low serum sodium, low CO_2-combining power with decreased alkaline reserve.

Serum potassium may be increased.

Blood pH is usually relatively normal but may be decreased. BUN and creatinine may be increased.

Urine examination

- Volume: Normovolemic patients have output ≥ 50 ml/hour; should investigate cause if < 25–30 ml/hour. In hypovolemia, normal kidney may lower 24-hour urine output to 300–400 ml.
- Specific gravity: > 1.020 with low urine output suggests patient is fluid-depleted. < 1.010 with low urine output suggests renal insufficiency. Specific gravity depends on weight rather than concentration of solutes; therefore is more affected than osmolarity by high-molecular-weight substances such as urea, albumin, and glucose.
- Osmolarity: Hypovolemia is suggested by high urine osmolarity and urine-plasma osmolarity ratio ≥ 1 : 2. Renal failure is suggested by low urine osmolarity with oliguria and urine-plasma osmolarity ratio ≤ 1 : 1.

Due To
(in neonates)

- Hypovolemia
  - Blood loss
    - Twin-to-twin or fetus-to-mother transfusion
    - Placental hemorrhage
    - Hemorrhage into GI tract, cerebral ventricles, lungs, trauma, or surgery
  - Plasma loss
    - Capillary leak (e.g., in sepsis, hypoxia, acidosis)
    - Hypoproteinemia
    - Peritonitis (e.g., necrotizing enterocolitis)
    - Pulmonary edema
  - Extravascular loss of fluid
    - Vomiting, diarrhea
    - Inappropriate diuresis
    - Excess insensible loss
- Excess vasodilatation
  - Sepsis
  - Drugs (e.g., certain anesthetics, muscle relaxants, sedatives, hypnotics, psychotropic drugs)
- Cardiovascular
  - Myocardial
    - Infections
    - Metabolic abnormalities (e.g., hypoglycemia)
    - Arrhythmias
  - Left-to-right shunt (e.g., patent ductus arteriosus)
  - Obstruction of blood flow (e.g., various congenital heart diseases)
- Laboratory monitoring of pH, blood gases, electrolytes, calcium

PHLEBOTHROMBOSIS OF LEG VEINS

Staphylococcal clumping test measures breakdown products of fibrin in serum; these indicate the presence of a clot that has begun to dissolve. Sensitivity = 88%, specificity = 66% using venography as "gold-standard."

Serial dilution protamine sulfate test measures the presence of a fibrin monomer that is one of the polymerization products of fibrinogen. It is less sensitive than the staphylococcal clumping test but indicates clotting earlier.

Tests indicate recent extensive clotting of any origin (e.g., postoperative status).

Laboratory findings of pulmonary infarction (see p. 148) should be sought as evidence of embolization.

SEPTIC THROMBOPHLEBITIS

Laboratory findings due to associated septicemia

- Increased WBC (often > 20,000/cu mm) with marked shift to left and toxic changes in neutrophils
- Disseminated intravascular coagulation may be present.
- Respiratory alkalosis due to ventilation-perfusion abnormalities with hypoxia. Significant acidosis indicates shock.
- Azotemia
- Positive blood culture

Laboratory findings due to complications (e.g., septic pulmonary infarction)

Laboratory findings due to underlying disease

CONGENITAL ANGIOMATOUS ARTERIOVENOUS FISTULAS

Platelet count may be decreased.

LABORATORY FINDINGS OF ACUTE HEART TRANSPLANT REJECTION AS GUIDE TO IMMUNOSUPPRESSIVE TREATMENT

Endocardial biopsy to determine acute rejection and follow effects of therapy has no substitute.

Increasing ESR and WBC

Increased isoenzyme LDH_1 as amount (> 100 IU) and percent (35%) of total LDH during first 4 weeks after surgery

These findings are reversed with effective immunosuppressive therapy. Total LDH continues to be increased even when LDH_1 becomes normal.

Chronic rejection is accelerated coronary artery atherosclerosis.

7

Respiratory Diseases

Laboratory Tests for Respiratory System Disease

SPUTUM

Color in various conditions

Rusty	Lobar pneumonia
Anchovy-paste (dark brown)	Amebic liver abscess rupture into bronchus
Red-currant jelly	*Klebsiella pneumoniae*
Red (pigment, not blood)	*Serratia marcescens;* rifampin overdose
Black	*Bacteroides melaninogenicus* pneumonia; anthracosilicosis
Green (with WBCs, sweet odor)	*Pseudomonas* infection
Milky	Bronchoalveolar carcinoma
Yellow (without WBCs)	Jaundice

Smears and cultures for infections (e.g., pneumonias, tuberculosis, fungi)—must be adequate samples of sputum (i.e., not just saliva)

Cytology for carcinoma

- Positive in 40% on first sample
- Positive in 70% with 3 samples
- Positive in 85% with 5 samples
- False positive in <1%

Cytology in bronchogenic carcinoma

- Positive in 67–85% of squamous cell carcinoma
- Positive in 64–70% of small-cell undifferentiated carcinoma
- Positive in 55% of adenocarcinoma

NEEDLE BIOPSY OF PLEURA (CLOSED CHEST)
(whenever cannot diagnose otherwise)

Positive for tumor in ~6% of malignant mesothelioma and ~60% of other cases of malignancy

Positive for tubercles in two-thirds of cases on first biopsy with increased yield on second and third biopsies; therefore repeat biopsy if suspicious clinically. Can also culture biopsy material for tuberculosis. Fluid culture alone establishes diagnosis of tuberculosis in 25% of cases.

SCALENE LYMPH NODE BIOPSY
(biopsy of scalene fat pad even without palpable lymph nodes)

Positive in 15% of bronchogenic carcinoma. May also be positive in various granulomatous diseases (e.g., tuberculosis, sarcoidosis, pneumoconiosis).

BRONCHOSCOPY

For biopsy of endobronchial tumor in which obstruction may cause secondary pneumonia with effusion but still be resectable carcinoma

To obtain bronchial washings for malignant cells

To diagnose nonresectable tumors that should be treated with irradiation (e.g., oat cell carcinoma, Hodgkin's disease)

BRONCHOALVEOLAR LAVAGE (BAL)*

(saline lavage of lung subsegment via nasal fiberoptic bronchoscope; performing quantitative bacterial culture and cytocentrifugation for staining slides provides overall diagnostic accuracy of 79% for pulmonary infection)

Giemsa stain

- Normal persons show <3% neutrophils, 8–18% lymphocytes, 80–89% alveolar macrophages.
- >10% neutrophils: acute inflammation—e.g., bacterial infection (including *Legionella,* adult respiratory distress syndrome [ARDS], drug reaction)
- >1% squamous epithelial cells: indicates that a positive culture may reflect oral contamination
- >80% macrophages: common in pulmonary hemorrhage. Aspergillosis is the only infection associated with significant alveolar hemorrhage, which may also be found in >10% of patients with hematologic malignancies
- >30% lymphocytes: may indicate hypersensitivity pneumonitis (often up to 50–60% with more cytoplasm and large irregular nucleus)
- >10% neutrophils and >3% eosinophils is characteristic of idiopathic pulmonary fibrosis; alveolar macrophages predominate. Lymphocyte percentage may be increased.
- $>10^5$ colony-forming bacteria/ml indicates bacterial infection if <1% squamous epithelial cells are present on Giemsa stain.

Gram's stain

- Many bacteria suggest bacterial infection if there are <1% squamous epithelial cells, especially if culture shows $>10^4$ bacteria/ml.
- No bacteria suggests bacterial infection is unlikely but should rule out *Legionella* with direct fluorescent antibody (DFA) if Giemsa stain shows increased neutrophils
- Combined with methenamine silver or Papanicolaou's (Pap) stain, 94% sensitivity for diagnosis of *Pneumocystis* infection in AIDS; increased to 100% when combined with transbronchial biopsy

Acid-fast stain positive may indicate *Mycobacterium tuberculosis* or *Mycobacterium avium intracellulare* infection

Toluidine blue stain may show *Pneumocystis carinii* cysts in *Pneumocystis* pneumonia or *Aspergillus* hyphae in immunocompromised host with invasive aspergillosis

Prussian blue–nuclear red stain strongly positive indicates severe alveolar hemorrhage; moderate positive indicates some hemorrhage; absent indicates no evidence of alveolar hemorrhage

DFA stain for *Legionella,* herpes simplex I and II (stains bronchial epithelial cells and macrophages), and cytomegalovirus (CMV) (stains mononuclear cells) may indicate infection with corresponding organism

Pap stain: atypical cytology: may be due to cytotoxic drugs, radiation therapy, viral infection (intranuclear inclusions of herpes or CMV), tumor

Oil red O stain shows many large intracellular fat droplets in one-third to one-half of cells in some patients with fat embolism due to bone fractures but in <3% of patients without embolism.

PLEURAL FLUID

Normal Values

Specific gravity	1.010–1.026
Total protein	
Albumin	0.3–4.1 gm/dl
Globulin	50–70%
Fibrinogen	30–45%
pH	6.8–7.6

*Data from FW Kahn and JM Jones, Bronchoalveolar lavage in the rapid diagnosis of lung disease. *Laboratory Management,* June 1986, p. 31.

Table 7-1. Pleural Fluid Findings in Various Diseases

Disease	Appearance	Total WBC (1000/cu mm)	Predominant Type WBC	Total RBC (1000/cu mm)	pH	Glucose	
						mg/dl	PF/S
Transudates							
Congestive heart failure	Clear, straw	<1	M	0–1	>7.4	>60	1
Cirrhosis	Clear, straw	<0.5	M	<1	>7.4	>60	1
Pulmonary embolus: atelectasis	Clear, straw	5–15	M	<5	>7.3	>60	1
Exudates							
Pulmonary embolus: infarction	Turbid to hemorrhagic	5–15	P	Bloody	>7.3	>60	1
Pneumonia	Turbid	5–40	P	<5	≧7.3	>60	1

Empyema	Turbid to purulent	25–100	P	<5	5.50–7.29	<60	<0.5
Tuberculosis	Straw; serosanguineous in 15%	5–10	M	<10	<7.3 in 20%	30–60 in 20%	1
Carcinoma	Straw to turbid to bloody	<10	M	1–>100	<7.3 in 30%	<60 in 30%	1
Rheumatoid arthritis effusion	Turbid or green or yellow	1–20	P in acute M in chronic	<1	<7.3; usually ≅ 7.0	<30 in 95%	
SLE	Straw to turbid		P in acute M in chronic		<7.3 in 30%	<60 in 30%	
Rupture of esophagus	Purulent		P		6.0	N or D	
Pancreatitis	Serous to turbid to serosanguineous	5–20	P	1–10	>7.3	>60	1

Table 7-1 (continued)

Disease	Protein PF/S	LDH PF/S	LDH IU/L	Amylase PF/S	Comment
Transudates					
Congestive heart failure	<0.5	<0.6	<200	≤1	
Cirrhosis	<0.5	<0.6	<200	≤1	Occurs in ≅ 5% of cirrhotics with clinical ascites.
Pulmonary embolus: atelectasis	<0.5	<0.6		≦1	
Exudates					
Pulmonary embolus: infarction	>0.5	>0.6		≦1	
Pneumonia	>0.5	>0.6		≦1	Occurs in 50% of bacterial pneumonias and Legionnaires' disease, 10% of viral and mycoplasma pneumonias.

Empyema	>0.5	>0.6	May be >1000/L	≦1	Most commonly due to anaerobic bacteria, *S. aureus*, gram-negative aerobic bacteria.
Tuberculosis	>0.5	>0.6		≦1	AFB stain + in 15–20% & culture of fluid + in 30% of cases. Biopsy for histologic exam & culture of pleura are diagnostic in 75–85% of cases.
Carcinoma	>0.5	>0.6		≦1	Cytology of fluid plus biopsy are diagnostic in about 90% of cases.
Rheumatoid arthritis effusion	>0.5	>0.6	Often >1000/L	≦1	Biopsy is useful, especially in men with rheumatoid nodules & high RF titer.
SLE	>0.5	>0.6		>2	PF may show LE cells, antinuclear antibody titer, and low complement. Usually found only when lupus is active.
Rupture of esophagus	>0.5	>0.6		Salivary type	
Pancreatitis	>0.5	>0.6		>2	Occurs in 15% of acute cases. Left-sided in 70% of cases.

PF/S = ratio of pleural fluid to serum; M = mononuclear cells; P = polynuclear leukocytes; N = normal; D = decreased.

SOME CAUSES OF PLEURAL EFFUSION

The underlying cause of an effusion is usually determined by first classifying the fluid as an exudate or a transudate. A transudate does not usually require additional testing, but exudates always do.

Transudate

Congestive heart failure (causes 15% of cases)
Cirrhosis with ascites (pleural effusion in ~5% of these cases)
Nephrotic syndrome
Pulmonary embolism (some cases)
Hypoalbuminemia
Early mediastinal malignancy
Myxedema (rare cause)
Early (acute) atelectasis
Superior vena cava obstruction
Peritoneal dialysis
Misplaced subclavian catheter

Exudate

- Infection (causes 25% of cases)
  - Parapneumonic effusion (empyema)
  - Viral, mycoplasmal, rickettsial
  - Tuberculous empyema
  - Parasitic (amoeba, hydatid cyst, filaria)
  - Fungal effusion (*Coccidioides, Cryptococcus, Histoplasma, Blastomyces, Aspergillus;* in immunocompromised host, *Aspergillus, Candida, Mucor*)
- Pulmonary embolism/infarction
- Neoplasms (metastatic carcinoma, especially breast, ovary, lung, lymphoma, leukemia, mesothelioma, pleural endometriosis) (causes 42% of cases)
- Meigs' syndrome (protein and specific gravity are often at transudate-exudate border but usually not transudate)
- Trauma (penetrating or blunt)
  - Hemothorax
  - Empyema
  - Chylothorax
  - Associated with rupture of diaphragm
- Immunologic mechanisms
  - Rheumatoid arthritis (5% of cases)
  - Systemic lupus erythematosus (SLE)
  - Other collagen vascular diseases occasionally cause effusions (e.g., Wegener's granulomatosis, Sjögren's syndrome, familial Mediterranean fever)
  - Following myocardial infarction or cardiac surgery
  - Vasculitis
  - Sarcoidosis (rare cause)
  - Hepatitis
  - Familial recurrent polyserositis
  - Drug reaction (e.g., nitrofurantoin hypersensitivity, methysergide)
- Chemical mechanisms
  - Uremic
  - Pancreatic (pleural effusion occurs in ~10% of these cases)
  - Subphrenic abscess
  - Esophageal rupture
- Lymphatic abnormality
  - Irradiation
  - Milroy's disease
  - Yellow nail syndrome (rare condition of generalized hypoplasia of lymphatic vessels)

Injury
  Asbestosis
Altered pleural mechanics
  Late (chronic) atelectasis
  Trapped lung
Unknown (~15% of all exudates)

Cirrhosis, pulmonary infarct, trauma, and connective tissue diseases compose ~9% of all cases.

Pleural fluid analysis results in definitive diagnosis in ~20% and a probable diagnosis in 50% of patients; may help to rule out a suspected diagnosis in 30%.

Location

Typically left-sided—ruptured esophagus, acute pancreatitis. Pericardial disease is left-sided or bilateral; rarely exclusively right-sided.

Typically right-sided or bilateral—congestive heart failure (if only on left, consider that right pleural space may be obliterated or patient has another process, e.g., pulmonary infarction)

Table 7-2. Comparison of "Typical"[a] Findings in Transudates and Exudates

Findings	Transudates	Exudates
Specific gravity[b]	<1.016	>1.016
Protein (gm/dl)[c]	<3.0	>3.0
Pleural fluid–serum ratio[d]	<0.5	>0.5
LDH[e]		
IU	<200	>200
Pleural fluid–serum ratio[d]	<0.6	>0.6
Ratio pleural fluid–upper limit normal serum[d]	<2/3	>2/3
Isoenzymes not useful for differentiating		
WBC count	<1000/cu mm Mainly lymphocytes	>1000/cu mm May be grossly purulent
RBCs	Few	Variable; few or may be grossly bloody
Glucose	Equivalent to serum	May be decreased because of bacteria or many WBCs
pH	Usually 7.4–7.5	Usually 7.35–7.45
Appearance	Clear	Usually cloudy
Color	Pale yellow	Variable

[a]"Typical" means 67–75% of patients.
[b]Long-standing transudates, however, can produce a high specific gravity.
[c]Protein level of 3.0 gm/dl misclassifies ~15% of effusions if it is the only criterion.
[d]Each one of these three criteria has been used to define pleural fluid exudate and transudate. *All* three constitute the best differential of exudate and transudate. Transudate meets none of these criteria, and exudates meet at least one criterion. Unequivocal criteria of transudate precludes the need for pleural biopsy in most cases unless two mechanisms are suspected (e.g., nephrotic syndrome with miliary tuberculosis, congestive heart failure with malignancy). It would be uncommon for use of diuretics in congestive heart failure to change characteristics of transudate to that of exudate.
[e]If nonhemolyzed, nonbloody effusion.

Gross Appearance

Clear, straw-colored fluid is typical of transudate.

Cloudy, opaque appearance indicates more cell components.

Blood fluid suggests malignancy, pulmonary infarct, trauma, postcardiotomy syndrome. Bloody fluid from traumatic thoracentesis should clot within several minutes, but blood present more than several hours has become defibrinated and does not form a good clot. Nonuniform color during aspiration and absence of hemosiderin-laden macrophages and some crenated RBCs also suggest traumatic aspiration.

Chylous (milky) is usually due to trauma (e.g., auto accident, postoperative) but may be obstruction of duct (e.g., lymphoma, metastatic carcinoma, granulomas). Pleural fluid triglyceride >110 mg/dl or triglyceride pleural fluid—serum ratio >2 occurs only in chylous effusion (seen especially within a few hours after eating). After centrifugation, supernatant is white due to chylomicrons, which also stain with Sudan III. Equivocal triglyceride levels (60–110 mg/dl) may require a lipoprotein electrophoresis of fluid. Triglyceride <30 mg/dl in nonchylous effusions.

White fluid suggests chylothorax, cholesterol effusion, or empyema.

Black fluid suggests *Aspergillus niger* infection.

Greenish fluid suggests biliopleural fistula.

Purulent fluid indicates infection.

Foul odor suggests anaerobic empyema.

Anchovy (dark red-brown) color is seen in amebiasis.

Turbid and greenish yellow fluid is classic for rheumatoid effusion.

Turbidity may be due to lipids or increased WBCs; after centrifugation, a clear supernatant indicates WBCs as cause; white supernatant is due to chylomicrons.

Very viscous (clear or bloody)—characteristic of mesothelioma

Debris in fluid suggests rheumatoid pleurisy; food particles indicate esophageal rupture.

Protein, Albumin, Lactic Dehydrogenase (LDH)

See Table 7-2.

Glucose

Same value as serum in transudate

Usually normal, but 30–55 mg/dl or pleural fluid–serum ratio <0.5 and pH <7.30 may be found in tuberculosis, malignancy, systemic lupus erythematosus (SLE); also esophageal rupture; lowest levels may occur in empyema and rheumatoid arthritis. Therefore, only helpful if very low level (e.g., <30). 0–10 mg/dl highly suspicious for rheumatoid arthritis.

pH

Low pH (<7.30) always means exudate, especially empyema, malignancy, rheumatoid pleurisy, SLE, tuberculosis, esophageal rupture. Esophageal rupture is only cause of pH close to 6.0; collagen vascular disease is only other cause of pH <7.0. pH <7.10 in parapneumonic effusion indicates need for tube drainage. In malignant effusion pH, pH <7.30 is associated with short survival time, poorer prognosis, and increased positive yield with cytology and pleural biopsy; tends to correlate with pleural fluid glucose <60 mg/dl.

Amylase

Increased in acute pancreatitis, perforated peptic ulcer, necrosis of small intestine (e.g., mesenteric vascular occlusion); sometimes in pancreatic pseudocyst; 10% of cases of metastatic cancer and esophageal rupture. Pleural fluid–serum ratio >1 strongly favors pancreatitis (normal ratio = 1); may be >5. Isoenzyme studies show pancreatic-type amylase in acute pancreatitis (often <10,000 Somogyi units/dl) and pancreatic pseudocyst (often >10,000 Somogyi units/dl); salivary-type amylase is found in esophageal rupture (often >10,000 Somogyi units/dl) and occasionally in carcinoma of ovary or lung or salivary gland tumor (often <10,000 Somogyi units/dl). Should be determined in undiagnosed left pleural effusions.

Other Chemical Determinations

Carcinoembryonic antigen (CEA), $beta_2$ microglobulin, etc., have been suggested for diagnosis of cancer, but value not established. Also acid phosphatase in prostatic cancer, hyaluronic acid in mesothelioma, etc.

Acid mucopolysaccharides (especially hyaluronic acid) may be increased (>120 μg/ml) in mesotheliomas.

Cholesterol <60 mg/dl is said to be found in transudates and >60 mg/dl in exudates.

Immune complexes (measured by Raji cell, C1q component of C, radioimmunoassay [RIA], etc.) are often found in exudates due to collagen vascular diseases (SLE, rheumatoid arthritis [RA]). RA latex agglutination tests show frequent false positives and should not be ordered.

Cell Count
(performed in counting chamber)

Total WBC count is almost never diagnostic.

- >10,000/cu mm indicates inflammation, most commonly with pneumonia, pulmonary infarct, pancreatitis, postcardiotomy syndrome.
- >50,000/cu mm is typical only in parapneumonic effusions, usually empyema.
- Malignancy and tuberculosis are usually <5,000/cu mm.
- Transudates are usually <1,000/cu mm.

5000–6000 RBCs/cu mm are needed to give red appearance to pleural fluid.

- Can be caused by needle trauma producing 2 ml of blood in 1000 ml of pleural fluid

>100,000 RBCs/cu mm is grossly hemorrhagic and suggests malignancy, pulmonary infarct, or trauma but occasionally seen in congestive heart failure alone.

Hemothorax (pleural fluid hematocrit ≥50% venous hematocrit) suggests trauma, bleeding from a vessel, bleeding disorder, or malignancy but may be seen in same conditions as above.

Smears

Wright's stain differentiates polymorphonuclear leukocytes (PMNs) from mononuclear cells; cannot differentiate lymphocytes from monocytes.

Mononuclear cells predominate in transudates and early effusions and chronic exudates (lymphoma, carcinoma, tuberculosis, rheumatoid, uremia). >50% is seen in two-thirds of cases due to cancer. >85–90% suggests tuberculosis, lymphoma, sarcoidosis, rheumatoid causes.

PMNs predominate in early inflammatory effusions (e.g., pneumonia, pulmonary infarct, pancreatitis, subphrenic abscess).

After several days, mesothelial cells, macrophages, lymphocytes may predominate.

Large mesothelial cells >5% are said to rule out tuberculosis (must differ from macrophages).

Eosinophilia in pleural fluid (>10% of total WBCs) is not diagnostically significant. May mean blood or air in pleural space (e.g., repeated thoracenteses, pneumothorax, traumatic hemothorax), infection. Also said to be associated with asbestosis, pulmonary infarction, polyarteritis nodosa, parasitic or fungal disease, drug-related (e.g., nitrofurantoin or dantrolene) and idiopathic effusion, but not unusual with malignant effusions and rules out tuberculosis. Not usually accompanied by striking blood eosinophilia. Many diseases associated with blood eosinophilia infrequently cause pleural effusion eosinophilia.

Occasionally LE cells make the diagnosis of SLE. Gram's stain for early diagnosis of bacterial infection. Occasionally countercurrent immunoelectrophoresis (CIE) or latex agglutination for bacterial antigens is useful. Gas-liquid chromatography has been reported to show butyric, isobutyric, propionic, and isovaleric acids in anaerobic acute bacterial infection and increased lactic and acetic acid levels in aerobic infections.

Acid-fast smears are positive in 20% of tuberculous pleurisy.

Cytology

Positive in 60% of malignancies on first tap, 80% by third tap. Therefore should repeat taps with cytologic examinations if cancer is suspected. Is more sensitive than needle biopsy. Combining with needle biopsy increases sensitivity by <10%.* (See also Bronchogenic Carcinoma, p. 146.) High yield with adenocarcinoma, low yield with Hodgkin's disease.

Assay for DNA aneuploidy and staining with monoclonal antibodies (e.g., CEA, cytokeratin) to distinguish malignant mesothelioma, metastatic tumor, and reactive mesothelial cells can be performed. (*Some malignant cells may be diploid.*)

PLEURAL FLUID FINDINGS IN VARIOUS CLINICAL CONDITIONS

Tuberculous effusion: Has high protein content and lymphocytes; acid-fast smears are positive in <20%, and culture is positive in ~67% of cases; culture combined with histologic examination establishes the diagnosis in 95% of cases. Needle biopsy can be done without hesitation. Tuberculosis often presents as effusion, especially in youth; pulmonary disease may be absent; risk of active pulmonary tuberculosis within 5 years is 60%. Large mesothelial cells >5% are said to rule out tuberculosis (must differ from macrophages).

Malignancy: Can cause effusion by metastasis to pleura, causing exudate type of fluid, or by metastasis to lymph nodes obstructing lymph drainage, giving transudate-type fluid. Low pH and glucose indicate a poor prognosis with short survival time. "Characteristic" effusion is moderate to massive, frequently hemorrhagic, moderate WBC count with predominance of mononuclear cells; however only half of malignant effusions have RBC >10,000/cu mm. Lung and breast cancer and lymphoma cause 75% of malignant effusions; in 6%, no primary tumor is found. Combined cytology and pleural biopsy give positive results in 90%. Pleural or ascitic effusion occurs in 20–30% of patients with malignant lymphoma; cytology establishes the diagnosis in approximately 50% of patients. In rare instances of suspected lymphoma with negative conventional test results, flow cytometric analysis of pleural fluid showing a monoclonal lymphocyte population can establish the diagnosis. Mucopolysaccharide level may be increased (normal <17 mg/dl) in mesothelioma.

Rheumatoid effusion: "Classic picture" is cloudy greenish fluid with 0 glucose level. Is <30 mg/dl in 25% of patients.

Rheumatoid arthritis cells may be found. Rheumatoid factor may also be found in other effusions (e.g., tuberculosis, cancer, bacterial pneumonia). Needle biopsy usually shows nonspecific chronic inflammation but may show characteristic rheumatoid nodule microscopically. *Nonpurulent, nonmalignant effusions not due to tuberculosis or rheumatoid arthritis almost always have glucose level >70 mg/dl.*

Pulmonary infarct effusion: Small volume, serous or bloody, predominance of PMNs, may show many mesothelial cells; this "typical pattern" is seen in

*Data from UBS Prakesh and HM Reiman, Comparison of needle biopsy with cytologic analysis for the evaluation of pleural effusion: Analysis of 414 cases. *Proc Mayo Clin* 60:158, 1985.

Table 7-3. Comparison of Pleural Fluid in Rheumatoid Arthritis and SLE

Test	Rheumatoid Arthritis	SLE
pH	≤7.2	>7.2
Glucose	<30 mg/dl	Normal
LDH	>700 IU/L	<700 IU/L
Rheumatoid factor (RF)	Strongly +	– or weakly +
Ratio pleural fluid–serum RF	>1.0	<1.0
Lupus cells	Absent	May be present
Rheumatoid arthritis cells (ragocytes)	May be present	Absent
Epithelioid cells	Present	Absent
C4	Markedly decreased (<10 × 10^5 gm/gm of protein)	Moderately decreased (<30 × 10^6 gm/gm of protein)
C1q-binding assay	Moderately +	Weakly +
Ratio pleural fluid–serum	>1.0	<1.0

only 25% of patients. Effusion occurs in 50% of patients with pulmonary infarct; is bloody in one-third to two-thirds of patients; often no characteristic diagnostic findings occur.

Congestive heart failure: Effusion is predominantly right-sided or bilateral. If unilateral or left-sided in patients with congestive heart failure, rule out pulmonary infarct.

Pneumonias: Parapneumonic effusion is exudate type of effusion occurring in course of pneumonia.

Empyema: Usually WBCs >50,000/cu mm, low glucose, and low pH.

Suspect clinically when effusion develops during adequate antibiotic therapy.

Aerobic gram-negative organisms (*Klebsiella, Escherichia coli, Pseudomonas*) are associated with a high incidence of exudates (with 5000–40,000/cu mm, high protein, normal glucose, normal pH) and resolve with antibiotic therapy. Nonpurulent fluid with positive Gram's stain or positive blood culture or low pH suggests that effusion will become or behave like empyema.

Streptococcus pneumoniae causes parapneumonic effusions in 50% of cases, especially with positive blood culture.

Staphylococcus aureus has effusion in 90% of infants, 50% of adults; usually widespread bronchopneumonia.

Streptococcus pyogenes usually has massive effusion, greenish color.

If pleural effusion occurs early in course of bacterial pneumonia, suspect Streptococcus *or* Staphylococcus, *since it takes 4–5 days to develop effusion in pneumococcus pneumonia.*

In parapneumonic effusions, pH < 7.0 and glucose < 40 mg/dl indicate need for closed chest tube drainage even without grossly purulent fluid. pH of 7.0–7.2 is questionable indication and should be repeated in 24 hours, but tube drainage is favored if pleural fluid LDH >1000 IU/L. Tube drainage is also indicated if there is grossly purulent fluid or positive Gram's stain or culture. Normal pH is alkaline and may approach 7.6. In *Proteus mirabilis* empyema, high ammonia level may cause a pH ~8.0.

Viral or mycoplasma pneumonia: Pleural effusions develop in 20% of cases.

Legionnaires' disease: Pleural effusion occurs in up to 50% of patients; may be bilateral.

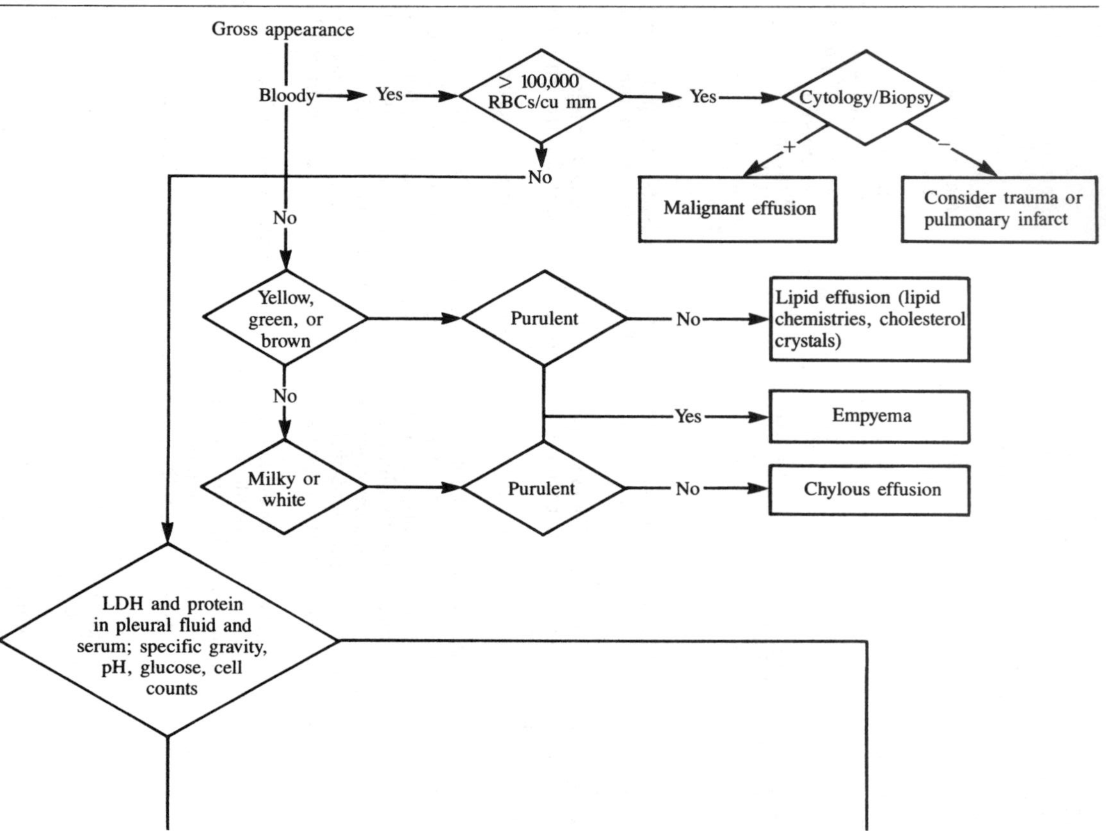

Gross appearance
Bloody
Yes
> 100,000 RBCs/cu mm
Yes
Cytology/Biopsy
+
−
Malignant effusion
Consider trauma or pulmonary infarct
No
No
Yellow, green, or brown
Purulent
No
Lipid effusion (lipid chemistries, cholesterol crystals)
Yes
Empyema
No
Milky or white
Purulent
No
Chylous effusion
LDH and protein in pleural fluid and serum; specific gravity, pH, glucose, cell counts

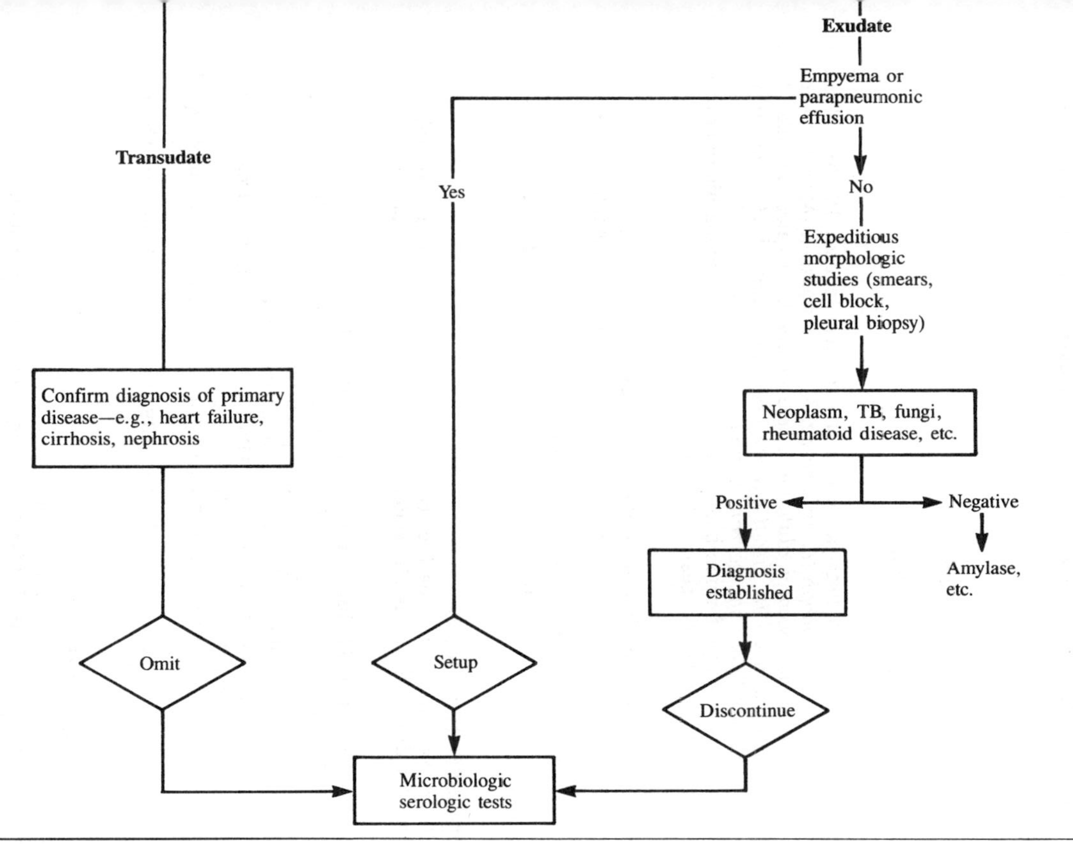

Fig. 7-1. Flow chart for pleural effusion.

Blood specimens should always be drawn at the same time as serous fluid for determination of glucose, protein, LDH, amylase, pH, etc. Pleural fluid for pH should be collected in the same way as arterial blood samples (i.e., heparinized syringe, maintained anaerobically on ice, analyzed promptly). Pleural fluid pH should normally be at least 0.15 greater than arterial blood pH.

Respiratory Diseases

ACUTE NASOPHARYNGITIS

Due To

Bacteria (e.g., Group A beta-hemolytic streptococci [causes 10–30% of cases seen by doctors], *Hemophilus influenzae, M. pneumoniae*). (*Mere presence of staphylococci, pneumococci, alpha- and beta-hemolytic streptococci [other than groups A, C, and G] in throat culture does not establish them as cause of pharyngitis and does not warrant antibiotic treatment.*)

Virus, fungus, allergy, foreign body, trauma, neoplasm, idiopathic (no cause is identified in ~50% of cases)

Microscopic Examination of Stained Nasal Smear

Large numbers of eosinophils suggest allergy. Does not correlate with blood eosinophilia.

Large numbers of neutrophils suggest infection.

Eosinophils and neutrophils suggest chronic allergy with superimposed infection.

DISEASES OF LARYNX

Cultures and smears for specific organisms (e.g., tubercle bacilli, fungi)

Biopsy for diagnosis of visible lesions (e.g., leukoplakia, carcinoma)

CROUP (EPIGLOTTITIS, LARYNGOTRACHEITIS)

Group B *H. influenzae* causes >90% of cases of epiglottitis; other bacteria include beta-hemolytic streptococci and pneumococci.

Cultures, smears, and tests for specific causative agents

Blood cultures should be taken at the same time as throat cultures.

Neutrophilic leukocytosis is present.

Clinical picture in infectious mononucleosis or diphtheria may resemble epiglottitis.

Laryngotracheitis is usually viral (especially parainfluenza) but rarely bacterial in origin.

CHRONIC BRONCHITIS

WBC and ESR normal or increased

Eosinophil count increased if there is allergic basis or component

Sputum bacterial smears and cultures (most common pathogens: pneumococcus, *H. influenzae;* occasionally *S. aureus* or gram-negative rods)

Smears and cultures of bronchoscopic secretions

Laboratory findings due to associated or coexisting diseases (e.g., emphysema, bronchiectasis)

ACUTE BRONCHITIS (ASTHMATIC BRONCHITIS)

WBC and ESR may be increased.

BRONCHIAL ASTHMA

Sputum is white and mucoid without blood or pus (unless infection is present).

Eosinophils, crystals (Curschmann's spirals), and mucus casts of bronchioles may be found.

Eosinophilia may be present.

Blood CO_2 may be decreased in early stages and may be increased in later stages.

With severe respiratory distress, rapid deterioration of patient's condition may be associated with precipitous fall in arterial PO_2 and rise in PCO_2.

When patient requires hospitalization, arterial blood gases should be measured frequently to assess his status.

Laboratory findings due to underlying diseases that may be primary and that should be ruled out, especially polyarteritis nodosa, parasitic infestation, bronchial carcinoid, drug reaction (especially aspirin), poisoning (especially cholinergic drugs and pesticides), hypogammaglobulinemia.

BRONCHIECTASIS

WBC usually normal unless pneumonitis is present

Mild to moderate normocytic normochromic anemia with chronic severe infection

Sputum abundant and mucopurulent (often contains blood); sweetish smell

Sputum bacterial smears and cultures

Laboratory findings due to complications (pneumonia, pulmonary hemorrhage, brain abscess, sepsis, cor pulmonale)

Rule out cystic fibrosis of the pancreas and hypogammaglobulinemia or agammaglobulinemia.

OBSTRUCTIVE PULMONARY EMPHYSEMA

Laboratory findings of underlying disease that may be primary (e.g., pneumoconiosis, tuberculosis, sarcoidosis, kyphoscoliosis, marked obesity, fibrocystic disease of pancreas, alpha_1 antitrypsin deficiency)

Laboratory findings of associated conditions, especially duodenal ulcer

Laboratory findings due to decreased lung ventilation

- Arterial blood oxygen decreased and CO_2 increased
- Ultimate development of respiratory acidosis
- Secondary polycythemia
- Cor pulmonale

ADULT RESPIRATORY DISTRESS SYNDROME (ARDS)

Arterial blood gases show profound hypoxemia ($PaO_2 < 50$ mm Hg on room air)

or

- $PaO_2 < 50$ mmHg on an FIO_2 (fractional inspired O_2 concentration) of >40% and positive end-expiratory pressure (PEEP) of >5 cm H_2O
- New bilateral and changing chest x-ray infiltrates

plus

- Pulmonary capillary wedge pressure < 15–19 mm Hg

plus

- Static pulmonary compliance < 50 ml/cm H_2O that markedly reduces vital capacity, total lung capacity, functional residual capacity

plus

- No other explanation for the above findings

plus

- Presence of a preceding or associated event (e.g., sepsis [most common], aspiration, infection, pneumonia, pancreatitis, shock, fat emboli, trauma, disseminated intravascular coagulation [DIC]; more than one cause is often present). Infection due to gram-negative is more likely than due to gram-positive organisms. Occurs in 23% of cases of gram-negative bacteremia.

PNEUMONIA

Due To

Bacteria—pneumococcus, staphylococcus, *K. pneumoniae, H. influenzae,* streptococcus, enterobacteria, tularemia, plague, tubercle bacilli

Diplococcus pneumoniae causes 60–70% of bacterial pneumonia in patients requiring hospitalization. May cause ~25% of hospital-acquired cases of pneumonia. Blood culture positive in 25% of untreated cases during first 3–4 days.

Staphylococcus causes <1% of all acute bacterial pneumonia with onset outside the hospital but more frequent after outbreaks of influenza; may be secondary to measles, mucoviscidosis, prolonged antibiotic therapy, debilitating diseases (e.g., leukemia, collagen diseases). Bacteremia in <20% of patients.

H. influenzae is important in 6- to 24-month age group; rare in adults except for middle-aged men with chronic lung disease and/or alcoholism. Can mimic pneumococcal pneumonia; may be isolated with *S. pneumoniae.*

Gram-negative bacilli (e.g., *K. pneumoniae,* enterobacteria, *E. coli, P. mirabilis, P. aeruginosa*) are common causes of hospital-acquired pneumonia but unlikely outside the hospital. *K. pneumoniae* causes 1% of primary bacterial pneumonias, especially in alcoholics and upper lobe pneumonia; tenacious red-brown sputum is typical.

Legionella pneumophila

Anaerobic lung abscess—marked increase in sputum that is foul smelling. Gram's stain is diagnostic—sheets of PMNs with a bewildering variety of organisms.

Mycoplasma pneumoniae—is most common in young adult male population (e.g., armed forces camps).

Viruses—influenza, parainfluenza, adenoviruses, respiratory syncytial virus, echovirus, Coxsackievirus, reovirus, cytomegalic inclusion virus, viruses of exanthems, herpes simplex

Rickettsiae—Q fever is most common in endemic areas; typhus fungi—*Histoplasma* and *Coccidioides* in particular; protozoans—*Toxoplasma, P. carinii*

Laboratory Findings

WBC is frequently normal or slightly increased in nonbacterial pneumonias; considerable increase in WBC is more common in bacterial pneumonia. *In severe bacterial pneumonia, WBC may be very high or low or normal. Since individual variation is considerable, there is limited value in distinguishing bacterial and nonbacterial pneumonia.*

In the urine, protein, WBCs, hyaline and granular casts in small amounts are common. Ketones may occur with severe infection. *Check for glucose to rule out underlying diabetes mellitus.*

Sputum reveals abundant WBCs in bacterial pneumonias. Gram's stain shows abundant organisms in bacterial pneumonias (e.g., pneumococcus, staphylococcus). Culture sputum for appropriate bacteria.

In all cases of pneumonia, blood and sputum cultures and smear for Gram's stain should be performed before antibiotic therapy is started. Optimum specimen of sputum shows >25 PMNs and <10 squamous epithelial cells/lpf (10 times normal), but >10 PMNs and <25 epithelial cells may be considered acceptable sputum specimen. >25 epithelial cells indicate unsatisfactory specimen from oropharynx and should not be submitted for culture.

Nasopharyngeal aspirate may identify *S. pneumoniae* with few false positives but *S. aureus* and gram-negative bacilli often represent false positive findings.

In *H. influenzae* pneumonia, sputum culture is negative in >50% of patients with positive cultures from blood, pleural fluid, or lung tissue and may be present in the sputum in the absence of disease.

Sputum that contains many organisms and WBCs on smear but no pathogens on aerobic culture may indicate aspiration pneumonia.

Sputum is not appropriate for anaerobic culture.

Transtracheal aspiration (puncture of cricothyroid membrane) generally yields a faster, more accurate diagnosis.

Testing urine for capsular antigen from *S. pneumoniae* or type B. *H. influenzae* by CIE or latex agglutination may be helpful. Latex agglutination is positive in ~90% of bacteremic pneumococcal and 40% of nonbacteremic pneumonias. Is particularly useful when antibiotic therapy has already begun.

Acute-phase serum should be stored at onset. If etiologic diagnosis is not established, a convalescent-phase serum should be taken. A 4-fold increase in antibody titer establishes the etiologic diagnosis (e.g., *Legionella pneumophila, Chlamydia* species, respiratory viruses [including influenza and respiratory syncytial virus (RSV)], *M. pneumoniae*). Serologic tests to determine whether pneumonia is due to *Histoplasma, Coccidioides,* etc.

Pleural effusions that are aspirated should also have Gram's stain and culture performed.

Respiratory pathogens isolated from blood, pleural fluid, or transtracheal aspirate (except patients with chronic bronchitis) or identified by bacterial polysaccharide antigen in urine may be considered the definite etiologic agent.

Diagnostic lung puncture to determine specific causative agent as a guide to antibiotic therapy may be indicated in critically ill children.

LEGIONNAIRES' DISEASE (*LEGIONELLA PNEUMOPHILA*)

Gram's stain of sputum shows few to moderate number of PMNs; bacteria are not seen because the gram-negative *Legionella* stains poorly in clinical specimens.

Direct immunofluorescent microscopy or DNA probe on sputum, pleural fluid, lung, or other tissue is extremely useful for rapid specific diagnosis (sensitivity ~70%; specificity >99%); may be negative with few organisms present, especially after erythromycin therapy.

Special culture technique of normally sterile material (pleural fluid, lung, transtracheal aspirate of lower respiratory secretions) may show growth in 2–3 days.

Urine antigen assay can detect infection. Kits will probably become available.

Antibody titers (by indirect fluorescent, ELISA, or agglutination) show 4-fold increase to 1:128 in two-thirds of patients in 3 weeks and all patients in 6 weeks or single titer of 1:256; most useful for retrospective diagnosis or epidemiologic study.

Increased WBC is typical; leukopenia is a bad prognostic sign.

Mild to moderate increase of serum glutamic-oxaloacetic transaminase (SGOT), alkaline phosphatase, LDH, or bilirubin in serum is found in ~50% of patients.

Hypoalbuminemia <2.5 gm/dl

Decreased serum phosphorus and sodium occur in ~50% of patients.

Proteinuria occurs in ~50% of patients; microscopic hematuria.

Renal failure and DIC are unusual complications.

Pleural effusions in up to 50% of patients may be bilateral; organism has been isolated from pleural fluid.

CSF is normal.

LIPID PNEUMONIA

Sputum shows fat-containing macrophages that stain with Sudan.

They may be present only intermittently; therefore, examine sputum more than once.

DIFFUSE INTERSTITIAL PNEUMONITIS

Serum LDH is increased.

LUNG ABSCESS

Sputum—abundant, foul, purulent; may be bloody; contains elastic fibers
- Bacterial cultures (including tubercle bacilli)—anaerobic as well as aerobic; rule out amebas, parasites
- Cytologic examination for malignant cells

Blood culture—may be positive in acute stage
Increased WBC in acute stages (15,000–30,000/cu mm)
Increased ESR
Normochromic normocytic anemia in chronic stage
Albuminuria is frequent
Findings of underlying disease—especially bronchogenic carcinoma; also drug addiction, postabortion state, coccidioidomycosis, amebic abscess, tuberculosis, alcoholism

BRONCHOGENIC CARCINOMA

Cytologic examination of sputum for malignant cells—positive in 40% of patients on first sample, 70% with three samples, 85% with five samples. False positive tests are <1%.

Sputum cytology gives highest positive yield with squamous cell carcinoma (67–85%), intermediate with small-cell undifferentiated carcinoma (64–70%), lowest with adenocarcinoma (55%).

Biopsy of scalene lymph nodes for metastases to indicate inoperable status—positive in 15% of patients

Findings of complicating conditions (e.g., pneumonitis, atelectasis, lung abscess)

Findings due to metastases (e.g., Addison's disease, diabetes insipidus, liver metastases with functional hepatic changes; malignant cells in pleural fluid

Findings due to secretion of active hormone substances (e.g., Cushing's syndrome, hypercalcemia, serotonin production by carcinoid of bronchus)

Biopsy of bronchus, pleura, lung, metastatic sites in appropriate cases

Transthoracic needle aspiration provides definitive cytologic diagnosis of cancer in 80–90% of cases; useful when other methods (e.g., sputum cytology, bronchoscopy) fail to provide a microscopic diagnosis.

Cancer cells in bone marrow and rarely in peripheral blood

Hypercalcemia occurs in <5% of all types of lung cancer and correlates with large tumor mass that is often incurable and quickly fatal (see Humoral Hypercalcemia of Malignancy, pp. 471, 475).

Biochemical tumor markers (see pp. 706–707)
- Serum CEA is increased in one-third to two-thirds of patients with all four types of lung cancer. Principal uses are for monitoring response to therapy and to correlate with staging. Levels <5 ng/ml correlate with survival over 3 years compared to level >5 ng/ml. Levels >10 ng/ml correlate with higher incidence of extensive disease and extrathoracic metastases. A fall to normal suggests complete tumor removal. A fall to a still elevated level may indicate residual tumor. An elevated unchanged level suggests residual progressive disease. A level that falls and then rises during chemotherapy suggests that resistance to drugs has occurred.
- Serum neuron-specific enolase (NSE) may be increased in some patients with small-cell cancer. May be used to monitor disease progression and response to therapy but not useful for screening.

PULMONARY ALVEOLAR PROTEINOSIS

Serum LDH increases when protein accumulates in lungs and drops to normal when infiltrate resolves.
Periodic acid–Schiff (PAS)–positive material appears in sputum.
Phenolsulfonphthalein (PSP) dye injected intravenously is excreted in sputum for long periods of time.
Biopsy of lung for histologic examination is in order.

PNEUMOCONIOSIS

Biopsy of lung, scalene lymph node—histologic, chemical, spectrographic, and x-ray diffraction studies (e.g., silicosis, berylliosis; also metastatic tumor, sarcoidosis, tuberculosis, fungus infection)
Increased WBC if associated infection
Secondary polycythemia or anemia
Bacterial smears and cultures of sputum (especially for tubercle bacilli)
Cytologic examination of sputum and bronchoscopic secretions for malignant cells, especially squamous cell carcinoma of bronchus and mesothelioma of pleura
Asbestos bodies sometimes in sputum after exposure to asbestos dust even without clinical disease
Acute beryllium disease may show occasional transient hypergammaglobulinemia
Chronic beryllium disease
- Secondary polycythemia
- Increased serum gamma globulin
- Increased urine calcium
- Increased beryllium in urine long after beryllium exposure has ended

GOODPASTURE'S SYNDROME

(malignant hypertension associated with pulmonary hemorrhages)

Eosinophilia absent and iron deficiency anemia more marked than in idiopathic pulmonary hemosiderosis
Proteinuria and RBCs and RBC casts in urine
Renal function may deteriorate rapidly
Renal biopsy may show characteristic linear immunofluorescent deposits and focal or diffuse proliferative glomerulonephritis
Serum may show antiglomerular basement membrane antibodies by enzyme immunoassay (EIA); may be found in cases without pulmonary hemorrhage.
Other causes of combined pulmonary hemorrhage and glomerulonephritis are
- Wegener's granulomatosis
- Hypersensitivity vasculitis
- SLE
- Polyarteritis nodosa
- Endocarditis
- Mixed cryoglobulinemia
- Allergic angiitis and granulomatosis (Churg-Strauss syndrome)
- Schönlein-Henoch purpura

HISTIOCYTOSIS X

(see also p. 442)

Pulmonary disorder is the major manifestation of this disease; bone involvement in minority of cases with lung disease.
Bronchoalveolar lavage shows increase in total number of cells; 2–20% are Langerhans' cells, small numbers of eosinophils, neutrophils, and lymphocytes, and 70% macrophages.
Most adults do not have positive ^{67}Ga scans.
Mild decrease in PO_2, which falls with exercise

PULMONARY EMBOLISM AND INFARCTION

No single laboratory test is diagnostic.

Arterial blood gases (obtained when patient is breathing room air) is the most sensitive and specific laboratory test.

PO_2 < 80 mm Hg in 88% of cases, but normal PaO_2 does not rule out pulmonary embolus. In appropriate clinical setting, PO_2 < 88 mm Hg (even with a normal chest x-ray) is indication for lung scans and search for deep vein thromboses. PO_2 > 90 mm Hg with a normal chest x-ray suggests a different diagnosis. Normal complete lung scans exclude the diagnosis.

Hypocapnia and slightly elevated pH

Increased WBC in 50% of patients is rarely >15,000/cu mm (whereas in acute bacterial pneumonia is often >20,000/cu mm)

Increased ESR

"Triad" of increased LDH and bilirubin with normal SGOT is found in only 15% of cases.

Increased serum LDH (due to isoenzymes 2 and 3) in 80% of patients rises on first day, peaks on second, normal by tenth day.

Serum SGOT is usually normal or only slightly increased. Serum enzymes differ from acute myocardial infarction.

Serum bilirubin is increased (as early as fourth day) to ~5 mg/dl in 20% of cases.

Fibrin degradation products and soluble fibrin complexes are higher in blood of patients with thromboembolism.

Measurements of CK, LDH, and fibrin products are not indicated as they do not have sufficient sensitivity or specificity to be of diagnostic value.

Pleural effusion occurs in one-half of patients; bloody in one-third to two-thirds of cases; typical pattern in only one-fourth of cases.

These laboratory findings depend on the size and duration of the infarction, and the tests must be performed at the appropriate time to detect abnormalities.

RHEUMATOID PLEURISY WITH EFFUSION

Decreased glucose level (<30 mg/dl in 25% of patients) is the most useful finding clinically. Nonpurulent nonmalignant effusions other than those due to tuberculosis or rheumatoid arthritis almost always have glucose levels >60 mg/dl.

Exudate is frequently turbid and may be milky.

Smears and cultures for bacteria, tubercle bacilli, and fungi are negative.

Cytologic examination for malignant cells is negative. Rheumatoid arthritis cells may be found.

Protein level is >3 gm/dl.

Increased LDH (usually higher than in serum) is commonly found in other chronic pleural effusions and is not useful in differential diagnosis.

Rheumatoid factor may be present but may also be found in other types of pleural effusion (e.g., with carcinoma, tuberculosis, bacterial pneumonia).

Needle biopsy of pleura usually shows nonspecific chronic inflammation, but characteristic changes of rheumatoid pleuritis may be found histologically.

Other laboratory findings of rheumatoid arthritis are found (see pp. 250–251).

DIAPHRAGMATIC HERNIA

Microcytic anemia (due to blood loss) may be present.

Stool may be positive for blood.

Gastrointestinal Diseases

Laboratory Tests of Gastrointestinal Function

GASTRIC ANALYSIS

1-hour basal acid

<2 mEq	Normal, gastric ulcer, or carcinoma
2–5 mEq	Normal, gastric or duodenal ulcer
>5 mEq	Duodenal ulcer
>20 mEq	Zollinger-Ellison (Z-E) syndrome

1 hour after stimulation (histamine or betazole hydrochloride)

0 mEq	Achlorhydria, gastritis, gastric carcinoma
1–20 mEq	Normal, gastric ulcer or carcinoma
20–35 mEq	Duodenal ulcer
35–60 mEq	Duodenal ulcer, high normal Z-E syndrome
>60 mEq	Z-E syndrome

Ratio of basal acid to post-stimulation outputs

20%	Normal, gastric ulcer, or carcinoma
20–40%	Gastric or duodenal ulcer
40–60%	Duodenal ulcer, Z-E syndrome
>60%	Z-E syndrome

Achlorhydria*

Occurs in normal persons: 4% of children, increasing to 30% of adults over age 60.

Chronic atrophic gastritis (serum gastrin is frequently increased)

Pernicious anemia	100% of patients
Vertiligo	20–25%
Alopecia areata	6%
Rheumatoid arthritis	10–20%
Thyrotoxicosis	10%

Gastric carcinoma (50% of patients) even following histamine or betazole stimulation. Hypochlorhydria occurs in 25% of patients with gastric carcinoma; hydrochloric acid is normal in 25% of patients with gastric carcinoma; hyperchlorhydria is rare in gastric carcinoma.

Gastric ulcer	Common
Adenomatous polyps of stomach	85% of patients
Menetrier's disease	75%
Chronic renal failure	13% (usually normal; occasionally increased)
Iatrogenic	
Postvagotomy, postantrectomy	>90%

(Measure acid output after IV insulin to demonstrate adequacy of vagotomy [see Insulin Test Meal, p. 151].)

*Data from MM Wolfe and AH Soll, The physiology of gastric acid secretion. *N Engl J Med* 319:1707, 1988.

Medical (e.g., potent H_2-receptor antagonists, substituted benzimidazoles)	>80%

True achlorhydria excludes duodenal ulcer.

Hyperchlorhydria and Hypersecretion*

Duodenal ulcer	40–45%
Z-E syndrome (see pp. 492–493)	100%

12-hour night secretion shows acid of >100 mEq/L and volume >1500 ml. Basal secretion is >60% of secretion caused by histamine or betazole stimulation.

Hyperplasia/hyperfunction of antral gastrin cells	>90%

(Unusual condition with marked hyperchlorhydria, severe peptic ulceration, moderately increased fasting serum gastrin with exaggerated postprandial increase [>200% above fasting levels], no gastrin-secreting tumors])

Hypertrophic hypersecretory gastropathy	100%
Massive resection of small intestine (transient)	50%
Systemic mastocytosis	Rare

When basal serum gastrin level is equivocal, serum gastrin level should be measured following stimulation with infusion of secretin or calcium.

Serum Gastrin
Normal levels: 0 to ≤200 pg gastrin/ml serum
Elevated levels: >500 pg/ml

Condition	**Serum Gastrin**	**Serum Gastrin After Intragastric Administration of 0.1N HCl**
Peptic ulcer without Z-E syndrome	Normal range	—
Z-E syndrome	Very high	No change
Pernicious anemia	High level may approach that in Z-E syndrome	Marked decrease

Secretin infusion† (IV of 2 units/kg body weight) with blood specimens drawn before and at intervals. Normal patients and patients with duodenal ulcer show no increase in serum gastrin. Patients with Z-E syndrome show increased serum gastrin that usually peaks in 45–60 minutes. With fasting gastrin <1000 pg/ml, sensitivity = 85% for an increased serum gastrin >200 pg/ml. Secretin test is the preferred first test because of greater sensitivity and simplicity.
Calcium infusion (IV calcium gluconate, 5 mg/kg body weight/hour for 3 hours) with preinfusion blood specimen compared to specimens every 30 minutes for

*Data from MM Wolfe and AH Soll, The physiology of gastric acid secretion. *N Engl J Med* 319:1707, 1988.

†Data from H Frucht et al., Secretin and calcium provocative tests in the Zollinger-Ellison syndrome. *Ann Intern Med* 111:713, 1989.

up to 4 hours. Normal patients show minimal serum gastrin response to calcium. Patients with Z-E syndrome show excessive increase in serum gastrin in 2–3 hours (sensitivity = 43% for an increase of 395 pg/ml in serum gastrin). Positive in one-third of patients with a negative secretin test. Recommended when secretin test is negative in patients suspicious for Z-E syndrome.

Indications for measurement of serum gastrin and gastric analysis include:

- Atypical peptic ulcer of stomach, duodenum, or proximal jejunum, especially if multiple, unusual location, poorly responsive to therapy, or multiple, rapid, or severe recurrence after adequate therapy
- Unexplained chronic diarrhea with or without peptic ulcer
- Peptic ulcer disease with associated endocrine conditions (see Multiple Endocrine Neoplasia, pp. 553–554).

Serum gastrin levels are indicated with any of the following:

- Basal acid secretion >10 mEq/hour in patients with intact stomachs
- Ratio of basal to post-stimulation output >40% in patients with intact stomachs
- All patients with recurrent ulceration after surgery for duodenal ulcer
- All patients with duodenal ulcer for whom elective gastric surgery is planned
- Measurement for screening of all peptic ulcer patients would not be practical or cost-effective.

Increased Serum Gastrin Without Gastric Acid Hypersecretion

Atrophic gastritis, especially when associated with circulating parietal cell antibodies

Pernicious anemia in ~75% of patients

Some patients have carcinoma of body of stomach, a reflection of the atrophic gastritis that is present.

Chronic renal failure with serum creatinine >3 mg/dl; occurs in 50% of patients

Increased Serum Gastrin with Gastric Acid Hypersecretion

Z-E syndrome

Hyperplasia of antral gastrin cells

Isolated retained antrum—a condition of gastric acid hypersecretion and recurrent ulceration following antrectomy and gastrojejunostomy that occurs when the duodenal stump contains antral mucosa

Pyloric obstruction with gastric distention

Short-bowel syndrome due to massive resection or extensive regional enteritis

INSULIN TEST MEAL

Aspirate gastric fluid every 15 minutes for 2 hours after IV administration of sufficient insulin (usually 15–20 units) to produce blood sugar of <50 mg/dl.

Normal: Hypoglycemia increases free HCl.

Successful vagotomy produces achlorhydria.

CHOLECYSTOKININ-SECRETIN TEST

The test measures the effect of IV administration of cholecystokinin and secretin on volume, bicarbonate concentration, and amylase output of duodenal contents and increase in serum lipase and amylase.

This is the most sensitive and reliable test ("gold standard") for chronic pancreatitis, especially in the early stages. It is technically difficult and is often not performed accurately; gastric contamination must be avoided. Normally serum lipase and amylase do not rise above normal limits.

Normal duodenal contents

- Volume: 95–235 ml/hour
- Bicarbonate concentration: 74–121 mEq/L
- Amylase output: 87,000–267,000 mg

BENTIROMIDE

Bentiromide (Chymex), 500 mg taken orally after overnight fast, is acted upon by pancreatic chymotrypsin, releasing PABA, which is readily absorbed and then excreted where it can be measured in a 6-hour urine sample (normal value is >50%) and (in some procedures) a 1- to 2-hour serum sample that gauges pancreatic exocrine activity if there is normal kidney function, gastric emptying, and gut function. Is a useful initial test to rule out pancreatic disease in patients with chronic diarrhea, weight loss, or steatorrhea. Can be used in conjunction with D-xylose tolerance test for differentiation of pancreatic exocrine insufficiency from intestinal mucosal disease. False negatives may occur due to drugs (e.g., thiazides, chloramphenicol, sulfonamides, acetaminophen, phenacetin, sunscreens, procaine anesthetics). Sensitivity of 6-hour test is 70–95% in severe chronic pancreatitis (with steatorrhea) and 40–50% in mild to moderate chronic pancreatitis (without steatorrhea).

D-XYLOSE TOLERANCE TEST

Give 25 gm of D-xylose in water orally. Collect a total 5-hour urine specimen (normal is >4 gm in 5 hours; <4 gm is consistent with malabsorption). May also measure 1- or 2-hour blood levels (normal is >25 mg/dl; <20 mg/dl is consistent with malabsorption). (Up to age 12 years, use 5-gm dose and 1-hour serum sample; urine collection is unreliable.) (Reference ranges may vary between laboratories.) The test reflects intestinal malabsorption. Chief value is in distinguishing proximal small intestinal malabsorption, which has decreased values, from pancreatic steatorrhea, which has normal values.

Decreased In

Steatorrhea due to proximal small-intestinal malabsorption (e.g., sprue, some patients with *Giardia lamblia* infestation, small-intestine bacterial overgrowth, viral gastroenteritis; may not be useful in adult celiac disease)
Elderly persons
Patients with decreased urinary excretion, although absorption is normal (e.g., renal insufficiency, myxedema, delayed gastric emptying, vomiting, dehydration). With mild renal insufficiency, use only serum test (normal > 20 mg/dl). Do not use with severe renal insufficiency.
Patients with ascites (urine values are low)

Normal In

Steatorrhea due to pancreatic disease
Cirrhosis of liver
Postgastrectomy state
Malnutrition

TRIOLEIN ^{131}I ABSORPTION TEST

The patient fasts overnight after taking 30 drops of Lugol's iodine solution on the previous day.
Administer 15–20 μc of triolein ^{131}I. Collect blood every 1–2 hours for the next 6–8 hours.
Collect stools for 48–72 hours until radioactivity disappears.
Normal: ≥10% of administered radioactivity appears in the blood within 6 hours; <5% appears in the feces.
The test is useful for screening patients with steatorrhea.
Normal values indicate that digestion of fat in the small bowel and absorption of fat in the small bowel are normal.
If results are abnormal, do an oleic acid ^{131}I absorption test.

OLEIC ACID ^{131}I ABSORPTION TEST

Methodology and normal values are the same as for the triolein absorption test.

An abnormal result indicates a defect in small-bowel mucosal absorption function (e.g., sprue, Whipple's disease, regional enteritis, tuberculous enteritis, collagen diseases involving the small bowel, extensive resection).

Abnormal pancreatic function does not affect the test.

POLYVINYLPYRROLIDONE (PVP-^{131}I)

Give 15–25 μc of PVP-^{131}I IV, and collect all stools for 4–5 days.

Normal: <2% is excreted in feces when the mucosa of the GI tract is intact. In protein-losing enteropathy, >2% of administered radioactivity appears in the stool.

^{51}Cr TEST FOR GASTROINTESTINAL BLEEDING

Tag 10 ml of the patient's blood with 200 μc of ^{51}Cr, and administer it IV. Collect daily stools for radioactivity measurement and also measure simultaneous blood samples.

Radioactivity in the stool establishes GI blood loss. Comparison with radioactivity measurements of 1 ml of blood indicates the amount of blood loss.

The test is useful in ulcerative diseases (e.g., ulcerative colitis, regional enteritis, peptic ulcer).

CAROTENE TOLERANCE TEST

Low values for serum carotene levels are usually associated with steatorrhea. Measure serum carotene following daily oral loading of carotene for 3–7 days.

Normal

Increase of serum carotene by >35 μg/dl indicates previously low dietary intake of carotene and/or fat.

Decreased In

Steatorrhea. Serum carotene increases >30 μg/dl. Patients with sprue in remission with normal fecal fat excretion may still show low carotene absorption.

Mineral oil interferes with carotene absorption. On a fat-free diet, only 10% is absorbed.

LABORATORY EXAMINATION OF STOOL

Normal Values

Bulk	100–200 gm
Water	Up to 75%
Total osmolality	200–250 mOsm
pH	7.0–7.5 (may be acid with high lactose intake)
Nitrogen	<2.5 gm/day
Coproporphyrin	400–1000 mg/24 hours
Trypsin	20–950 units/gm

Color

Brown: normal
Clay color (gray-white): biliary obstruction
Tarry: if >100 ml of blood in upper GI tract
Red: blood in large intestine or undigested beets or tomatoes
Black: blood or iron or bismuth medication
Various colors: depending on diet

OCCULT BLOOD IN STOOL*

Kits (e.g., Hemoccult cards) utilize guaiac; will detect blood losses of ~20 ml/day; "normal" amount of blood lost in stool daily is <2 ml/day or 2 mg of hemoglobin/gm of stool, but sensitivity is only 20% at this level and 90% at hemoglobin concentration >25 mg/gm of stool. ~50% of colon cancers shed enough blood to produce a positive test. Hemoccult will give 1–3% false positives even with strict protocol for stool collection.

Chief usefulness is for screening for asymptomatic ulcerated lesions of GI tract, especially carcinoma of the colon that is beyond the reach of routine sigmoidoscopy.

In various screening programs, 2–6% of participants have positive tests; of these, carcinoma is found in 5–10% and adenoma in 20–40%.

Adenomas <2 cm in size are less likely to bleed. Upper GI tract bleeding is less likely than lower GI tract bleeding to cause a positive test.

Long distance running is associated with positive guaiac test in up to 23% of runners.

Recommendations for testing:

- Test two areas from each of three consecutive stools to sample
- Test all samples within 4 days of collection
- Do not rehydrate slide prior to development
- For 3 days before test, avoid large doses of ascorbic acid, oral iron, aspirin, and other nonsteroidal anti-inflammatory drugs; red meat and certain fruits and vegetables that contain catalases and peroxidases (e.g., cucumbers, horseradish, cauliflower), especially if slides are rehydrated.
- Even one positive should be considered a positive test even without dietary restriction.

Other tests:

- Quantitative HemoQuant test kit (uses fluorescence to assay stool-derived porphyrins) doubles sensitivity of guaiac tests; may be affected by red meat and aspirin (for up to 4 days) but not by the other substances; manual test performed in a laboratory requiring 90 minutes; (normal <2 mg/gm; >4 mg/gm is increased; 2–4 mg/gm is borderline).
- Immunochemical tests (e.g., HemeSelect) specifically detect human hemoglobin, do not require diet or chemical restrictions (do not react with animal heme or foods), are stable for up to 30 days, detect ~0.3 mg Hb/gm of stool compared to 5–10 times this amount to cause a positive guaiac test.

Samples from *upper* GI tract should not be tested for blood using urine dipsticks or stool occult blood test kits (low pH may cause false negative and oral drugs false positive results).

QUALITATIVE SCREENING TEST FOR FAT IN STOOL

Microscopic examination for neutral fat (ethyl alcohol + Sudan III) and free fatty acids (acetic acid + Sudan III + heat) is made.

Random specimen is collected on diet of >60 gm of fat daily.

4+ fat in stool means excessive fecal fat loss.

Increased neutral fat

- Mineral and castor oil ingestion
- Dietetic low-calorie mayonnaise ingestion
- Rectal suppository use
- Steatorrhea

*Data from KK Knight et al., Occult blood screening for colorectal cancer. *JAMA* 261:587, 1989; DE Fleischer et al., Detection and surveillance of colorectal cancer. *JAMA* 261:580, 1989.

QUANTITATIVE DETERMINATION OF FECAL FAT

Is "gold standard" test to establish the diagnosis of malabsorption.

Normal is <7 gm/24 hours when a 3-day stool sample is collected on diet of 60–100 gm of fat daily. <5 gm/24 hours (or <4% of measured fat intake) on diet of <50 gm of fat/day for a 3-day period.

Determination parallels but is more sensitive than triolein ^{131}I test in chronic pancreatic disease.

Increased In

Chronic pancreatic disease (>9.5 gm/24 hours).

May also be increased in

- High-fiber diet (>100 gm/day)
- When dietary fat is ingested in solid form (e.g., whole peanuts)
- In neonatal period.

UROBILINOGEN IN STOOL

(normal = 50–300 mg/24 hours; 100–400 Ehrlich units/100 gm)

Increased In

Hemolytic anemias

Decreased In

Complete biliary obstruction
Severe liver disease
Oral antibiotic therapy altering intestinal bacterial flora
Decreased hemoglobin turnover (e.g., aplastic anemia, cachexia)

MICROSCOPIC EXAMINATION

Normal

RBCs absent

Epithelial cells present (increased with GI tract irritation); absence of epithelial cells in meconium of newborn may aid in diagnosis of intestinal obstruction in the newborn

Few WBCs present (increased with GI tract inflammation)

Crystals of calcium oxalate, fatty acid, and triple phosphate commonly present

Hematoidin crystals sometimes found after GI tract hemorrhage

Charcot-Leyden crystals sometimes found in parasitic infestation (especially amebiasis)

Some undigested vegetable fibers and muscle fibers sometimes found normally

Neutral fat globules (stained with Sudan), normal 0–2+

MICROSCOPIC EXAMINATION OF DIARRHEAL STOOLS FOR FECAL LEUKOCYTES

Primarily polymorphonuclear leukocytes (PMNs)

- Shigellosis
- Salmonellosis
- Invasive *Escherichia coli* colitis
- *Yersinia* infection
- Ulcerative colitis

Primarily mononuclear leukocytes

- Typhoid

Leukocytes absent

- Cholera
- Noninvasive *E. coli* diarrhea
- Other bacterial toxins (e.g., *Staphylococcus, Clostridium perfringens*)
- Viral diarrheas
- Parasitic infestations (e.g., *Giardia lamblia, Entamoeba histolytica, Dientamoeba fragilis*)

FECAL ELECTROLYTES

	Sodium (mEq/24 hours)	Chloride (mEq/24 hours)	Potassium (mEq/24 hours)
Normal*	7.8 ± 2.0	3.2 ± 0.7	18.2 ± 2.5
Idiopathic proctocolitis	22.3	19.8	Normal
Ileostomy	30	19.0	4.1
Cholera	Increased	Increased	

Normal calcium ~0.6 gm/24 hours

OTHER PROCEDURES

Alkalinization of stool to pH of 10 turns blue in presence of phenolphthalein in cases of laxative overuse (hypokalemia, low urine potassium)

Examination for ova and parasites

Trypsin digestion (see Cystic Fibrosis of Pancreas, pp. 214–215)

Microscopic examination (see Laboratory Diagnosis of Malabsorption, pp. 162–164)

Diseases of the Gastrointestinal Tract

BULIMIA

Laboratory findings due to induced vomiting, starvation, misuse of diuretics or laxatives

Increased serum bicarbonate with metabolic alkalosis suggests vomiting

Decreased serum bicarbonate with metabolic acidosis suggests laxative misuse

Hypochloremia

Hypokalemia

Hyponatremia

Serum amylase increased (<2 times normal level) in one-fourth of patients; possibly of mostly salivary type

MALLORY-WEISS SYNDROME

(spontaneous cardioesophageal laceration following retching)

Laboratory findings due to hemorrhage from cardioesophageal laceration

SPONTANEOUS PERFORATION OF ESOPHAGUS

Gastric contents in thoracocentesis fluid

PLUMMER-VINSON SYNDROME

Hypochromic anemia associated with dysphagia and cardiospasm in women

CARCINOMA OF ESOPHAGUS

Cytologic examination of esophageal washings is positive for malignant cells in 75% of patients. It is falsely positive in <2% of patients.

DIAPHRAGMATIC HERNIA

Microcytic anemia (due to blood loss) may be present.

Stool may be positive for blood.

*Average values for 8 healthy individuals. Variable but considerably lower than simultaneous concentrations in serum.

SOME CONDITIONS OF GASTROINTESTINAL TRACT IN WHICH NO USEFUL ABNORMAL LABORATORY FINDINGS OCCUR

Chronic esophagitis
Diverticula of esophagus and stomach
Esophageal spasm
Prolapse of gastric mucosa
Foreign bodies in stomach

PEPTIC ULCER OF STOMACH

Laboratory findings due to underlying conditions
- Administration of adrenocorticotropic hormone (ACTH) and adrenal steroids
- Acute burns (Curling's ulcer)
- Cerebrovascular accidents and trauma and inflammation (Cushing's ulcer)
- Various drugs (e.g., salicylates)
- Uremia
- Cirrhosis

Laboratory findings due to complications
- Gastric retention—dehydration, hypokalemic alkalosis
- Perforation—increased WBC with shift to the left, dehydration, increased serum amylase, increased amylase in peritoneal fluid
- Hemorrhage

See also pp. 149–151.

Curling's ulcer—hemorrhage 8–10 days and perforation 30 days after burn, causes death in 15% of fatal burn cases.

CHRONIC GASTRITIS

Diagnosis depends on biopsy of gastric mucosa. (Other forms of chronic gastritis include hypertrophic [see next section], eosinophilic, granulomatous.)

Anemia due to iron deficiency and malabsorption may occur.

Gastric acid studies are of limited value. Severe hypochlorhydria or achlorhydria after maximal stimulation usually denotes mucosal atrophy.

Fasting serum gastrin is greatly increased in chronic gastritis with achlorhydria and relative sparing of antral mucosa but may be normal with severe antral involvement even with achlorhydria.

Parietal cell antibodies and intrinsic factor antibodies help define the autoimmune type of chronic gastritis and those patients prone to pernicious anemia; absence does not rule out significant chronic gastritis.

Chronic antral gastritis is consistently present in patients with benign gastric ulcer.

Campylobacter pylori appears to be associated with chronic gastritis and peptic ulcers by biopsy; culture has low sensitivity.

BENIGN GIANT HYPERTROPHIC GASTRITIS (MENETRIER'S DISEASE)

Serum protein and albumin decreased in 80% of cases due to loss of plasma proteins through gastric mucosa; gamma globulins may be decreased. Serum calcium may be low due to decreased serum albumin. Protein loss is nonselective in contrast to loss through glomerular membrane in which there is greater loss of low- than high-molecular-weight proteins.

Hypochlorhydria by gastric analysis in 75% of cases. Gastric fluid taken during endoscopy shows increased protein concentration (normal = 0.8–2.5 gm/L), and protein electrophoresis resembles pattern of serum electrophoresis. Increased pH of gastric fluid (normal <2).

Protein loss can also be determined by injecting radiolabeled ^{51}Cr-albumin and measuring radioactivity in stool. Can also use alpha$_1$ antitrypsin clearance (calculated by measuring trypsin in blood and stool; normal <13) to measure protein loss since this resists digestion by trypsin; can only be used if there is acid hyposecretion, since it is destroyed by pH <3.

Diagnosis is confirmed by full-thickness gastric biopsy showing thickening of gastric mucosa due to hyperplasia of mucus-secreting glands (parietal and chief cells are usually diminished or absent); superficial biopsy may appear normal.

Laboratory findings due to complications (e.g., iron deficiency anemia due to chronic GI hemorrhage, edema due to hypoalbuminemia).

Liver function tests are normal.

Proteinuria is absent.

ADENOMATOUS POLYP OF STOMACH

Gastric analysis—achlorhydria in 85% of patients

Sometimes evidence of bleeding

Polyps occur in 5% of patients with pernicious anemia and 2% of patients with achlorhydria.

CARCINOMA OF STOMACH

Anemia due to chronic blood loss

Occult blood in stool

Gastric analysis
- Achlorhydria following histamine or betazole in 50% of patients
- Hypochlorhydria in 25% of patients
- Normal in 25% of patients
- Hyperchlorhydria rare

Exfoliative cytology positive in 80% of patients; false positive in <2%

Lymph node biopsy for metastases; needle biopsy of liver, bone marrow, etc.

Carcinoma of the stomach should always be searched for by periodic prophylactic screening in high-risk patients, especially those with pernicious anemia, gastric atrophy, gastric polyps.

CHRONIC DUODENAL ULCER

Laboratory findings due to associated conditions
- Z-E syndrome (ulcerogenic tumor of pancreas)
- Chronic pancreatitis
- Mucoviscidosis
- Rheumatoid arthritis
- Chronic pulmonary disease (e.g., pulmonary emphysema)
- Cirrhosis
- Certain drugs (e.g., ACTH)
- Hyperparathyroidism
- Polycythemia vera

Laboratory findings due to treatment
- Milk-alkali (Burnett's) syndrome—alkalosis, hypercalcemia, azotemia, renal calculi, or nephrocalcinosis
- Inadequate vagotomy—use insulin test meal (see p. 151)
- Gastric acidity shows late response >4.5 mEq total free acid in 30 minutes or any early response.

To obtain valid collection, tube must be correctly placed fluoroscopically.

DUMPING SYNDROME

(occurs in ≤70% of post–subtotal gastrectomy patients)

During symptoms may have
- Rapid prolonged alimentary hyperglycemia

Decreased plasma volume
Decreased serum potassium
Increased blood and urine serotonin
Hypoglycemic syndrome (occurs in $<5\%$ of post–subtotal gastrectomy patients)
Prolonged alimentary hyperglycemia followed after 2 hours by precipitous hypoglycemia
Late hypoglycemia shown by 6-hour oral glucose tolerance test
Stomal gastritis—anemia due to chronic bleeding
Postgastrectomy malabsorption
Postgastrectomy anemia (e.g., due to chronic blood loss, malabsorption, vitamin B_{12} deficiency)
Afferent-loop obstruction—marked increase in serum amylase to >1000 units
Laboratory findings due to complications of gastric or duodenal ulcer, e.g., hemorrhage, perforation, obstruction
Gastric analysis
True achlorhydria following maximum stimulation rules out duodenal ulcer.
Normal secretion or hypersecretion does not prove the presence of an ulcer.

Duodenal ulcer is absent in patients with ulcerative colitis (unless under steroid therapy), carcinoma of stomach, pernicious anemia, pregnancy.

ACUTE APPENDICITIS

Increased WBC (12,000–14,000/cu mm) with shift to the left in acute catarrhal stage; higher and more rapid rise with suppuration or perforation
Erythrocyte sedimentation rate (ESR) may be normal during first 24 hours
Later—laboratory findings due to complications (e.g., dehydration, abscess formation, perforation with peritonitis)

ACUTE DIVERTICULITIS

Increased WBC and ESR
Hypochromic microcytic anemia (some patients)
Occult blood in stool
Cytologic examination of stool—negative for malignant cells
Laboratory findings due to complications (e.g., hemorrhage, perforation, obstruction)

GASTROINTESTINAL INVOLVEMENT IN AIDS

Candida—oropharyngeal or esophageal thrush
Mycobacterium avium intracellulare—diarrhea, malabsorption, or hepatitis
Cytomegalovirus—esophagitis or colitis or hepatitis
Isosporosis—diarrhea
Cryptosporidiosis
Increased susceptibility to many bacteria, viruses, parasites, etc.

AGENTS OF INFECTIOUS GASTROENTERITIS

Agent	**Frequency (%) in Traveler's Diarrhea**
Enterotoxigenic *Escherichia coli*	40–60
Shigella species	5–10
Salmonella species	<5
Campylobacter species	<5
Unknown agents	30–40
Giardia lamblia	Rare

Entamoeba histolytica	Rare
Enteropathogenic *E. coli*	NA
Enteroinvasive *E. coli*	NA
Enterohemorrhagic *E. coli*	NA
Rotavirus, groups A, B, C	NA
Norwalk viruses	NA
Enteric adenovirus	
Astrovirus	
Calicivirus	
Cryptosporidium species	NA
Balantidium coli	
Isospora belli	
Other bacteria to consider	
Yersinia enterocolitica	
Vibrio cholerae, Vibrio parahaemolyticus	
Aeromonas hydrophila	
Clostridium difficile, Clostridium perfringens type A	
Staphylococcus aureus	
Bacillus cereus	

NA = data on frequency not available

MOST COMMON AGENTS OF FOODBORNE DISEASE OUTBREAKS (GASTROENTERITIS)*

	% of Cases (known etiology)
Viral	5.5
Parasitic	0.8
Chemical (scroboid)	5.1
Bacterial*	88.6
Salmonella	31.9
Staphylococcus aureus	16.5
Clostridium botulinum	0.4
Clostridium perfringens	18.5
Shigella	18.0
Vibrio parahaemolyticus	0.03
Bacillus cereus	0.03
Streptococcus, Group A	3.2
Brucella melitensis	0.1

CAMPYLOBACTERIOSIS

See p. 626.

VIRAL GASTROENTERITIS

Agent	Proportion of Childhood Hospitalizations for Diarrhea	Peak Age	Comment
Rotavirus	1/3	6 months–2 years	Produces long-term immunity to serious infection
Adenoviruses	5–20%	<2 years	Not seasonal
Calicivirus	3%	3 months–6 years	Not seasonal

*Confirm by culture of food, patient's stool, or food handler's stool.

Astrovirus	3–5%		
Norwalk-like viruses (heterogeneous group)		≥School age	Usually occurs in outbreaks
Others (e.g., pestivirus, picobirnavirus, parvovirus, enteroviruses, torovirus, coronavirus)			

Antigen detection

Commercial kits for rotavirus are inexpensive, permit rapid diagnosis, require only small amounts of stool, which may be frozen until testing. Sensitivities of 70–100% and specificities of 50–100% are reported. False positive rates high in newborn and breast-feeding children. Less useful in adults and outside of rotavirus season when confirmatory testing should be performed. Kits also available for adenovirus. Rapid assays for other viruses are under development.

Antibody detection (e.g., Norwalk agent)

Fourfold rise in specific titers drawn at the first week (acute-phase serum) and the third to sixth week (convalescent serum). Patient has long since recovered from self-limited illness.

Electron microscopy (e.g., rotaviruses, adenoviruses, astroviruses, caliciviruses, Norwalk virus)

Identifies virus by characteristic morphology

Detection requires ≥1 million viruses/ml of stool; usually present only during first 48 hours of viral diarrhea. Immune electron microscopy improves sensitivity by 10–100 times, but technology limits this to few laboratories.

Culture

Rotavirus, adenoviruses, astrovirus culture available in research centers; not useful for routine diagnosis. Other viruses cannot be cultured.

Electropherotyping

Detection of rotavirus RNA in stool by gel electrophoresis pattern is 100% specific and >90% sensitive in first days of illness; chiefly research tool in USA.

Dot-hybridization probes for rotavirus are more sensitive and specific than antigen detection but only available in research centers.

Polymerase chain reaction techniques are being developed.

WHIPPLE'S DISEASE (INTESTINAL LIPODYSTROPHY)

Characteristic biopsy of intestine and mesenteric lymph nodes establishes the diagnosis by light and electron microscopy

Malabsorption syndrome

Arthritis

CELIAC DISEASE (GLUTEN-SENSITIVE ENTEROPATHY, NONTROPICAL SPRUE, IDIOPATHIC STEATORRHEA)

Malabsorption syndrome; return to normal on gluten-free diet

Biopsy of small intestine

TUMORS OF SMALL INTESTINE

Laboratory findings due to complications, e.g., hemorrhage, obstruction, intussusception, malabsorption

Laboratory findings due to underlying condition, e.g., Peutz-Jeghers syndrome, malignant lymphoma, carcinoid syndrome

MULTIPLE DIVERTICULA OF JEJUNUM

Laboratory findings due to malabsorption syndrome

MECKEL'S DIVERTICULUM

Laboratory findings due only to complications
- Gastrointestinal hemorrhage
- Intestinal obstruction
- Perforation or intussusception (~20% of patients; the other 80% of patients are asymptomatic)

CLASSIFICATION OF MALABSORPTION

Inadequate mixing of food with bile salts and lipase (e.g., pyloroplasty, subtotal or total gastrectomy, gastrojejunostomy)

Inadequate lipolysis due to lack of lipase (e.g., cystic fibrosis of the pancreas, chronic pancreatitis, cancer of the pancreas or ampulla of Vater, pancreatic fistula, vagotomy)

Inadequate emulsification of fat due to lack of bile salts (e.g., obstructive jaundice, severe liver disease)

Primary absorptive defect in small bowel

Inadequate absorptive surface due to extensive mucosal disease (e.g., regional enteritis, tumors, amyloid disease, scleroderma, irradiation)

Biochemical dysfunction of mucosal cells (e.g., celiac-sprue syndrome, severe starvation, intestinal infections, infestations, or administration of drugs such as neomycin sulfate, colchicine, or para-aminosalicylic acid)

Obstruction of mesenteric lymphatics (e.g., by lymphoma, carcinoma, Whipple's disease, intestinal tuberculosis)

Inadequate length of normal absorptive surface (e.g., surgical resection, fistula, shunt)

Miscellaneous (e.g., "blind loops" of intestine, diverticula, Z-E syndrome, agammaglobulinemia, endocrine and metabolic disorders)

Chronic infection (e.g., in common variable hypogammaglobulinemia, 50–55% of patients have chronic diarrhea and malabsorption due to specific pathogen such as *Giardia lamblia* or overgrowth of bacteria in small bowel)

LABORATORY DIAGNOSIS OF MALABSORPTION

Direct stool examination
- Gross—oil droplets, egg particles, buttery materials
- Sudan III stain for qualitative screening for fat (see p. 154)
- Quantitative test for fat is "gold standard" to establish the diagnosis of malabsorption (see p. 155)
  - Normal is <7 gm of fat/24 hours as average of 3-day collection when diet includes 60–100 gm of fat/day
  - Increased in chronic pancreatic disease >9.5 gm/24 hours. May also be increased in high-fiber diet, when fat is ingested in solid form (e.g., peanuts), in neonatal period.
- Weight—much heavier (>300 gm/24 hours) than normal (normal weight is <200 gm/24 hours or normal solids of 25–30 gm/24 hours)
- Na_2CO_3 and Nile blue dye give blue color to stool proportional to the concentration of oleates.

Indirect indices of fat absorption; these lack sensitivity and specificity for routine screening.
- Serum cholesterol may be decreased.
- Prothrombin time (PT) may be prolonged due to malabsorption of vitamin K.
- Serum carotene is always abnormal in steatorrhea unless therapy is successful. Not recommended for screening; poor precision at lower end of reference range. May also be low in liver disease, high fever, hyperthyroidism, chronic illness, and decreased dietary intake (blood level falls within 1 week, but vitamin A level is unaffected by dietary change for 6 months because of much larger body stores). May be increased in hyper-

lipidemia and hypothyroidism. Normal is 70–290 μm/ml. 30–70 μg/dl indicates mild depletion; <30 indicates severe depletion.

Vitamin A tolerance test (for screening steatorrhea)

Measure plasma vitamin A level 5 hours after ingestion.

Normal rise is 9 times fasting level.

Flat curve in liver disease

Not useful after gastrectomy

With vitamin A as ester of long-chain fatty acid, flat curve occurs in both pancreatic disease and intestinal mucosal abnormalities; when water-soluble forms of vitamin A are used, the curve becomes normal in patients with pancreatic disease but remains flat in intestinal mucosal abnormalities.

Triolein ^{131}I and oleic acid ^{131}I absorption with measurement of blood and fecal radioactivity; sensitive and specific for screening but may not be routinely available.

Carbohydrate absorption indices

Oral glucose tolerance test—limited value

Flat curve or delayed peak occurs in celiac disease and nontropical sprue.

Curve is normal in pancreatic insufficiency.

D-Xylose tolerance test of carbohydrate absorption

Measure total 5-hour urine excretion; may also measure serum levels at 2 hours. Accuracy is 90% in distinguishing normal levels in pancreatic disease from decreased levels in intestinal mucosal disease and intestinal bacterial overgrowth, but opinions vary on usefulness. Also decreased in renal disease, myxedema, and the elderly, although absorption is normal.

Protein absorption indices

Normal nitrogen is <2 gm/day. There is marked increase in sprue and severe pancreatic deficiency.

Measure plasma glycine or urinary excretion of hydroxyproline after gelatin meal. Plasma glycine increases 5 times in 2 hours in normal persons. In those with cystic fibrosis of the pancreas, the increase is <2.5 times.

Serum albumin may be decreased.

Serum trypsinogen (radioimmunoassay) <10 ng/ml in 75–85% of patients with severe chronic pancreatitis (those with steatorrhea) and 15–20% of those with mild to moderate disease; occasionally low in cancer of pancreas; normal (10–75 ng/ml) in nonpancreatic causes of malabsorption.

Bentiromide used to differentiate pancreatic exocrine insufficiency (abnormal result) from intestinal mucosal disease (normal result). Sensitivity of 70–95% in severe chronic pancreatitis (with steatorrhea).

Secretin-cholecystokinin is the most sensitive and reliable test of chronic pancreatic disease

Schilling test. Performed before and after administration of antibiotics, is the most useful adjunct to intestinal culture to detect bacterial overgrowth.

Electrolyte absorption indices

Serum calcium, magnesium, potassium, and vitamin D may be decreased.

PVP-^{131}I test is indicated.

^{51}Cr albumin test (IV dose of 30–50 μCi) shows increased excretion in 4-day stool collection due to protein-losing enteropathy.

Biopsy of small-intestine mucosa is excellent for verification of sprue, celiac disease, and Whipple's disease.

Culture for bacterial overgrowth should be considered in malabsorption associated with abnormal intestinal motility (e.g., scleroderma) or anatomic abnormalities (e.g., diverticuli). Positive if $>10^6$ organisms/ml of intestinal contents but may vary from one location to another. Perform with peroral intestinal biopsy. If breath tests using ^{14}C bile acid and xylose or hydrogen are available, they are more sensitive and specific for bacterial overgrowth.

Anemia is due to deficiency of iron, folic acid, vitamin B_{12}, or various combinations, depending on their decreased absorption.

Most common laboratory abnormalities are decreased serum carotene, albumin, and iron, increased ESR, increased stool weight (>300 gm/24 hours) and stool fat (>7 gm/24 hours), anemia.

Normal D-xylose test, low serum trypsinogen, and pancreatic calcification on x-ray of abdomen establishes diagnosis of chronic pancreatitis. If calcification is absent (as occurs in 70–80% of cases), abnormal contents of pancreatic secretion after secretin-cholecystokinin stimulation or abnormal bentiromide tests establish diagnosis of chronic pancreatitis.

DISACCHARIDE MALABSORPTION

Oral Disaccharide Tolerance Test

Administer 1 gm/kg body weight of the test carbohydrate (disaccharide).
Determine blood glucose at fasting, 1/2-, 1-, 2-, and 3-hour intervals.
Normal: Blood glucose increases >24 mg/dl above fasting level.
Abnormal in disaccharide malabsorption: Blood glucose increases 0–21 mg/dl above fasting level. False abnormal test may be due to delayed gastric emptying or delayed blood collection.
Confirm disaccharide malabsorption by
- Repeating tolerance test using constituent monosaccharides
- Testing stool for
  - pH: ≤5 is abnormal.
  - Sugar: >0.5% is abnormal; 0.25–0.5% is suspicious; 0.25% is normal.
  - Taking intestinal biopsy for histologic study and disaccharidase activity assay

Due To

Primary malabsorption (congenital or acquired) due to absence of specific disaccharidase in brush border of small-intestine mucosa
- Sucrose-isomaltose malabsorption (inherited recessive defect)
  - Oral sucrose tolerance curve is flat, but glucose plus fructose tolerance test is normal. Occasionally there is an associated malabsorption with increased stool fat and abnormal D-xylose tolerance test, although intestinal biopsy is normal.
- Isolated lactase deficiency (also called milk allergy, milk intolerance, congenital familial lactose intolerance, lactase deficiency; is most common of these defects; occurs in ~10% of whites and 60% of blacks; infantile type shows diarrhea, vomiting, failure to thrive, malabsorption, etc.; often appears first in adults; becomes asymptomatic when lactase is removed from diet)
  - Oral lactose tolerance curve is flat (blood glucose rises <20–25 mg/dl in blood drawn 15, 30, 60, 90 minutes after 50–100 gm dose of lactose), but glucose plus galactose (25 gm of each) tolerance test is normal, indicating isolated lactase deficiency rather than general mucosal absorptive defect.
    - In diabetics, blood sugar may increase >20–25 mg/dl despite impaired lactose absorption. Test may also be influenced by impaired gastric emptying or small bowel transit.
  - Hydrogen breath test measures amount of H_2 exhaled at 2 hours after ingestion of 50 gm of lactose in fasting state. Normal = 0–0.11 ml/minute; in lactase deficiency = 0.31–2.50 ml/minute. Peak or cumulative 4-hour values also differentiate these patients. Based on production of H_2 by bacteria in colon from unabsorbed lactose. False negative test due to absence of H_2-producing bacteria in colon or prior antibiotic therapy in ~20% of patients.

Peroral intestinal biopsy to prove decreased lactase activity is now considered obsolete.

After 50–100 gm of lactose, frothy diarrheal stools typically show low pH (4.5–6.0; normal >7.0), high osmolality, positive test for reducing substances (e.g., Clinitest tablets). Fecal studies are of limited value.

Glucose-galactose malabsorption (inherited autosomal recessive defect that affects kidney and intestine)

Oral glucose or galactose tolerance curve is flat, but intravenous tolerance curves are normal. Glucosuria is common. Fructose tolerance test is normal.

Secondary malabsorption

Resection of >50% of disaccharidase activity

Lactose is most marked, but there may also be sucrose.

Oral disaccharide tolerance (especially lactose) is abnormal, but intestinal histology and enzyme activity are normal.

Diffuse intestinal disease—especially celiac disease in which activity of all disaccharidases may be decreased, with later increase as intestine becomes normal on gluten-free diet; also cystic fibrosis of pancreas, severe malnutrition, ulcerative colitis, severe *Giardia* infestation, blind-loop syndrome, beta-lipoprotein deficiency, effect of drugs (e.g., colchicine, neomycin, birth control pills)

Oral tolerance tests (especially lactose) are frequently abnormal, with later return to normal with gluten-free diet. Tolerance tests with monosaccharides may also be abnormal because of defect in absorption as well as digestion.

LABORATORY FINDINGS

Oral carbohydrate (disaccharide) tolerance test is abnormal (blood glucose rises 0–21 mg/dl above fasting level).

Oral tolerance test using constituent monosaccharides. Normal result demonstrates normal absorption of monosaccharides.

Examine stool during disaccharide tolerance test.

pH of ≤5 is abnormal.

Measure disaccharide (Clinitest tablet).

>0.5% is abnormal.

0.25–0.5% is suspicious.

<0.25% is normal.

Biopsy of small-intestine mucosa will reveal activity of specific disaccharidase.

PROTEIN-LOSING ENTEROPATHY

Secondary (i.e., disease states in which clinically significant protein-losing enteropathy may occur as a manifestation)

- Giant hypertrophy of gastric rugae (Menetrier's disease)
- Gastric neoplasms
- Regional enteritis
- Whipple's disease
- Nontropical sprue
- Inflammatory and neoplastic diseases of small and large intestine
- Ulcerative colitis
- Constrictive pericarditis

Primary (i.e., hypoproteinemia is the major clinical feature)

- Intestinal lymphangiectasia
- Nonspecific inflammatory or granulomatous disease of small intestine

Serum total protein, albumin, and gamma globulin decreased

Serum alpha and beta globulins normal

Serum cholesterol usually normal

Mild anemia

Eosinophilia (occasionally)
Serum calcium decreased
Steatorrhea with abnormal tests of lipid absorption
Increased permeability of GI tract to large molecular substances shown by IV PVP-^{131}I test (see p. 153)
Proteinuria absent

INTESTINAL LYMPHANGIECTASIA

May manifest abnormal lymph nodes (inguinal, pelvic, retroperitoneal) and lymphedema between early infancy and childhood
Decreased serum protein
IV infusion of ^{51}Cr-labeled albumin demonstrates excessive protein loss in stools.
Biopsy of small bowel or lymphangiography will confirm the diagnosis.

REGIONAL ENTERITIS (CROHN'S DISEASE)

No pathognomonic findings for this disease or to distinguish from ulcerative colitis
Increased WBC, ESR, C-reactive protein (CRP), other acute-phase reactants
Anemia due to iron deficiency or vitamin B_{12} or folate deficiency
Decreased serum albumin, increased gamma globulins
Diarrhea may cause hyperchloremic metabolic acidosis, dehydration, decreased sodium, potassium, magnesium.
Mild liver function test changes due to pericholangitis (especially increased alkaline phosphatase)
Serum carcinoembryonic antigen (CEA) may be increased.

ACUTE MEMBRANOUS ENTEROCOLITIS

Laboratory findings due to antecedent condition
- Disease for which antibiotics are administered
- Myocardial infarction
- Surgical procedure
- Other

Laboratory findings due to shock, dehydration
Culture of staphylococci from stool or rectal swab

PSEUDOMEMBRANOUS COLITIS

Antibiotic-related diarrhea and colitis related to *Clostridium difficile*
Stool culture is the most sensitive test (86% with one culture and 96% with two cultures), but the false positive rate may be >20%.
Detection of cytotoxin by tissue culture (found in 62–90% of cases)
Demonstration of toxins by antibodies (e.g., ELISA, latex agglutination) show good sensitivity (64–90%) but poor specificity. Rapid results make these useful for screening.
One stool culture plus latex agglutination or tissue culture increases sensitivity to 96%.
Countercurrent immunoelectrophoresis, gas-liquid chromatography (GLC), and Gram's stain of stool have high false negative and positive results.

CHRONIC NONSPECIFIC ULCERATIVE COLITIS

Laboratory findings parallel severity of the disease
- Anemia due to blood loss (frequently Hb = 6 gm/dl)
- WBC usually normal unless complication occurs (e.g., abscess)
- ESR often normal or only slightly increased

Stools
- Positive for blood (gross and/or occult)
- Negative for usual enteric bacterial pathogens and parasites; high total bacterial count

Changes in liver function
- Microscopic changes in needle biopsy of liver
- Serum alkaline phosphatase often increased slightly
- Other liver function tests usually normal

Changes in serum electrolytes due to diarrhea or to therapy with adrenal steroids or ACTH

Laboratory changes due to complications or sequelae (e.g., malabsorption due to involvement of small intestine, perforation, abscess formation, hemorrhage, carcinoma, arthritis)

Rectal biopsy

COLLAGENOUS COLITIS

Diagnosis is established by biopsy of colon in patients thought to have irritable bowel syndrome. Incidence ~3/1000 in such patients.

ESR may be increased in some patients.

Eosinophil count may be increased in some patients.

ACUTE PROCTITIS

Rectal Gram's stain shows >1 PMN/hpf (1000×).

In homosexual men, specific etiology can be found in 80% of cases completely studied. The most common causes are *Chlamydia trachomatis* (non–lymphogranuloma venereum strains) in >75% of cases, *Neisseria gonorrhoeae,* lymphogranuloma venereum, herpes simplex virus type 2, *Treponema pallidum.*

Histopathology of rectal biopsy in acute proctocolitis due to C. trachomatis *is indistinguishable from Crohn's disease; culture and serologic tests for* C. trachomatis *and serologic tests for lymphogranuloma venereum strains should be performed in such cases. Primary or secondary syphilitic proctitis may be very severe and of variable appearance; serologic test for syphilis should be performed in such cases.*

CARCINOMA OF COLON

Blood in stool (occult or gross)

Evidence of inflammation
- Increased WBC and ESR

Anemia—usually hypochromic
- May be the only symptom of carcinoma of right side of colon (present in >50% of these patients)
- Stools sometimes negative for occult blood

Laboratory evidence of liver metastases

Biopsy of colon lesion

Serum CEA

Villous tumor of rectum may cause secretory diarrhea with potassium loss and decreased serum potassium.

Carcinoid tumors may cause increased 5-hydroxyindoleacetic acid (5-HIAA) in urine.

Laboratory findings due to complications (e.g., hemorrhage, perforation, obstruction)

Laboratory findings due to underlying condition (e.g., hereditary polyposis, chronic nonspecific ulcerative colitis)

VILLOUS ADENOMA OF RECTUM

Stool contains large amount of mucus tinged with blood; frequent watery diarrhea.

Serum potassium sometimes decreased

Biopsy of lesion

MESENTERIC VASCULAR OCCLUSION

Chronic (mesenteric arterial insufficiency)

Laboratory findings due to malabsorption and starvation

Acute

Marked increase in WBC (≥15,000–25,000/cu mm) with shift to the left

Laboratory findings due to intestinal hemorrhage, obstruction, metabolic acidosis, shock

Infarction of intestine may cause increased LDH, SGOT, CK, BUN, and phosphorus.

INTESTINAL OBSTRUCTION

WBC is normal early. Later it tends to rise, with increase in PMNs; 15,000–25,000/cu mm suggests strangulation; >30,000/cu mm suggests mesenteric thrombosis.

Hemoglobin and hematocrit levels are normal early but later increase, with dehydration.

Urine specific gravity increases, with deficit of water and electrolytes unless preexisting renal disease is present. Urinalysis helps rule out renal colic, diabetic acidosis, etc.

Gastric contents

Positive guaiac test suggests strangulation; there may be gross blood if strangulated segment is high in jejunum.

Rectal contents—gross rectal blood suggests carcinoma of colon or intussusception.

Decreased serum sodium, potassium, chloride, and pH and increased CO_2 are helpful indications for following the course of the patient and to guide therapy.

Increased BUN suggests blood in intestine or renal damage. Serum amylase may be moderately increased in absence of pancreatitis.

Increased serum LDH, SGOT, CK, and phosphorus may indicate strangulation (infarction) of small intestine.

ACUTE PERITONITIS

Primary

Gram's stain of direct smear of peritoneal fluid shows streptococci or pneumococci in absence of *E. coli.*

Marked increase in WBC (≤50,000/cu mm) and PMN (80–90%)

Secondary

Laboratory findings due to underlying condition (e.g., appendicitis, perforated ulcer, volvulus)

ASCITES

Chronic liver disease: To differentiate ascites due to malignancy from that due to chronic liver disease, gradient (= serum albumin minus ascitic fluid albumin) <1.1 in >90% of cases of malignancy and almost always >1.1 in hepatic ascites. Total protein is often not useful because of high protein content in 12–19% of these ascites as well as changes due to albumin infusion and diuretic therapies. Total WBC is usually <300/cu mm (one-half of cases) and PMN <25% (two-thirds of cases).

Cardiac ascites is associated with a blood-ascitic fluid albumin gradient >1.1 gm/dl, but malignant ascites shows blood-ascitic fluid albumin gradient <1.1 gm/dl in 93% of cases.

Infected ascites: WBC >500/cu mm and neutrophils >50% are presumptive of bacterial peritonitis. pH <7.35 and arterial-ascitic fluid pH difference >0.10; both these findings are virtually diagnostic of bacterial peritonitis, and absence of these findings virtually excludes bacterial peritonitis. Ascitic fluid lactate >25 mg/dl and arterial-ascitic fluid difference >20 mg/dl are often present. Ascitic fluid glucose is unreliable for diagnosis. Gram's stain is positive in 25% of cases. Acid-fast stains and culture establish the diagnosis of tuberculosis in only 25–50% of cases.

To monitor peritoneal dialysate in continuous ambulatory peritoneal dialysis: Patients monitor outflow bags for turbidity and when peritonitis is defined as WBC >100/cu mm usually with >50% PMNs, or positive culture (most prevalent: coagulase negative staphylococci, *Staphylococcus aureus, Streptococcus* species; multiple organisms, especially mixed aerobes and anaerobes occur with bowel perforation). Successful therapy causes fall in WBC within first 2 days and return to <100/cu mm in 4–5 days; differential returns to predominance of monocytes in 4–7 days with increased eosinophils in 10% of cases. Turbid dialysate can occasionally occur without peritonitis during first few months of placing catheter (due to catheter hypersensitivity) with WBC 100–8000/cu mm and 10–95% eosinophils and sometimes increased PMNs and negative cultures. Occasional RBCs may be seen during menstruation or with ovulation at midcycle. *Because of low WBC decision level, manual hemocytometer count rather than an automated instrument must be used.*

Pancreatic disease: Ascitic fluid amylase > serum amylase is virtually specific for pancreatic disease, but both levels are normal in 10% of cases. Methemalbumin in serum or ascitic fluid and total protein >4.5 gm/dl indicate poor prognosis.

Chylous ascites: Triglyceride is 2–8 times serum level. Protein = 2–3 gm/dl. Due to lymphatic obstruction, e.g., lymphoma or carcinoma (60% of cases), inflammation or obstruction of small intestine, trauma to chest or abdomen, filariasis; in pediatric patients, is often due to congenital lymphatic defects.

Criteria to diagnose penetrating abdominal wounds by peritoneal lavage
- >10,000 RBC/cu mm (>5000 RBC/cu mm for gunshot wounds)
- >500 WBC/cu mm
- or the presence of bile, vegetable matter, or bacteria on Gram's stain

Criteria to diagnose blunt abdominal trauma by peritoneal lavage
- Grossly bloody fluid or
- >100,000 RBC/cu mm or
- <500 WBC/cu mm or
- Amylase >2.5 times normal

To differentiate urine from ascitic or pleural fluid (in cases of possible GU tract fistula or accidental aspiration of bladder)
- Urine creatinine is >2 times the serum level
- Uncontaminated ascitic or pleural fluid is usually same as serum level but always <2 times serum level.

Increased serum inorganic phosphate in 25% of cases of ischemic bowel disease; >5.5 mg/dl indicates extensive bowel injury, acute renal failure, metabolic acidosis, and poorer prognosis.

9

Hepatobiliary Diseases and Diseases of the Pancreas

Liver Function Tests

GENERALIZATIONS ON LIVER FUNCTION TEST INTERPRETATION

Patterns of abnormalities rather than single test changes are particularly useful despite sensitivities of only 65% in some cases.

Tests may be abnormal in many conditions that are not primarily hepatic (e.g., heart failure, sepsis, infections such as brucellosis, subacute bacterial endocarditis), and individual tests may be positive in other conditions than liver disease. Individual tests are normal in high proportions of patients with proven specific liver diseases, and normal values may not rule out liver disease.

SOME COMMON PATTERNS (TEST COMBINATIONS) OF LIVER FUNCTION CHANGES

Serum bilirubin (direct-total ratio)

< 20%	Constitutional hyperbilirubinemias (e.g., Gilbert's disease, Crigler-Najjar syndrome) Hemolytic states
20–40%	Favors hepatocellular disease rather than extrahepatic obstruction
40–60%	Occurs in either hepatocellular or extrahepatic type
> 50%	Favors extrahepatic obstruction rather than hepatocellular disease

Total serum bilirubin must exceed 2.5 mg/dl to produce clinical jaundice.

Total serum bilirubin > 5 mg/dl seldom occurs in uncomplicated hemolysis unless hepatobiliary disease is also present.

Total serum bilirubin level is generally less markedly elevated in hepatocellular jaundice (≤ 10 mg/dl) than in periampullary carcinomas (≤ 20 mg/dl) or intrahepatic cholestasis. In extrahepatic biliary obstruction, bilirubin may rise progressively to a plateau of 30–40 mg/dl (due in part to balance between renal excretion and diversion of bilirubin to other metabolites). Such a plateau tends not to occur in hepatocellular jaundice, and bilirubin may exceed 50 mg/dl (partly due to concomitant renal insufficiency and hemolysis).

Serum bilirubin levels are generally higher in obstruction due to carcinoma than due to stones.

Increased serum bilirubin with normal alkaline phosphatase suggests constitutional hyperbilirubinemias or hemolytic states.

Normal serum bilirubin with increased alkaline phosphatase (of liver origin) suggests obstruction of one hepatic duct or metastatic or infiltrative disease of liver. Metastatic and granulomatous lesions of liver cause 1.5–3.0 times increase of serum alkaline phosphatase.

Mild increase of serum glutamic-oxaloacetic (SGOT) and glutamic-pyruvic transaminases (SGPT) (usually < 500 IU/L) with alkaline phosphatase increased > 3 times normal indicates cholestatic jaundice, but more marked increase of SGOT and SGPT (especially > 1000 IU/L) with alkaline phosphatase increased < 3 times normal indicates hepatocellular jaundice.

SGOT and SGPT are most markedly increased in viral hepatitis, drug injury, carbon tetrachloride poisoning (100–2000 IU/L). SGOT > 10 times normal indicates acute hepatocellular injury, but lesser increases are nonspecific and may occur with virtually any other form of liver injury. Levels are usually < 200 IU/L in posthepatic jaundice and intrahepatic cholestasis. Levels are usually < 50 IU/L in fatty liver, < 100 IU/L in alcoholic cirrhosis, < 150 IU/L in alcoholic hepatitis (may be higher if patient has delirium tremens), < 200 IU/L in 65% of patients with cirrhosis, < 200 IU/L in 50% of patients with metastatic liver disease, lymphoma, and leukemia.

SGOT-SGPT ratio > 1 with SGOT < 300 IU/L favors alcoholic hepatitis in cases of liver disease. Increased SGOT > SGPT also occurs in cirrhosis and metastatic liver disease. Increased SGOT < SGPT favors viral hepatitis, posthepatic jaundice, intrahepatic cholestasis. *SGOT is increased in acute myocardial infarction and in muscle diseases, but SGPT is normal. SGPT is more specific for liver disease than SGOT.*

SGOT soaring to peak of 1000–9000 IU/L, declining by 50% within 3 days and to < 100 IU/L within a week suggests shock liver with centrolobular necrosis (e.g., due to congestive heart failure, arrhythmia, sepsis, GI hemorrhage); serum bilirubin and alkaline phosphatase reflect underlying disease. Rapid rise of SGOT and SGPT to very high levels (e.g., > 600 IU/L and often > 2000 IU/L) followed by a sharp fall in 12–72 hours is said to be typical of acute biliary duct obstruction. Abrupt SGOT rise may also be seen in acute fulminant viral hepatitis (rarely > 4000 IU and decline more slowly; positive serologic tests) and acute chemical injury.

Gamma-glutamyl transpeptidase (GGT)–alkaline phosphatase ratio > 5 favors alcoholic liver disease.

Isolated elevation of GGT is a sensitive screening and monitoring test for alcoholism.

Serum 5′-nucleotidase and leucine aminopeptidase (LAP) parallel the increase in alkaline phosphatase in obstructive type of hepatobiliary disease, but the 5′-nucleotidase is increased only in the latter and is normal in pregnancy and bone disease, whereas the LAP is increased in pregnancy but usually normal in bone disease. GGT is normal in bone disease and pregnancy. Therefore, these enzymes are useful in determining the source of increased serum alkaline phosphatase.

Serum Enzyme	Biliary Obstruction	Pregnancy	Bone Disease
Alkaline phosphatase	I	I	I
5′-Nucleotidase	I	N	N
LAP	I	I	N
GGT	I	N	N

I = increased; N = normal.

Serum alkaline phosphatase is the best indicator of biliary obstruction but does not differentiate intrahepatic cholestasis from extrahepatic obstruction. High values (> 5 times normal) favor obstruction, and normal levels virtually exclude this diagnosis. Is markedly increased in infants with congenital intrahepatic bile duct atresia but is much lower in extrahepatic atresia.

Bilirubin ("bile") in urine implies increased serum direct bilirubin and excludes hemolysis as the cause. Often precedes clinical icterus. May occur without jaundice in anicteric or early hepatitis, early obstruction, or liver metastases. (Tablets detect 0.05–0.1 mg/dl; dipsticks are less sensitive; test is negative in normal persons.)

Complete absence of urine urobilinogen strongly suggests complete bile duct obstruction; normal in incomplete obstruction. Decreased in some phases of hepatic jaundice. Increased in hemolytic jaundice and subsiding hepatitis.

Increase may evidence hepatic damage even without clinical jaundice (e.g., some patients with cirrhosis, metastatic liver disease, congestive heart failure). Presence in viral hepatitis depends on phase of disease. (Normal is < 1 mg or 1 Ehrlich unit/2-hour specimen.)

Serum cholesterol

- May be normal or slightly decreased in hepatitis.
- Markedly decreased in severe hepatitis or cirrhosis.
- Increased in posthepatitic jaundice or intrahepatic cholestasis.
- Markedly increased in primary biliary cirrhosis.

Prothrombin time (PT) may be prolonged due to lack of vitamin K absorption in obstruction or lack of synthesis in hepatocellular disease. Corrected by parenteral administration of vitamin K (10 mg/day for 3 days) in obstructive but not in hepatocellular disease. Markedly prolonged PT is a good index of severe liver cell damage in hepatitis and cirrhosis; not useful when only slightly prolonged.

Serum gamma globulin tends to increase with most forms of chronic liver disease; marked increases (e.g., > 3 gm/dl) are suggestive of chronic active hepatitis. Serum albumin is slow to reflect liver damage. Is usually normal in hepatitis and cholestasis.

Unusual patterns:

- Some patients do not present the usual pattern: SGOT and SGPT are < 200 units in 20% of acute viral hepatitis. Serum alkaline phosphatase is increased > 3 times in 5% of acute hepatitis.
- Normal values may not rule out liver disease: SGPT is normal in 50% and SGOT is normal in 25% of patients with alcoholic cirrhosis.
- Liver function test abnormalities may occur in systemic diseases, e.g., systemic lupus erythematosus (SLE), sarcoidosis, tuberculosis, subacute bacterial endocarditis, brucellosis, sickle cell disease
- A confusing pattern may occur in mixed forms of jaundice, e.g., sickle cell disease producing hemolysis and complicated by pigment stones causing duct obstruction.

SEROLOGIC TESTS FOR VIRAL HEPATITIS A (HAV)

Anti-HAV-IgM appears at the same time as symptoms and is detectable for 3–12 weeks after symptoms subside. Presence confirms the diagnosis of recent acute infection.

Anti-HAV-IgG appears after the acute period and is usually detectable for life; found in 45% of adult population. Indicates previous exposure to HAV, recovery, and immunity to type A hepatitis. Usually order anti-HAV-total and anti-HAV-IgM tests simultaneously; positive anti-HAV-total and negative anti-HAV-IgM indicates anti-HAV-IgG and immunity.

Serial testing is usually not indicated.

SEROLOGIC TESTS FOR VIRAL HEPATITIS B (HBV)

Hepatitis B Surface Antigen (HB_sAg)

Earliest indicator of HBV infection. Usually appears in 27–41 days (as early as 14 days). Appears 7–26 days before biochemical abnormalities. Persists during the acute illness. Usually disappears 1–13 weeks after onset of laboratory abnormalities. Is the most reliable serologic marker of HBV infection. May also be found in chronic infection. HB vaccination does not cause a positive HB_sAg. Titers are not of clinical value. Present sensitive assays detect < 1.0 ng/ml of circulating antigen, which is the level needed to find 10–15% of reactive blood donors who carry antigen but express only low levels.

Table 9-1. Increased Serum Enzyme Levels in Liver Diseases

	Acute Viral Hepatitis		Complete Biliary Obstruction		Cirrhosis		Liver Metastases	
Serum Enzyme	Frequency	Amplitude	Frequency	Amplitude	Frequency	Amplitude	Frequency	Amplitude
SGOT	>95%	14	>95%	3	75%	2	50%	1–2
SGPT	>95%	17	>95%	4	50%	1	25%	1–2
Alkaline phosphatase	60%	1–2	>95%	4–14	55%	1–2	50% 40% 80% Frequently	1–10 (tuberculosis) 1–3 (sarcoidosis) 1–14 (carcinoma) 1–20 (amyloidosis)
Leucine amino-peptidase	80%	1–2	85%	3	30%	1	70%	2–3
Isocitric dehy-drogenase	>95%	6	10%	1	20%	1	40%	2
5′-Nucleotidase	70%	1–2	>95%	6	50%	1–2	65%	3–4
Aldolase	90%	10		Normal		Normal	20%	

Frequency = average % frequency of patients with increased serum enzyme level when blood taken at optimal time.
Amplitude = average number of times normal that serum level is increased.

Table 9-2. Serum Enzymes in Differential Diagnosis of Various Liver Diseases

Disease	Alkaline Phosphatase	SGOT	SGPT	ICD
Acute viral hepatitis	N to 3 × N (15–70 BU during obstructive phase)	Both rise during preicteric phase to peaks (up to 50 × N) by the time jaundice appears; then rapid fall in several days; become normal 2–5 weeks after onset of jaundice		500–2000 units in first week; <800 units after 2 weeks; slightly elevated in third week
Alcoholic hepatitis	Rarely > 5 × N	SGOT rarely > 10 × N; SGOT/SGPT > 2:1		
Portal cirrhosis	<2 × N (5–15 BU in 40–50% of cases)	≦ 300 units in 65–75% of patients	≦200 units in 50% of patients; wide fluctuation	<500 units; poor prognosis if higher
Primary biliary cirrhosis	3–20 × N	<5 × N (≦200 units) in 90% of cases		
Cholestasis (e.g., drugs)	2–10 × N	N to 5 × N (<300 units)	N to 5 × N (<300 units)	

Incomplete biliary obstruction (or obstruction of 1 duct)	Frequently 10–14 BU (≦70 BU in 100% of patients)	
Complete biliary obstruction		
Stones*	≦10 × N	May *abruptly* rise to 10 × N
Periampullary CA*	Many × > stones	Often N
Metastatic focal disease		
Metastatic CA	≦70 BU in 80% of cases	
Tuberculosis	≦50 BU in 50% of cases	
Sarcoidosis	≦18 BU in 40% of cases	
Amyloidosis	≦100 BU frequently	

BU = Bodansky units; N = normal; CA = carcinoma.
*Serum bilirubin ≦ 20 mg/dl (mostly direct) due to CA; < 10 mg/dl due to stones causing complete biliary obstruction.

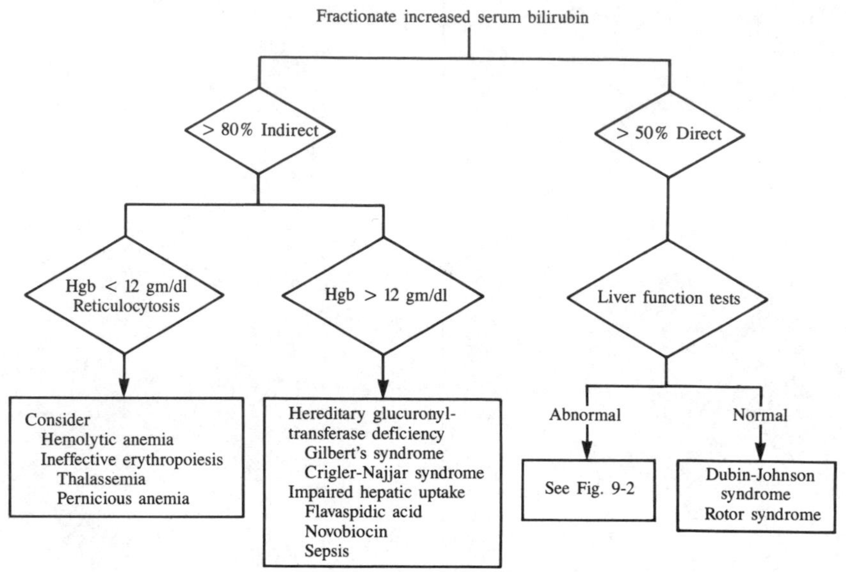

Fig. 9-1. Flow chart illustrating workup for jaundice.

HB_sAg and Blood Transfusions

Transfusion of blood containing HB_sAg causes hepatitis or appearance of HB_sAg in blood in > 70% of recipients; needle-stick from such blood causes hepatitis in 45% of cases. Transfusion of blood not containing HB_sAg caused anicteric hepatitis in 16% of recipients and icteric hepatitis in 2%.

Screening out of blood donors with HB_sAg will reduce posttransfusion hepatitis by 25–40%.

When HB_sAg carrier is discovered (e.g., in screening program), 60–80% show some evidence of hepatic damage.

Persons with a positive test for HB_sAg should never be permitted to donate blood or plasma.

HB_sAg is found in

Chronic persistent hepatitis	50%
Chronic active hepatitis	25%
Cirrhosis	3%
Prevalence in U.S.	0.25%
Multiple transfused patients	3.8%
Drug addicts	4.2%
Blood donor population	< 0.1%

Antibody to HB_sAg (Anti-HB_sAg)

Indicates clinical recovery and immunity to HBV. May also occur after transfusion by passive transfer. Found in 80% of patients after clinical cure. Appearance may take several weeks or months after HB_sAg has disappeared and after SGPT has returned to normal, causing a "serologic gap" during which time (usually 2–6 weeks) this system cannot identify patients who are recovering but may still be infectious.

In fulminant hepatitis—antibody is produced early and may coexist with low antigen titer.

In chronic carriers—no antibody is present, but antigen titers are very high.

Presence of antibody (without HB_sAg detectable) indicates recovery from HBV infection, absence of infectivity, immunity from future HBV infection, no need for gamma globulin administration if exposed to infection; this blood can be transfused. Presence can be used to show efficiency of immunization program.

Hepatitis B "e" Antigen (HB_eAg)

Indicates highly infectious state. Appears within 1 week after HB_sAg; in acute cases disappears prior to disappearance of HB_sAg; is found only when HB_sAg is found. Occurs early in disease before biochemical changes. Usually lasts 3–6 weeks. Persistence > 10 weeks suggests progression to chronic carrier state and possible chronic hepatitis.

Antibody to HB_e (Anti-HB_e)

Indicates decreasing infectivity, suggesting good prognosis for resolution of acute infection. Association with anti-HB_c in absence of HB_sAg and anti-HB_s confirms recent acute infection (2–16 weeks).

Antibody to Core Antigen–Total (Anti-HB_c-Total)

Occurs early in acute infection, 4–10 weeks after appearance of HB_sAg, at same time as clinical illness; persists for years or for lifetime. Anti-HB_c-IgM may be the only serologic marker present after HB_sAg and HB_eAg have subsided but before these antibodies have appeared; this period is called the "serologic gap" or "window."

The earliest specific anti-HB_c is IgM. This anti-HB_c-IgM is found in high titer for a short time during the acute disease stage that covers the serologic window and then declines to low levels during recovery (see Fig. 9-4). Since this is the only test unique to recent infection, it can differentiate acute from chronic HBV. It is the only serologic test that can differentiate recent and remote infection with one specimen.

Anti-HB_c detects persons who have been previously infected with HBV and can therefore serve as surrogate test for other infectious agents (e.g., NANB). Exclusion of anti-HB_c-positive donors reduces the incidence of posttransfusion hepatitis and possibly of other virus infection (e.g., AIDS) due to the frequency of dual infection. Present without other serologic markers and with normal SGOT in ~2% of routine blood donors; 70% of these are due to recovery from subclinical HBV (and may be infectious), and the rest are considered false positive. False positive anti-HB_c can be confirmed by immune response pattern to hepatitis B vaccination.

SEROLOGIC TESTS FOR VIRAL HEPATITIS D (DELTA) (HDV)*

Hepatitis D is due to a transmissible virus that depends on HBV for expression and replication. It consists of hepatitis D antigen (HDAg) within the external coat of HB_sAg. It may be found for 7–14 days in the serum during acute infection. Delta agent can be an important cause of acute or chronic hepatitis.

*Data from JH Hoofnagle, Type D (delta) hepatitis. *JAMA* 261:1321, 1989.

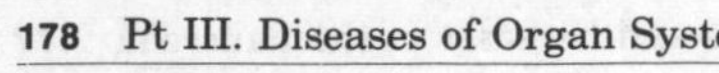

SGOT > ALP
ALP I/N
Bil I/N

Yes

Alb D
Glob I

Yes
No

LDH > 2N
or
LDH/SGOT > 2

LDH > 2N
or
LDH/SGOT > 2

Yes
No
No
Yes

Chronic active necrosis

Acute necrosis or chronic persistent inflammation

GGT/ALP > 5 : 1

GGT/ALP > 5 : 1

Yes
No
No
Yes

Alcoholic chronic liver disease

Nonalcoholic chronic liver disease

Acute hypoxic liver disease

Acute alcoholic liver disease

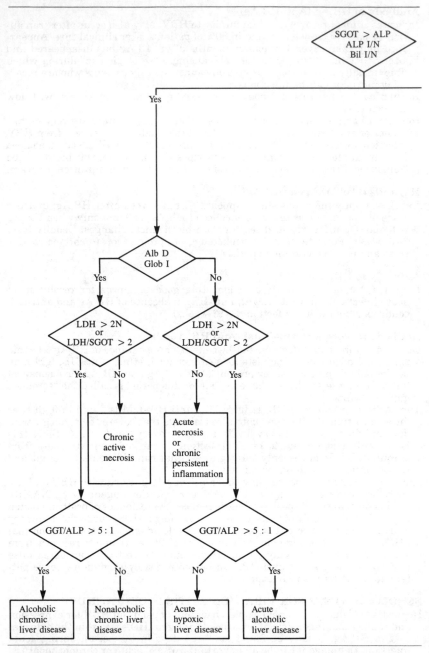

Fig. 9-2. Flow chart illustrating sequential abnormal liver function test interpretation. (N = normal; I = increased; Bil = bilirubin; Alb = albumin; glob = globulin; ALP = alkaline phosphatase. Enzymes all in same U/L.) (Adapted from JB Henry, *Clinical Diagnosis and Management by Laboratory Methods* [16th ed.]. Philadelphia: Saunders, 1979.)

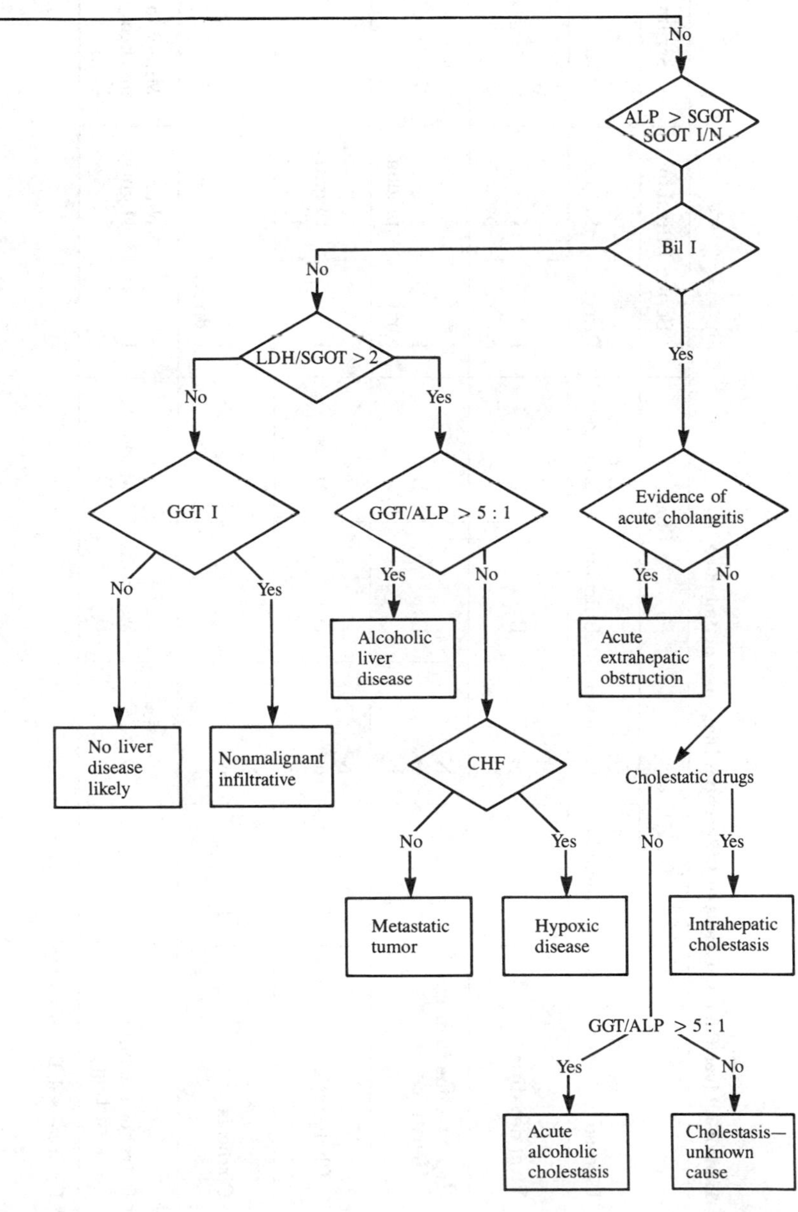
No
ALP > SGOT
SGOT I/N
Bil I
No
Yes
LDH/SGOT > 2
No
Yes
GGT I
GGT/ALP > 5 : 1
Evidence of acute cholangitis
No
Yes
Yes
No
Yes
No
Alcoholic liver disease
Acute extrahepatic obstruction
No liver disease likely
Nonmalignant infiltrative
CHF
Cholestatic drugs
No
Yes
No
Yes
Metastatic tumor
Hypoxic disease
Intrahepatic cholestasis
GGT/ALP > 5 : 1
Yes
No
Acute alcoholic cholestasis
Cholestasis—unknown cause

Table 9-3. Liver Function Tests in Differential Diagnosis of Jaundice

	Urine		Stool		Serum Bilirubin		Serum Cholesterol	
Disease	Bilirubin	Uro-bilinogen	Bilirubin	Uro-bilinogen	Direct	Indirect	Total	Esters
Viral hepatitis	I	N or I	D	D	I early	I predom.	N or D	Mildly to markedly D
Hepatitis due to drugs Hepatitic type	I	N or I	D	D	I early	I predom.	N	
Cholestatic type	I	N or D	D	D	I	Slightly I	I	
Cirrhosis	I	N or I			I < indirect	I > direct	N or D	Mildly to markedly D
Extrahepatic biliary obstruction	I	D	Markedly D	Markedly D	I	N or slightly I	Mildly to markedly I	

I = increased; D = decreased; N = normal.

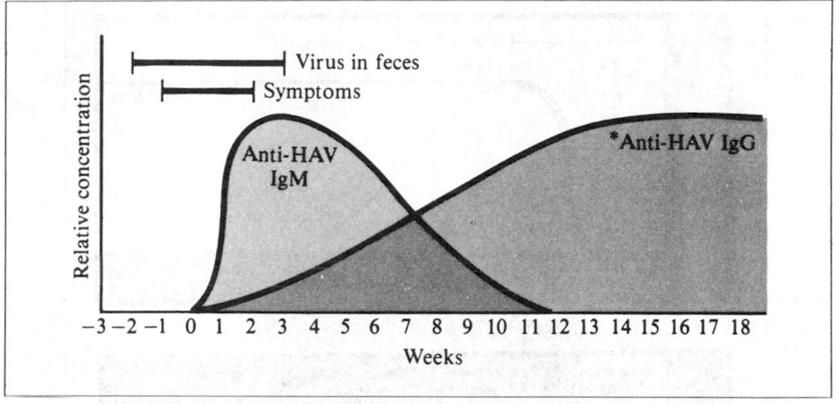

Fig. 9-3. Antibody markers in HAV. (Reproduced with permission of Abbott Laboratories, So. Pasadena, CA.)

The course depends on the presence of HBV infection. HDV hepatitis is often severe, with relatively high mortality in acute disease and frequent development of cirrhosis in chronic disease.

Coinfection means simultaneous acute HBV and acute HDV infection usually causes acute limited illness with additive liver damage due to each virus followed by recovery. Usually is self-limited; < 5% become chronic. Serum HDAg and HDV-RNA appear during incubation period after HB_sAg and before rise in SGOT, which often shows a biphasic elevation. HB_sAg and HDAg are transient; HDAg resolves with clearance of HB_sAg. Anti-HDV appears soon after clinical symptoms, but titer is often low and short-lived.

Superinfection means acute HDV infection in a chronic HBV carrier. > 80% develop chronic hepatitis. Serum anti-HDV appears and rises to high sustained titers, indicating continuing replication of HDV; intrahepatic HDAg is present. HDV-RNA persists in low titers.

Diagnosis of HDV hepatitis by presence of serum anti-HDV in patient with HB_sAg-positive hepatitis.

Acute coinfection is distinguished from superinfection by presence of serum anti-HB_c-IgM, which indicates acute HBV.

Chronic HDV infection shows presence of HB_sAg and high titer of anti-HDV in serum (radioimmunoassay [RIA] titer > 1 : 100 suggests chronic HDV hepatitis). Confirm by liver biopsy showing HDAg by immunofluorescence or immunoperoxidase.

New tests that will become available:

- Serum anti-HDV-IgM will document acute HDV infection; low levels will remain in persistent infection.
- Western blot can demonstrate serum HDAg when RIA is negative. Persistence correlates with development of chronic HDV hepatitis and viral antigen in liver biopsy.
- DNA probe for HDV-RNA in serum to monitor HDV replication.

Serum anti-HDV may be sought in patients with HB_sAg-positive chronic or acute hepatitis in high-risk group or with severe disease or with biphasic acute hepatitis or acute onset in chronic hepatitis.

In populations positive for HB_sAg, a high prevalence of HDV markers is found in drug addicts (43%) and hemophiliacs (25%) but not in homosexual men

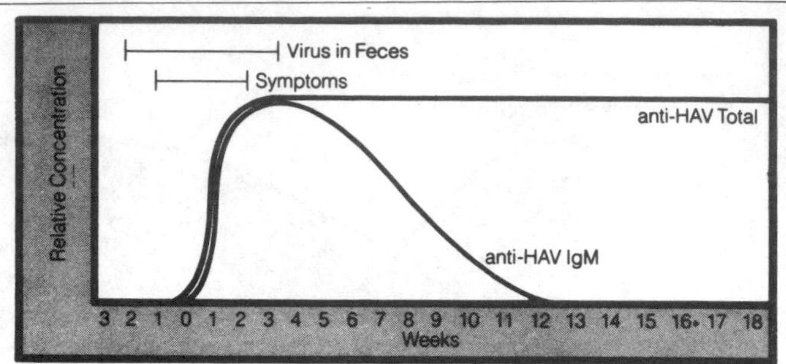

Virus in Feces
Symptoms
anti-HAV Total
anti-HAV IgM
Relative Concentration
3 2 1 0 1 2 3 4 5 6 7 8 9 10 11 12 13 14 15 16 17 18
Weeks

A

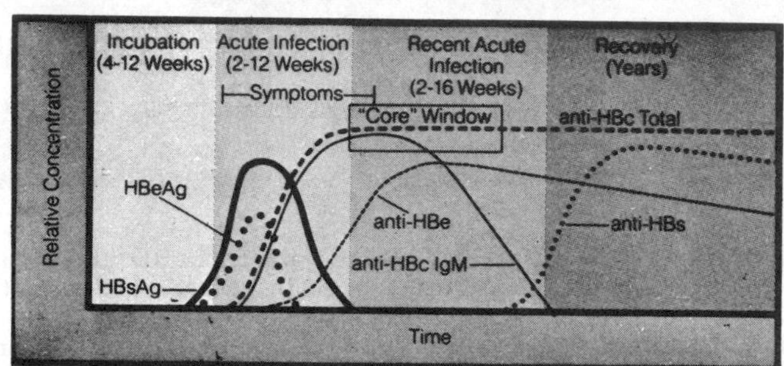

Incubation (4-12 Weeks)
Acute Infection (2-12 Weeks)
Recent Acute Infection (2-16 Weeks)
Recovery (Years)
Symptoms
"Core" Window
anti-HBc Total
HBeAg
anti-HBe
anti-HBs
anti-HBc IgM
HBsAg
Relative Concentration
Time

B

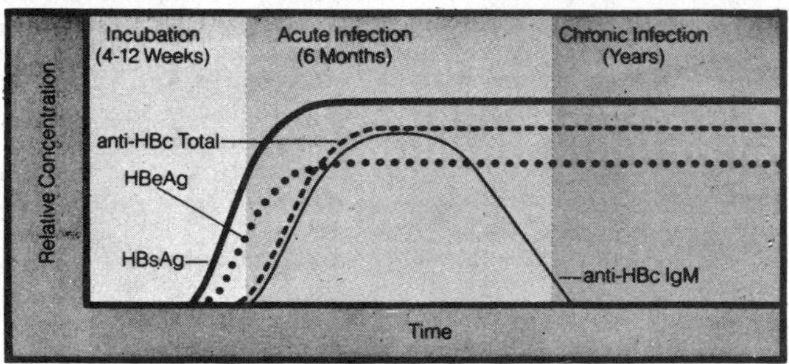

Incubation (4-12 Weeks)
Acute Infection (6 Months)
Chronic Infection (Years)
anti-HBc Total
HBeAg
HBsAg
anti-HBc IgM
Relative Concentration
Time

C

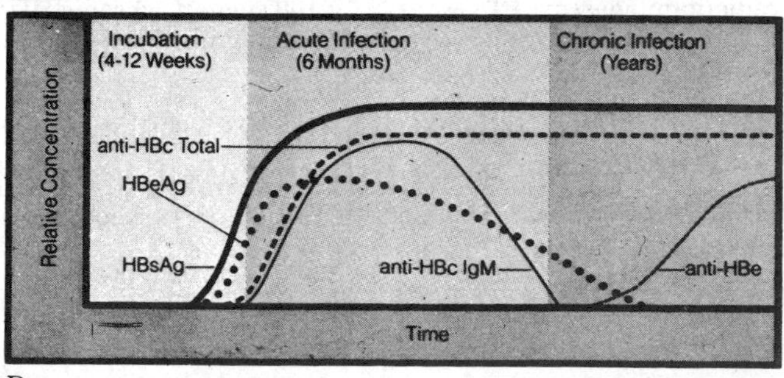

Incubation (4-12 Weeks)
Acute Infection (6 Months)
Chronic Infection (Years)
anti-HBc Total
HBeAg
HBsAg
anti-HBc IgM
anti-HBe
Relative Concentration
Time

D

Table 9-4. Serologic Diagnosis of Acute Viral Hepatitis

Test			
HB_sAg	Anti-HB_c-IgM	Anti-HAV-IgM	Interpretation
−	−	+	Recent HAV infection
+	+	−	Acute HBV infection
+	−	−	Early acute HBV infection or chronic HBV
−	+	−	Confirms recent HBV infection
−	−	−	Hepatitis C, or other causes of hepatitis (e.g., infectious mononucleosis, cytomegalovirus), or liver toxins
+	+	+	Recent HAV and simultaneous acute HBV (uncommon pattern)

If diagnosis is HBV, further testing should be done.

(< 1%); 8% of commercial blood donors and 4% of volunteer donors had such markers. Detection of HDAg is not a practical method; commercial testing for anti-HDV-total and anti-HDV-IgM will soon become available in kit form.

ANTIBODY TO HEPATITIS C VIRUS (ANTI-HCV)

Very specific for hepatitis C virus (HCV). Sensitivity ~80% in chronic carriers; ~15% for first 6 months following acute HCV infection. Is not seen until 2–6 months after infection or 2–3 months after increase in SGOT, so serial specimens (as well as SGOT) may be needed for diagnosis.

Present in 70–85% of cases of chronic posttransfusion NANB hepatitis but is relatively infrequent in acute cases.

Present in 20% of donors with anti-HB_c or increased SGOT and in > 60% of donors who transmitted NANB hepatitis. Only one-third of anti-HCV donors had increased SGOT and 54% were positive for anti-HB_c. Thus surrogate markers fail to detect one-third to one-half of blood units positive for anti-HCV. Found in 7–10% of transfusion recipients.

Present in 6% of patients with autoimmune chronic active hepatitis.

Prevalence in normal blood donors is 0.5–2.0%. In routine blood donor screening, it is estimated that 40–70% of initial reactors will prove not to be true positives.

In one study, anti-HCV was positive in 75% of patients with hepatocellular carcinoma, 56% of patients with cirrhosis, and 7% of controls.

Fig. 9-4. Hepatitis serological profiles. A. Antibody response to hepatitis A. B. Hepatitis B core window identification. C, D. Hepatitis B chronic carrier profiles: no seroconversion (C); late seroconversion (D). (Reproduced with permission of Hepatitis Information Center, Abbott Laboratories, Abbott Park, IL.)

Table 9-5. Serologic Tests for Viral Hepatitis B (HBV)

Test						
HB_sAg	Anti-HB_s	HB_eAg	Anti-HB_e	Anti-HB_c-Total	Anti-HB_c-IgM	Interpretation
+	–	–	–	–	–	Late incubation or early acute HBV
+	–	+	–	–	–	Early acute HBV
+	–	+	–	+	+	Acute HBV
+	–	–	+	+	+	"Serologic window/gap" or acute HBV
–	–	–	–	+	+	Serologic gap
–	–	–	+	+	+	Convalescence
–	+	–	+	+	+	Early recovery
–	+	–	+	+	–	Recovery[a]
+	–	±	±	+	–	Chronic infection (chronic carrier)[a]
–	+	–	–	–	–	Old previous HBV with recovery and immunity or HBV vaccination or passive transfer antibody[b]
–	–	–	–	–	–	Not HBV infection

[a] Chronic carriers of HBV may have clinical hepatitis due to non-A, non-B hepatitis rather than HBV.
[b] Various serologic patterns may occur following blood transfusion or injection of immune (gamma) globulin by passive transfer. Anti-HB_s can be found for up to 6–8 months after injection of high-titer HB immunoglobulin because of 25-day half-life.

Table 9-6. Serologic Diagnosis of HBV/HDV Hepatitis

Test				
HB_sAg	Anti-HB_c-IgM	Anti-D-IgM	Anti-D-IgG	Interpretation
Transient +	+ High titer	Transient +	Transient low titer	Acute HBV and acute HDV[a]
Transient decrease due to inhibitory effect of HDV on HBV synthesis	Negative or low titers	High titer first, low titer later	Increasing titers	Acute HDV and chronic HBV[b]
May remain + in chronic HBV	Replaced by anti-HB_c-IgG in chronic HBV	+ correlates with HDAg in hepatocytes	High titers correlate with active infection; may remain + for years after infection resolves	Chronic HDV and chronic HBV[c]

[a] Clinically resembles acute viral hepatitis; fulminant hepatitis is rare, and progression to chronic hepatitis is unlikely. If HBV does not resolve, HDV can continue to replicate indefinitely.
[b] Clinically resembles exacerbation of chronic liver disease or of fulminant hepatitis with liver failure.
[c] Clinically resembles chronic liver disease progressing to cirrhosis.

Table 9-7. Comparison of Acute HDV Coinfection and Superinfection

	Coinfection	Superinfection
HBV infection	Acute	Chronic
HDV infection	Acute	Acute to chronic
Chronicity rate	< 5%	> 80%
Serum HB_sAg	Transient positive	Usually persistent
Serum anti-HB_c-IgM	Positive	Negative
Serum anti-HDV	May be transient positive	Usually persistent
Serum anti-HDV-IgM	Transient positive	Usually persistent
Serum HDV-RNA	Transient positive	Usually persistent
Liver HDAg	Transient positive	Usually persistent

Disorders of the Liver, Gallbladder, Biliary Tree, and Pancreas

ACUTE VIRAL HEPATITIS

In the U.S., about 60% of acute viral hepatitis is type B (HBV), about 20% is type A (HAV), and about 20% is non-A, non-B (NANB).

Prodromal Period

Serologic markers appear in serum.
Bilirubinuria occurs before serum bilirubin increases.
There is an increase in urinary urobilinogen and total serum bilirubin just before clinical jaundice occurs.
Serum SGOT and SGPT both rise during the preicteric phase and show very high peaks (> 500 units) by the time jaundice appears.
ESR is normal.
Leukopenia (lymphopenia and neutropenia) is noted with onset of fever, followed by relative lymphocytosis and monocytosis; may find plasma cells and < 10% atypical lymphocytes (in infectious mononucleosis is > 10%).

Asymptomatic Hepatitis

Biochemical evidence of acute hepatitis is scant and often absent.

Acute Icteric Period

(tests show parenchymal cell damage)

Serum bilirubin is 50–75% direct in the early stage; later, indirect bilirubin is proportionately more.
Serum SGOT and SGPT fall rapidly in the several days after jaundice appears and become normal 2–5 weeks later.
In *hepatitis associated with infectious mononucleosis,* peak levels are usually < 200 units, and peak occurs 2–3 weeks after onset, becoming normal by the fifth week. *In toxic hepatitis,* levels depend on severity; slight elevations may be associated with therapy with anticoagulants, anovulatory drugs, etc.; poisoning (e.g., carbon tetrachloride) may cause levels ≤ 300 units. *In severe toxic hepatitis (especially carbon tetrachloride poisoning),* serum enzymes may be 10–20 times higher than in acute hepatitis and show a different pattern, i.e., increase in lactic dehydrogenase (LDH) > SGOT > SGPT. *In acute hepatitis,* SGPT > SGOT > LDH.
Serum aldolase is increased in 90% of patients, ≤ 10 times normal. It parallels transaminase with a sharp rise before serum bilirubin and a return to normal 2–3 weeks after jaundice begins.
Serum isocitric dehydrogenase (ICD) is usually elevated in the early stage (5–10 times normal) but returns to normal in 2–3 weeks; increase persists in chronic hepatitis.
Other liver function tests are often abnormal, depending on severity of the disease—e.g., bilirubinuria, abnormal serum protein electrophoresis, alkaline phosphatase
Serum cholesterol-ester ratio is usually depressed early; total serum cholesterol is decreased only in severe disease.
Serum phospholipids are increased in mild but decreased in severe hepatitis.
Plasma vitamin A is decreased in severe hepatitis.
Urine urobilinogen is increased in the early icteric period; at peak of the disease it disappears for days or weeks; urobilinogen simultaneously disappears from stool.
Erythrocyte sedimentation rate (ESR) is increased; falls during convalescence.

Serum iron is often increased.

Urine: Cylindruria is common; albuminuria occurs occasionally; concentrating ability is sometimes decreased.

In acute viral hepatitis B, very high SGOT and serum bilirubin are not reliable indicators of patient's clinical course, but prolonged PT, especially > 20 seconds, indicates the likely development of acute hepatic insufficiency; therefore the PT should be performed when patient is first seen. Triad of prolonged PT, increased polymorphonuclear leukocytes (PMN), and nonpalpable liver is omen of massive hepatic necrosis and likely development of coma.

Acute viral hepatitis B completely resolves in 90% of patients within 12 weeks with disappearance of HB_sAg and development of anti-HB_s. Up to 10% of patients have disease for > 6 months (chronic hepatitis); 70% of these have benign chronic persistent hepatitis and 30% have chronic active hepatitis that can progress to cirrhosis and liver failure (see Table 9-8). Fulminant hepatitis occurs in 1–2% of patients with HBV, and 90% die within 2–4 weeks. Relapse, usually within 1 year, has been recognized in 20% of patients by some elevation of SGOT and changes in liver biopsy.

Defervescent Period

Diuresis occurs at onset of convalescence.

Bilirubinuria disappears while serum bilirubin is still increased.

Urine urobilinogen increases.

Serum bilirubin becomes normal after 3–6 weeks.

ESR falls.

Anicteric Hepatitis

Laboratory findings are the same as in the icteric type, but abnormalities are usually less marked and there is slight or no increase of serum bilirubin.

Acute Fulminant Hepatitis With Hepatic Failure

Develops in ~1–3% of adults with acute icteric type B hepatitis with resultant death.

Findings are the same as in acute hepatitis but more severe.

There are findings of hepatic failure (see p. 205).

Serum bilirubin is very high unless death occurs in the prodromal period.

Serum cholesterol and esters are markedly decreased.

Aminoaciduria occurs.

Patient may show anemia, leukocytosis, thrombocytopenia, etc.

Serologic markers are similar in cases of typical acute hepatitis, but seroconversion from HB_eAg to anti-HB_e or from HB_sAg to anti-HB_s is uncommon. As patient deteriorates, titers of HB_sAg and HB_eAg may often fall and disappear.

Cholangiolitic Hepatitis

Same as acute hepatitis, but evidence of obstruction is more prominent (e.g., increased serum alkaline phosphatase and direct serum bilirubin), and tests of parenchymal damage are less marked (e.g., SGOT increase may be 3–6 times normal).

Chronic Hepatitis

(see Table 9-8)

Occurs in 5–10% of adults with acute HBV.

HBV hepatitis is generally divided into three stages:

1. Stage of acute hepatitis: usually lasts 1–6 months with mild or no symptoms.

   SGOT and SGPT are increased > tenfold.

Table 9-8. Two Forms of Chronic Hepatitis

	Chronic Active Liver Disease		Benign Persistent Hepatitis	
Synonyms	Lupoid hepatitis, subacute hepatitis, plasma cell hepatitis, chronic active hepatitis, chronic liver disease in young women, autoimmune hepatitis, juvenile cirrhosis, chronic aggressive hepatitis, active chronic hepatitis		Chronic persistent hepatitis, chronic lobular hepatitis, chronic portal hepatitis, triaditis, transaminitis, unresolved hepatitis	
Criteria for diagnosis	After 12 weeks of hepatitis, tenfold increase in SGOT or fivefold increase in SGOT, with a twofold increase in gamma globulin			
		% of Patients		*% of Patients*
Laboratory abnormalities in serum	Increase in SGOT	100	Increase in SGOT may be stable or fluctuate widely, from < 6 times normal to > 10 times normal	75
	Increase in gamma globulin	90	Other liver function tests are near normal	10
	Increase in alkaline phosphatase	90	Twofold increase in alkaline phosphatase	50
	Increase in bilirubin	90		
	Increase in immunoglobulin G	80		
	Smooth muscle antibody	80		

	Prolonged prothrombin time	50		
	Increase in immunoglobulin M	50	Increase in bilirubin ≦ 4 mg/dl	20
	Decrease in albumin	50	Increase in gamma globulin twofold	50
	Increase in immunoglobulin A	33		
	Antinuclear antibody	33		
	Antisalmonella antibody	33		
	Antimitochondrial antibody	20		
	HB_sAg	10–60	HB_sAg	≦50
	Laboratory findings of associated diseases (e.g., Hashimoto's thyroiditis, Sjögren's syndrome, primary biliary cirrhosis, pernicious anemia, idiopathic thrombocytopenic purpura)	25	No associated autoimmune diseases present	
Liver biopsy	Different histologic criteria for diagnosis of each condition			
Laboratory findings of sequelae	Cirrhosis, portal hypertension, or liver failure may occur; primary hepatocellular carcinoma is uncommon in U.S. but very important elsewhere		Do not occur	

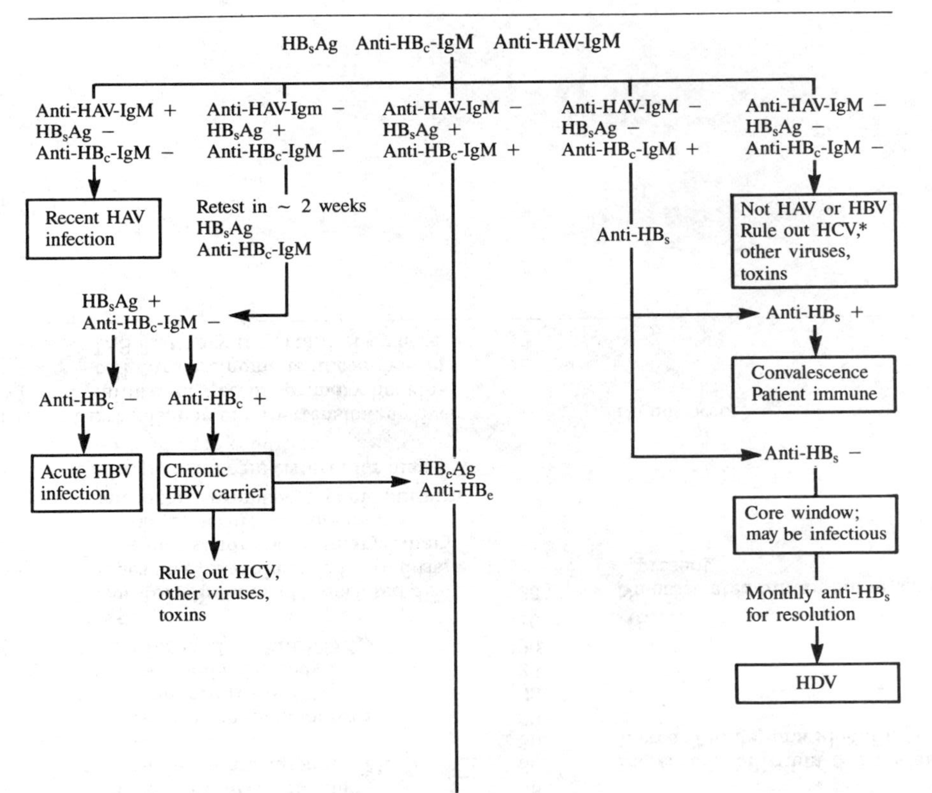

HB_sAg Anti-HB_c-IgM Anti-HAV-IgM
Anti-HAV-IgM + HB_sAg − Anti-HB_c-IgM −
Anti-HAV-Igm − HB_sAg + Anti-HB_c-IgM −
Anti-HAV-IgM − HB_sAg + Anti-HB_c-IgM +
Anti-HAV-IgM − HB_sAg − Anti-HB_c-IgM +
Anti-HAV-IgM − HB_sAg − Anti-HB_c-IgM −
Recent HAV infection
Retest in ~ 2 weeks HB_sAg Anti-HB_c-IgM
HB_sAg + Anti-HB_c-IgM −
Anti-HB_c −
Anti-HB_c +
Acute HBV infection
Chronic HBV carrier
Rule out HCV, other viruses, toxins
HB_eAg Anti-HB_e
Anti-HB_s
Not HAV or HBV Rule out HCV,* other viruses, toxins
Anti-HB_s +
Convalescence Patient immune
Anti-HB_s −
Core window; may be infectious
Monthly anti-HB_s for resolution
HDV

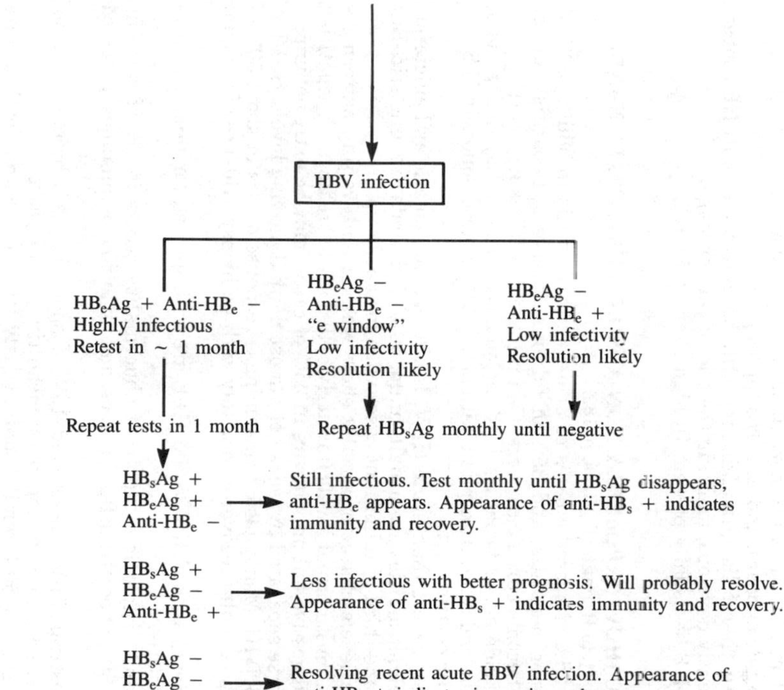

*Do anti-HCV (see pp. 183, 186).

Fig. 9-5. Flow chart illustrating use of serologic tests for diagnosis of acute hepatitis.

Serum bilirubin is usually normal or only slightly increased.
HB_sAg gradually arises to high titers and persists; HB_eAg also appears.
Gradually merges with next stage.

2. Stage of chronic hepatitis: transaminases increased > 50% for > 6 months' duration; may last only 1 year or for several decades with mild or severe symptoms; most cases resolve, but some develop cirrhosis and liver failure.
   SGOT and SGPT fall to 2–10 times normal range.
   HB_sAg usually remains high, and HB_eAg remains present.
3. Chronic carrier stage: are usually, but not always, healthy and asymptomatic.
   SGOT and SGPT fall to normal or < 2 times normal.
   HB_eAg disappears, and anti-HB_e appears.
   HB_sAg titer falls although may still be detectable; anti-HB_s subsequently develops, marking the end of carrier stage.
   Anti-HB_c is usually present in high titer (> 1 : 512).

HEPATITIS C (HCV) (FORMERLY NON-A, NON-B HEPATITIS [NANB])

(see also Antibody to Hepatitis C Virus, p. 183)

Causes up to 25% of sporadic cases of acute viral hepatitis in adults, 90% of posttransfusion hepatitis, and 35% of fulminant cases of hepatitis. 50% of acute cases become chronic carriers. Can remain infectious for years.

Should be considered in hepatitis in drug addicts, hemophilia, thalassemia, hemodialysis, and renal transplant patients. 3–7% of blood donors in U.S. are asymptomatic carriers.

Typically is less severe than acute HBV. Is often asymptomatic and anicteric.

Biochemical abnormalities are usually mild; 50% of patients are anicteric. But may cause one-third of fulminant cases with mortality up to 90%.

Transaminase levels characteristically show waxing and waning pattern returning to almost normal levels (formerly called acute "relapsing" hepatitis); is highly suggestive but only occurs in 25% of cases; may be extreme, unpredictable course separated by weeks of almost normal enzyme levels. SGPT is usually < 800 IU. Monophasic transaminase response occurs in about 50% of patients, who usually recover completely with no biopsy evidence of residual disease.

Anicteric patients with SGPT > 300 IU/L are at high risk for progressing to chronic hepatitis.

Biochemical and histologic evidence of abnormality occurs in 7% of sporadic cases, up to 60% of posttransfusion cases, and up to 80% of immunosuppressed patients.

40–60% of posttransfusion cases and 10% of sporadic cases become chronic. Cirrhosis develops in ~20% of cases; mean time = 17 years.

In chronic disease, > 50% remit spontaneously within 3 years; death is rare due to chronic disease. Appreciable risk for development of hepatocellular carcinoma; mean time = 20 years.

FATTY LIVER

Laboratory findings are due to underlying conditions (most commonly alcoholism; also diabetes mellitus, poor nutritional state, toxic chemicals).

Needle biopsy of liver establishes the diagnosis.

Liver function tests are normal in at least 50% of patients; others may show abnormalities of one or several tests, including clinical jaundice.

Mild anemia and increased WBC may occur.

Not infrequently, fatty liver is the only postmortem finding in cases of sudden, unexpected death.

ALCOHOLIC HEPATITIS

Increased serum GGT and mean corpuscular volume (MCV) > 100 together or separately are useful clues for occult alcoholism.

SGOT is increased (rarely > 300 IU), but SGPT is normal or only slightly elevated. SGOT and SGPT are more specific but less sensitive than GGT. Levels of SGOT and SGPT do not correlate with severity of liver disease.

SGOT/SGPT ratio > 1 associated with SGOT < 300 mU/ml will identify 90% of patients with alcoholic liver disease; is particularly useful for differentiation from viral hepatitis, in which increase of SGOT and SGPT are about the same.

In acute alcoholic hepatitis, GGT level is usually higher than SGOT level. GGT is often abnormal in alcoholics even with normal liver histology. Is more useful as index of occult alcoholism or to indicate that elevated serum alkaline phosphatase is of bone or liver origin than to follow course of patient for which SGOT and SGPT are most useful.

Serum alkaline phosphatase may be normal or increased and is not useful as a diagnostic test.

Serum bilirubin is not useful as a diagnostic test. However, if bilirubin continues to increase during a week of therapy in the hospital, it indicates a poor prognosis.

Decreased serum albumin means long-standing or relatively severe disease. Decreased serum albumin and increased serum globulin (polyclonal) are frequent.

Increased IgA

Increased PT that is not corrected by parenteral administration of 10 mg/day of vitamin K for 3 days is best indicator of poor prognosis.

Increased WBC (> 15,000) in up to one-third of patients with shift to left (WBC is decreased in viral hepatitis); normal WBC may indicate folic acid depletion.

Anemia in > 50% of patients may be macrocytic (folic acid or vitamin B_{12} deficiency), microcytic (iron or pyridoxine deficiency), mixed, or hemolytic.

Metabolic alkalosis may occur due to K^+ loss with pH normal or increased, but pH < 7.2 often indicates disease is becoming terminal.

In terminal stage (last week before death) of chronic alcoholic liver disease, there is often decrease of serum sodium and albumin and increase of PT and serum bilirubin; SGOT and LDH decrease from previously elevated levels.

Indocyanine green (50 mg/kg) is abnormal in 90% of patients.

Liver biopsy should be done in any alcoholic with enlarged liver as the only way to make definite diagnosis of alcoholic hepatitis. Many have normal liver biopsy; others show characteristic alcoholic hyalin.

Compared to nonalcoholics, alcoholics as a group show an increase in a number of blood components (e.g., SGOT, phosphorus, alkaline phosphatase, GGT, MCV, mean corpuscular hemoglobin [MCH], hemoglobin, WBC) and a decrease in others (e.g., total protein, urea nitrogen [BUN]); however these variations usually remain within the reference range. These changes may last for > 6 weeks after abstaining from alcohol.

COMPARISON OF CHOLESTATIC AND HEPATOCELLULAR JAUNDICE

	Hepatocellular	**Cholestasis**	**Infiltration**
Disease example	Acute viral hepatitis	Common duct stone	Metastatic tumor
Serum bilirubin (mg/dl)	4–8	6–20*	Usually < 4, often normal

*Serum bilirubin > 10 mg/dl is rarely seen with common duct stone and usually indicates carcinoma.

SGOT, SGPT (IU/ml)	Markedly increased, often 500–1000	May be slightly increased < 200	May be slightly increased < 100
Serum alkaline phosphatase	1–2 times normal	3–5 times normal*	2–4 times normal
Prothrombin time	Increased in severe disease	Increased in chronic cases	Normal
Response to parenteral vitamin K	No	Yes	—

Occasionally SGOT and LDH are markedly increased in biliary obstruction or liver cancer.

CHOLESTASIS

Increased serum alkaline phosphatase
Increased 5′-nucleotidase and LAP parallel alkaline phosphatase and confirm the hepatic source of alkaline phosphatase.
Increased GGT (also increased in many other conditions; see pp. 57–58)
Increased serum cholesterol and phospholipids but not triglycerides
Increased fasting serum bile acid (> 1.5 μg/ml) with ratio of cholic acid–chenodeoxycholic acid > 1 in primary biliary cirrhosis and many intrahepatic cholestatic conditions but < 1 in most chronic hepatocellular conditions (e.g., Laennec's cirrhosis, chronic active hepatitis). *(There is relatively little experience with this test.)*

Cholestasis may occur without hyperbilirubinemia.

Due To

Canalicular

Drugs (e.g., estrogens, anabolic steroids)—most common cause (see Table 9-9)
Normal pregnancy
Alcoholic hepatitis
Acute viral hepatitis
Sickle cell crisis
Postoperative state following long procedure and multiple transfusions
Benign recurrent familial intrahepatic cholestasis—rare condition
Hodgkin's disease (some cases)
Gram-negative sepsis

Interlobular Bile Ducts

Sclerosing pericholangitis (associated with inflammatory bowel disease)
Primary biliary cirrhosis
Postnecrotic cirrhosis (20% of cases)
Congenital intrahepatic biliary atresia

Interlobular and Larger Intrahepatic Bile Ducts

Multifocal lesions (e.g., metastases, lymphomas, granulomas)

Larger Intrahepatic Bile Ducts

Sclerosing cholangitis
Intraductal stones
Intraductal papillomatosis

*Increased serum alkaline phosphatase < 3 times normal in 15% of patients with extrahepatic biliary obstruction, especially if obstruction is incomplete or due to benign conditions.

Table 9-9. Comparison of Three Main Types of Liver Disease Due to Drugs

	Predominantly Cholestatic	Predominantly Hepatitic	Mixed Biochemical Pattern
Laboratory findings	Obstructive type of jaundice (see pp. 194, 196)		Some aspects of each type, but one may be more marked
	Average duration of jaundice = 2 weeks; may last for years		
	Serum bilirubin may be > 30 mg/dl		
	Alkaline phosphatase and LAP are markedly increased; may remain increased for years after jaundice has disappeared	Less markedly increased	
	SGOT, SGPT, LDH show mild to moderate increase	More markedly increased	
Some causative drugs	Organic arsenicals	Cinchophen	Phenytoin
	Anabolic steroids*	Monoamine oxidase inhibitors (particularly iproniazid)	Phenylbutazone
	Estrogens*		
	Sulfonylurea derivatives (including sulfonamides, phenothiazine tranquilizers, antidiabetic drugs, oral diuretics)	Isonicotinic acid hydrazide	Para-Aminosalicylic acid (PAS) and other anti-tuberculosis agents
	Antithyroid drugs (e.g., methimazole)		
	Chlorpromazine		
	PAS (usually this type but may be mixed)		
	Erythromycin		
Pathology	Centrilobular bile stasis	Same as acute viral hepatitis	
	Low incidence		
	High mortality (20%)		

*Alkaline phosphatase, SGOT, and SGPT are not increased as much compared with other drugs.

Cholangiocarcinoma
Caroli's disease (congenital biliary ectasia)

Extrahepatic Ducts (Surgical or Extrahepatic Jaundice)
Carcinoma (e.g., pancreas, ampulla, bile ducts, gallbladder)
Stricture, stone, cyst, etc., of ducts
Pancreatitis (acute, chronic), pseudocysts

CIRRHOSIS OF LIVER

Serum bilirubin is often increased; may be present for years. Fluctuations may reflect liver status due to insults to the liver (e.g., alcoholic debauches). Most bilirubin is of the indirect type unless cirrhosis is of the cholangiolitic type. Higher and more stable levels occur in postnecrotic cirrhosis; lower and more fluctuating levels occur in Laennec's cirrhosis. Terminal icterus may be constant and severe.

Serum SGOT is increased (≤ 300 units) in 65–75% of patients. Serum SGPT is increased (≤ 200 units) in 50% of patients. Transaminases vary widely and reflect activity or progression of the process (i.e., hepatic parenchymal cell necrosis).

Serum ICD is normal or only slightly increased (< 500 units) in 20% of patients. A large increase suggests a poorer prognosis.

Serum 5′-nucleotidase is increased in 50% of patients.

Serum alkaline phosphatase is increased (≤ 15 Bodansky units) in 40–50% of patients.

Serum LAP is slightly increased in 30% of patients.

Total serum protein is usually normal or decreased. Serum albumin parallels functional status of parenchymal cells and may be useful for following progress of liver disease; but it may be normal in the presence of considerable liver cell damage. Lowering of serum albumin may reflect development of ascites or hemorrhage. Serum globulin level is usually increased; it reflects inflammation and parallels the severity of the inflammation. Increased serum globulin (usually gamma) may cause increased total protein, especially in chronic (viral) hepatitis and posthepatitic cirrhosis.

Total serum cholesterol is normal or decreased. Decreased esters reflect more severe parenchymal cell damage. Urine bilirubin is increased; urobilinogen is normal or increased.

Laboratory findings due to complications or sequelae
- Ascites
- Bleeding esophageal varices
- Hypersplenism
- Hepatoma
- Portal vein thrombosis
- Hepatic coma

BUN is often decreased (< 10 mg/dl); increased with GI hemorrhage.

Serum uric acid is often increased.

Electrolytes and acid-base balance are often abnormal and reflect various combinations of circumstances at the time, such as malnutrition, dehydration, hemorrhage, metabolic acidosis, respiratory alkalosis. In cirrhosis with ascites, the kidney retains increased sodium and excessive water, causing dilutional hyponatremia.

Anemia reflects increased plasma volume and some increased destruction of RBCs. If more severe, rule out hemorrhage in GI tract, folic acid deficiency, excessive hemolysis, etc.

WBC is usually normal with active cirrhosis; increased (≤ 50,000/cu mm) with massive necrosis, hemorrhage, etc.; decreased with hypersplenism.

Blood ammonia level is increased in liver coma and cirrhosis and with portacaval shunting of blood.

Abnormalities of coagulation mechanisms

- Prolonged PT (does not respond to parenteral vitamin K as frequently as in patients with obstructive jaundice)
- Abnormal thromboplastin generation test (TGT) reflecting various abnormalities

Biopsy of liver is valuable.

Laboratory findings due to associated diseases or conditions

- Alcoholism
- Wilson's disease
- Hemochromatosis
- Mucoviscidosis
- Glycogen-storage diseases
- Galactosemia
- Alpha$_1$ antitrypsin deficiency
- Porphyria
- Fructose intolerance
- Tyrosinosis
- Schistosomiasis
- Gaucher's disease
- Ulcerative colitis
- Osler-Weber-Rendu disease

PRIMARY BILIARY CIRRHOSIS (CHOLANGIOLITIC CIRRHOSIS, HANOT'S HYPERTROPHIC CIRRHOSIS, CHRONIC NONSUPPURATIVE DESTRUCTIVE CHOLANGITIS)

Laboratory findings of cholestatic pattern of long duration (may last for years) associated with antimitochondrial antibodies make the diagnosis likely; patency of bile ducts should be confirmed (e.g., with ultrasound or CT scan).

Serum bilirubin is normal in early phase but increases in 60% of patients with progression of disease and is a reliable prognostic indicator; an elevated level is a poor prognostic sign. Direct serum bilirubin is increased in 80% of patients; levels > 5 mg/dl in only 20% of patients; levels > 10 mg/dl in only 6% of patients. Indirect bilirubin is normal or slightly increased.

Serum alkaline phosphatase is markedly increased; in 50% of cases, > 70 King-Armstrong units (normal is ≤ 13). Be wary of making this diagnosis with values < 40. Reaches a plateau early in the course and then fluctuates within 20% thereafter; changes in serum level have no prognostic value. 5′-Nucleotidase and GGT parallel the alkaline phosphatase. This is one of the few conditions that will elevate both serum alkaline phosphatase and GGT to striking levels.

Serum IgM is increased in ~75% of patients; levels may be very high (4–5 times normal). Other serum immunoglobulins are also increased.

Serum mitochondrial antibody titer is strongly positive in 90–95% of patients (1 : 40–1 : 80); similar titers occur in 5% of patients with chronic hepatitis; low titers occur in 10% of patients with other liver disease. Many other circulating antibodies are present (e.g., antinuclear [ANA], antithyroid) although not useful diagnostically.

Biopsy of liver categorizes the four stages and helps assess prognosis, but needle biopsy is subject to sampling error since the lesions may be spotty; findings consistent with all four stages may be found in one specimen.

Marked increase in total cholesterol and phospholipids with normal triglycerides; serum is not lipemic; serum triglycerides become elevated in late stages. Associated with xanthomas and xanthelasmas. In early stages, LDL and VLDL are mildly elevated and HDL is markedly elevated (thus atherosclerosis is rare). In advanced stage, LDL is markedly elevated with decreased HDL and lipoprotein-X.

Table 9-10. Serum Protein Electrophoretic Patterns in Various Diseases*

Condition	Total Protein	Albumin	Alpha$_1$ Globulin	Alpha$_2$ Globulin	Beta Globulin	Gamma Globulin	Comment
Multiple myeloma	I	D	Dyscrasia of beta$_{2A}$ or gamma$_2$ Ig				Total globulin, marked I Variable location of M globulin
Macroglobulinemia	I	D	Dyscrasia of beta$_{2M}$			Marked I	Electrophoresis same as multiple myeloma
Hodgkin's disease	D	D	I	I		V	
Lymphatic leukemia and lymphoma		D			D	D	
Myelogenous and monocytic leukemia	D	D			D	I	Gamma globulin to differentiate types of acute leukemias
Hypogammaglobulinemia	D	N	N	N	N	D	
Analbuminemia	Marked D	Marked D	N	I	I	I	
Gastrointestinal diseases							
Peptic ulcer	D	D	May be I	May be I			

Ulcerative colitis	D	D	May be I	May be I	D		
Protein-losing enteropathy		Marked D	I	I		D	
Acute cholecystitis	D	D				N	
Nephrosis	D	D		D	D, I(N)	D(N, I)	Typical pattern
Chronic glomerulonephritis	D	D	N	I	N	N	
Laennec's cirrhosis	D, N, I	D	N	D	Characteristic pattern of beta-gamma "bridging"		
Acute viral hepatitis	D, N	D	D (means acute hepato-cellular damage)	D	D	V, I	
Stress		D	I	I			"Three-fingered" pattern
Hypersensitivity						I	
Sarcoidosis	I	D			Stepwise increase of alpha$_2$, beta, and gamma		"Sarcoid steps" help differentiate from other lung disease

Table 9-10 (continued)

Condition	Total Protein	Albumin	Alpha$_1$ Globulin	Alpha$_2$ Globulin	Beta Globulin	Gamma Globulin	Comment
Collagen disease Lupus erythematosus (SLE)		D		I		I	Gamma globulin levels of prognostic value
Polyarteritis nodosa		D		I		N	
Rheumatoid arthritis		D		I	I	I	
Scleroderma						V	No significant changes
Acute rheumatic fever		D		I	No significant changes		Albumin D due to hemodilution
Essential hypertension Congestive heart failure	D	D		No significant changes			(Hemodilution, diminished hepatic synthesis, and possible excessive enteric loss)

Metastatic carcinomatosis	D	I	I	D		Nonspecific pattern
Certain infections (meningitis, pneumonia, osteomyelitis)	D		I			
Myxedema						Changes due to hemodilution
Hyperthyroidism	D	N	N	N	N	
Diabetes mellitus	D		I	I		

I = increased or elevated; D = decreased or diminished; V = variable; N = normal; blank = no significant change.
*Nonspecific changes of decreased albumin and increased globulin occur in many conditions (e.g., infections, neoplasms, metabolic diseases).
Source: Data from FW Sunderman, Jr., Recent Advances in Clinical Interpretation of Electrophoretic Fractionations of the Serum Proteins. In FW Sunderman and JC Sunderman (Eds), *Serum Proteins and the Dysproteinemias*. Philadelphia: Lippincott, 1964; HH Harrison and MH Levitt, Serum Protein Electrophoresis: Basic Principles, Interpretations, and Practical Considerations. *ASCP Check Sample*. Core Chemistry No. PTS 87-7 (PTS-25). ASCP: Chicago, 1987.

Laboratory findings show relatively little evidence of parenchymal damage.

SGOT and SGPT may be normal or slightly increased (up to 1–5 times normal), fluctuate within a narrow range, and have no prognostic significance.

Serum albumin, globulin, and PT normal early; abnormal values not corrected by therapy indicate advanced disease and poor prognosis.

Serum ceruloplasmin is characteristically elevated (in contrast to Wilson's disease), and liver copper may be increased 10–100 times normal.

ESR is increased 1–5 times normal in 80% of patients.

There are laboratory findings of steatorrhea.

Serum 25-hydroxyvitamin D and vitamin A are usually low.

PT is normal or restored to normal by parenteral vitamin K.

Urine contains urobilinogen and bilirubin.

Laboratory findings due to associated diseases

> 80% have one and > 40% have at least two other autoimmune diseases (e.g., rheumatoid arthritis, autoimmune thyroiditis, Sjögren's syndrome, scleroderma).

Laboratory findings due to complications (e.g., portal hypertension, treatment-resistant osteoporosis, hepatic encephalopathy). Increased susceptibility to urinary tract infection is associated with advanced disease. Renal tubular acidosis is frequent but usually subclinical.

HEMOCHROMATOSIS*

Due To

Idiopathic hemochromatosis (IH) (autosomal recessive defect in ability of duodenum) to block excess iron absorption; abnormal gene present in 10% of Americans; frequency of homozygosity ~3 : 1000)

Secondary

Increased intake (e.g., excessive medicinal iron ingestion, Bantu siderosis, long-term frequent transfusions)

Anemias with increased erythropoiesis (especially thalassemia major; also thalassemia minor, some other hemoglobinopathies, paroxysmal nocturnal hemoglobinuria, sideroblastic anemias, refractory anemias with hypercellular bone marrow)

Porphyria cutanea tarda

Following portal-systemic shunt

Congenital atransferrinemia

Serum iron (SI) is increased (usually 200–300 μg/dl) but should not be only screening test because of many other conditions in which it occurs. Confirm by repeat fasting sample at least 2 more times.

Total iron-binding capacity (TIBC) is decreased (~200 μg/dl; often approaches zero; generally higher in secondary than primary type).

Best screening method is increased transferrin saturation (100 × SI/TIBC); usually > 70% and frequently approaches 100%; > 62% in fasting men warrants further evaluation of iron status (by serum ferritin) if have ruled out other causes of increased SI (e.g., ingestion of iron, especially in form of vitamin supplements). Levels of 50–62% usually indicate heterozygous state but occasionally found in homozygous persons. Most heterozygous persons have no detectable changes. An elevated value should be repeated twice at weekly intervals. *SI may show marked diurnal variation, with lowest values in evening and highest between 7* A.M. *and noon.* Confirmed elevation of SI, serum ferritin, and transferrin saturation is indication for needle biopsy of liver to

*Data from WH Crosby, Hemochromatosis: Current concepts and management. *Hospital Practice,* Feb. 15, 1987, p. 173; DL Witte, Hemochromatosis. CAP Seminar, Oct. 24, 1990.

confirm or refute diagnosis, grade amount of iron, and assess tissue damage. Screening will discover hemochromatosis in 2–3/1000 persons; should be sought especially in patients with diabetes mellitus, congestive heart failure, idiopathic cardiomyopathy, rheumatoid arthritis, alcoholic cirrhosis, hypogonadism. If serum ferritin is not increased, liver biopsy may be deferred and serum ferritin should be repeated periodically.

Increased serum ferritin (usually > 1000 μg/L); elevated in ~two-thirds of patients with idiopathic type. Is good index of total body iron but has limited value for screening because may be increased in acute inflammatory conditions (e.g., rheumatoid arthritis) and less sensitive than transferrin saturation in early cases. May not be increased in young patients who have not yet accumulated excess amounts of iron. > 5000 μg/L indicates tissue damage (e.g., liver degeneration) with release of ferritin into circulation.

Test	Sensitivity	Specificity
Serum iron > 177 μg/dl	0.68	0.83
Saturation > 50%	0.82	0.88
Ferritin (> 200 ng/ml in males, > 150 ng/ml in females)	0.85	0.95
Ferritin + saturation	0.94	0.86

Liver biopsy is needed to confirm the diagnosis. Increased stainable iron in perilobular hepatocytes in idiopathic type with little in Kupffer cells or bone marrow. Liver iron is increased (normal < 200 μg/100 mg of dry liver by atomic absorption or UV spectroscopy). > 1000 μg/100 mg of dry liver is consistent with homozygous state but may reach 5000. Some heterozygotes may reach 1000 μg/100 mg but do not progress beyond this level. Fibrosis or cirrhosis usually does not occur at levels < 2000 μg/100 mg of dry liver unless alcoholism is also present. For chemical analysis of iron, should use acid-washed needle and place specimen in iron-free container.

Presence of excess iron in other tissue biopsy sites (e.g., synovia, GI tract) should arouse suspicion of IH; iron stains should be done.

Bone marrow biopsy stained for iron is not useful for diagnosis of idiopathic hemochromatosis.

Urinary iron following deferoxamine (0.5 gm administered IM) is increased to 5–20 mg/24 hours (normal is < 2 mg/24 hours); not a useful diagnostic test.

Liver function tests depend on presence and degree of liver damage (e.g., cirrhosis).

Laboratory findings due to involvement of various organs (e.g., diabetes mellitus, glucose intolerance, cirrhosis, arthralgia, congestive heart failure, hypogonadism); underlying diseases (see above), associated alcoholism. Hepatocellular carcinoma develops in ~30% of cases and has become the chief cause of death in idiopathic hemochromatosis.

When diagnosis of idiopathic hemochromatosis is established, other family members should be screened; one-fourth of siblings will have the disease; 5% of patient's children will be homozygous for hemochromatosis gene. Negative relatives should be rescreened every 5 years.

HLA-A3 is not used for screening to discover sporadic cases but may be useful to identify patient's siblings at risk, since HLA-identical siblings will almost always also be homozygous for hemochromatosis gene and at high risk for developing clinical disease.

Increased susceptibility to *Yersinia* sepsis (also in other iron overload conditions).

Adequate treatment with phlebotomy (1–3 units/week) sufficient to maintain a mild anemia is determined by hematocrit (37–39%) prior to each phlebotomy. If > 40%, an additional treatment may be scheduled. Serum iron and ferritin are only used when anemia becomes refractory to establish whether iron stores are exhausted. Maintenance phlebotomy (4–6 units/year) can be monitored with serum ferritin to indicate normal amount of storage iron. Insulin requirement decreases in > one-third of diabetics; liver function tests often improve; arthritis, impotence, and sterility usually do not improve.

WILSON'S DISEASE

Serum ceruloplasmin is decreased (< 20 mg/dl). (*It is normal in 2–5% of patients with overt Wilson's disease.*) It may also be decreased in normal infants (therefore cannot use test for Wilson's disease in first year of life). Moderate transient deficiencies occur in some patients with nephrosis, sprue, kwashiorkor.

Serum ceruloplasmin is increased in pregnancy and patients taking estrogen or birth control pills, thyrotoxicosis, cirrhosis, cancer, acute inflammatory reactions (e.g., infection, rheumatoid arthritis (may cause green color of plasma).

Measure ceruloplasmin in any patient under age 30 with hepatitis, hemolysis, or neurologic symptoms to allow early diagnosis and treatment of Wilson's disease.

Decreased serum ceruloplasmin (< 20 mg/dl) with increased hepatic copper (> 250 μg/gm) occurs only in Wilson's disease or normal infants aged < 6 months.

Heterozygous gene for Wilson's disease occurs in 1 of 200 in the general population; 10% of these have decreased serum ceruloplasmin; liver copper is not increased (< 250 μg/gm of dry liver). Serum copper and ceruloplasmin and urine copper are inadequate to detect heterozygous state.

Homozygous gene (clinical Wilson's disease) occurs in 1 of 200,000 in the general population.

Total serum copper is decreased and generally parallels serum ceruloplasmin.

Nonceruloplasmin copper in serum is increased.

Urinary copper is increased (> 100 μg/24 hours); may be normal in presymptomatic patients and increased in other types of cirrhosis.

Liver biopsy shows high copper concentration (> 250 μg/gm of dry liver; normal = 20–45). (Should use special copper-free needle.)

Liver biopsy may show no abnormalities, moderate to marked fatty changes with or without fibrosis, or active or inactive cirrhosis.

Findings of liver function tests may not be abnormal, depending on the type and severity of disease.

Aminoaciduria (especially cystine and threonine), glucosuria, hyperphosphaturia, hypercalciuria, uricosuria, and decreased serum uric acid may occur due to renal proximal tubular dysfunction; distal renal tubular acidosis is less common.

Coombs-negative nonspherocytic hemolytic anemia may occur.

Other tests that have been used in diagnosis of heterozygotes may not be available locally:

- D-Penicillamine administration induces increased urinary copper excretion.
- Excretion of radioactive copper
- Conversion of ionic radiocopper to radioceruloplasmin
- Copper content of cultured fibroblasts

LIVER FUNCTION ABNORMALITIES IN CONGESTIVE HEART FAILURE

Pattern of abnormal liver function tests is variable depending on severity of heart failure; the mildest show only slightly increased alkaline phosphatase and slightly decreased serum albumin; moderately severe also show slightly increased serum bilirubin and GGT; one-fourth to three-quarters of the most severe will also show increased SGOT and SGPT (up to ≈ 200 U/L) and LDH (up to ≈ 400 U/L). All will return to normal when heart failure responds to treatment. Serum alkaline phosphatase is usually the last to become normal, and this may be weeks to months later.

Serum bilirubin is frequently increased (indirect more than direct); usually 1–5 mg/dl. It usually represents combined right- and left-sided failure with hepatic engorgement and pulmonary infarcts. Serum bilirubin may suddenly rise rapidly if superimposed myocardial infarction occurs.
SGOT and SGPT are disproportionately increased compared with other liver function tests in left-sided heart failure.
Increased serum alkaline phosphatase and LDH (mild to moderate).
PT may be slightly increased, with increased sensitivity to anticoagulant drugs.
Serum cholesterol and esters may be decreased.
Urine urobilinogen is increased. Urine bilirubin is increased in the presence of jaundice.

These findings may occur with marked liver congestion due to other conditions (e.g., Chiari's syndrome [occlusion of hepatic veins] and constrictive pericarditis).

HEPATIC FAILURE

Serum bilirubin progressively increases; may become very high.
Decreased albumin and also total protein
Previously elevated SGOT and SGPT that fall abruptly with onset of hepatic failure
Decreased blood glucose
Prolonged PT; is never normal in acute hepatic failure
Blood ammonia level usually increased
Laboratory findings of hemorrhage, especially in GI tract

HEPATIC ENCEPHALOPATHY

(neurologic and mental abnormalities in some patients with liver failure)

Blood ammonia is increased in 90% of patients but does not reflect the degree of coma. Normal level in comatose patient suggests another cause of coma. Not reliable for diagnosis but may be useful to follow individual patients. May be increased by tight tourniquet or vigorously clenched fist; thus arterial specimen may be preferable.
Respiratory alkalosis due to hyperventilation is frequent.
Hyponatremia and iatrogenic hypernatremia are frequent complications and are associated with a higher mortality rate.
Hypokalemic metabolic alkalosis may occur due to diuretic excess.
Serum amino acid profile is abnormal. All serum amino acids are markedly increased in coma due to acute liver failure.
CSF is normal except for increased glutamine level.
Diagnosis is clinical; characteristic laboratory findings are supportive but not specific.

SPACE-OCCUPYING LESIONS OF LIVER

Increased serum alkaline phosphatase is the most useful index of partial obstruction of the biliary tree in which serum bilirubin is usually normal and urine bilirubin is increased.
- Increased in 80% of patients with metastatic carcinoma (≤ 70 Bodansky units)
- Increased in 50% of patients with tuberculosis (≤ 50 Bodansky units)
- Increased in 40% of patients with sarcoidosis (≤ 18 Bodansky units)
- Increased frequently in patients with amyloidosis (≤ 100 Bodansky units)

Increased serum LAP parallels alkaline phosphatase but is not affected by bone disease.
Whenever the alkaline phosphatase is increased, a simultaneous increase of 5′-nucleotidase establishes biliary disease as the cause of the elevated alkaline phosphatase.

SGOT is increased in 50% of patients (≤ 300 units).
SGPT is increased less frequently (≤ 150 units).
ICD may show a moderate increase.
Detection of metastases by panel of blood tests (alkaline phosphatase, LDH, transaminase, bilirubin) has sensitivity of 85%. Alkaline phosphatase or GGT alone has sensitivity of 25–33% and specificity of up to 75%. Serum LDH is often increased in cancer even without liver metastases.
Radioactive scanning of the liver has 65% sensitivity.
Blind needle biopsy of the liver is positive in 65–75% of patients.
Laboratory findings due to primary disease are noted. See also
 Carcinoid syndrome
 Pyogenic liver abscess
 Other
Laboratory findings due to primary disease (e.g., increased serum carcinoembryonic antigen (CEA) in colon carcinoma).

Hepatoma

Serum alpha-fetoprotein present in 50% of white and 75–90% of nonwhite patients; may be present for up to 18 months before symptoms; is sensitive indicator of recurrence in treated patients, but a normal postoperative level does not ensure absence of metastases. Levels > 500 ng/dl in adults strongly suggest primary carcinoma of liver.
Laboratory findings associated with underlying disease (> 60% occur with preexisting cirrhosis).
 Hemochromatosis (≤ 20% of patients die of hepatoma).
 More frequent in postnecrotic than in alcoholic cirrhosis.
 Cirrhosis associated with $alpha_1$ antitrypsin deficiency and other inborn errors of metabolism (e.g., tyrosinemia).
 Clonarchis sinensis infection is associated with cholangiosarcoma.
 Relative absence of hepatoma associated with cirrhosis of Wilson's disease.
Sudden progressive worsening of laboratory findings of underlying disease (e.g., increased alkaline phosphatase, LDH, SGOT, serum bilirubin).
Hemoperitoneum—ascites in ~50% of patients but tumor cells found irregularly.
Laboratory findings due to obstruction of hepatic (Budd-Chiari syndrome) or portal veins or inferior vena cava may occur.
Occasional marked hypoglycemia unresponsive to epinephrine injection; occasional hypercalcemia.
ESR and WBC sometimes increased.
Anemia is common; polycythemia occurs occasionally.
Serologic markers of HBV frequently present.

OBSTRUCTION OF ONE HEPATIC BILE DUCT

Serum bilirubin that remains normal in the presence of serum alkaline phosphatase that is markedly increased is characteristic pattern.

COMPLETE BILIARY OBSTRUCTION (INTRAHEPATIC OR EXTRAHEPATIC)

Typical pattern of extrahepatic obstruction includes increased serum alkaline phosphatase (> 2–3 times normal), SGOT < 300 U/L, increased direct serum bilirubin.
Serum alkaline phosphatase is markedly increased (> 2–3 times normal). In extrahepatic type, the increase is related to the completeness of obstruction. Normal alkaline phosphatase is extremely rare in extrahepatic obstruction. Very high levels may also occur in cases of intrahepatic cholestasis.
Serum LAP parallels alkaline phosphatase.
SGOT is increased (≤ 300 units), and SGPT is increased (≤ 200 units); they usually return to normal in 1 week after relief of obstruction. In *acute* biliary duct obstruction (e.g., due to common bile duct stones or acute pancreatitis),

SGOT and SGPT are increased > 300 IU (and often > 2000 IU) and decline 58–76% in 72 hours without treatment; simultaneous serum total bilirubin shows less marked elevation and decline, and alkaline phosphatase changes are inconsistent and unpredictable.

Direct serum bilirubin is increased; indirect serum bilirubin is normal or slightly increased.

Serum cholesterol is increased (acute, 300–400 mg/dl; chronic, ≤ 1000 mg/dl).

Serum phospholipids are increased.

PT is prolonged, with response to parenteral vitamin K more frequent than in hepatic parenchymal cell disease.

Urine bilirubin is increased; urine urobilinogen decreased.

There are decreased stool bilirubin and urobilinogen (clay-colored stools).

Laboratory findings due to underlying causative disease are noted (e.g., stone, carcinoma of duct, metastatic carcinoma to periductal lymph nodes).

PRIMARY SCLEROSING CHOLANGITIS

Chronic fibrosing inflammation of intra- and extrahepatic bile ducts predominantly in men under age 45; 52–74% are associated with inflammatory bowel disease, especially ulcerative colitis, and up to 4% of ulcerative colitis patients have this disease; also associated with syndrome of retroperitoneal and mediastinal fibrosis, characteristic cholangiography image; slow, relentless, progressive course of chronic cholestasis to death (usually from liver failure). Diagnosis should not be made if previous bile duct surgery, gallstones, or suppurative cholangitis. Radiologic studies distinguish from primary biliary cirrhosis (see preceding section); diagnosis is best established by characteristic cholangiogram.

Cholestatic biochemical profile

- Serum alkaline phosphatase may fluctuate but is always increased (usually ≥ 3 times upper limit of normal).
- SGOT is mildly increased in > 90%. SGPT > SGOT in three-fourths of cases.
- Bilirubin is increased in one-half of patients; occasionally is very high; may fluctuate markedly.
- Serum albumin is decreased in one-third of cases.

No serologic markers in serum (in contrast to primary biliary cirrhosis; antimitochondrial antibody, smooth-muscle antibody, rheumatoid factor, ANA are negative in > 90% of patients. HB_sAg is negative.

Liver biopsy provides only confirmatory evidence in patients with compatible history, laboratory, and x-ray findings.

Adenocarcinoma of bile ducts and colon develops in some patients.

GILBERT'S DISEASE (UNCONJUGATED HYPERBILIRUBINEMIA WITHOUT OVERT HEMOLYSIS)

Mildly symptomatic, benign, familial, nonhemolytic unconjugated hyperbilirubinemia with an evanescent increase of indirect serum bilirubin, which is usually discovered on routine laboratory examinations due to defective uptake, transportation, and conjugation of unconjugated bilirubin. Jaundice is usually accentuated by pregnancy, fever, exercise, and various drugs, including alcohol and birth control pills.

Indirect serum bilirubin is increased. It may rise to 18 mg/dl but usually is < 4 mg/dl. Fasting (< 400 calories/day) for 72 hours causes elevated indirect bilirubin to increase > 100% in Gilbert's disease but not in normal persons or those with liver disease or hemolytic anemia. Direct serum bilirubin is normal but may give elevated results using liquid diazo methods but not by dry methods or chromatography.

Liver function tests are usually normal.

Fecal urobilinogen may be decreased.

Urine shows no increased bilirubin.

LIVER TRAUMA

Serum LDH is frequently increased (> 1400 units) 8–12 hours after major injury. Shock due to any injury may also increase LDH.

Other serum enzymes and liver function tests are not generally helpful.

Findings of abdominal paracentesis

- Bloody fluid (in ~75% of patients) confirming traumatic hemoperitoneum and indicating exploratory laparotomy
- Nonbloody fluid (especially if injury occurred > 24 hours earlier)
  - Microscopic—some red and white blood cells
  - Determine amylase, protein, pH, presence of bile.

SUPPURATIVE CHOLANGITIS

Marked increase in WBC (≤ 30,000/cu mm) with increase in granulocytes

Blood culture often positive

Laboratory findings of incomplete duct obstruction due to inflammation or of preceding complete duct obstruction that caused the cholangitis (e.g., stone, tumor, scar)

Laboratory findings of parenchymal cell necrosis and malfunction

- Increased serum SGOT, SGPT, etc.
- Increased urine urobilinogen

SEPTIC PYLEPHLEBITIS

Increased WBC and PMNs in > 90% of patients; usually > 20,000/cu mm

Anemia of varying severity

Moderate increase in serum bilirubin in ~33% of patients

Other liver function tests positive in ~25% of patients

Needle biopsy of liver not helpful—contraindicated

Blood culture sometimes positive

Laboratory findings due to preceding disease (e.g., acute appendicitis, diverticulitis, ulcerative colitis)

Laboratory findings due to complications (e.g., portal vein occlusion)

PYOGENIC LIVER ABSCESS

Increase in WBC due to increase in granulocytes

Abnormalities of liver function tests

- Decreased serum albumin, increased serum globulin
- Increased serum alkaline phosphatase
- Increased serum bilirubin (> 10 mg/dl usually indicates pyogenic rather than amebic and suggests poorer prognosis because of more tissue destruction)
- Other laboratory findings (see Space-Occupying Lesions of Liver, p. 205)

Anemia frequent

Laboratory findings due to complications (e.g., subphrenic abscess, pneumonia, empyema, bronchopleural fistula)

Patients with amebic abscess of liver due to *Entamoeba histolytica* also show positive serologic tests for ameba (see p. 683).

- Stools may be negative for cysts and trophozoites.
- Needle aspiration of abscess may show *E. histolytica* in 50% of patients. *(Characteristic brown or anchovy-sauce color may be absent; secondary bacterial infection may be superimposed.)*

ACUTE CHOLECYSTITIS

Increased ESR, WBC (average 12,000/cu mm; if > 15,000, suspect empyema or perforation), and other evidence of acute inflammatory process

Increased serum bilirubin in 20% of patients (usually > 4 mg/dl; if higher, suspect associated choledocholithiasis)

Increased serum alkaline phosphatase (some patients) even if serum bilirubin is normal

Increased serum amylase and lipase in some patients

Laboratory findings of associated biliary obstruction if such obstruction is present
Laboratory findings of preexisting cholelithiasis (some patients)
Laboratory findings of complications (e.g., empyema of gallbladder, perforation, cholangitis, liver abscess, pylephlebitis, pancreatitis, gallstone ileus)

Serum SGOT is increased in 75% of patients.

CHRONIC CHOLECYSTITIS

May be mild laboratory findings of acute cholecystitis or no abnormal laboratory findings
May be laboratory findings of associated cholelithiasis

CHOLELITHIASIS

Laboratory findings of underlying conditions causing hypercholesterolemia (e.g., diabetes mellitus)
Laboratory findings of causative chronic hemolytic disease (e.g., hereditary spherocytosis)
Laboratory findings of resultant cholecystitis or choledocholithiasis, etc.

CHOLEDOCHOLITHIASIS

During or soon after an attack of biliary colic
- Increased WBC
- Increased serum bilirubin in ~one-third of patients
- Increased urine bilirubin in ~one-third of patients
- Increased serum and urine amylase

Laboratory evidence of fluctuating cholestases (see p. 194)
Laboratory findings due to secondary cholangitis
In duodenal drainage, crystals of both calcium bilirubinate and cholesterol (some patients); 50% accurate (only useful in nonicteric patients)

CANCER OF GALLBLADDER AND BILE DUCTS

Laboratory findings reflect varying location and extent of tumor infiltration that may cause partial intrahepatic duct obstruction or obstruction of hepatic or common bile duct, metastases in liver, or associated cholangitis (see pp. 205, 206, 208); 50% of patients have jaundice at the time of hospitalization.
Laboratory findings of duct obstruction are of progressively increasing severity in contrast to the intermittent or fluctuating changes due to duct obstruction caused by stones. A papillary intraluminal duct carcinoma may undergo periods of sloughing, producing the findings of intermittent duct obstruction.
Stool is frequently positive for occult blood.
Anemia is present.
Cytologic examination of aspirated duodenal fluid may demonstrate malignant cells.
Laboratory findings of the preceding cholelithiasis are present (gallbladder cancer occurs in ~3% of patients with gallstones).

Tests for Differential Diagnosis of Pancreatic Diseases

SERUM AMYLASE

(composed of pancreatic and salivary types of isoamylases; distinguished by various methodologies; nonpancreatic etiologies are almost always salivary; both types may be increased in renal insufficiency)

Increased In

Acute pancreatitis. Increase begins in 3–6 hours; reaches maximum in 20–30 hours; may persist for 48–72 hours. May increase up to 40 times normal.

Level should be at least 500 Somogyi units/dl to be significant evidence of acute pancreatitis. Urine levels reflect serum changes by a time lag of 6–10 hours.

Acute exacerbation of chronic pancreatitis

Obstruction of pancreatic duct by

- Stone or carcinoma
- Drug-induced spasm of sphincter (e.g., opiates, codeine, methyl choline, chlorothiazide) to levels 2–15 times normal
- Partial obstruction + drug stimulation (see Cholecystokinin-Secretin Test, p. 151)

Complications of pancreatitis (pseudocyst, ascites, abscess)

Pancreatic trauma (abdominal injury; following endoscopic retrograde cholangiopancreatography [ERCP])

Altered GI permeability

- Ischemic bowel disease or frank perforation
- Esophageal rupture
- Perforated or penetrating peptic ulcer
- Postoperative upper abdominal surgery, especially partial gastrectomy (up to 2 times normal in one-third of patients)
- Acute alcohol ingestion or poisoning
- Salivary gland disease (mumps, suppurative inflammation, duct obstruction due to calculus, radiation)
- Malignant tumors (especially lung, ovary, pancreas; also breast, colon); usually > 25 times upper limit of normal, which is rarely seen in pancreatitis

Advanced renal insufficiency. Often increased even without pancreatitis

Macroamylasemia

Increased Serum Amylase With Low Urine Amylase

May be seen in renal insufficiency and macroamylasemia

May also be increased in ruptured tubal pregnancy, ovarian cyst, burns, diabetic acidosis

It has been suggested that a level > 1000 Somogyi units is usually due to surgically correctable lesions (most frequently stones in biliary tree), the pancreas being negative or showing only edema; but 200–500 units is usually associated with pancreatic lesions that are not surgically correctable (e.g., hemorrhagic pancreatitis, necrosis or pancreas)

Decreased In

Extensive marked destruction of pancreas (e.g., acute fulminant pancreatitis, advanced chronic pancreatitis, advanced cystic fibrosis)

Severe liver damage (e.g., hepatitis, poisoning, toxemia of pregnancy, severe thyrotoxicosis, severe burns)

Decreased levels are clinically significant only in occasional cases of fulminant pancreatitis.

Amylase-creatinine clearance ratio =

$$\frac{\text{urine amylase concentration}}{\text{serum amylase concentration}} \times \frac{\text{serum creatinine concentration}}{\text{urine creatinine concentration}} \times 100$$

- Normal: 1–5%
- Macroamylasemia: < 1%; very useful for this diagnosis
- Acute pancreatitis: > 5%; use is presently discouraged for this diagnosis

False Positives

Burns, chronic renal failure, pregnancy, diabetic ketoacidosis, duodenal perforation, recent thoracic surgery, myoglobinuria, or presence of myeloma proteins

SERUM LIPASE

Increased In

Acute pancreatitis. Reported sensitivity of 80% and specificity of 60%. May remain elevated for as long as 14 days after amylase returns to normal.

Perforated or penetrating peptic ulcer, especially with involvement of pancreas

Obstruction of pancreatic duct by

- Stone
- Drug-induced spasm of sphincter (e.g., by opiates, codeine, methyl choline) to levels 2–15 times normal
- Partial obstruction + drug stimulation

Usually Normal In

Mumps

Diseases of the Pancreas

ACUTE PANCREATITIS*

Serum amylase increase begins in 3–6 hours, rises to > 250 Somogyi units within 8 hours in 75% of patients, reaches maximum in 20–30 hours, and may persist for 48–72 hours. > 95% sensitivity during first 12–24 hours. The increase may be ≤ 40 times normal, but the height of the increase and rate of fall do not correlate with the severity of the disease, prognosis, or rate of resolution; however, an increase > 7–10 days suggests an associated cancer of pancreas or pseudocyst, pancreatic ascites, nonpancreatic etiology. The level should be ≥ 500 Somogyi units/dl to be significant of acute pancreatitis. *Similar high values may occur in obstruction of pancreatic duct; they tend to fall after several days. > 10% of patients with acute pancreatitis (especially when seen more than 2 days after onset of symptoms) may have normal values, even when dying of acute pancreatitis.* May also be normal in relapsing chronic pancreatitis and patients with hypertriglyceridemia (technical interference with test). Frequently normal in acute alcoholic pancreatitis. Acute abdomen due to GI infarction or perforation rather than acute pancreatitis is suggested by only moderate increase in serum amylase and lipase (< 3 times ULN), evidence of bacteremia. 10–40% of patients with acute alcoholic intoxication have elevated serum amylase (about half are salivary type); they often present with abdominal pain, but increased serum amylase is usually < 3 times ULN. Levels > 25 times ULN indicates metastatic tumor rather than pancreatitis.

Serum pancreatic isoamylase can distinguish elevations due to salivary amylase that may account for 25% of all elevated values. (In healthy persons, 40% of total serum amylase is pancreatic type, and 60% is salivary type.)

Serum lipase increases in 50% of patients and may remain elevated for as long as 14 days after amylase returns to normal. (*Lipase should always be determined whenever amylase is determined, since the amylase may have already returned to normal values.*) New methodology may improve clinical utility. Urinary lipase is not clinically useful.

*Data from Ranson JHC., Etiological and prognostic factors in human acute pancreatitis: A review. *Am. J. Gastroenterol.* 77:633, 1982.

Serum calcium is decreased in severe cases 1–9 days after onset (due to binding to soaps in fat necrosis). The decrease usually occurs after amylase and lipase levels have become normal. Tetany may occur. (*Rule out hyperparathyroidism if serum calcium is high or fails to fall in hyperamylasemia of acute pancreatitis.*)

Increased urinary amylase tends to reflect serum changes by a time lag of 6–10 hours, but sometimes increased urine levels are higher and of longer duration than serum levels. The 24-hour level may be normal even when some of the 1-hour specimens show increased values. Amylase levels in hourly samples of urine may be useful (> 40 Somogyi units/hour). Ratio of amylase clearance to creatinine clearance is increased (> 5%) and avoids the problem of timed urine specimens; also increased in any condition that decreases tubular reabsorption of amylase (e.g., severe burns, diabetic ketoacidosis, chronic renal insufficiency, multiple myeloma, acute duodenal perforation). Considered not specific and now discouraged by some, but still recommended by others.

Serum bilirubin may be increased when pancreatitis is of biliary tract origin but is usually normal in alcoholic pancreatitis. Serum alkaline phosphatase, SGPT, and SGOT may increase and parallel serum bilirubin rather than amylase, lipase, or calcium levels.

Serum trypsin (RIA test) is increased. High sensitivity makes a normal value useful for excluding acute pancreatitis. But low specificity (increased in large proportion of patients with hepatobiliary, bowel, and other diseases and renal insufficiency; increased in 13% of patients with chronic pancreatitis, 50% with pancreatic carcinoma) and RIA technology limit utility.

WBC is slightly to moderately increased (10,000–20,000/cu mm).

Hemoconcentration occurs (increased hematocrit). Hematocrit may be decreased in severe hemorrhagic pancreatitis.

Glycosuria appears in 25% of patients.

Ascites may develop, cloudy or bloody or "prune juice" fluid, 0.5–2.0 L in volume, containing increased amylase with a level higher than that of serum amylase. No bile is evident (unlike in perforated ulcer). Gram's stain shows no bacteria (unlike infarct of intestine).

Methemalbumin may be increased in serum and ascitic fluid in hemorrhagic (severe) but not edematous (mild) pancreatitis; may distinguish these two conditions but not useful in diagnosis of acute pancreatitis.

Adult respiratory distress syndrome (with pleural effusion, alveolar exudate, or both) may occur in ~40% of patients; arterial hypoxemia is present.

Hypokalemia, metabolic alkalosis, or lactic acidosis may occur.

Laboratory findings due to predisposing conditions
- Alcoholism and biliary tract disease account for 65–90% of cases.
- Idiopathic (up to 25% of cases)
- Infections (especially viral such as mumps and Coxsackie)
- Trauma and postoperative
- Drugs (e.g., steroids, thiazides, azathioprine)
- Tumors (pancreas, ampulla)
- Hereditary
- Hypertriglyceridemia (hyperlipidemia—Types I, IV, V)
- Miscellaneous (collagen vascular disease, pregnancy, ischemia)

Prognostic laboratory findings:
- On admission
  - WBC > 16,000/cu mm
  - Blood glucose > 200 mg/dl
  - Serum LDH > 350 IU/L
  - SGOT > 250 units/L
  - Age > 55 years
- Within 48 hours
  - Decreased serum calcium < 8.0 mg/dl

Fall in hematocrit > 10%
Rise in BUN > 5 mg/dl
Arterial PO_2 < 60 mmHg
Metabolic acidosis with base deficit > 4 mEq/L

Mortality = 1% if 3 signs are positive
15% if 3–4 signs are positive
40% if 5–6 signs are positive
100% if ≥ 7 signs are positive

Degree of amylase elevation has no prognostic significance.

Diagnostic Efficiency of Amylase and Lipase in Acute Pancreatitis*

	Sensitivity	Specificity	Efficiency
Serum amylase	95%	88%	89%
Serum lipase	86%	99%	96%
Pancreatic isoamylase	92%	85%	87%
Serum trypsinogen	97%	83%	87%

Based on upper limit of normal.

Absence of a "gold standard" for diagnosis of acute pancreatitis makes all of these values unclear.

CHRONIC PANCREATIC DISEASE (CHRONIC PANCREATITIS; CARCINOMA OF PANCREAS)

(see also Laboratory Diagnosis of Malabsorption, p. 162)

Examine duodenal contents (volume, bicarbonate concentration, amylase output) after IV administration of cholecystokinin and secretin. Some abnormality occurs in > 85% of patients with chronic pancreatitis. Amylase output is the most frequent abnormality. When all three are abnormal, there is a greater frequency of abnormality in the tests listed below.

Serum amylase and lipase increase after administration of cholecystokinin and secretin in ~20% of patients with chronic pancreatitis. They are more often abnormal when duodenal contents are normal.

Fasting serum amylase and lipase increased in 10% of patients with chronic pancreatitis.

There will be a diabetic oral glucose tolerance test (GTT) in 65% of patients with chronic pancreatitis and frank diabetes in > 10% of patients with chronic relapsing pancreatitis. When GTT is normal in the presence of steatorrhea, the cause should be sought elsewhere than in the pancreas.

Chemical determination of fecal fat demonstrates steatorrhea. It is more sensitive than tests using triolein ^{131}I.

Triolein ^{131}I is abnormal in one-third of patients with chronic pancreatitis.

Starch tolerance test is abnormal in 25% of patients with chronic pancreatitis.

Radioactive scanning of pancreas (selenium) yields variable findings in different clinics.

Laboratory findings due to causes of chronic pancreatitis and pancreatic exocrine insufficiency are noted (e.g., alcohol, cystic fibrosis, pancreatic cancer, trauma, heredity, pancreas divisum, idiopathic, protein caloric malnutrition, miscellaneous [Zollinger-Ellison syndrome, Schwachman syndrome, primary hyperparathyroidism, $alpha_1$ antitrypsin deficiency, trypsinogen deficiency, enterokinase deficiency, hemochromatosis, parenteral hyperalimentation). No cause is found in 25% of cases.

*Data from Steinberg WM, et al., Diagnostic assays in acute pancreatitis. *Ann Intern Med* 102:576, 1985.

PSEUDOCYST OF PANCREAS

Serum direct bilirubin is increased (> 2 mg/dl) in 10% of patients.

Serum alkaline phosphatase is increased (> 5 Bodansky units) in 10% of patients.

Fasting blood sugar is increased in < 10% of patients.

Laboratory findings of preceding acute pancreatitis are present (this is mild and unrecognized in one-third of patients).

Persistent increase of serum amylase and lipase after an acute episode may indicate formation of a pseudocyst.

Duodenal contents after secretin-pancreozymin stimulation usually show decreased bicarbonate content (< 70 mEq/L) but normal volume and normal content of amylase, lipase, and trypsin.

Laboratory findings due to conditions preceding acute pancreatitis are noted (e.g., alcoholism, trauma, duodenal ulcer, cholelithiasis).

CYSTIC FIBROSIS OF PANCREAS (MUCOVISCIDOSIS)

(incidence of 1 : 1500 to 1 : 2000 in Caucasians with a carrier frequency of 1 : 20; 1 : 17,000 in American blacks)

Quantitative pilocarpine iontophoresis sweat test (properly performed) shows a striking increase in sweat sodium and chloride (> 60 mEq/L), and to a lesser extent, potassium is present in virtually all homozygous patients; level is 3–5 times higher than in healthy persons or other diseases. It is consistently present throughout life from time of birth, and degree of abnormality is not related to severity of disease or organ involvement. There is a broad range of values in this disease and in normal but minimal overlap. *Sweat chloride is somewhat more reliable than sodium for diagnostic purposes.* Sensitivity = 98%, specificity = 83%, positive predictive value = 93%. Sweat sodium and chloride increase is not useful for detection of heterozygotes (who have normal values) or genetic counseling. In children, chloride > 60 mEq/L is considered positive for cystic fibrosis; 40–60 mEq/L is considered borderline and requires further investigation. Up to 80 mEq/L may be normal for adults. *Sweat testing is fraught with problems, and technical and laboratory errors are very frequent; pilocarpine iontophoresis should be performed in duplicate and repeated at least once on separate days on samples > 100 mg of sweat.* Rare patients with borderline values have only mild disease. On occasion, 1–2% of cystic fibrosis patients have normal, borderline, or variable values. Sweat potassium is not diagnostically valuable because of overlap with normal controls. Values may be increased to cystic fibrosis range in healthy persons when sweat rate is rapid (e.g., exercise, high temperature), but pilocarpine test does not increase sweating rate. Sweat electrolytes may also be increased in untreated adrenal insufficiency (Addison's disease) and some unusual disease syndromes (e.g., glucose-6-PD deficiency, glycogen storage disease, vasopressin-resistant diabetes insipidus). *Sweat sodium is reduced by administration of mineralocorticoids (e.g., aldosterone) by ~50% in normal subjects and 10–20% in cystic fibrosis patients whose final sodium concentration remains abnormally high.*

Sweat values (mEq/L)

	Chloride		Sodium		Potassium	
	Mean	**Range**	**Mean**	**Range**	**Mean**	**Range**
Cystic Fibrosis	115	79–148	111	75–145	23	14–30
Normal	28	8–43	28	16–46	10	6–17

Abnormal sweat colors

- Brown: ochronosis.
- Red: rifampin overdose.
- Blue: occupational exposure to copper.
- Blue-black: idiopathic chromhidrosis (in black persons, axillary chromhidrosis may also be yellow, blue-green).

Serum chloride, sodium, potassium, calcium, and phosphorus are normal unless complications occur (e.g., chronic pulmonary disease with accumulation of CO_2, massive salt loss due to sweating). Urine electrolytes are normal.

Submaxillary saliva has slightly increased chloride and sodium but not potassium; however, considerable overlap with normal persons prevents diagnostic use. Submaxillary saliva also is more turbid, with increased calcium, total protein, and amylase. These changes are not generally found in parotid saliva.

Serum protein electrophoresis shows increasing gamma globulin with progressive pulmonary disease, mainly due to immunoglobulins G and A; M and D are not appreciably increased.

Glucose intolerance in ~40% of patients with glycosuria and hyperglycemia in 8%

Serum albumin is often decreased (because of hemodilution due to cor pulmonale; may be found before cardiac involvement is clinically apparent). In late stages of chronic lung disease, decreased serum electrolytes, hemoglobin, hematocrit level, etc., may also reflect hemodilution.

Bacteriology: Special culture techniques should be used in these patients. Hemolytic *Staphylococcus aureus* is the most frequent and important organism in the respiratory tract; *Pseudomonas aeruginosa* is found increasingly often after treatment of *Staphylococcus*, and special identification and susceptibility tests should be performed on *P. aeruginosa*. *Pseudomonas cepacia* is becoming more important in older children.

Adrenal and pituitary function tests are normal.

Laboratory changes secondary to complications (e.g., pancreatic deficiency, chronic pulmonary disease, sinusitis, nasal polyps, excessive loss of electrolytes in sweat, biliary cirrhosis, cholelithiasis, aspermia in 98%, intestinal obstruction)

- Pancreas (see Laboratory Diagnosis of Malabsorption, p. 162)
  - 80% of patients show loss of all pancreatic enzyme activity.
  - 10% of patients show decrease of pancreatic enzyme activity.
  - 10% of patients show normal pancreatic enzyme activity.
- Cirrhosis (in > 25% of patients at autopsy)
- Chronic lung disease (especially upper lobes) with laboratory changes due to accumulation of CO_2, severe recurrent infection, secondary cor pulmonale, etc.
- Meconium ileus during early infancy; causes 20–30% of cases of neonatal intestinal obstruction; present at birth in 8% of these children. Almost all of them will develop the clinical picture of cystic fibrosis.

Stool and duodenal fluid show lack of trypsin digestion of x-ray film gelatin; this is a useful screening test up to age 4; decreased chymotrypsin production gauged by bentiromide test (see p. 152).

CARCINOMA OF BODY OR TAIL OF PANCREAS

Laboratory tests are often normal.

Serum markers for tumor CA 19-9, CEA, etc. (see pp. 709–711)

- In carcinoma of pancreas, CA 19-9 sensitivity = 70%, specificity = 87%, positive predictive value = 59%, negative predictive value = 92%. No difference in sensitivity between local disease and metastatic disease.*

Serum amylase and lipase may be slightly increased in early stages (< 10% of cases); with later destruction of pancreas, they are normal or decreased. They may increase following secretin-pancreozymin stimulation before destruction is extensive; therefore, the increase is less marked with a diabetic glucose tolerance curve. Serum amylase response is less reliable.

Glucose tolerance curve is of the diabetic type, with overt diabetes in 20% of patients with pancreatic cancer. Flat blood sugar curve with IV tolbutamide

*Data from DK Pleskow et al., Evaluation of a serologic marker CA19-9, in the diagnosis of pancreatic cancer. *Ann Intern Med* 110:704, 1989.

tolerance test indicates destruction of islet cell tissue. *Unstable, insulin-sensitive diabetes that develops in an older man should arouse suspicion of carcinoma of the pancreas.*

Secretin-cholecystokinin stimulation evidences duct obstruction when duodenal intubation shows decreased volume of duodenal contents (< 10 ml/10-minute collection period) with usually normal bicarbonate and enzyme levels in duodenal contents. Acinar destruction (as in pancreatitis) shows normal volume (20–30 ml/10-minute collection period), but bicarbonate and enzyme levels may be decreased. Abnormal volume, bicarbonate, or both are found in 60–80% of patients with pancreatitis or cancer. In carcinoma, the test result depends on the relative extent and combination of acinar destruction and of duct obstruction. Cytologic examination of duodenal contents shows malignant cells in 40% of patients. Malignant cells may be found in up to 80% of patients with periampullary cancer.

Serum leucine aminopeptidase (LAP) is increased (> 300 units) in 60% of patients with carcinoma of pancreas due to liver metastases or biliary tract obstruction. *It may also be increased in chronic liver disease.*

Triolein ^{131}I test demonstrates pancreatic duct obstruction with absence of lipase in the intestine, causing flat blood curves and increased stool excretion.

Radioisotope scanning of pancreas may be done (^{75}Se) for lesions > 2 cm.

CARCINOMA OF HEAD OF PANCREAS

The abnormal pancreatic function tests that occur with carcinoma of the body of the pancreas may be evident.

Laboratory findings due to complete obstruction of common bile duct

- Serum bilirubin increased (12–25 mg/dl), mostly direct (increase persistent and nonfluctuating)
- Serum alkaline phosphatase increased (usually 12–30 Bodansky units)
- Urine and stool urobilinogen absent
- Increased PT; normal after IV vitamin K administration
- Increased serum cholesterol (usually > 300 mg/dl) with esters not decreased
- Other liver function tests are usually normal.

The most useful diagnostic tests are ultrasound or CAT scanning followed by endoscopic retrograde cholangiopancreatography (ERCP) (at which time fluid is also obtained for cytologic and pancreatic function studies). This combination will correctly diagnose or rule out cancer of pancreas in ≥ 90% of cases.

CEA level in bile (obtained by percutaneous transhepatic drainage) was reported elevated in 76% of a small group of cases.

Needle biopsy (with radiologic guidance) may be positive.

MACROAMYLASEMIA

Serum amylase persistently increased without apparent cause

Urine amylase normal or low

Amylase-creatinine clearance ratio < 1% with normal renal function is very useful for this diagnosis; should make the clinician suspect this diagnosis.

Macroamylase is identified in serum by special gel filtration or ultracentrifugation technique.

May be found in ~1% of randomly selected patients and 2.5% of persons with increased serum amylase. Same findings may also occur in patients with normal-molecular-weight hyperamylasemia in which excess amylase is principally salivary gland isoamylase types 2 and 3.

When associated with pancreatic disease, the serum lipase may be elevated.

10

Central and Peripheral Nervous System Diseases

Laboratory Tests for Disorders of the Nervous System

NORMAL CSF VALUES

Measurement of these components should always be performed on simultaneously drawn blood samples.

Appearance	**Clear, colorless: no clot**
Total cell count	
Adults, children	0–6/cu mm (all mononuclear cells)
Infants	$<$19/cu mm
Neonates	$<$30/cu mm
Glucose	45–80 mg/dl (20 mg/dl less than blood level) Ventricular fluid 5–10 mg/dl $>$ lumbar
Total protein	
Cisternal	15–25 mg/dl
Ventricular	5–15 mg/dl
Lumbar	
Neonates	15–100 mg/dl
3 months–60 years	15–45 mg/dl
$>$60 years	15–60 mg/dl
Albumin	10–30 mg/dl
Protein electrophoresis	
Prealbumin	2–7%
Albumin	56–76%
Alpha$_1$ globulin	2–7%
Alpha$_2$ globulin	4–12%
Beta globulin	8–18%
Gamma globulin	3–12%
IgG	$<$10% of total CSF protein
Chloride	120–130 mEq/L (20 mEq/L $>$ serum)
Sodium	142–150 mEq/L
Potassium	2.2–3.3 mEq/L
Carbon dioxide	25 mEq/L
pH	7.35–7.40
Glutamic-oxaloacetic transaminase (GOT)	7–49 units
Lactic dehydrogenase (LDH)	~10% of serum level
Creatine kinase (CK)	0–3 IU
Bilirubin	0
Urea nitrogen	5–25 mg/dl
Amino acids	30% of blood level
Xanthochromia	0

ENZYMES IN CSF

Normal CSF is not permeable to serum enzymes. Changes in GOT are irregular and generally of limited diagnostic value. If GOT, LDH, and CK in CSF are all performed, at least one shows marked increase in 80% of cortical stroke (usually due to emboli) but not in lacunar strokes (usually due to small-vessel hypertensive disease).

Glutamic-Oxaloacetic Transaminase (GOT)

Increased In

Large infarcts of brain during first 10 days. (In severe cases, SGOT may also be increased; occurs in ~40% of patients.)
~40% of CNS tumors (various benign, malignant, and metastatic), depending on location, growth rate, etc.; chiefly useful as indicator of organic neurologic disease
Some other conditions (e.g., head injury, subarachnoid hemorrhage)

Lactic Dehydrogenase (LDH)

Increased In

Cerebrovascular accidents—increase occurs frequently, reaches maximum level in 1–3 days, and is apparently not related to xanthochromia, RBC, WBC, protein, sugar, or chloride levels.
CNS tumors (primary and metastatic), depending on location, growth rate, etc.
Meningitis—is sensitive indicator of meningitis (in specimen with no blood); normal or mild increase in viral meningitis due to LDH_1 and LDH_2; more marked increase in bacterial meningitis due to LDH_4 and LDH_5.

Creatine Kinase (CK)

Not Useful Because

It does not consistently increase in various CNS diseases
No relationship to CSF protein, WBC, or RBC values
No pattern of relationship to LDH and GOT in CSF
No correlation of serum CK and CSF CK

In ischemic brain disease, total CK and CK-BB are reported to be increased.

NORMAL CSF

Found In

Korsakoff's syndrome
Wernicke's encephalopathy
Alzheimer's disease (diffuse cerebral atrophy)
Jakob-Creutzfeldt disease
Tuberous sclerosis (protein rarely increased)
Idiopathic epilepsy (If protein is increased, rule out neoplasms; if cell count is increased, rule out neoplasm or inflammation.)
Narcolepsy, cataplexy, etc.
Parkinson's disease
Hereditary cerebellar degenerations
Huntington's disease
Migraine
Ménière's syndrome
Psychiatric conditions (e.g., neurocirculatory asthenia, hysteria, depression, anxiety, schizophrenia) (*Rule out psychiatric condition as a manifestation of primary disease, e.g., drugs, porphyria, primary endocrine diseases.*)
Transient cerebral ischemia
Amyotrophic lateral sclerosis
Muscular dystrophy
Progressive muscular atrophy
Syringomyelia
Vitamin B_{12} deficiency with subacute combined degeneration of spinal cord
Pellagra
Beriberi
Subacute myelo-opticoneuropathy (SMON)
Minimal brain dysfunction of childhood

Cerebral palsies
Febrile convulsions of childhood

See Chapter 13 for metabolic and hereditary diseases that affect the nervous system (e.g., gangliosidosis, mucopolysaccharidoses, glycogen storage disease).

ABNORMAL CSF

Viscous CSF may occur with metastatic mucinous adenocarcinoma (e.g., colon), large numbers of cryptococci, or rarely, injury to annulus fibrosus with release of nucleus pulposus fluid.

Turbidity may be due to presence of microorganisms (bacteria, fungi, amebae), contrast media, epidural fat aspirated during lumbar puncture, as well as increased WBC or RBC.

WBC of 200–300/cu mm causes cloudiness of CSF.

Protein >100 mg/dl usually causes CSF to look faintly yellow.

CSF with RBC >6000/cu mm appears grossly bloody; with RBC = 500–6000/cu mm, appears cloudy, xanthochromic, or pink-tinged (in bright light in clear glass tubes containing >1 ml of CSF).

Xanthochromia may be due to prior (at least 2–4 hours) bleeding, or markedly elevated protein (>150 mg/dl), or serum bilirubin >6 mg/dl.

CSF WBC may be corrected for presence of blood (e.g., traumatic tap, subarachnoid hemorrhage) by subtracting 1 WBC for each 700 RBCs/cu mm counted in CSF if the CBC is normal. If there is significant anemia or leukocytosis (all values are cells per cu mm):

$$\text{Corrected WBC} = \text{WBC in bloody CSF} - \frac{\text{WBC (blood)} \times \text{RBC (CSF)}}{\text{RBC (blood)}}$$

In normal CSF, minimal blood contamination may cause ≤2 polymorphonuclear leukocytes (PMNs)/25 RBCs, ≤10 PMNs/25–100 RBCs.

CSF total protein may be corrected for presence of blood by subtracting 1 mg/dl of protein for each 1000 RBCs/cu mm (if serum protein and CBC are normal and CSF protein and cell count are performed on same tube of CSF).

High WBC count (>3000/cu mm) predominantly PMNs strongly suggests bacterial cause, but when WBC <1000/cu mm in bacterial meningitis, one-third of patients have >50% lymphocytes or mononuclear cells. However, WBCs are usually PMNs in early stages of all types of meningitis; mononuclear cells only appear in a second specimen 18–24 hours later. Similarly, protein may not be increased in early stages of many types of meningitis.

Neutrophilic leukocytes are found in
- Bacteria (e.g., *Nocardia, Actinomyces, Arachnia, Brucella*)
- Fungi (*Blastomyces, Coccidioides, Candida, Aspergillus, Zygomycetes, Cladosporium, Pseudoallescheria*)
- Chemical (see p. 234)
- Other (e.g., systemic lupus erythematosus [SLE])

Lymphocytic cells are found in
- Bacteria (e.g., *Treponema pallidum, Leptospira, Actinomyces israelii, Arachnia propionica,* 90% of *Brucella* cases, *Borrelia burgdorferi* [Lyme disease], *Mycobacterium tuberculosis*)
- Fungi (e.g., *Cryptococcus neoformans, Candida* species, *Coccidioides immitis, Histoplasma capsulatum, Blastomyces dermatitides, Sporothrix schenckii, Pseudoallescheria boydii, Cladosporium trichoides*)
- Parasites (e.g., toxoplasmosis, cysticercosis)
- Viral (e.g., mumps, lymphocytic choriomeningitis, HTLV-III, echovirus)
- Parameningeal (e.g., brain abscess)
- Noninfectious (e.g., neoplasms, sarcoidosis, multiple sclerosis, granulomatous arteritis)

CSF glucose is decreased by utilization by bacteria (pyogens or tubercle bacilli) or occasionally cancer cells in CSF. Normally is ~50–65% of blood glucose, which should be drawn simultaneously. CSF glucose lags behind blood glucose by about 1 hour. In pyogenic meningitis, is usually <50% of blood level; may rapidly become normal after onset of antibiotic therapy; is decreased in only ~50% of cases of bacterial meningitis. May be decreased in 10–20% of cases of lymphocytic choriomeningitis, encephalitis due to mumps, or herpes simplex, but generally rare in viral infections or parameningeal processes. May also be decreased in rheumatoid meningitis, lupus myelopathy, chemical meningitis, meningeal parasites, hypoglycemia, granulomatous meningitis (e.g., sarcoid), some cases of subarachnoid hemorrhage. CSF glucose (40–45 mg/dl) is almost always abnormal; <40 mg/dl is always abnormal.

CSF lactic acid is increased (>35 mg/dl; normal = 10–25 mg/dl and up to 45 mg/dl in premature newborn) in both bacterial and fungal meningitis but *not in viral meningitis*. Level is still high after 1–2 days of antibiotic therapy in bacterial meningitis. Is increased whenever CSF glucose is very low or CSF WBC is elevated.

CSF protein, glucose, and WBC levels may not return to normal in ~50% of patients clinically cured of bacterial meningitis and therefore are not recommended as a test of cure.

CSF protein is normal in 10% of patients with bacterial meningitis (20% of meningococcal meningitis). CSF protein is usually >150 mg/dl; >500 mg/dl is infrequent and occurs chiefly in bacterial meningitis, bloody CSF, or cord tumor with spinal block and occasionally in polyneuritis and brain tumor. >1000 mg/dl suggests subarachnoid block; with complete spinal block, the lower the level of cord tumor, the higher the protein concentration. Rarely >200 mg/dl in viral meningitis. With antibiotic treatment of bacterial meningitis before CSF obtained, protein may be only slightly elevated.

CSF protein may show mild to moderate elevation in myxedema (25% of cases), uremia, connective tissue disorders, Cushing's syndrome.

Decreased CSF protein (3–20 mg/dl) may occur in hyperthyroidism, one-third of patients with benign intracranial hypertension, after removal of large volumes of CSF (e.g., during pneumoencephalography), in children 6–24 months old.

Serum protein levels must be normal in order to interpret any CSF protein values and should therefore always be done concurrently.

CSF chloride reflects only blood chloride level, although in tuberculous meningitis a decrease of 25% may exceed the decrease of serum chloride due to dehydration and electrolyte loss. Is not useful in diagnosis of tuberculous meningitis.

CSF glutamine >35 mg/dl is associated with hepatic encephalopathy (due to conversion from ammonia).

Blood and CSF serology is positive in CNS syphilis (see pp. 638–639); positive in 7–10% of active cases of infectious mononucleosis

Colloidal gold test is no longer used and replaced by protein electrophoresis of CSF. IgG in CSF is increased 14–35% in two-thirds of patients with neurosyphilis. IgG oligoclonal bands are seen in neurosyphilis as well as in multiple sclerosis.

Smears for Gram's and acid-fast stains must be made routinely, since the other findings may be normal in meningitis. Occasionally animal inoculations may be required. Gram's stain of CSF sediment is negative in 20% of cases of bacterial meningitis because at least 10^5 bacteria/ml of CSF must be present to demonstrate 1–2 bacteria/100 × microscopic field. Gram's stain is positive in 70–80% of cases due to pneumococci, *Hemophilus influenzae,* and meningococci but only 30–50% of cases due to gram-negative enteric bacilli. If antibiotics have been given before CSF is obtained, Gram's stain may be negative.

Stains are positive in <60% of treated bacterial meningitis, <5% of tubercular meningitis, 20–70% of fungal meningitis, and <2% of brain abscess. Sensitivity of Gram's stain is increased using fluorescent techniques with acridine orange.

Positive CSF culture has sensitivity of 92%, specificity of 95%, false negative rate of 8%, false positive rate of 5%.

Limulus amebocyte lysate is a rapid specific indicator of endotoxin produced by gram-negative bacteria (*Neisseria meningitidis, H. influenzae* type B, *Escherichia coli, Pseudomonas*). Is not affected by prior antibiotic therapy; is more rapid and sensitive than countercurrent immunoelectrophoresis (CIE). Is often not routinely available.

CIE detects bacterial antigens in CSF; identifies *H. influenzae* and meningococci but does not recognize *N. meningitidis* group B.

Agglutination kits (e.g., latex particle, coagglutination) for *H. influenzae* type B, *Cryptococcus neoformans, N. meningitidis, Streptococcus pneumoniae, Streptococcus agalactiae* (group B streptococcus) are simpler rapid methods that are now replacing CIE. Negative results are not considered conclusive; positive results should be confirmed by culture, especially to determine antibiotic susceptibility. Use to complement smear and culture. Antigen may be detected also in urine and serum but less sensitive than CSF specimens. Specific antigens have also been detected in urine and other body fluids in nonmeningeal infections (e.g., pneumococcal pneumonia, *H. influenzae* epiglottitis, Legionnaires' disease).

Serologic methods are often preferred (e.g., positive in 85% of coccidioidal cases compared to 37% positive for culture) especially in syphilis, brucella, Lyme disease.

In eclampsia, CSF shows gross or microscopic blood and increased protein (up to 200 mg/dl) in most patients. Glucose is normal. Uric acid is increased (to 3 times normal level) in all patients, reflecting the marked increase in serum level. (In normal pregnancy, CSF values have same reference range as in nonpregnant women.)

Tumor markers:

- Increased CSF carcinoembryonic antigen (CEA) has been reported helpful in diagnosis of suspected metastatic carcinoma (from breast, lung, bowel) with negative cytology.
- Beta-glucuronidase has been reported to be increased in 75% of patients with metastatic adenocarcinoma and 60% of patients with acute myeloblastic leukemia involving CNS.
- Lysozyme (muramidase) is increased in various CNS tumors, especially myeloid and monocytic leukemias, but is also increased when there are increased neutrophils present (e.g., bacterial meningitis).

Gamma-aminobutyric acid is decreased in CSF in Huntington's disease.

DEXAMETHASONE SUPPRESSION TEST (DST)

Blood is drawn at 11 P.M., 8 A.M., 12 noon, 4 P.M., and 11 P.M. for plasma cortisol levels. 1 mg of dexamethasone is given immediately after the first sample is taken. An abnormal test result is failure of suppression of plasma cortisol to level ≤5 μg/dl in any sample after the first.

A positive DST will "rule in" the diagnosis of melancholia (endogenous depression), but a negative DST will not rule it out, since it may be positive in only 40–50% of such patients.

In the presence of a positive DST, appropriate drug treatment (e.g., tricyclic antidepressants) that results in normalization of DST with clinical recovery is a good prognostic sign, whereas failure of normalization of DST suggests a poor prognosis and the need for continued antidepressant therapy. Despite clinical improvement, treatment should be continued until DST becomes negative. With relapse, DST may become abnormal when symptoms are still mild, before fully developed syndrome develops. The need to continue treatment is indicated if a positive DST that became negative with therapy reverts to positive after discontinuation of drug treatment or lowering of drug dosage.

Interference with DST may be caused by

- Certain drugs that cause nonsuppression, especially phenytoin, barbiturates, meprobamate, carbamazepine, alcohol (chronic high doses or withdrawal within 3 weeks)
- Enhanced suppression may be caused by benzodiazepines (high doses), corticosteroids (spironolactone, cortisone, artificial glucocorticoids such as prednisone, topical and nasal forms), dextroamphetamine.
- Other drugs that are said to interfere include estrogens (not birth control pills), reserpine, narcotics, and indomethacin.
- Medical conditions including weight loss to 20% below ideal body weight, pregnancy or abortion within 1 month, endocrine diseases, systemic infections, serious liver disease, cancer, other severe physical illnesses may also cause false positive test results.

Lithium maintenance therapy will not interfere with DST.

With a 50% prevalence of melancholia in the population studied and fulfillment of certain medical criteria, DST has sensitivity of 67%, specificity of 96%, and confidence level of 94% in diagnosis. Using only the 4 P.M. blood, sensitivity is ~50%. However, there are still no clear indications for routine use of DST in clinical psychiatry, and many of the routine methods are not accurate at the decision level.

Response of thyroid-stimulating hormone (TSH) to administration of thyrotropin-releasing hormone (TRH) has also been suggested as useful in the diagnosis of unipolar depression and prediction of relapse. These patients have a maximum rise in serum TSH level of <7 μU/ml (normal = 17 ± 9). Use of this test with DST is said to add confidence to diagnosis of major unipolar depression; abnormal response to either test before treatment suggests that patient is particularly liable to early relapse unless there is laboratory as well as clinical recovery after treatment.

Diseases of the Nervous System

HEAD TRAUMA

Laboratory findings due to single or various combinations of brain injuries

- Contusion, laceration, subdural hemorrhage, extradural hemorrhage, subarachnoid hemorrhage

Laboratory findings due to complications (e.g., pneumonia, meningitis)

In possible skull fractures, it has been recommended that nasal secretions may be differentiated from CSF by absence of glucose (using test tapes or tablets) in latter, but this is not reliable since nasal secretions may normally contain glucose. If enough (100 μl) fluid can be obtained to perform immunoelectrophoresis, CSF transferrin shows a double band, but only a single transferrin band is seen in other fluids (serum, nasal secretions, saliva, tears, lymph). In CSF, IgM is 5 times higher, prealbumin is 12 times higher, and transferrin is 2 times higher than in serum.

ACUTE EPIDURAL HEMORRHAGE

CSF is usually under increased pressure; clear unless there is associated cerebral contusion, laceration, or subarachnoid hemorrhage.

SUBDURAL HEMATOMA

CSF findings are variable—clear, bloody, or xanthochromic, depending on recent or old associated injuries (e.g., contusion, laceration).

Table 10-1. Differentiation of Bloody CSF due to Subarachnoid Hemorrhage and Traumatic Lumbar Puncture

CSF Findings	Subarachnoid Hemorrhage	Traumatic Lumbar Puncture
CSF pressure	Often increased	Low
Blood in tubes for collecting CSF	Mixture with blood is uniform in all tubes	Earlier tubes more bloody than later tubes
CSF clotting	Does not clot	Often clots
Xanthochromia	Present if >8–12 hours since cerebral hemorrhage	Absent unless patient is icteric
Immediate repeat of lumbar puncture at higher level	CSF same as initial puncture	CSF clear

Chronic subdural hematoma fluid is usually xanthochromic; protein content is 300–2000 mg/dl.
Anemia is often present in infants.

CEREBROVASCULAR ACCIDENT (NONTRAUMATIC)

Due To

Occlusion (e.g., thrombosis, embolism) in 80% of patients
Hemorrhage
- Ruptured berry aneurysm (45% of patients)
- Hypertension (15% of patients)
- Angiomatous malformations (8% of patients)
- Miscellaneous (e.g., brain tumor, blood dyscrasia)—infrequent
- Undetermined (rest of patients)

CSF
- In early subarachnoid hemorrhage (<8 hours after onset of symptoms), the test for occult blood may be positive before xanthochromia develops. After bloody spinal fluid occurs, WBC/RBC ratio may be higher in CSF than in peripheral blood.
- Bloody CSF clears by tenth day in 40% of patients. CSF is persistently abnormal after 21 days in 15% of patients. ~5% of cerebrovascular episodes due to hemorrhage are wholly within the parenchyma with normal CSF.

CEREBRAL THROMBOSIS

Laboratory findings due to some diseases that may be causative
- Hematologic (e.g., polycythemia, sickle cell disease, thrombotic thrombopenia, macroglobulinemia)
- Arterial (e.g., polyarteritis nodosa, Takayasu's syndrome, dissecting aneurysm of aorta, syphilis, meningitis)
- Hypotension (e.g., myocardial infarction, shock)

CSF
- Protein normal or may be increased ≤100 mg/dl
- Cell count normal or ≥10 WBC/cu mm during first 48 hours and rarely ≥2000 WBC/cu mm transiently on third day

CEREBRAL EMBOLISM

Laboratory findings due to underlying causative disease
- Bacterial endocarditis
- Nonbacterial thrombotic vegetations on heart valves

Chronic rheumatic mitral stenosis.
Mural thrombus due to underlying myocardial infarction
Myxoma of left atrium
Fat embolism in fracture of long bones
Air embolism in neck, chest, or cardiac surgery

CSF

Usually findings are the same as in cerebral thrombosis. One-third of patients develop hemorrhagic infarction, usually producing slight xanthochromia several days later; some of these patients may have grossly bloody CSF (10,000 RBCs/cu mm). Septic embolism (e.g., bacterial endocarditis) may cause increased WBC (≤200/cu mm with variable lymphocytes and PMNs), increased RBC (≤1000/cu mm), slight xanthochromia, increased protein, normal sugar, negative culture.

INTRACEREBRAL HEMORRHAGE

Increased WBC (15,000–20,000/cu mm) (higher than in cerebral occlusion, e.g., embolism, thrombosis)

Increased erythrocyte sedimentation rate (ESR)

Urine

Transient glycosuria
Laboratory findings of concomitant renal disease

Laboratory findings due to other causes of intracerebral hemorrhage (e.g., leukemia, aplastic anemia, purpuras, hemophilias, anticoagulant therapy, SLE, polyarteritis nodosa)

CSF

See Table 10-1, p. 223.
See Table 10-2, pp. 226–230.
See Cerebrovascular Accident (Nontraumatic), p. 223.

Especially if blood pressure is normal, always rule out ruptured berry aneurysm, hemorrhage into tumor, angioma.

Laboratory findings due to other diseases that occur with increased frequency in association with berry aneurysm (e.g., coarctation of the aorta, polycystic kidneys, hypertension)

HYPERTENSIVE ENCEPHALOPATHY

Laboratory findings due to changes in other organ systems

Cardiac
Renal
Endocrine
Toxemia of pregnancy

Laboratory findings due to progressive changes that may occur (e.g., focal intracerebral hemorrhage)

CSF frequently shows increased pressure and protein ≤100 mg/dl.

PSEUDOTUMOR CEREBRI

(benign intracranial hypertension with neurologic complex of headache and papilledema without mass lesion or ventricular obstruction)

CSF normal except for increased pressure

Laboratory findings due to associated conditions (only obesity has been reported consistently) (e.g., Addison's disease, infection, metabolic [acute hypocalcemia and other "electrolyte disturbances," empty sella syndrome, pregnancy]), drugs (e.g., psychotherapeutic drugs, sex hormones and oral contraceptives, corticosteroid administration [usually after reduction of dosage or change to different preparation]), immune diseases (e.g., SLE, periarteritis nodosa, serum sickness), others (e.g., sarcoid, Guillain-Barré syndrome, head trauma, various anemias)

BRAIN TUMOR

CSF findings

- CSF is clear, occasionally xanthochromic or bloody if there is hemorrhage into the tumor.
- WBC may be increased ≤150 cells/cu mm in 75% of patients; normal in others.
- Protein is usually increased.
- Tumor cells may be demonstrable in 20–40% of patients with all types of solid tumors, but failure to find malignant cells does not exclude meningeal neoplasm.
- Glucose may be decreased if cells are present.

CSF protein is particularly increased with meningioma of the olfactory groove and with acoustic neurinoma.

Brain stem gliomas, which are characteristically found in childhood, usually show normal CSF.

"Diencephalic syndrome" of infants due to glioma of hypothalamus usually shows normal CSF.

Laboratory findings due to underlying causative disease (e.g., primary brain tumors, metastatic tumors, leukemias and lymphomas, infections [e.g., tuberculoma, schistosomiasis, torulosis, hydatid cyst], pituitary adenomas [CSF protein and pressure usually normal])

LEUKEMIC INVOLVEMENT OF CNS

Intracranial hemorrhage—principal cause of death in leukemia (may be intracerebral, subarachnoid, subdural)

More frequent when WBC is >100,000/cu mm and with rapid increase in WBC, especially in blastic crises

Platelet count frequently decreased

Evidence of bleeding elsewhere

CSF findings of intracranial hemorrhage (see p. 224)

Meningeal infiltration of leukemic cells: CNS is involved in 5% of patients with acute lymphoblastic leukemia (ALL) at diagnosis and is the major site of relapse. Meninges are involved in up to 30% of patients with malignant lymphoma; most prevalent in diffuse large cell ("histiocytic"), lymphoblastic, immunoblastic, and one-third to one-half of Burkitt's lymphoma patients; 15–20% of cases of non-Hodgkin's lymphoma. Hodgkin's disease seldom involves CNS. Involvement by chronic lymphocytic leukemia, well-differentiated lymphocytic lymphoma, and plasmacytoid lymphomas is exceedingly rare. Malignant cells are found in CSF in 60–80% of patients with meningeal involvement.

- CSF may show
  - Increased pressure and protein
  - Glucose decreased to <50% of blood level
  - Increased cells that are often not recognized as blast cells because of poor preservation may be identified with cytochemical, immunoenzymatic, immunofluorescent, and flow cytometry techniques.

Complicating meningeal infection (e.g., various bacteria, opportunistic fungi)

BACTERIAL MENINGITIS

75% of cases are due to *N. meningitidis,* pneumococcus, *H. influenzae.* Bacteria can be identified in only 90% of cases; culture is more reliable than Gram's stain, although the stain offers a more immediate guide to therapy. Gram's stain is positive in ~70% of cases. When Gram's stain is positive, CSF is more likely to show decreased glucose, increased protein, and increased RBC count.

Detection of bacterial antigen (by CIE) in CSF for *Streptococcus pneumoniae, H. influenzae,* some strains of *N. meningitidis.*

Table 10-2. Cerebrospinal Fluid Findings in Various Diseases

Disease	Appearance	Initial Pressure (mm of water)	Protein (mg/dl)	Fasting Sugar (mg/dl)	WBC/cu mm
Normal					
Ventricular	Clear, colorless, no clot	70–180	5–15	45–80	0–10
Cisternal			10–25		
Lumbar			15–45		
Tuberculous meningitis	O, slightly yellow, delicate clot	Usually I	45–500	10–45	25–1000, chiefly L
Acute pyogenic meningitis	O–Pu, slightly yellow, coarse clot	Usually I	50–1500	0–45	25–10,000, chiefly P
Aseptic meningeal reaction	C or T or X	Often N	20–200 +	N	≦ 500, occasionally 2000
Syphilis					
Tabes dorsalis	N	N	25–100	N	10–80
General paresis	N	N	50–300	N	10–150
Meningovascular syphilis	N	N	45–150, N in 30% of patients	N	10–100, N in 45%

Acute anterior poliomyelitis	C or slightly O, may be slightly yellow, may be delicate clot	Usually N, may be I	20–350	N	10–500 +, L > P
Other virus Mumps	N or O	N or slightly I	20–125	N	0–2000 +
Measles	N or O	N or slightly I	Slightly I	N	≦500
Herpes zoster	N	N	20–110	N	≦300, 40% of patients
Equine, St. Louis encephalitis, choriomeningitis	N or slightly T	N or I	20–200 +	N	10–200, occasionally to 3000
Postinfectious encephalitis	N	May be slightly I	15–75	N	5–200, rarely to 1000
Toxoplasmosis (congenital)	X	I	≦2000		50–500, chiefly monocytes
Cryptococcal meningitis	N	I	≦500 in 90%	Moderately decreased in 55%	≦800 (L > P)
Coccidioidomycosis		I	I	N early, then D	≦200 early; may be higher later

Table 10-2 (continued)

Disease	Appearance	Initial Pressure (mm of water)	Protein (mg/dl)	Fasting Sugar (mg/dl)	WBC/cu mm
Primary amebic meningoencephalitis (due to free-living *Naegleria*)	Sanguino-purulent, may be T or Pu	I	I	Usually D	400–21,000 (predominantly P). Usually RBCs are also found. Amebas seen on Wright's stain
Tumor					
Cord	C, occasionally X	N or D	≦3500 in 85%, N in 15%	N	≦100, chiefly L; N in 60%
Brain	C, occasionally X	I	≦500	N	≦150, N in 75%
Pseudotumor cerebri	N	I	N	N	N
Cerebral thrombosis	N	25% I, 75% N	≦100+, N in 60%	N	≦50, N in 75%
Cerebral hemorrhage	N in 15%, X in 10%, B in 75%	80% I, 20% N	≦2000, usually I	N	Same as in blood, N in 10%
Subarachnoid hemorrhage (ruptured berry aneurysm)	B, X in 24 hours, no clot	Usually I	≦1000+, usually I	N	Same as in blood

Bloody tap (traumatic)	B	N or D	I by blood	N	Same as in blood
Head trauma	N, B, or X	Often I	I if bloody	N	Same as in blood
Subdural hematoma	N, B only with contusion	80% I, 20% N	N or slightly I	N	Same as in blood
Multiple sclerosis (see pp. 236–237)	N	N	≦130, N in 75%; IgG I in 75%	N	≦40, N in 70%
Polyneuritis Polyarteritis	N; X if protein is very I	N	Usually N	N	N, but albuminocytologic dissociation in Guillain-Barré syndrome that may occur in heavy metal poisoning, infection, etc.
Porphyria		N	Usually N	N	
Beriberi		N	Usually N	N	
Alcohol		N	Usually N	N	
Arsenic		N	Usually N	N	
Diabetes mellitus		N	Often ≦300	N	
Acute infections		N	≦1500	N	
Lead encephalopathy	N or slightly yellow	I	≦100	N	0–100

Table 10-2 (continued)

Disease	Appearance	Initial Pressure (mm of water)	Protein (mg/dl)	Fasting Sugar (mg/dl)	WBC/cu mm
Alcoholism	N	May be I	N	N	Usually N
Diabetic coma	N	D	N	I	Usually N
Uremia	N	Usually I	N or I	N or I	Usually N
Epilepsy	N	N	N	N	N

C = clear; O = opalescent; T = turbid; N = normal; X = xanthochromic; B = bloody; Pu = purulent; I = increased; D = decreased; P = polymorphonuclear leukocyte; L = lymphocyte.

Laboratory findings due to preceding diseases
- Pneumonia, otitis media, sinusitis, skull fracture prior to pneumococcal meningitis
- *Neisseria* epidemics prior to this meningitis
- Bacterial endocarditis, septicemia, etc.
- Pneumococci in alcoholism, myeloma, sickle cell anemia, splenectomy, immunocompromised state
- *Cryptococcus* and *Mycobacterium* tuberculosis in steroid therapy and immunocompromised state
- Gram-negative bacilli in immunocompromised state
- *H. influenzae* in splenectomy

Laboratory findings due to complications (e.g., Waterhouse-Friderichsen syndrome, subdural effusion)

Most frequent and important differential is between acute bacterial meningitis (ABM) and acute viral meningitis (AVM). The most useful tests that favor the diagnosis of ABM rather than AVM are as follows:*
- CSF positive by bacterial stain, culture, or antigen detection
- Decreased CSF glucose (not <30 mg/dl in AVM but in 43% of ABM)
- Decreased CSF/serum ratio of glucose (<0.25 in <1% of AVM cases and 44% of ABM cases) even if CSF glucose is normal
- Increased CSF protein >1.72 gm/L (1% of AVM and 50% of ABM but may be normal in 10% of ABM cases). Increase occurs especially with *S. pneumoniae*
- CSF WBC >2000/cu mm in 38% of ABM cases and PMN >1180/cu mm, but low counts do not rule out ABM.
- Peripheral WBC is only useful if very high WBC (>27,200) and total PMN (>21,000/cu mm), which occurs in relatively few patients; leukopenia is common in infants and elderly.
- Combination of findings can exclude AVM and rule in ABM, but none of them can establish the diagnosis of AVM, and absence of these findings cannot exclude ABM.

NEUROLOGIC MANIFESTATIONS OF INFECTION WITH HUMAN IMMUNODEFICIENCY VIRUS (HIV) (ACQUIRED IMMUNE DEFICIENCY SYNDROME [AIDS])

(see also Acquired Immune Deficiency Syndrome [AIDS], pp. 653–655)

Dementia (also called subacute encephalitis) is most common neurologic syndrome with AIDS; in >50% of patients; may be initial or later manifestation.
- CSF abnormalities in 85%
    - Increased protein (50–100 mg/dl) in 60% of cases
    - Mild mononuclear pleocytosis (5–50 cells/cu mm) in 20% of cases
    - HIV antibodies

Aseptic meningitis—may occur early, late, or chronic recurrent
- CSF may show
    - 20–300 cells/cu mm
    - Protein may be 50–100 mg/dl.
    - HIV culture is usually positive.
    - Increased CSF/serum antibody ratio indicates local antibody production

Myelopathy—gradual onset; usually associated with dementia. Polymyositis is most common type.

Peripheral neuropathies, some of which may resemble Guillain-Barré syndrome
- CSF may show
    - Increased protein (50–100 mg/dl)
    - Pleocytosis of 10–50 cells/cu mm

*Data from A Spands, FE Harrell, and DT Durack, Differential diagnosis of acute meningitis: An analysis of the predictive value of initial observations. *JAMA* 262:2700, 1989.

Table 10-3. Etiology of Bacterial Meningitis by Age

	Newborns	Less Than 1 Year	1–5 Years	5–14 Years	More Than 15 Years	Elderly
Most frequent	*Escherichia coli*	*Hemophilus influenzae*		*Neisseria meningitidis*	Pneumococcus	Pneumococcus *Neisseria meningitidis*
Common	*Klebsiella-Aerobacter* Beta-hemolytic streptococcus *Listeria monocytogenes* *Staphylococcus aureus*	*Neisseria meningitidis* Pneumococcus		*Hemophilus influenzae* Pneumococcus	*Neisseria meningitidis* *Staphylococcus aureus*	Gram-negative bacilli *Listeria monocytogenes*
Uncommon	Paracolon bacilli *Pseudomonas* species *Hemophilus influenzae*	*Pseudomonas* species *Staphylococcus aureus* Beta-hemolytic streptococcus *Escherichia coli*	Beta-hemolytic streptococcus		Beta-hemolytic streptococcus *Escherichia coli* *Pseudomonas* species	
Rare	*Neisseria meningitidis*	*Klebsiella-Aerobacter*, paracolons, various other gram-negative organisms			*Hemophilus influenzae*	

The frequency of different organisms may vary from year to year, in presence of epidemics, or by geographic location.

Occasionally more than one organism is recovered.

Hemophilus influenzae (almost always type B) causes most cases between age 6 months and 3 years but is unusual before age 2 months. Enteric bacteria are so rarely found in older children that in their presence immunologic defect or congenital dermal sinus should be ruled out. If surgery has not been performed, congenital dermal sinus should be ruled out if *Staphylococcus aureus* is present.

A Gram's stain of CSF should always be done in addition to a culture because it provides a more immediate clue to the causative agent and the proper therapy and because the culture may be negative if the patient received antibiotics soon before the lumbar puncture. Cultures should also be obtained from blood and petechial skin lesions if present. Gram stain of buffy coat of blood is often useful.

CSF glucose is very useful in differentiating bacterial and viral meningitis and is a good index to the severity of the infection, with a lower level in more severe infections. *Newborns with overwhelming pneumococcal infections may have no decrease in glucose or increase of cells.*

CSF should be reexamined in 24 hours as a guide to therapeutic response; a good response shows negative gram-stained smear and culture, increased glucose level, and a changing cell count from predominance of polymorphonuclear cells to predominance of mononuclear cells; total cell count and protein may show an initial rise. CSF should be reexamined when therapy is to be stopped; treatment should not be stopped unless CSF is normal except for slight increase of cells ($\leqq$ about 20 lymphocytes).

Opportunistic infections
- Viral (e.g., cytomegalovirus [CMV], herpes simplex virus [HSV] I and II, papovavirus)
- Nonviral (e.g., cryptococcal, toxoplasmosis, *Aspergillus fumigatus, Candida albicans, Coccidioides immitis, Mycobacterium avium-intracellulare* and *tuberculosis, Nocardia asteroides, Listeria*)

Neoplasms (e.g., Kaposi's sarcoma, non-Hodgkin's lymphoma)
Vascular (e.g., infarction, hemorrhage, vasculitis)
Associated diseases (e.g., neurosyphilis)

ASEPTIC MENINGITIS

CSF
- Protein is normal or slightly increased.
- Increased cell count shows predominantly PMNs at first, mononuclear cells later.
- Glucose is normal.
- Bacterial cultures are negative.

If glucose levels are decreased, rule out tuberculosis, cryptococcosis, leukemia, lymphoma, metastatic carcinoma, sarcoidosis.

Due To
(clinically most important types)

Viral infections (especially poliomyelitis, Coxsackievirus, echovirus, lymphocytic choriomeningitis, infectious mononucleosis, and many others)
Leptospirosis, syphilis
Tuberculosis, cryptococcosis (CSF glucose levels may not be decreased until later stages.)
Brain abscess, incompletely treated bacterial meningitis
Neoplasm (leukemia, carcinoma)

PRIMARY AMEBIC MENINGOENCEPHALITIS
(due to free-living amebas—*Naegleria*)

Increased WBC, predominantly neutrophils
CSF findings
- Fluid may be cloudy, purulent, or sanguinopurulent.
- Protein is increased.
- Glucose is usually decreased; may be normal.
- Increased WBCs are chiefly PMNs. RBCs are frequently present also. Motile amebas are seen in hemocytometer chamber.
- Amebas are seen on Wright's stain. Gram's stain and cultures are negative for bacteria and fungi.

ACUTE VIRAL ENCEPHALOMYELITIS
(infectious, postvaccinal, postexanthematous, postinfectious)

In U.S., HSV and rabies are most common endemic causes of encephalitis; outside of North America, Japanese B encephalitis is most common epidemic infection. Postinfectious encephalomyelitis patients have an invariable, irreversible demyelinating syndrome; is most commonly associated with varicella and upper respiratory infection (especially influenza) in U.S., but measles is the most common worldwide cause.
Vaccination has reduced the incidence of acute and postinfectious encephalitis due to measles, mumps, rubella, and yellow fever.
Vaccination has greatly decreased incidence of poliomyelitis, but a few cases of vaccine-associated infections occur.
Coxsackie and echoviruses usually cause benign aseptic meningitis.
CSF shows increased protein and lymphocytes.
Laboratory findings due to preceding condition (e.g., measles) are noted.

Paired serum samples during acute and convalescent periods may show seroconversion or 4-fold rise in specific antibody titers.

ELISA to detect IgM in CSF is sensitive and specific for Japanese B encephalitis; is usually present at hospitalization and almost always present by third day of illness.

Detection of HSV antigen in CSF is reported to be 80% sensitive and 90% specific if performed within 3 days of onset of illness. Brain biopsy is most sensitive and specific for HSV and its mimics.

HSV can be cultured from CSF in ~50% of babies with encephalitis or disseminated disease but uncommon in older patients; therefore viral culture is indicated in newborns.

Brain biopsy is presently reserved for patients who do not respond to acyclovir therapy and have unknown abnormality on CAT scan or MRI.

MOLLARET'S MENINGITIS

Numerous recurrent episodes (2–7 days each) of aseptic meningitis occur over a period of several years with symptom-free intervals showing mild leukopenia and eosinophilia. Other organ systems are not involved. There is frequently a history of previous severe trauma with fractures and concussions.

CSF during first 12–24 hours may contain ≤several thousand cells/cu mm, predominantly PMNs and 66% of a large type of mononuclear cell. The mononuclear cells (sometimes called "endothelial" cells) are of unknown origin and significance and are characterized by vague nuclear and cytoplasmic outline with rapid lysis even while being counted in the hemocytometer chamber; they may be seen only as "ghosts" and are usually not detectable after the first day of illness. After the first 24 hours, the PMNs disappear and are replaced by lymphocytes, which in turn rapidly disappear when the attack subsides.

CSF protein may be increased ≤100 mg/dl. CSF glucose is normal or may be slightly decreased.

CHEMICAL MENINGITIS

(due to injection of anesthetic, antibiotic, radiopaque dye, etc., or to rupture into CSF of contents of epidermoid tumor or craniopharyngioma)

CSF

- Pleocytosis is mild to moderate, largely lymphocytic.
- Protein shows variable increase.
- Glucose is usually normal.

GUILLAIN-BARRÉ SYNDROME

CSF shows albuminocytologic dissociation with normal cell count and increased protein (average 50–100 mg/dl). Protein increase parallels increasing clinical severity; increase may be prolonged.

Laboratory findings due to preceding disease may be present (e.g., acute infections of respiratory or GI tract [e.g., Epstein-Barr virus, *Campylobacter jejuni,* varicella zoster, *Mycoplasma pneumoniae,* CMV, hepatitis, other viral and rickettsial infections], Refsum's disease, immune disorders, endocrine disturbances, exposure to toxins, neoplasms).

SENILE DEMENTIA (ALZHEIMER-PICK DISEASE; CEREBRAL ATROPHY)*

There are no abnormal laboratory findings, but laboratory tests are useful to rule out other diseases that may resemble these syndromes but are amenable to therapy.

*Data from EB Larson et al., Diagnostic tests in the evaluation of dementia: A prospective study of 200 elderly outpatients. *Arch Intern Med* 146:1917, 1986.

Recommended tests in all patients with new onset of dementia should include CBC, urinalysis, electrolyte and blood chemistry panel, screening metabolic panel, serum vitamin B_{12} and folate, thyroid function tests (chemistry panel screens for some other endocrine disorders), serologic test for syphilis.
In 200 patients > age 60 with dementia, the causes were

Alzheimer's type	74.5%
Due to drugs	9.5%
Alcohol related	4.0%
Hypothyroidism	3.0%
Multi-infarct	1.5%
Hyperparathyroidism	1.0%
Hyponatremia	1.0%
Hypoglycemia	0.5%
Unknown cause	3.5%
Not demented	7.5%

Other newly recognized conditions were low serum iron, folate or cobalamin (8%), urinary tract infection (2.5%). Serum urea nitrogen (BUN) was also useful.

NEUROPSYCHIATRIC DISORDERS DUE TO COBALAMIN DEFICIENCY

(see also Pernicious Anemia, p. 285)

More than 25% may present with neuropsychiatric findings (e.g., paresthesias, sensory loss, abnormal gait and ataxia, mental or psychiatric disturbances) with some normal hematologic findings (e.g., hematocrit, mean corpuscular volume [MCV], WBC, platelet count, serum bilirubin, serum LDH) and some abnormal findings (e.g., hypersegmentation of PMNs, macroovalocytes, mild megaloblastic bone marrow).
Serum cobalamin and Schilling test may occasionally be only borderline decreased or even normal.
Increased serum methylmalonic acid and total homocysteine, which return to normal after cyanocobalamin therapy, confirms diagnosis.

REFSUM'S DISEASE

This is a rare hereditary recessive lipidosis of the nervous system with retinitis pigmentosa, peripheral neuropathy, cerebellar ataxia, nerve deafness, and ichthyosis.
CSF shows albuminocytologic dissociation (normal cell count with protein usually increased to 100–700 mg/dl).

METACHROMATIC LEUKODYSTROPHY

Urine sediment may contain metachromatic lipids (from breakdown of myelin products).
CSF protein may be normal or elevated $\leq$200 mg/dl.
Biopsy of dental or sural nerve with demonstration of accumulated metachromatic sulfatide is diagnostic.

PROGRESSIVE CEREBELLAR ATAXIA WITH SKIN TELANGIECTASIAS (LOUIS-BAR SYNDROME)

This is an autosomal recessive multisystem disease with cerebellar ataxia and oculocutaneous telangiectasia.
Some patients have
- Glucose intolerance
- Abnormal liver function tests
- Decreased or absent serum IgA and IgE causing recurrent pulmonary infections; IgM present
- Increased serum alpha-fetoprotein

See also Table 12-22, pp. 354–355.

BASSEN-KORNZWEIG SYNDROME

Abnormal RBCs (acanthocytes) are present in the peripheral blood smear.

There may be

- Marked deficiency of serum beta-lipoprotein and cholesterol
- Abnormal pattern of RBC phospholipids
- Marked impairment of GI fat absorption
- Low serum carotene levels (see pp. 162–163)

LINDAU–VON HIPPEL DISEASE (HEMANGIOBLASTOMAS OF RETINA AND CEREBELLUM)

Laboratory findings due to associated conditions (e.g., polycythemia, pheochromocytomas), various tumors (e.g., kidney)

MULTIPLE SCLEROSIS (MS)*

No changes of diagnostic value in peripheral blood or routine CSF tests.

CSF WBC is slightly elevated in ~25% of patients but usually <20 mononuclear cells/cu mm; >25 cells/cu mm in <1% of cases. >50 cells/cu mm should be interpreted with extreme caution. Albumin, glucose, and pressure are normal.

CSF total protein may be mildly elevated in ~25% of cases. Levels >100 mg/dl should cast doubt on diagnosis. CSF gamma globulin is increased in 60–75% of patients regardless of whether the total CSF protein is increased. Gamma globulin ≥12% of CSF total protein is abnormal without corresponding increase in serum gamma globulin but may also be increased in other CNS disorders (e.g., syphilis, subacute panencephalitis, meningeal carcinomatosis) and may also be increased when serum electrophoresis is abnormal due to non-CNS diseases (e.g., rheumatoid arthritis, sarcoidosis, cirrhosis, myxedema, multiple myeloma).

CSF IgG is increased in ~70% of cases, often when total protein is normal. Increase of IgG is expressed as ratio of CSF to serum total protein or albumin to rule out increased IgG due to disruption of blood-brain barrier. CSF IgG does not correlate with duration, activity, or course of MS. Increase may also be found in neurosyphilis, acute Guillain-Barré syndrome, 5–15% of miscellaneous neurologic diseases, and a few normal persons; recent myelogram is said to invalidate the test.

CSF IgM and IgA may also be elevated but are not useful for diagnosis.

Agar or agarose gel electrophoresis of CSF shows discrete bands of oligoclonal proteins (due to abnormal gamma globulins) in 85–95% of patients with definite MS and 30–40% with possible MS; is the most sensitive marker of MS. Positive results also occur in ≤10% of noninflammatory neurologic disease and ≤40% of inflammatory CNS disorders (e.g., neurosyphilis, viral encephalitis, subacute sclerosing panencephalitis, progressive rubella encephalitis, cryptococcal meningitis, inflammatory neuropathies). Not known to correlate with severity, duration, or course of MS. During steroid treatment, prevalence of oligoclonal bands and other gamma globulin abnormalities may be reduced by 30–50%.

A few patients with definite MS may have normal CSF immunoglobulins and lack oligoclonal bands.

Myelin basic protein is elevated in 70–90% of MS patients during an acute exacerbation and usually returns to normal within 2 weeks. Is frequently elevated in other causes of demyelination and tissue destruction (e.g., encephalitis, leukodystrophies, metabolic encephalopathies, CNS lupus, cranial irradiation and intrathecal chemotherapy, 45% of patients with recent stroke).

*Data from H Markowitz and E Kokmen, Neurologic diseases and the cerebrospinal fluid immunoglobulin profile. *Proc Mayo Clin* 58:273, 1983; JW Swanson, Multiple sclerosis: Update in diagnosis and review of prognostic factors. *Proc Mayo Clin* 64:577, 1989.

Increased association with certain histocompatibility antigens (e.g., whites with B7 and Dw2 antigen)
Abnormal CSF IgG values in MS:

$$\text{CSF IgG index} = \frac{(\text{CSF IgG/CSF albumin})}{(\text{serum IgG/serum albumin})} \qquad (\text{normal} \leq 0.77)$$

CSF IgG: normal $\leq$8.4 mg/dl
CSF albumin: normal $\leq$26.0 mg/dl

$$\text{IgG synthesis rate (mg/day)} = \left[\left(\text{CSF IgG} - \frac{\text{serum IgG}}{341}\right) - \left(\text{CSF albumin} - \frac{\text{serum albumin}}{169}\right)\left(\frac{\text{serum IgG}}{\text{serum albumin}}\right)0.43\right] \times 5$$

>90% of patients with definite MS have rate >3 mg/day.

CSF IgG index >0.77 in 80–90% of definite MS cases, 33% of inflammatory neurologic diseases, 12% of other neurologic disorders.
CSF IgG index has sensitivity of 88%, specificity of 95% in MS.
Oligoclonal bands have sensitivity of 88%, specificity of 79%.

Diagnosis should not be made on CSF findings unless there are multiple clinical lesions in time and anatomic location.

CRANIAL ARTERITIS

ESR is markedly increased.

CAVERNOUS SINUS THROMBOPHLEBITIS

CSF is usually normal unless there is associated subdural empyema or meningitis, or it may show increased protein and WBC with normal glucose, or it may be hemorrhagic. In the diabetic patient, mucormycosis may cause this clinical appearance.
Laboratory findings due to preceding infections, complications (e.g., meningitis, brain abscess) or other causes of venous thromboses (e.g., sickle cell disease, polycythemia, dehydration)

ACUTE SUBDURAL EMPYEMA

CSF
- Cell count is increased to a few hundred, with predominance of PMNs.
- Protein is increased.
- Glucose is normal.
- Bacterial smears and cultures are negative.

WBC is usually increased ($\leq$25,000/cu mm).
Laboratory findings due to preceding diseases
- Ear, nose, and throat infections, especially acute sinusitis
- Intracranial surgery

Streptococci are the most common organisms when preceding condition is sinusitis. Staphylococcus aureus *or gram-negative organisms are the most common organisms following trauma or surgery.*

BRAIN ABSCESS

CSF shows increased neutrophils, lymphocytes, RBCs, and WBC ~25–300/cu mm.
There may be increased protein level (75–300 mg/dl). The sugar level is normal. Bacterial cultures are negative. Findings depend on stage and duration of abscess.

Associated primary disease
- Ear, nose, and throat infections
- Primary septic lung disease (e.g., lung abscess, bronchiectasis, empyema)
- Congenital heart disease (e.g., septal defects)

Due To

Usually mixed anaerobic (e.g., streptococci or *Bacteroides*) and aerobic organisms (e.g., streptococci, staphylococci, or pneumococci)

May be caused by almost any organism, including fungi, *Nocardia*

TUBERCULOMA OF BRAIN

CSF shows increased protein with small number of cells. The tuberculoma may be transformed into tuberculous meningitis with increased protein and cells (50–300/cu mm), decreased sugar and chloride.

Laboratory findings due to tuberculosis elsewhere are noted.

TUBERCULOUS MENINGITIS

See p. 643.

SPINAL CORD TUMOR

CSF protein is increased. It may be very high and associated with xanthochromia when there is a block of the subarachnoid space.

With complete block, lower levels of cord tumor are associated with higher protein concentration.

See Table 10-2, p. 226.

EPIDURAL ABSCESS OF SPINAL CORD/INTRACRANIAL EXTRADURAL ABSCESS

CSF protein is increased (usually 100–400 mg/dl), and WBCs (lymphocytes and neutrophils) are relatively few in number.

Most common organism is *S. aureus,* followed by streptococci and gram-negative bacilli.

Laboratory findings due to preceding condition (e.g., adjacent osteomyelitis, bacteremia due to dental, respiratory, or skin infections)

MYELITIS

CSF may be normal or may show increased protein and cells (20–1000/cu mm—lymphocytes and mononuclear cells).

Laboratory findings due to causative condition (e.g., poliomyelitis, herpes zoster, tuberculosis, syphilis, parasites, abscess, multiple sclerosis, postvaccinal myelitis)

INFARCTION OF SPINAL CORD

CSF changes same as in cerebral hemorrhage or infarction

Laboratory findings due to causative condition
- Polyarteritis nodosa
- Dissecting aneurysm of aorta
- Arteriosclerosis of aorta with thrombus formation
- Iatrogenic (e.g., aortic arteriography, clamping of aorta during cardiac surgery)

CHRONIC ADHESIVE ARACHNOIDITIS

(due to spinal anesthesia, syphilis, etc.)

CSF protein may be normal or increased.

CERVICAL SPONDYLOSIS
CSF shows increased protein in some cases.

RETROBULBAR NEUROPATHY
CSF is normal or may show increased protein and $\leq$200 lymphocytes.

75% of these patients ultimately develop multiple sclerosis.

GLOMUS JUGULARE TUMOR
CSF protein may be increased.

11

Musculoskeletal and Joint Diseases

Laboratory Tests for Musculoskeletal Diseases

SERUM ENZYMES IN SOME MUSCULOSKELETAL DISEASES*

Creatine kinase (CK) is the measurement of choice. It is more specific and sensitive than serum glutamic-oxaloacetic transaminase (SGOT) and lactic dehydrogenase (LDH) and more discriminating than aldolase (ALD).

Increased In

Polymyositis
Muscular dystrophy (see p. 244)
Myotonic dystrophy (see p. 245)
Some metabolic disorders (see p. 245)

Normal In

Rheumatoid arthritis
Scleroderma
Acrosclerosis
Discoid lupus erythematosus
Muscle atrophy of neurologic origin (e.g., old poliomyelitis, polyneuritis)
Hyperthyroid myopathy

CK-Isoenzymes

Duchenne's dystrophy—increased CK-MB (10–15% of total) in 60–90% of cases; CK-BB may be slightly increased; CK-MM is chief fraction. CK-MB may be slightly increased (usually <4%) in carriers with increased total CK.

CK-MB is sometimes seen in Becker's and limb-girdle dystrophy in up to 10% of total.

Hypothyroidism rare; increases CK-MB up to 6% of total.

CREATINE AND CREATININE

Increased blood creatinine, decreased creatinine excretion, increased creatine excretion

Occurs In

Progressive muscular dystrophy
Decreased muscle mass in
- Neurogenic atrophy
- Polymyositis
- Addison's disease
- Hyperthyroidism
- Male eunuchoidism

CREATINE TOLERANCE TEST

(ingestion of 1–3 gm creatine)

Normal: Creatine is not increased in blood or urine.
Decreased muscle mass: Blood and urine creatine increases in
- Neurogenic atrophy
- Polymyositis
- Addison's disease
- Hyperthyroidism
- Male eunuchoidism

*Data from SB Rosalki, Serum enzymes in diseases of skeletal muscle. *Clin Lab Med* 9:767, 1989.

Table 11-1. Laboratory Findings in the Differential Diagnosis of Some Muscle Diseases

Disease	Complete Blood Count	ESR	Thyroid Function Tests	Percent of Patients with Increase in Various Serum Enzyme Levels	Muscle Biopsy	Comment
Myasthenia gravis	N	N	N	N	Lymphorrhages	Cancer of lung should always be ruled out; high frequency of associated diabetes mellitus, especially in older patients Serum electrolytes N
Polymyositis	Total eosinophil count frequently I	Moderately to markedly I; occasionally N	N	CK in 65%; levels may vary greatly and become N with steroid therapy; markedly I may occur in children ALD in 75%, LDH in 25%, SGOT in 25%; α-HBD parallels LDH; MDH offers no additional diagnostic value	Necrosis of muscle with phagocytosis of muscle fibers, infiltration of inflammatory cells	Associated cancer in ≦ 17% of cases (especially lung; also breast) LE preparation and latex fixations occasionally positive; serum $alpha_2$ and gamma globulin may be increased.
Muscular dystrophy	N	N	N	In active phase; CK in 50%, ALD in 20%, LDH in 10%, SGOT in 15%	Various degenerative changes in muscle; late muscle atrophy; no cellular infiltration	

N = normal; I = increased.

Table 11-2. Increased Serum Enzyme Levels in Muscle Diseases

	Muscular Dystrophy							
	Duchenne		Limb-Girdle		Facioscapulohumeral		Myotonic Dystrophy	Polymyositis
Enzyme	Frequency	Amplitude	Frequency	Amplitude	Frequency	Amplitude	Frequency	Frequency
CK	>95%	65	75%	25	80%	5	50%	70%
ALD	90%	9	25%	3	30%	2	20%	75%
SGOT	90%	4	25%	2	25%	1½	15%	25%
LDH	90%	4	15%	1½	10%	1	10%	25%

Frequency = average % frequency of patients with increased serum enzyme level when blood is taken at optimal time.
Amplitude = average number of times normal that serum level is increased.

Diseases of Musculoskeletal System

MYASTHENIA GRAVIS

Fluorescent antibodies to skeletal muscle cross-striations have been reported in 30–40% of patients.

Antibodies to acetylcholine receptor (AChR) occur in >85% of patients, but normal levels do not rule out myasthenia gravis. False positive results have been seen in some patients with amyotrophic lateral sclerosis, especially those treated with cobra venom, and in a small percentage of patients treated with penicillamine who develop myasthenia-like symptoms. Titers only correspond roughly to clinical status of patients as a group but correlate better with the course of an individual patient and are particularly useful for monitoring during plasmapheresis therapy. Approximately 9% of patients with clinical myasthenia gravis lack detectable anti-AChR antibodies; these are of recent onset or mild and only involve extraocular muscles.

Serum enzymes and electrolytes are normal.

CBC and erythrocyte sedimentation rate (ESR) are normal (occasional cases of associated macrocytic anemia).

Thyroid function tests are normal (disease may be associated with, but independent of, hyperthyroidism or hypothyroidism).

High frequency of associated diabetes mellitus is seen, especially in older patients; therefore glucose tolerance test (GTT) should be performed with or without cortisone.

Other immunologic abnormalities are frequent.

- Anti-DNA antibodies in 40% of cases
- Antinuclear antibody (ANA), anti–parietal cell, anti–smooth muscle, antimitochondrial, antithyroid antibodies, rheumatoid factor, etc., may be found.

Always rule out cancer of lung.

Thymic tumor is present in up to 10% of patients; 70% of patients have thymic hyperplasia with germinal centers in medulla (see p. 358).

POLYMYOSITIS

(nongenetic primary inflammatory myopathy; may be due to infection or idiopathic; may be associated with skin disease [dermatomyositis] or collagen or malignant disease)

Serum enzymes

- Serum CK is the most useful. Increased in 70% of patients. Levels may vary greatly. Degree of increase is highest in children and reflects the activity of the disease; decrease usually occurs 3–4 weeks before improvement in muscle strength and increase 5–6 weeks before clinical relapse; the level frequently becomes normal with steroid therapy (in ~3 months) or in chronic myositis.
- Serum aldolase is increased in 75% of patients.
- Serum LDH is increased in 25% of patients.
- Serum SGOT is increased in ~25% of the patients.
- Serum alpha-hydroxybutyric dehydrogenase (α-HBD) may be increased, paralleling the increased LDH.
- Serum MDH may be increased but offers no additional diagnostic value.

Muscle biopsy shows necrosis of muscle, with phagocytosis of muscle fibers and infiltration of inflammatory cells.

Total eosinophil count is frequently increased. WBC may be increased in fulminant disease.

Mild anemia may occur.

ESR is moderately to markedly increased; may be normal; not clinically useful.

Thyroid function tests are normal.

Urine shows a moderate increase in creatine and a decrease in creatinine. Myoglobinuria occurs occasionally in severe cases.

Increased ANA titers are found in 20% of cases. Rheumatoid factor (RA) tests may be positive in 50% of patients.

Serum gamma globulins may be increased.

Associated carcinoma is present in ≤20% of the patients and in ≤5% of patients over age 40 (especially cancer of lung and cancer of breast). The polymyositis may antedate the neoplasm by up to 2 years.

MUSCULAR DYSTROPHY

(genetic primary myopathies)

Serum enzymes (CK is most useful) are increased, especially in

- Young patients. Highest levels (≤50 times normal) are found at onset of infancy and childhood, with gradual return to normal.
- The more rapidly progressive dystrophies (such as the Duchenne type) and may be slightly or inconsistently increased in the limb-girdle and facioscapulohumeral types
- The active early phase. Increased levels are not constant and are affected by patient's age and duration of disease. Enzymes may be increased before disease is clinically evident. Elevated serum enzyme levels are not affected by steroid therapy.

Serum CK is useful for

- **Preclinical diagnosis** of Duchenne's and Becker's dystrophy in families with history of disease or for screening. Always increased in affected children (5–100 times upper limit of normal [ULN] of adults) to peak by age 2 years; then begin to fall as disease becomes manifest. Persistent normal CK virtually rules out this diagnosis. Begin testing at 2–3 months of age. (*Normal children have CK level that is very high during first few days, falls to 3 times ULN by fourth day, falls to 2–3 times adult level during first month of life, and levels remain > adults during first 2 years.*) Neonatal screening that is positive with whole blood should be confirmed with serum. CK > 3 times ULN for age in all boys with Duchenne's dystrophy and >2 times in Becker's dystrophy. Sex-linked dystrophy is virtually only cause of high values in normal neonates. High values persist in dystrophy but not with false-positives. Neonatal screening of girls has been discontinued. Prenatal screening at 18–20 weeks' gestation by placental aspiration of fetal blood has been abandoned due to false negative and false positive results.
- **Clinical diagnosis.** CK is increased in almost all cases of Duchenne's (average 30 times ULN) and Becker's (average 10 times ULN) dystrophies. Diagnosis is in doubt if CK is normal. Highest in young patients and falls with age by ~50% at age 7 years; usually remains >5 times ULN but in terminal cases may decline further. Except for polymyositis, other myopathies and neurogenic atrophy show normal CK or <5 times ULN. Serum aldolase is increased in ~20% of patients. Serum LDH is increased in ~10% of patients. SGOT is increased in ~15% of patients.
- **Identifying female carriers.** CK is increased in carriers with two affected sons or one son and one affected male relative in ~70% of Duchenne's and 50% of Becker's dystrophy. Highest levels and greatest frequency in younger carriers; may only be present during childhood and not in later life. Levels may be up to 10 times ULN but usually <3 times and average

= 1.5 times ULN; values overlap with normal females. Therefore special precautions are needed: Draw blood after normal activity in afternoon or evening but not after severe or long exercise or IM injections or during pregnancy; recheck at weekly intervals 3 times; values are higher in blacks than whites.

Muscle biopsy shows muscle atrophy but no cellular infiltration.

Urine creatine is increased; urine creatinine is decreased. These changes are less marked in limb-girdle and facioscapulohumeral types than in the Duchenne type.

ESR is usually normal.

Thyroid function tests are normal.

Recently developed test for antibodies to a muscle protein (dystrophin) establishes diagnosis by showing dystrophin to be absent in Duchenne's and qualitatively abnormal in Becker's dystrophies.

Recombinant DNA technology allows

- Prenatal diagnosis by chorionic villous sampling at 12th week of gestation
- Diagnosis of carriers
- Diagnosis and differential diagnosis (e.g., from limb-girdle dystrophy)

Limb-Girdle Dystrophy

(heterogeneous group of disorders in both sexes; autosomal recessive that begins in second decade and progresses to disability by age 30 and death by age 50)

Serum CK is increased in 70% of patients to average 10 times ULN. Not useful to detect carriers. Not useful to distinguish from other autosomal recessive forms of dystrophy, myopathy, or neurologic disorders (e.g., hereditary proximal spinal muscular atrophy).

Fascioscapulohumeral Dystrophy

(begins in late adolescence; normal life span)

Serum CK is increased in 75% of patients to average 3 times ULN. Frequently normal by age 50.

MYOTONIC DYSTROPHY

(autosomal dominant disorder presents in adolescence)

Serum CK is increased in 50% of cases to average 3 times ULN.

Increased creatine in urine may occur irregularly.

Findings due to atrophy of testicle and androgenic deficiency are noted.

Urine 17-ketosteroids are decreased.

Thyroid function may be decreased.

METABOLIC DISEASES OF MUSCLE

Hypothyroidism (rarely associated with myotonia)

- Increased serum CK in 60–80% of cases to average 4–8 times ULN; becomes normal 4–6 weeks after treatment. CK-MB is rarely increased up to 6% of total.
- Decreased urine creatine
- Increased creatine tolerance
- Other serum enzyme levels normal
- Hyperthyroidism
- Normal serum enzyme levels
- Increased urine creatine
- Decreased creatine tolerance
- Normal muscle biopsy
- *Causes some cases of hypokalemic periodic paralysis.*

Acromegaly

- Serum CK may be increased to average of 2 times ULN.

Associated with administration of adrenal corticosteroids and with Cushing's syndrome
- Increased serum enzymes—uncommon, and may be due to the primary disease
- Muscle biopsy—degenerative and regenerative changes in scattered muscle fibers; no inflammatory cell infiltration
- Increased urine creatine

MYOTUBULAR MYOPATHY, MITOCHONDRIAL MYOPATHY, NEMALINE (ROD) MYOPATHY

Routine laboratory studies including measurement of serum enzymes are normal.

Biopsy of muscle with histochemical staining reaction establishes the diagnosis.

MYOPATHY ASSOCIATED WITH ALCOHOLISM

Acute
- Increased serum CK, SGOT, and other enzymes. Serum CK increased in 80% of patients; rises in 1–2 days; reaches peak in 4–5 days; lasts ~2 weeks. CK in CSF is normal, even when serum level is elevated.
- Gross myoglobinuria
- Acute renal failure (some patients)

Chronic—may show some or all of the following changes
- Increased serum CK in 60% of patients to average of 2 times ULN
- SGOT and other enzymes may also be increased due to liver as well as muscle.
- Increased urine creatine
- Diminished ability to increase blood lactic acid with ischemic exercise
- Abnormalities on muscle biopsy (support the diagnosis)
- Myoglobinuria

FAMILIAL PERIODIC PARALYSIS

Serum potassium is decreased during the attack.

Urine potassium excretion decreases at the same time.

Serum enzymes are normal.

ADYNAMIA EPISODICA HEREDITARIA (GAMSTORP'S DISEASE)

Transient increase in serum potassium occurs during the attack; attack is induced by administration of potassium.

Urine potassium excretion is unchanged during or before the attack.

MALIGNANT HYPERTHERMIA

(autosomal dominant syndrome triggered by potent inhalational anesthetic agents, local anesthetic agents in large doses [e.g., lidocaine], muscle relaxants [e.g., succinylcholine, tubocurarine], various types of stress)

Combined metabolic and respiratory acidosis is the most consistent abnormality and is diagnostic in the presence of muscle rigidity or rising temperature. pH is often <7.2, base excess (BE) > -10, and $PaCO_2$ 70–120 mmHg. *Immediate* arterial blood gas analysis should be performed.

Increased serum potassium and calcium initially, with below-normal values later.

Serum CK, LDH, and SGOT are markedly increased with peak in 24–48 hours following surgery; CK levels are often 20,000–100,000 units/L.

Myoglobinemia and myoglobinuria may be present early.

Oliguria with acute renal shutdown may occur later.

Coagulopathy, including disseminated intravascular coagulation (DIC), may occur later but is infrequent.

Table 11-3. Types of Periodic Paralysis

	Hypokalemic (familial, sporadic, associated with hyperthyroidism)	Hyperkalemic (adynamia episodica hereditaria)	Normokalemic
Induced by	Glucose and insulin, ACTH, DOCA, epinephrine	KCl	KCl
Serum potassium during attack	Decreased	Increased	Normal or slightly decreased
Urine potassium excretion	Decreased	Normal	Decreased

OSTEOMYELITIS

WBC may be increased, especially in acute cases.

ESR is increased in <50% of patients but may be important clue in occult cases (e.g., intervertebral disk space infection).

Bacteriology

Staphylococcus aureus causes almost all infections of hip and two-thirds of infections of skull, vertebrae, and long bones. Other bacteria may simultaneously be present and contribute to infection.

Gram-negative bacteria cause most infections of mandible, pelvis, and small bones.

Salmonella is more commonly found in patients with sickle hemoglobinopathy.

Laboratory findings due to underlying conditions, e.g., postoperative status, irradiation therapy, foreign body, tissue gangrene, contiguous infection.

RICKETS

Serum alkaline phosphatase is increased. This is the earliest and most reliable biochemical abnormality; parallels severity of the rickets. It may remain elevated until bone healing is complete.

Serum calcium is usually normal or slightly decreased.

Serum phosphorus is usually decreased. In some persons, serum calcium and phosphorus may be normal.

Generalized renal aminoaciduria is present; it disappears when adequate vitamin D is given.

Serum calcium and phosphorus rapidly become normal after institution of vitamin D therapy.

Serum 25-hydroxyvitamin D is low (usually <5 ng/ml; normal = 10–20 ng/ml)

Vitamin D–deficient state is suggested by

Low serum phosphorus
Severe liver disease
Malabsorption
Anticonvulsant therapy

OSTEOPENIA

(generic term for decreased mineralized bone on x-ray, but x-ray cannot distinguish osteomalacia from osteoporosis in most patients unless pseudofractures are seen)

All serum chemistries may be normal in any form of osteopenia.

All chemistries are commonly normal in osteomalacia, especially with coexisting osteoporosis that occurs in 20%.

Serum vitamin D that is below normal (e.g., 15 ng/ml of 25-hydroxyvitamin D) suggests osteomalacia.

Diagnosis is established with bone biopsy that may be combined with tetracycline labeling.

During therapeutic trial of calcium and vitamin D, serum and urine calcium should be monitored monthly to avoid toxicity.

Urine calcium is maintained <300 mg/gm of creatinine and serum calcium <10.2 mg/dl by reducing dose of vitamin D.

PRIMARY HYPOPHOSPHATEMIA (FAMILIAL VITAMIN D–RESISTANT RICKETS)

(hereditary metabolic defect in phosphate transport in renal tubules and possibly intestine)

Serum phosphorus is markedly decreased.

Serum calcium is relatively normal.

Serum alkaline phosphatase is moderately increased.

Stool calcium is increased, and urine calcium is decreased.

Administration of vitamin D does not cause serum phosphorus to rise (in contrast to ordinary rickets), but urine and serum calcium may be increased with sufficiently large dose.

Renal aminoaciduria is absent, in contrast to ordinary rickets.

Treatment is monitored by choosing dose of vitamin D that will not increase serum calcium >11 mg/dl or urine calcium >200 mg/day.

Serum phosphorus usually remains low; increase >4 mg/dl may indicate renal injury due to vitamin D toxicity.

VITAMIN D–DEPENDENT RICKETS

Serum calcium is frequently decreased, sometimes causing tetany.

Serum phosphorus is decreased but not as markedly or as consistently as in hypophosphatemic rickets.

Serum alkaline phosphatase is increased.

Urine calcium is decreased.

Generalized renal aminoaciduria is present; it disappears when adequate vitamin D is given.

Serum chemistries return to normal after adequate vitamin D is given (may require very large doses).

May be due to familial genetic pattern.

FAMILIAL OSTEOECTASIA

(uncommon inherited disorder of membranous bone showing painful swelling of the periosteal soft tissue and spontaneous fractures)

Serum alkaline phosphatase is increased.

Serum acid phosphatase and aminopeptidase are also increased.

OSTEOPETROSIS (ALBERS-SCHÖNBERG DISEASE; MARBLE BONE DISEASE)

Normal serum calcium, phosphorus, alkaline phosphatase

Serum acid phosphatase increased (some patients)

Myelophthisic anemia (some patients)

Laboratory findings due to complications, e.g., osteomyelitis

PAGET'S DISEASE OF BONE (OSTEITIS DEFORMANS)

Marked increase in serum alkaline phosphatase directly related to severity and extent of disease; sudden additional increase with development of osteogenic sarcoma

Normal serum calcium increased during immobilization (e.g., due to intercurrent illness or fracture)
Normal or slightly increased serum phosphorus
Frequently increased urine calcium; renal calculi common
Increase in hydroxyproline in urine may be marked.

OSTEOGENIC SARCOMA

Marked increase in serum alkaline phosphatase (≤40 times normal); reflects new bone formation and parallels clinical course (e.g., development of metastases, response to therapy); is said to occur in only 50% of patients.
Laboratory findings due to metastases—80% of patients have lung metastases at time of diagnosis.
Laboratory findings due to preexisting (e.g., Paget's) disease

OSTEOLYTIC TUMORS OF BONE

(e.g., Ewing's sarcoma)

Usually normal serum calcium, phosphorus, alkaline phosphatase

METASTATIC CARCINOMA OF BONE

Osteolytic metastases (especially from primary tumor of bronchus, breast, kidney, thyroid)
- Urine calcium is often increased; marked increase may reflect increased rate of tumor growth.
- Serum calcium and phosphorus may be normal or increased.
- Serum alkaline phosphatase is usually normal or slightly to moderately increased.
- Serum acid phosphatase is often slightly increased, especially in prostatic metastases.

Osteoblastic metastases (especially from primary tumor in prostate)
- Serum calcium is normal; it is rarely increased.
- Urine calcium is low.
- Serum alkaline phosphatase is usually increased.
- Serum acid phosphatase is increased in prostatic carcinoma.
- Serum phosphorus is variable.

FAT EMBOLISM

Occurs after trauma (e.g., fractures, insertion of femoral head prosthesis)
Unexplained fall in hemoglobin in 30–60% of patients
Decreased platelet count in 80% of patients
Free fat in urine in 50% of patients
Fat globules in sputum (some patients)
Decreased arterial PO_2 with normal or decreased PCO_2
Increased serum lipase in 30–50% of patients; increased free fatty acids; not of diagnostic value
Increased serum triglycerides
Fat globulinemia in 42–67% of patients and in 17–33% of controls
Normal CSF
Hypocalcemia is a common nonspecific finding (due to binding to free fatty acids).
Arterial blood gas values are always abnormal in clinically significant fat embolism syndrome; are the most useful and important laboratory data. Show decreased lung compliance, abnormal ventilation-perfusion ratios, increased shunt effect.

Laboratory findings alone are inadequate for diagnosis.

Normal Values—Synovial Fluid

Volume	1.0–3.5 ml
pH	Parallels serum
Appearance	Clear, pale yellow or straw-colored Viscous, does not clot
Fibrin clot	0
Mucin clot	Good
WBC	<200/cu mm (even in presence of leukocytosis in blood)
Neutrophils	<25%
Crystals	
Free	0
Intracellular	0
Fasting uric acid, bilirubin	Approximately the same as serum
Total protein	~25–30% of serum protein Mean = 1.8 gm/dl Abnormal if >2.5 gm/dl; inflammation is moderately severe if >4.5 gm/dl
Glucose	<10 mg/dl lower than simultaneously drawn serum level
Culture	No growth

Diseases of Joints

OSTEOARTHRITIS

Laboratory tests are all normal and not helpful.

ESR may be slightly increased (possibly because of soft-tissue changes secondary to mechanical alterations in joints).

RHEUMATOID ARTHRITIS (RA)

American Rheumatism Association has 11 criteria for diagnosis of RA; 7 are required for diagnosis of classic RA, 5 for definite RA, and 3 for probable RA. Four laboratory tests included in these criteria are positive serum test for rheumatoid factor (RF), poor mucin clotting of synovial fluid, characteristic histologic changes in synovium, characteristic histologic changes in rheumatoid nodules.

Serologic tests for RF (e.g., using latex, bentonite, or sheep or human RBCs)

- Use slide test only for screening; confirm positive test with tube dilution. Significant titer is ≥1:80. In RA, titers are often 1:640 to 1:5120 and sometimes ≤1:320,000. Titers in conditions other than RA are usually <1:80. Becomes positive after disease is active for 6 months. Various methods show sensitivity of 50–75% and specificity of 75–90%. Positive in 80% of "typical" cases; high titers in patients with splenomegaly, vasculitis, subcutaneous nodules or neuropathy. Positive test early in course of disease and progressive increases in titer during the first 2 years indicate a more severe course.
- Gives useful objective evidence of RA, but a negative test does not rule out RA. Negative in one-third of patients with definite RA. Positive in 5–10% of normal population; progressive increase with age up to 25–50% of persons over age 70.
- Positive in 5% of rheumatoid variants (arthritis associated with psoriasis, ulcerative colitis, regional enteritis, Reiter's syndrome, juvenile rheumatoid arthritis, rheumatoid spondylitis).
- May be positive in 20–30% of patients with systemic lupus erythematosus (SLE), scleroderma, mixed connective tissue disease, polymyositis.
- May be positive in 90% of patients with primary Sjögren's syndrome or cryoglobulinemic purpura.

May be positive in 10–40% of patients with Waldenström's macroglobulinemia, chronic infections (e.g., syphilis, leprosy, brucellosis, tuberculosis, subacute bacterial endocarditis), viral infections (e.g., infectious hepatitis, Epstein-Barr virus, influenza, vaccinations), parasitic diseases (e.g., malaria, schistosomiasis, trypanosomiasis, filariasis), sarcoidosis, chronic liver disease, infectious hepatitis, chronic pulmonary interstitial fibrosis, etc.

Negative in osteoarthritis, gout, ankylosing spondylitis, rheumatic fever, suppurative arthritis, arthritis associated with ulcerative colitis.

Positive LE test in ≤20% of patients is usually weakly reactive. ANA present in up to 28% of patients (see Table 11-5). Serum complement is usually normal except in patients with vasculitis; depressed level is usually associated with very high levels of RF and immune complexes.

Immune complexes—monoclonal rheumatoid factors and C1q binding assays are positive more frequently in RA than other assays but correlated poorly with disease activity. Positive test for mixed cryoglobulins indicates presence of immune complexes and is associated with increased incidence of extra-articular manifestations, especially vasculitis.

Increased ESR, positive C-reactive protein (CRP) and other acute-phase reactants. Westergren ESR is often used as guide to activity and to therapy, but ESR is normal in 5% of cases. Very high ESR (>100 mm/hour) is distinctly unusual in early cases.

Serum protein electrophoresis shows increase in globulins, especially in gamma and $alpha_2$ globulins, and decreased albumin.

Moderate normocytic hypochromic anemia of chronic disease; not responsive to iron, folic acid, vitamin B_{12}, or splenectomy. If hematocrit <26%, search for other cause of anemia (e.g., GI bleeding). Anemia diminishes as patient goes into remission or responds to therapy.

Serum iron is decreased; total iron-binding capacity (TIBC) is normal. Normal iron stores (serum ferritin and bone marrow iron).

WBC is usually normal; there may be a slight increase early in the active disease.

Serum calcium, phosphorus, alkaline phosphatase, uric acid, and antistreptolysin-O titer (ASOT) are normal.

Synovial biopsy is especially useful in monoarticular form to rule out tuberculosis, gout, etc.

Synovial fluid glucose may be greatly decreased (<10 mg/dl); mucin clotting is fair to poor (see Table 11-4, pp. 252–253).

See Amyloidosis, pp. 702–704.

FELTY'S SYNDROME

Occurs in 5–10% of patients with far-advanced RA associated with splenomegaly and leukopenia and rheumatoid nodules

Serologic tests for RF are positive in high titers.

Positive LE test is more frequent than in RA.

ANA tests are usually present. Higher titer of immune complexes and lower complement levels than RA patients.

Leukopenia (<2500/cu mm) and granulocytopenia are present.

Anemia and thrombocytopenia due to hypersplenism may occur and respond to splenectomy.

SJÖGREN'S SYNDROME*

May be secondary to connective tissue disease in one-half to two-thirds of cases or primary; immunologic abnormality associated with decreased secretion of salivary and lacrimal glands. 90% of patients are female.

*Data from RD Collins and GV Ball, *J Musculoskeletal Med,* April 1984, pp. 42–51.

Table 11-4. Synovial Fluid Findings in Various Diseases of Joints

Property	Normal	Noninflammatory[a]	Hemorrhagic[b]		Acute Inflammatory[c]			Septic		
Volume	3.5 ml	I	I		I			I		
Appearance	Clear, colorless	Clear, straw	Bloody or xanthochromic		Turbid yellow			Turbid yellow		
Viscosity	High	High	V		D			D		
Fibrin clot	0	Usually 0	Usually 0		+			+		
Mucin clot	Good	Good	V		Fair to poor			Poor		
					Acute Gouty Arthritis	Rheumatic Fever	Rheumatoid Arthritis	Tuberculous Arthritis	Gonorrheal Arthritis	Septic Arthritis[d,e]
WBC (no./cu mm)[f]	<200	<5000	<10,000	Range	750–45,000	300–98,000	300–75,000	2500–105,000	1500–108,000	15,600–213,000
				Average	13,500	17,800	15,500	23,500	14,000	65,400

Neutrophils (%)	<25	<25	<50	Range	48–94	8–98	5–96	29–96	2–96	75–100
				Average	83	46	65	67	64	95
Blood-synovia glucose difference (mg/dl)[g]	<10	<10	<25	Range	0–41		0–88	0–108	0–97	40–122
				Average	12	6	31	57	26	71
Culture[h]	0	0	0		0	0	0		See p. 259	

I = increased; D = decreased; 0 = absent; + = positive; V = variable.
[a]For example, degenerative joint disease, traumatic arthritis, some cases of pigmented villonodular synovitis.
[b]For example, tumor, hemophilia, neuroarthropathy, trauma, some cases of pigmented villonodular synovitis.
[c]For example, rheumatoid arthritis, Reiter's syndrome, acute gouty arthritis, acute pseudogout, systemic lupus erythematosus, etc.
[d]For example, pneumococcal.
[e]In purulent arthropathy of undetermined cause, very high synovial fluid lactate (>2000 mg/dl) indicates a nongonococcal septic arthritis (gram-negative bacilli, gram-positive cocci, fungi). Lactate is < 100 mg/dl in gonococcal infection, gout, rheumatoid arthritis, osteoarthritis, trauma.
[f]Use saline instead of acetic acid, which clumps the joint fluid.
[g]Joint tap should be performed preferably after patient has been fasting for > 4 hours, and a blood glucose determination should be performed simultaneously.
[h]Material should be cultured aerobically and anaerobically. Culture for tubercle bacilli and guinea pig inoculation should be performed.

Synovial fluid analysis is primarily useful to diagnose or rule out infectious arthritis, gout, or pseudogout.
To distinguish inflammatory from noninflammatory conditions, synovial fluid WBC >2000/cu mm and >75% PMNs have sensitivities of 84% and 75% and specificities of 84% and 92% respectively.

Table 11-5. Serologic Tests in Various Rheumatoid Diseases

Disease[a]	ANA[b]	LE Clot[c]	RF[d]	Serum Complement
SLE	100 (H)	70–80	30–40	D
Rheumatoid arthritis				
Adult	50 (L–M)	5–15	80–90	N or I
Juvenile	< 5 (L–M)	< 5	15	N
Mixed connective tissue disease	100 (M–H)	20	50	N or I
Dermatomyositis	25	< 5	10–15	N
Scleroderma	25–40	< 5	33	N
Periarteritis nodosa	< 5 (L)	< 5	5–10	N or D
Sjögren's syndrome	95 (M–H)	20	75	N or D
Ankylosing spondylitis	5–10	< 5	< 5	N

Numbers = % of cases positive for each test. D = decreased; N = normal; I = increased.

[a]Normal ESR in patients with nonspecific rheumatic symptoms suggests fibromyositis rather than any of the above disorders.

[b]ANA = fluorescent antinuclear antibody; H = titer > 1:200; M–H = titer 1:100–1:200; L–M = titer 1:20–1:100; ANA titer ≧ 1:160 with suggestive pattern and clinical setting is very helpful diagnostically, but when titer is negative, other laboratory tests are not productive. Anti-DNA antibodies correlate best with a diagnosis of SLE; they are positive in < 5% of patients with other immunologic diseases. Diagnosis of SLE is barely credible without a positive ANA test.

[c]LE cells in peripheral blood clot preparation.

[d]Positive RF (rheumatoid factor) test in rheumatoid arthritis shows a significantly higher titer than in other collagen diseases, but diagnosis is primarily clinical rather than serologic. Serial titers are not helpful to follow response to treatment since antiglobulins remain at constant levels despite clinical status. Frequently positive at low to moderate titers in polyclonal hypergammaglobulinemia (e.g., SLE, sarcoidosis, cirrhosis, active viral hepatitis, some acute viral infections).

Diagnosis is established by biopsy of gland (minor salivary gland of lower lip is easiest).

Antinuclear antibodies in speckled or homogeneous pattern is present in 65% of patients, more frequently in primary type. Anti-SS-A is present in 70–88% of primary and <10% of secondary type. Anti-SS-B is present in 48–73% of primary and <5% of secondary type. Anti–salivary duct antibody is rare (<30%) in primary and frequent (76–83%) in secondary type. Also occurs in ≤25% of RA patients without Sjögren's syndrome. Patients with primary syndrome also have higher tissue antibodies (e.g., thyroid, gastric parietal, smooth muscle).

RF (latex agglutination) is present in ≤90% of primary and secondary types.

Mild normochromic, normocytic anemia in 50% of patients.

Leukopenia in up to one-third of cases

ESR is usually increased.

Serum protein electrophoresis shows increased gamma globulins (usually polyclonal) largely due to IgG.

Laboratory findings due to primary disease

Rheumatoid arthritis is found in 30–55% of patients with Sjögren's syndrome; Sjögren's syndrome is found in 20–100% of patients with RA.

SLE is found in 4–5% of patients with Sjögren's syndrome; Sjögren's syndrome is found in 50–98% of patients with SLE.

Table 11-6. Comparison of Rheumatoid Arthritis and Osteoarthritis

Rheumatoid Arthritis	Osteoarthritis
Synovial fluid has high WBC and low viscosity	Effusions infrequent Synovial fluid has low WBC and high viscosity
ESR more markedly increased	ESR may be mildly to moderately increased
Rheumatoid factor usually present	RF usually absent
Positive biopsy of subcutaneous rheumatoid nodule and synovia	Rheumatoid changes in tissue absent

Table 11-7. ESR in Differential Diagnosis of Juvenile Rheumatoid Arthritis

Disease	ESR Falls to Normal
Untreated acute rheumatic fever	9–12 weeks
Salicylate-treated acute rheumatic fever	5 weeks
Steroid-treated acute rheumatic fever	2 weeks
Chronic rheumatic fever	Occasionally shows persistent elevation
Juvenile rheumatoid arthritis	May remain elevated for months or years despite therapy

Primary biliary cirrhosis is found in 3% of patients with Sjögren's syndrome; Sjögren's syndrome is found in 50–100% of patients with primary biliary cirrhosis.

Other associated diseases include generalized scleroderma, mixed connective tissue disease, chronic active hepatitis.

Laboratory findings due to frequent concomitant diseases (e.g., pseudolymphoma, Waldenström's macroglobulinemia; incidence of B-cell lymphoma is 44 times greater).

Immune complex glomerulonephritis may occur, but chronic tubulointerstitial nephritis is more characteristic.

ANKYLOSING RHEUMATOID SPONDYLITIS (MARIE-STRUMPELL DISEASE)

ESR is increased in ≤80% of cases.

Mild to moderate hypochromic anemia appears in ≤30% of cases.

Serologic tests for rheumatoid factor are positive in <15% of patients with arthritis of only the vertebral region.

CSF protein is moderately increased in ≤50% of patients.

Secondary amyloidosis appears in 6% of patients.

Laboratory findings of carditis and aortitis with aortic insufficiency, which occur in 1–4% of patients, are noted.

Laboratory findings of frequently associated diseases (e.g., chronic ulcerative colitis, regional ileitis, psoriasis)

Histocompatibility antigen HLA-B27 is found in about 95% of these white pa-

Table 11-8. Synovial Fluid Findings in Acute Inflammatory Arthritis of Various Etiologies

Disease	WBC	Complement Activity	Rheumatoid Factor (RF)	Crystals*	Other Findings
Acute gouty arthritis	I	I	0	Monosodium urate; within PMNs during acute stage	
Acute chondrocalcinosis (pseudogout)	I	I	0	Calcium pyrophosphate	
Reiter's syndrome	Markedly I	Markedly I	0		Macrophages with ingested leukocytes
Rheumatoid arthritis	I	Low	Usually +		
Juvenile rheumatoid arthritis	I	Low	0		Abundant lymphocytes (sometimes > 50%); immature lymphocytes and monocytes present
Systemic lupus erythematosus	Usually very low	Low or 0	V	0	LE cells may be present
Arthritis associated with psoriasis, ulcerative colitis, ankylosing spondylitis	I	I			

I = increased; 0 = absent; V = variable; PMN = polymorphonuclear leukocyte; + = positive.
*Crystals should be identified using polarized light microscopy. Finding of characteristic crystals is diagnostic of gout and of chondrocalcinosis. Must be differentiated from crystals of corticosteroid esters and cholesterol or talc (after recent joint infections).

tients and in lesser numbers with variants of this condition. About 20% of persons carrying HLA-B27 have ankylosing spondylitis. Not helpful in establishing the diagnosis.

ARTHRITIS ASSOCIATED WITH PSORIASIS

Arthritis occurs in 2% of patients with psoriasis. There is no correlation between activity of skin and joint manifestations; either one may precede the other.

Increased serum uric acid is due to increased turnover of skin cells in psoriasis.

Serologic tests for rheumatoid factor are negative.

ARTHRITIS ASSOCIATED WITH ULCERATIVE COLITIS OR REGIONAL ENTERITIS

There may be rheumatoid arthritis, ankylosing spondylitis, or acute synovitis (monoarticular or polyarticular—absent rheumatoid factor).

Joint fluid is sterile bacteriologically and microscopically. It is similar to fluid of rheumatoid arthritis and Whipple's disease (cell count, differential count, specific gravity, viscosity, protein, sugar, poor mucin clot formation). Joint fluid examination is principally useful in monoarticular involvement to rule out suppurative arthritis.

Synovial biopsy is similar to rheumatoid arthritis biopsy.

Abnormal laboratory results (e.g., increased ESR, WBC, platelets) are related to activity of bowel disease.

Absent RA and ANA.

ARTHRITIS ASSOCIATED WITH WHIPPLE'S DISEASE

This is a nonspecific synovitis.

HEMOCHROMATOSIS-ASSOCIATED ARTHRITIS

Laboratory findings of hemochromatosis

Negative RA factor

No subcutaneous nodules

Biopsy of synovia—iron deposits in synovia lining but not in cartilage, little iron in deep macrophages

- Hemarthrosis—iron diffusely distributed in macrophages (e.g., in hemophilia, trauma, and pigmented villonodular synovitis)
- Osteoarthritis—small amount of iron that is limited to deep macrophages
- Rheumatoid arthritis—iron in both deep macrophages and lining cells

Chondrocalcinosis frequently associated

REITER'S SYNDROME

This triad of arthritis, urethritis, and conjunctivitis has additional features: dermatitis, buccal ulcerations, circinate balanitis, and keratosis blennorrhagica.

Increased ESR parallels the clinical course.

WBC is increased (10,000–20,000/cu mm), as are granulocytes.

Serum globulins are increased in long-standing disease.

Nonbacterial cystitis, prostatitis, or seminal vesiculitis is found (significance of culturing pleuropneumonia-like organisms is not determined).

HLA-B27 is found in up to 90% of white patients; not diagnostically useful.

GOUT

Presence of crystals of monosodium urate from tophi or joint fluid (viewed microscopically under polarized light) establishes the diagnosis and differentiates from pseudogout. Negative birefringent needle-shaped crystals are seen within polymorphonuclear leukocytes (PMNs) and also extracellularly. (In pseudogout, crystals are typically weakly positive birefringent, smaller, rhomboid crystals. Calcium oxalate crystals are positively birefringent, with a characteristic bipyramidal shape, inside or outside of cells.)

Increased serum uric acid does not establish the diagnosis of gout. Several determinations may be required to establish elevated values; beware of serum levels reduced to normal range by recent aspirin use. Changes in therapy may cause wide fluctuations in serum uric acid levels. The incidence of gout at various uric acid levels in men was found to be 1.1% at <6 mg/dl, 7.3% at 6.0–6.9 mg/dl, 14.2% at 7.0–7.9 mg/dl, 18.7% at 8.0–8.9 mg/dl, 83% at ≥9 mg/dl. Many gout patients have levels <8 mg/dl, and >one-third never have an elevated level. Since the mean interval between first and second gout attacks is 11.4 years and only 25% have a second attack within 12 years, therapy for this group may not be cost-effective.

Serum uric acid levels are increased in ~25% of asymptomatic relatives.

About 10% of adult males have elevated serum uric acid levels.

Only 1–3% of patients with hyperuricemia have gout.

Uric acid stones occur 3–10 times more frequently in gouty patients than in the general population, even though 75% of gouty patients have normal 24-hour excretion of uric acid. When serum uric acid is <9 mg/dl or urine level is <700 mg/24 hours, risk of renal calculi is <21%; when serum uric acid is >13 mg/dl or urine level is >1100 mg/24 hours, risk is >50%.

Secondary hyperuricemia usually produces much higher uric acid level than primary type. If serum uric acid is >10 mg/dl, underlying malignancy should be considered after renal failure has been ruled out.

24-hour urine for uric acid: If elevated (>600 mg/24 hours), it should be repeated after 3–5 days on purine-free diet. (If excretion <600 mg/day or urine uric acid–creatinine ratio <0.6 and no history of kidney or GU tract disease, treatment is with probenecid; if >600 mg/day or urine uric acid–creatinine ratio >0.8 or there is history of GU tract or kidney disease, allopurinol is drug of choice; ratios 0.6–0.8 are indeterminate; ratios of 0.2–0.6 are considered normal or underexcretors.) >1100 mg/24 hours in asymptomatic hyperuricemia is indication for treatment.

Drug-induced gout may cause up to 50% of all new cases of gouty arthritis; these occur later in life and are more common in women than primary gout.

Diseases associated with gout include hypertension (in one-third of patients with gout), diabetes mellitus, disorders causing ketosis or acidosis, familial hypercholesterolemia, acute intermittent porphyria, von Gierke's disease, sarcoidosis, parathyroid dysfunction, cardiovascular disease, myxedema, obesity, alcohol ingestion. Serum triglycerides are frequently increased, resulting in a high frequency of types IIb and IV lipoprotein patterns; HDL-cholesterol level is frequently decreased.

10–25% of primary gout patients develop uric acid stones; in 40% of these, the stones appear >5 years before an episode of gout.

Moderate leukocytosis and increased ESR occur during acute attacks; normal at other times.

Uric acid crystals and amorphous urates are normal findings in urinary sediment.

Low-grade proteinuria occurs in 20–80% of gouty persons for many years before further evidence of renal disease appears.

Histologic examination of gouty nodule.

RF detectable in low titers in 10% of patients with gout or pseudogout; but rheumatoid arthritis rarely coexists with these conditions.

See Tables 11-4, pp. 252–253, and 11-8, p. 256.
See also sections on renal diseases and serum uric acid.

SECONDARY GOUT

Occurs In

Lead intoxication

Neoplastic and hemolytic conditions (e.g., leukemia, polycythemia vera, second-

ary polycythemia, malignant lymphomas). Blood dyscrasias are found in ~10% of patients with clinical gout.
Cytotoxic drug therapy
Psoriasis

CHONDROCALCINOSIS ("PSEUDOGOUT")

Joint fluid contains crystals identified as calcium pyrophosphate dihydrate, inside and outside of WBCs; differentiated from urate crystals under polarized light distinguishes from gout (see Gout, p. 257). Crystals may also be identified by other means (e.g., chemical, x-ray diffraction).
Blood and urine findings are normal.
Laboratory findings due to more frequently associated conditions (e.g., hyperparathyroidism, hypothyroidism, hemochromatosis, hypomagnesemia)

See Tables 11-4, pp. 252–253, and 11-8, p. 256.

SEPTIC ARTHRITIS (SUPPURATIVE OR PURULENT ARTHRITIS)

Laboratory findings due to preexisting infections (e.g., subacute bacterial endocarditis, meningococcal meningitis, pneumococcal pneumonia, typhoid, gonorrhea, tuberculosis) are noted.
Joint fluid (see Table 11-4, pp. 252–253)
- In purulent arthritis
  - Gram's stain is particularly useful for establishing diagnosis promptly and in cases in which cultures are negative.
  - Culture may be negative because of prior administration of antibiotics.
- In tuberculous arthritis
  - Gram's stain and bacterial cultures are negative, but acid-fast stain, culture for tubercle bacilli, guinea pig inoculation, and biopsy of synovia confirm the diagnosis.

Infection of prosthetic joints is usually due to organisms introduced during surgery that multiply slowly (50% occur >1 year later). Most common are skin flora (e.g., Staphylococcus epidermidis, *other coagulase-negative staphylococci,* Corynebacterium *sp.).*

OCHRONOSIS

Lumbosacral spondylitis associated with scleral pigmentation and darkening of urine on alkalinization.

POLYMYALGIA RHEUMATICA

ESR is markedly increased; is a criterion for diagnosis.
Mild hypochromic or normochromic anemia is commonly found.
WBC may be increased in some patients.
Abnormalities of serum proteins are frequent, although there is no consistent or diagnostic pattern. Most frequently the albumin is decreased with an increase in $alpha_1$ and $alpha_2$ globulins and fibrinogen.
Cryoglobulins are sometimes present.
Rheumatoid factor is present in serum in 7.5% of patients.
LE test is negative.
Serum enzymes (e.g., SGOT, alkaline phosphatase) may be increased in one-third of patients.
Muscle biopsy is usually normal or may show mild nonspecific changes.
Temporal artery biopsy is often positive because one-third of patients with giant cell arteritis present with polymyalgia rheumatica, which ultimately develops in 50–90% of them (see Temporal Arteritis, pp. 699–700).

Hematologic Diseases

Hematologic Laboratory Tests

CAUSES OF NEUTROPENIA

(absolute neutrophil count [total WBC × % segmented neutrophils and bands] < 1800/cu mm; < 1000 in black persons)

- Infections, especially
  - Bacterial (e.g., overwhelming bacterial infection, septicemia, miliary tuberculosis, typhoid, paratyphoid, brucellosis, tularemia)
  - Viral (e.g., infectious mononucleosis, hepatitis, influenza, measles, rubella, psittacosis)
  - Rickettsial (e.g., scrub typhus, sandfly fever)
  - Other (e.g., malaria, kala-azar)
- Drugs and chemicals, especially
  - Sulfonamides
  - Antibiotics
  - Analgesics
  - Marrow depressants
  - Arsenicals
  - Antithyroid drugs
  - Many others
- Ionizing radiation
- Hematopoietic diseases
  - Pernicious anemia
  - Aleukemic leukemia
  - Aplastic anemia and related conditions
  - Hypersplenism
  - Gaucher's disease
  - Felty's syndrome
  - Myelophthisis
- Anaphylactic shock
- Cachexia
- Miscellaneous
  - Systemic lupus erythematosus (SLE)
  - Severe renal injury
  - Various neutropenias (e.g., cyclic neutropenia)
- Artifactual associated with automated WBC counters (artifact is corrected when manual WBC counts are performed)
  - Leukocyte fragility due to immunosuppressive and antineoplastic drugs
  - Lymphocyte fragility in lymphocytic leukemia
  - Excessive clumping of leukocytes in monoclonal gammopathies (e.g., multiple myeloma), cryofibrinogenemia (e.g., SLE), in presence of cold agglutinins

CAUSES OF NEUTROPHILIA

(absolute neutrophil count > 8000/cu mm)

- Acute infections
- Localized (e.g., pneumonia, meningitis, tonsillitis, abscess)
- Generalized (e.g., acute rheumatic fever, septicemia, cholera)
- Inflammation (e.g., vasculitis)
- Intoxications
  - Metabolic (uremia, acidosis, eclampsia, acute gout)

Poisoning by chemicals, drugs, venoms, etc. (e.g., mercury, epinephrine, black widow spider)
Parenteral (foreign protein and vaccines)

Acute hemorrhage
Acute hemolysis of red blood cells
Myeloproliferative diseases
Tissue necrosis

Acute myocardial infarction
Necrosis of tumors
Burns
Gangrene
Bacterial necrosis, etc.

Physiologic conditions (e.g., exercise, emotional stress, menstruation, obstetric labor)

Steroid administration (e.g., prednisone, 40 mg orally) causes increased polymorphonuclear neutrophil leukocytes of 1700–7500 (peak in 4–6 hours and return to normal in 24 hours); no definite shift to left. Lymphocytes decrease 70%, and monocytes decrease 90%.

Table 12-1. Some Common Causes of Leukemoid Reaction

Cause	Myelocytic	Lymphocytic	Monocytic
Infections	Endocarditis Pneumonia Septicemia Leptospirosis Other	Infectious mononucleosis Infectious lymphocytosis Pertussis Chickenpox Tuberculosis	Tuberculosis
Toxic conditions	Burns Eclampsia Poisoning (e.g., mercury)		
Neoplasms	Carcinoma of colon Embryonal carcinoma of kidney	Carcinoma of stomach Carcinoma of breast	
Miscellaneous	Treatment of megaloblastic anemia (of pregnancy, pernicious anemia) Acute hemorrhage Acute hemolysis Recovery from agranulocytosis	Dermatitis herpetiformis	
Myeloproliferative diseases			

Table 12-2. Comparison of Leukemia and Leukemoid Reaction

	Leukemia	Leukemoid Reaction
Causative disease	—	None
WBC	May be >100,000	Usually <50,000
Neutrophils	May have myeloid cells earlier than bands	Mature; <10% bands
Leukocyte alkaline phosphatase	Decreased in chronic myelogenous; variable in others	Increased
Basophilia, eosinophilia, monocytosis	Frequently present	Absent
Platelets	Frequently abnormal morphology Frequently >1 million Thrombocytopenia may occur	Usually small Rarely >600,000 No thrombocytopenia
Peripheral smear RBC	Nucleated RBC, abnormal forms (teardrop, polychromatophilia) may occur	Normal
Bone marrow	Abnormal	Hyperplastic

The WBC differential count is often ordered inappropriately and has almost no value as a screening test. The neutrophil and band counts may be useful in acute appendicitis and neonatal sepsis with moderate sensitivity and specificity, but there is little documentation of utility in other bacterial infections.

CAUSES OF LYMPHOCYTOSIS

(> 4000/cu mm in adults, > 7200/cu mm in adolescents, > 9000/cu mm in young children and infants)

- Infections
  - Pertussis
  - Infectious lymphocytosis
  - Infectious mononucleosis
  - Infectious hepatitis
  - Mumps
  - German measles
  - Toxoplasmosis
  - Chickenpox
  - Chronic tuberculosis
  - Undulant fever
  - Convalescence from acute infection
- Thyrotoxicosis (relative)
- Addison's disease
- Neutropenia with relative lymphocytosis
- Lymphatic leukemia
- Crohn's disease
- Ulcerative colitis
- Serum sickness
- Drug hypersensitivity
- Vasculitis

CAUSES OF LYMPHOCYTOPENIA

(< 1500/cu mm in adults, < 3000/cu mm in children)

- Increased destruction
  - Chemotherapy or radiation treatment
  - Corticosteroids (Cushing's syndrome, stress)
- Increased loss via GI tract
  - Intestinal lymphectasia

Thoracic duct drainage
Obstruction to lymphatic drainage (e.g., tumor, Whipple's disease, intestinal lymphangiectasia)
Congestive heart failure

Decreased production
Aplastic anemia
Malignancy, especially Hodgkin's disease
Inherited immunoglobulin disorders (e.g., Wiskott-Aldrich, combined immunodeficiency, ataxia-telangiectasia)
Infection (e.g., AIDS)

Others (e.g., SLE, renal failure, miliary tuberculosis, myasthenia gravis, aplastic anemia)

CD4 LYMPHOCYTES

(usually performed by flow cytometry; calculated as total WBC × % lymphocytes × % lymphocytes stained with CD4)

Decreased In

Immune dysfunction. Especially useful in AIDS, in which severely depressed count is the single best predictor of imminent opportunistic infection and an increase is associated with therapeutic effect of drugs. May also be expressed as CD4/CD8 lymphocyte ratio, but CD8 count is more labile and may diminish the value of the CD4 counts

Acute minor viral infections. Should recheck in 3 months.

Also diurnal variation with peak evening values may be 2 times morning values. Imprecision in total WBC and differential may cause 25% variability in CD4 values.

CAUSES OF ATYPICAL LYMPHOCYTES

Lymphatic leukemia
Viral infections
Infectious lymphocytosis
Infectious mononucleosis
Infectious hepatitis
Viral pneumonia and other exanthems of childhood
Mumps
Chickenpox
German measles
Cytomegalovirus
Pertussis
Brucellosis
Syphilis (in some phases)
Toxoplasmosis
Drug reactions and serum sickness
Normal persons may show up to 12% atypical lymphocytes.

"Heterophil negative" infectious mononucleosis is most often seen in
Early stage of infectious mononucleosis
Toxoplasmosis
Cytomegalovirus
Infectious hepatitis

BASOPHILIC LEUKOCYTES

Increased In

(> 50/cu mm or > 1%)

Chronic myelogenous leukemia (may be first sign of blast crisis or accelerated phase)
Basophilic leukemia

Polycythemia
Myeloid metaplasia
Hodgkin's disease
Postsplenectomy
Chronic hemolytic anemia (some patients)
Chronic sinusitis
Chickenpox
Smallpox
Myxedema
Nephrosis (some patients)
Foreign protein injection
Ionizing radiation

Decreased In
Hyperthyroidism
Pregnancy
Period following irradiation, chemotherapy, and glucocorticoids
Acute phase of infection

CAUSES OF MONOCYTOSIS

(> 10% of differential count; absolute count > 500/cu mm)

Monocytic leukemia, other leukemias
Myeloproliferative disorders (myeloid metaplasia, polycythemia vera)
Hodgkin's disease and other malignant lymphomas
Lipid storage diseases (e.g., Gaucher's disease)
Postsplenectomy
Tetrachlorethane poisoning
Recovery from agranulocytosis and subsidence of acute infection
Many protozoan infections (e.g., malaria, kala-azar, trypanosomiasis)
Some rickettsial infections (e.g., Rocky Mountain spotted fever, typhus)
Certain bacterial infections (e.g., subacute bacterial endocarditis, tuberculosis, brucellosis)
Chronic ulcerative colitis, regional enteritis and sprue
Sarcoidosis
Collagen diseases (e.g., rheumatoid arthritis, SLE)

Most common causes are indolent infections (e.g., *Mycobacterium,* subacute bacterial endocarditis) and recovery phase of neutropenia.

Monocyte phagocytosis of RBCs in peripheral smears from earlobe is said to occur often in subacute bacterial endocarditis.

PLASMA CELLS

Increased In
Plasma cell leukemia
Multiple myeloma
Hodgkin's disease
Chronic lymphocytic leukemia
Other neoplasias (cancer of liver, kidney, breast, prostate)
Cirrhosis
Rheumatoid arthritis
SLE
Serum reaction
Bacterial infections (e.g., syphilis, tuberculosis)
Parasitic infections (e.g., malaria, trichinosis)
Viral infections (e.g., infectious mononucleosis, rubella, measles, chickenpox, benign lymphocytic meningitis)

Decreased In
Not clinically significant

CAUSES OF EOSINOPHILIA

(> 250/cu mm; diurnal variation with highest levels in morning)

Allergic diseases (e.g., bronchial asthma, hay fever, urticaria, drug therapy, allergic rhinitis)
Parasitic infestation, especially with tissue invasion (e.g., trichinosis, *Echinococcus* disease, schistosomiasis, filariasis, fascioliasis)
Some infectious diseases (e.g., scarlet fever, erythema multiforme, *Chlamydia*)
Collagen-vascular diseases (e.g., periarteritis nodosa, SLE, rheumatoid arthritis, scleroderma, dermatomyositis)
Some diffuse skin diseases (e.g., pemphigus, dermatitis herpetiformis)
Some hematopoietic diseases (e.g., pernicious anemia, chronic myelogenous leukemia, polycythemia, Hodgkin's disease, T-cell lymphomas, eosinophilic leukemia); postsplenectomy
Some immunodeficiency disorders (e.g., Wiskott-Aldrich syndrome, graft-versus-host disease, cyclic neutropenia, IgA deficiency)
Some gastrointestinal diseases (e.g., eosinophilic gastroenteritis, ulcerative colitis, regional enteritis)
Some endocrine diseases (e.g., hypopituitarism, Addison's disease)
Postirradiation
Miscellaneous conditions
- Certain tumors (ovary, involvement of bone or serosal surfaces)
- Sarcoidosis
- Loeffler's parietal fibroplastic endocarditis
- Familial condition
- Poisoning (e.g., phosphorus, black widow spider bite)

Hypereosinophilic syndrome (see new section p. 329)

Highest levels occur in trichinosis, *Clonorchis sinensis* infection, and dermatitis herpetiformis.

LEUKOCYTE ALKALINE PHOSPHATASE STAINING REACTION

(in untreated diseases)

Usually Increased In
Leukemoid reaction
Polycythemia vera
Lymphoma (including Hodgkin's, reticulum cell sarcoma)
Acute and chronic lymphatic leukemia
Multiple myeloma
Myelosclerosis
Aplastic anemia
Agranulocytosis
Bacterial infections
Cirrhosis
Obstructive jaundice
Pregnancy and immediate postpartum period
Administration of Enovid
Mongolism (trisomy 21)
Klinefelter's syndrome (XXY)

Usually Decreased In
Chronic myelogenous leukemia
Paroxysmal nocturnal hemoglobinuria

Hereditary hypophosphatasia
Nephrotic syndrome
Progressive muscular dystrophy
Refractory anemia (siderotic)
Sickle cell anemia

Usually Normal In

Secondary polycythemia
Hemolytic anemia
Infectious mononucleosis
Viral hepatitis
Lymphosarcoma

Usually Variable In

Pernicious anemia
Idiopathic thrombocytopenic purpura
Iron deficiency anemia
Acute myelogenous leukemia
Acute undifferentiated leukemia

This test is clinically most useful in differentiating chronic myelogenous leukemia from leukemoid reaction.

NITROBLUE TETRAZOLIUM (NBT) REDUCTION IN NEUTROPHILS

Increased In

Bacterial infections, including miliary tuberculosis and tuberculous meningitis
Nocardia and other systemic fungal infections
Various parasitic infections
Malaria
Chédiak-Higashi syndrome
Idiopathic myelofibrosis
Normal infants up to age 2 months
Pregnancy
Patients taking birth control pills
Some patients with lymphoma suppressed by chemotherapy

Decreased Or Normal
(in absence of bacterial infection)

Normal persons
Postpartum state
Postoperative state (after 7–10 days)
Cancer
Tissue transplantation
Other conditions with fever or leukocytosis not due to bacterial infection (e.g., rheumatoid arthritis)

Decreased Or Normal
(in presence of bacterial infection)

Antibiotic therapy—effectiveness of treatment indicated by reduction of previous elevation, sometimes in < 6 hours
Localized infection
Administration of corticosteroids and immunosuppressive drugs (contrary findings with corticosteroids have also been reported)
Miscellaneous conditions, probably involving metabolic defects of neutrophil function
- Chronic granulomatous disease
- Neutrophilic deficiency of glucose 6-phosphate dehydrogenase (glucose-6-PD) or myeloperoxidase

SLE
Sickle cell disease
Chronic myelogenous leukemia
Lipochrome histiocytosis
Congenital and acquired agammaglobulinemia
Other

Increased
(from previously determined normal level)

May be used before other clinical parameters to monitor development of infection in chronically ill patients
Development of wound sepsis in burn patients
Development of infection in uremic patients on chronic hemodialysis
Other

Usual normal values reported are < 10%, but there is considerable variation (< 14%), and each laboratory should establish its own normal range.

NBT test has been used principally in differentiating untreated bacterial infection from other conditions that may simulate it and for the diagnosis of poor neutrophilic function, particularly in chronic granulomatous disease. In many studies, few patients are included, considerable variation in technical performance occurs, or inadequate data are presented for comparison. Further evaluation of the clinical usefulness of the test in many of the conditions in which contradictory findings have been reported must await more definitive studies.

FREE ERYTHROCYTE PROTOPORPHYRIN (FEP)
(normal < 100 μg/dl/packed RBCs)

Increased In

Iron deficiency
Lead poisoning
Acquired idiopathic sideroblastic anemia
Certain chronic disorders

Normal In

Thalassemia minor (therefore useful to differentiate from iron deficiency)

SERUM IRON

Increased In

Idiopathic hemochromatosis
Hemosiderosis of excessive iron intake (e.g., repeated blood transfusions, iron therapy)
Decreased formation of RBCs (e.g., thalassemia, pyridoxine-deficiency anemia, pernicious anemia in relapse)
Increased destruction of RBCs (e.g., hemolytic anemias)
Acute liver damage (degree of increase parallels the amount of hepatic necrosis); some cases of chronic liver disease
Progesteronal birth control pills
Falsely increased by hemolysis
Iron dextran administration causes increase for several weeks.

Decreased In

Iron deficiency anemia
Normochromic (normocytic or microcytic) anemias of infection and chronic diseases (e.g., neoplasms, active collagen diseases)
Nephrosis (due to loss of iron-binding protein in urine)
Pernicious anemia at onset of remission
Falsely decreased in lipemic specimens

Because of diurnal variation (6–7 A.M. specimen $< 50\ \mu g/dl >$ 6–8 P.M. specimen) and because reference ranges are for morning levels. Diurnal variation disappears at levels $< 45\ \mu g/dl$.

SERUM TOTAL IRON-BINDING CAPACITY (TIBC)

Increased In

Iron deficiency anemia
Acute and chronic blood loss
Acute liver damage
Late pregnancy

Decreased In

Hemochromatosis
Cirrhosis of the liver
Thalassemia
Anemias of infection and chronic diseases (e.g., uremia, rheumatoid arthritis, some neoplasms)
Nephrosis

TIBC (μmol/L) = transferrin (mg/L) × 0.025

SERUM TRANSFERRIN

Increased In

Iron deficiency anemia
Pregnancy, estrogen therapy, hyperestrogenism

Decreased In

Hypochromic microcytic anemia of chronic disease
Acute inflammation
Protein deficiency or loss
- Thermal burns
- Chronic infections
- Chronic diseases (e.g., various liver and kidney diseases, neoplasms)
- Nephrosis
- Malnutrition

Genetic deficiency

SERUM TRANSFERRIN SATURATION

(serum iron divided by TIBC; normal ≥ 16%)

Increased In

Hemochromatosis
Hemosiderosis
Thalassemia

Decreased In

Iron deficiency anemia (usually < 10% in established deficiency)
Anemias of infection and chronic diseases (e.g., uremia, rheumatoid arthritis, some neoplasms)

$$\text{Transferrin saturation (\%)} = \frac{\text{Serum iron } (\mu g/dl)}{\text{TIBC } (\mu g/dl)} \times 100$$

Unsaturated iron-binding capacity (UIBC) = TIBC − serum iron (μg/dl)

SERUM FERRITIN

Chief iron-storage protein in the body
Reflects reticuloendothelial storage of iron
Correlates with total body iron stores

Decreased In

Iron deficiency anemia. *May be decreased before anemia and other changes occur. No other condition causes a low level. Is more sensitive test than percent iron saturation (iron × 100 divided by TIBC) and/or RBC zinc protoporphyrin. Returns to normal range within few days after onset of oral iron therapy; failure to produce serum ferritin level > 50 μg/L suggests noncompliance or continued iron loss.* < 18 ng/ml is associated with absent stainable iron in marrow.

Increased In

Anemias other than iron deficiency (e.g., megaloblastic, hemolytic, sideroblastic, thalassemia major and minor)

Ferritin is an acute-phase reactant and thus is increased in many patients with various acute and chronic liver diseases, malignancies (e.g., leukemia, Hodgkin's disease), chronic inflammation (e.g., arthritis), hyperthyroidism, Gaucher's disease, acute myocardial infarction (AMI), etc. *Serum ferritin may not be decreased when these conditions coexist with iron deficiency, and bone marrow stain for iron may be the only way to detect the iron deficiency.*

Iron overload (e.g., hemosiderosis, idiopathic hemochromatosis) (can be used to monitor therapeutic removal of excess storage iron). Transferrin saturation is more sensitive to detect early iron overload in hemochromatosis; serum ferritin is used to confirm diagnosis and as indication to proceed with liver biopsy. Ratio of serum ferritin (in ng/ml) to serum glutamic-pyruvic transaminase (SGPT) (in IU/L) > 10 in iron-overloaded thalassemic patients but average ≤ 2 in viral hepatitis; ratio decreases with successful iron chelation therapy.

Indications For Serum Ferritin Measurements

Detect iron deficiency

Determine response to iron therapy

Differentiate iron deficiency from chronic disease as cause of anemia

Monitor iron status in patients with chronic renal disease with or without dialysis

Detect iron overload states and monitor rate of iron accumulation and response to therapy

Population studies of iron levels and response to iron supplement

STAINABLE IRON (HEMOSIDERIN) IN BONE MARROW

(present in reticuloendothelial cells and developing normoblasts [sideroblasts])

Increased In

Hemolytic anemias (decrease or absence may signify acute hemolytic crisis)

Megaloblastic anemias in relapse

Hemochromatosis and hemosiderosis

Uremia (some patients)

Chronic infection (some patients)

Chronic pancreatic insufficiency

Decreased In

Iron deficiency anemia (e.g., inadequate dietary intake, chronic bleeding, malignancy, acute blood loss)

Polycythemia vera (usually absent in polycythemia vera but usually normal or increased in secondary polycythemia)

Pernicious anemia in early phase of therapy

Collagen diseases (especially rheumatoid arthritis, SLE)

Infiltration of marrow (e.g., malignant lymphomas, metastatic carcinoma, myelofibrosis, miliary granulomas)

Uremia

Chronic infection (e.g., pulmonary tuberculosis, bronchiectasis, chronic pyelonephritis)
Miscellaneous conditions (e.g., old age, diabetes mellitus)
Myeloproliferative diseases—iron stores may be absent without other evidence of iron deficiency.

The absence of iron in marrow is the most reliable index of iron deficiency; its presence almost invariably rules out iron deficiency anemia. Only individuals with decreased marrow iron are likely to benefit from iron therapy.

Marrow iron disappears before the peripheral blood changes. It rapidly disappears after hemorrhage.

One may have a normal serum iron and TIBC in iron deficiency anemia, especially if hemoglobin is < 9 gm/dl.

EXCESSIVE IRON DEPOSITION IN DISEASES ASSOCIATED WITH IRON OVERLOAD

Idiopathic hemochromatosis
Hemochromatosis secondary to
- Increased intake (e.g., Bantu siderosis, excessive medicine ingestion)
- Anemias with increased erythropoiesis (especially thalassemia major; also thalassemia minor, some other hemoglobinopathies, paroxysmal nocturnal hemoglobinuria, "sideroachrestic" anemias, refractory anemias with hypercellular bone marrow, etc.)
- Liver injury (e.g., following portal shunt surgery)
- Atransferrinemia

RETICULOCYTES

Increased In

After blood loss or increased RBC destruction—normal response is 3- to 6-fold increase.
After iron therapy for iron deficiency anemia
After specific therapy for megaloblastic anemias

Increase indicates effective RBC production mechanisms. It is a useful index of therapeutic response in these diseases.

Possibly other hematologic conditions (e.g., polycythemia, metastatic carcinoma in bone marrow, Di Guglielmo disease)

Increased reticulocyte count can elevate mean corpuscular volume (MCV) in hemolytic disorders, hemorrhage, treatment of vitamin B_{12} deficiency.

Decreased In

Ineffective erythropoiesis or decreased RBC formation
- Severe autoimmune type of hemolytic disease
- Aregenerative crises
- Megaloblastic disorders

Alcoholism
Myxedema

Reticulocyte count can be corrected for degree of anemia:

$$\text{Reticulocyte count} \times \frac{\text{patient's Hct}}{45\ (\text{assumed normal Hct})} \times \frac{1}{1.85}$$

(1.85 is number of days for reticulocyte to mature into an RBC.)

FETAL HEMOGLOBIN

(alkali denaturation method; confirmed by examination of hemoglobin bands on electrophoresis)

Normal

< 2% over age 2
> 50% at birth; gradual decrease to ~5% by age 5 months

Increased In

Various hemoglobinopathies (see Table 12-7, p. 303). ~50% of patients with thalassemia minor have high levels of Hb F; even higher levels are found in virtually all patients with thalassemia major. In sickle cell disease, Hb F > 30% protects the cell from sickling; therefore, even infants with homozygous S have few problems before age 3 months.
Hereditary persistence of fetal hemoglobin
Nonhereditary refractory normoblastic anemia (one-third of patients)
Pernicious anemia (50% of untreated patients); increases after treatment and then gradually decreases during next 6 months; some patients still have slight elevation thereafter. Minimal elevation occurs in ~5% of patients with other types of megaloblastic anemia.
Some patients with leukemia, especially juvenile myeloid leukemia with Hb F of 30–60%, absence of Philadelphia chromosome, rapid fatal course, more pronounced thrombocytopenia, and lower total WBC count
Multiple myeloma
Molar pregnancy
Patients with an extra D chromosome (trisomy 13–15, D_1 trisomy) or an extra G chromosome (trisomy 21, Down's syndrome, mongolism)
Acquired aplastic anemia (due to drugs, toxic chemicals, or infections, or idiopathic); returns to normal only after complete remission and therefore is reliable indicator of complete recovery. Better prognosis in patients with higher initial level.

Decreased In

A rare case of multiple chromosome abnormalities (probably C/D translocation)

SERUM HEMOGLOBIN

(normal < 10 mg/dl; < 30 mg/dl is not accurate technically; > 150 mg/dl causes hemoglobinuria; > 200 mg/dl causes clear cherry red color to serum)

Slight Increase In

Sickle cell thalassemia
Hemoglobin C disease

Moderate Increase In

Sickle cell–hemoglobin C disease
Sickle cell anemia
Thalassemia major
Acquired (autoimmune) hemolytic anemia

Marked Increase In

Any rapid intravascular hemolysis

OSMOTIC FRAGILITY

Increased In

Hereditary spherocytic anemia (can be ruled out if there is a normal fragility after 24-hour sterile incubation)
Hereditary nonspherocytic hemolytic anemia
Acquired hemolytic anemia (usually normal in paroxysmal nocturnal hemoglobinuria)

Hemolytic disease of newborn due to ABO incompatibility
Some cases of secondary hemolytic anemia (usually normal)
After thermal injury
Symptomatic hemolytic anemia in some cases of
- Malignant lymphoma
- Leukemia
- Carcinoma
- Pregnancy
- Cirrhosis
- Infection (e.g., tuberculosis, malaria, syphilis)

Decreased In

Early infancy
Iron deficiency anemia
Thalassemia
Sickle cell anemia
Homozygous hemoglobin C disease
Nutritional megaloblastic anemia
Postsplenectomy
Liver disease
Jaundice

BLOOD VOLUME

Blood volume determination is usually done using albumin tagged with ^{125}I or ^{131}I; red cell mass may be measured by labeling RBCs with ^{51}Cr.

May Be Useful To

Determine the most appropriate blood component (whole blood, plasma, or packed cells) for replacement therapy. For example, normal total blood volume and decreased red cell mass indicate the need for packed red cell transfusion.

Evaluate the clinical course. For example, immediately after acute severe hemorrhage, the hemoglobin concentration, hematocrit value, and RBC may be normal and not indicate the severity of blood loss, whereas appropriate measurements will show decreased blood volume, plasma volume, and red cell mass. After hemorrhage, the subsequent fluid shift from extravascular to intravascular space may produce a "falling" value for hemoglobin concentration, hematocrit, and RBC and falsely suggest continuing hemorrhage.

Assess the real degree of anemia in chronic conditions in which other mechanisms may disguise or accentuate the extent of RBC deficiency. For example, anemia and hemoconcentration together may produce an apparently normal hemoglobin concentration, hematocrit reading, and RBC. Hemodilution in uremia may make the anemia more marked and apparently more severe.

Alert the surgeon who compares the preoperative and postoperative values in surgical patients to
- Unexpected blood loss
- Need for replacement of the appropriate blood component, which may vary with the surgical procedure (e.g., in thoracoplasty the blood loss may be 900 ml, representing approximately equal red cell and plasma losses; in gastrectomy the blood loss may be 1800 ml, representing an RBC loss of 400 ml and a plasma loss of 1400 ml)

Differentiate polycythemia vera (increased total blood volume, plasma volume, red cell mass) and secondary polycythemia (normal or decreased total blood volume and plasma volume) in most cases

Radioisotopes should not be administered to children or pregnant women. In the presence of active hemorrhage, the isotope is lost via the bleeding site, and a false value will be produced.

RBC UPTAKE OF RADIOACTIVE IRON (^{59}Fe)

^{59}Fe is injected IV, and blood samples are drawn in 3, 7, and 14 days for measurement of radioactivity.

In pure red cell anemia, the rate of uptake of ^{59}Fe is markedly decreased.

PLASMA IRON ^{59}Fe CLEARANCE

^{59}Fe is injected IV, and blood samples are drawn in 5, 15, 30, 60, and 120 minutes for measurement of radioactivity.

ERYTHROCYTE SURVIVAL IN HEMOLYTIC DISEASES (^{51}Cr)

Increased In

Thalassemia minor

Decreased In

Idiopathic acquired hemolytic anemia
Paroxysmal nocturnal hemoglobinuria
Association with chronic lymphatic leukemia
Association with uremia
Congenital nonspherocytic hemolytic anemia
Hereditary spherocytosis
Elliptocytosis with hemolysis
Hemoglobin C disease
Sickle cell–hemoglobin C disease
Sickle cell anemia
Pernicious anemia
Megaloblastic anemia of pregnancy
In the normal person, half of the radioactivity of plasma disappears in 1–2 hours.
In pure red cell anemia, half of the plasma radioactivity may not disappear for 7–8 hours.

Normal In

Sickle cell trait
Hemoglobin C trait
Elliptocytosis without hemolysis or anemia

COOMBS' (ANTIGLOBULIN) TEST

Positive Direct Antiglobulin Test (DAT) (Coombs' test)

(due to immunoglobulin antibodies and/or complement present on patient's RBC membrane)

Erythroblastosis fetalis
Most cases of autoimmune hemolytic anemia, including ≤ 15% of certain systemic diseases, especially acute and chronic leukemias, malignant lymphomas, collagen diseases. Strength of reaction may be of prognostic value in patients with lymphoproliferative disorders.
Delayed hemolytic transfusion reaction
Drug induced
- Alpha methyldopa (in 30% of patients but < 1% show hemolysis)
- L-Dopa
- Mefenamic acid
- Penicillin
- Cephalosporins
- Quinidine
- Digitalis
- Insulin

Healthy blood donors (1 : 4000–1 : 8000 persons)

May be *weakly* positive in renal disease, epithelial malignancies, rheumatoid arthritis, inflammatory bowel diseases. Weakly positive reactions are not usually clinically significant.
False positive may occur in multiple myeloma.
Negative in hemolytic anemias due to intrinsic defect in RBC (e.g., glucose-6-PD deficiency, hemoglobinopathies)
Negative in 2–9% of patients with hemolytic anemia (due to smaller amount of IgG bound to RBC but similar response to splenectomy or steroid therapy or to IgM, IgA, or IgD rather than IgG). This is a diagnosis of exclusion.

Positive Indirect Coombs' Test
(using patient's serum that contains antibody)
Specific antibody—usually isoimmunization from previous transfusion
"Nonspecific" autoantibody in acquired hemolytic anemia
Incompatible cross-matched blood prior to transfusion

Beware of false positive and false negative results due to poor quality test serum, not using fresh blood (must have complement), etc.

UNSATURATED VITAMIN B_{12}–BINDING CAPACITY (UBBC)
(normal range = 870–1800 ng/L)

Increased In
Myeloproliferative diseases (especially polycythemia vera and chronic myelocytic leukemia)
Pregnancy
Oral contraceptive drugs

Decreased In
Hepatitis and cirrhosis

Table 12-3. Red Blood Cell Indices

Type of Anemia	Mean Corpuscular Volume (MCV)[a] (fl)	Mean Corpuscular Hemoglobin (MCH)[b] (pg)	Mean Corpuscular Hemoglobin Concentration (MCHC)[c] (gm/dl)
Normal	82–92	27–31	32–36
Normocytic anemias	82–92	25–30	32–36
Macrocytic anemias	95–150	30–50	32–36
Microcytic (usually hypochromic) anemias	50–80	12–25	25–30

[a] Mean corpuscular volume (MCV) (fl) = hematocrit/RBC.
[b] Mean corpuscular hemoglobin (MCH) (pg) = hemoglobin/RBC; represents weight of hemoglobin in average RBC. Not as useful as MCHC.
[c] Mean corpuscular hemoglobin concentration (MCHC) (gm/dl) = hemoglobin/hematocrit; represents concentration of hemoglobin in average RBC.

MCHC is increased only in hereditary spherocytosis. MCHC is not increased in pernicious anemia.

RED BLOOD CELL INDICES IN VARIOUS ANEMIAS

Macrocytic (MCV > 95 fl; mean corpuscular hemoglobin concentration [MCHC] > 30 gm/dl)
- Megaloblastic anemia
  - Pernicious anemia
  - Sprue (e.g., steatorrhea, celiac disease, intestinal resection or fistula)
- Macrocytic anemia of pregnancy
- Megaloblastic anemia of infancy
- Fish tapeworm infestation
- Carcinoma of stomach, following total gastrectomy
- Drug therapy (e.g., estrogens, antimetabolites, phenytoin)
- Orotic aciduria
- Di Guglielmo disease
- Liver disease
- Alcohol intoxication

Miscellaneous macrocytic nonmegaloblastic anemias that are usually normocytic
- Anemia of hypothyroidism
- Hemolytic anemia
- Aplastic anemia

MCHC is not increased in pernicious anemia. MCHC is increased only in hereditary spherocytosis. Spurious increase in indices with automated cell counters may occur in presence of lipemia, cold agglutinins, microclots, rouleaux, or RBC agglutinates. MCHC may be impossibly high, e.g., > 36; any count with MCHC > 36 should be suspect.

Normocytic (MCV = 80–94 fl; MCHC > 30 gm/dl)
- Following acute hemorrhage
- Hemolytic anemias
- Anemias due to inadequate blood formation
  - Myelophthisic
  - Hypoplastic
  - Aplastic
- Endocrinopathies (hypopituitarism, hypothyroidism, hypoadrenalism, hypogonadism)
- Anemia of chronic disease (e.g., chronic infections, neoplasms, uremia)

Microcytic (usually hypochromic) (MCV < 80 fl; MCHC < 30 gm/dl)
- Iron deficiency
  - Inadequate intake
  - Poor absorption
  - Excessive iron requirements
  - Chronic blood loss
  - Other
- Pyridoxine-responsive anemia
- Thalassemia (major or combined with hemoglobinopathy)
- Sideroblastic anemia (hereditary)
- Lead poisoning
- Chronic inflammation

Microcytic (usually normocytic)
- Anemia of chronic diseases
- Hemoglobinopathies

MEAN CORPUSCULAR VOLUME (MCV)
(hematocrit divided by RBC count)

Decreased In

Microcytic anemias, especially iron deficiency, anemia of chronic disease, and certain hemoglobinopathies

Marked leukocytosis (> 50,000/cu mm)*
In vitro hemolysis or fragmentation of RBCs*
Warm autoantibodies*

Increased In
Macrocytic anemias
Chronic alcoholism (may be a useful screening test for this)
Infants and newborns
Methanol poisoning*
Marked hyperglycemia (> 600 mg/dl)*
Marked reticulocytosis (> 50%) due to any cause*
Marked leukocytosis (> 50,000/cu mm)*

RED CELL DISTRIBUTION WIDTH (RDW)

Normal = 11.5–14.5. No subnormal values have been reported.

Is coefficient of variation (CV) of the RBC size as determined by some newer automated blood cell counting instruments. Is quantitative measure of anisocytosis.

$$CV = \frac{\text{standard deviation of RBC size}}{\text{mean corpuscular volume (MCV)}}$$

Classification of anemias based on MCV and RDW is most useful to distinguish iron deficiency anemia from that of chronic disease or heterozygous thalassemia and to improve detection of early iron or folate deficiency. The RDW is more sensitive in microcytic than macrocytic RBC conditions. Not helpful for patients without anemia.

Classification Of RBC Disorders By MCV And RDW

RDW normal, MCV low	Thalassemia minor Anemia of chronic disease
RDW high, MCV low	Iron deficiency Hb H disease S-beta-thalassemia Fragmentation of RBCs Hemoglobinopathy traits (AC) Some patients with anemia of chronic disease
RDW normal, MCV normal	Normal Anemia of chronic disease Hereditary spherocytosis Some hemoglobinopathy traits (e.g., AS)
RDW high, MCV normal	Early deficiency of iron or vitamin B_{12} or folate sickle cell anemia Hb SC disease
RDW normal, MCV high	Aplastic anemia Myelodysplastic syndrome
RDW high, MCV high	Deficiency of vitamin B_{12} or folate Immune hemolytic anemia Cold agglutinins

MEAN CORPUSCULAR HEMOGLOBIN (MCH)
(hemoglobin divided by RBC count)

Limited value in differential diagnosis of anemias

Decreased In
Microcytic and normocytic anemias

*Due to methodologic interference.

Increased In

Macrocytic anemias
Infants and newborns
Conditions with cold agglutinins*
In vivo hemolysis*
Monoclonal proteins in blood*
High heparin concentration*

MEAN CORPUSCULAR HEMOGLOBIN CONCENTRATION (MCHC)

(hemoglobin divided by hematocrit)

Changes occur very late in the course of any disease process; therefore chief use is for laboratory quality control.

Decreased In

(< 30.1 gm/dl)

Microcytic anemias. *Normal value does not rule out any of these anemias. Low MCHC may not occur in iron deficiency anemia when performed with automated instruments.*
Marked leukocytosis (> 50,000/cu mm)*

Increased In

Hereditary spherocytosis should be considered whenever MCHC > 36 gm/dl.
Infants and newborns
In vivo hemolysis*
Conditions with cold agglutinins or severe lipemia of serum*
High heparin concentration*

PERIPHERAL BLOOD SMEAR IN DIFFERENTIAL DIAGNOSIS OF ANEMIAS

The smear may also confirm the RBC indices or indicate leukemia or other conditions.

RBC Inclusions

Basophilic or polychromatophilic macrocytes	Increased erythropoiesis in hemorrhage or hemolysis
Microcytes with stippling	Thalassemia, lead or heavy-metal poisoning
Cabot's rings	Occasional in severe hemolytic anemias and pernicious anemia
Howell-Jolly bodies (dark purple spherical bodies)	Occasionally in severe hemolytic anemias and pernicious anemia Occasionally in leukemia, thalassemia, postsplenectomy state
Pappenheimer bodies (siderotic granules) (purple coccoid granules at periphery)	Anemias with defect of incorporating iron into hemoglobin (e.g., sideroblastic anemia, thalassemia, lead poisoning, pyridoxine-unresponsive and responsive anemias)
Heinz-Ehrlich bodies†	Congenital glucose-6-PD deficiency Other drug-induced hemolytic anemias Unstable hemoglobin disorders after splenectomy
Plasmodium trophozoites	Malaria
Reticulocytes†	See p. 270

*Due to methodologic interference.
†Not seen with Wright's stain; requires supravital stain, e.g., cresyl violet.

Abnormally Shaped RBCs

Shape	Associated conditions
Round	
Macrocytes	Increased erythropoiesis Oval in megaloblastic anemia Round in liver disease
Microcytes	See pp. 290–296
Spherocytes	Hereditary spherocytosis Immunohemolytic anemia
Stomatocytes	Acute alcoholism (transient) Certain drugs (e.g., phenothiazines) Neoplastic, cardiovascular, hepatobiliary diseases Congenital stomatocytosis (see p. 315) Artifactual
Target cells	Hemoglobin C disease or trait Thalassemia minor Iron deficiency anemia Liver disease Postsplenectomy state Artifactual
Elongated	
Ovalocytes (elliptocytes)	Hereditary (> 25% in smear) (see p. 314) Microcytic anemia (< 25% in smear) (see Table 12-6, pp. 294–295) Megaloblastic anemia
Teardrop (dacrocyte)	Spent polycythemia Myelofibrosis Thalassemia (especially homozygous beta)
Sickle cells	Sickle cell disorders (not in S trait)
Hemoglobin C crystalloids	Hemoglobin C trait or disease
Spiculated	
Acanthocytes	Abetalipoproteinemia (many are present) (see p. 417) Postsplenectomy state (few are present) Fulminating liver disease (variable number)
Burr cells (echinocyte; crenated RBC)	Usually artifactual Uremia, GI bleeding, stomach carcinoma
Schistocytes (helmet, triangle)	Microangiopathic hemolytic anemia (e.g., disseminated intravascular coagulation [DIC], thrombotic thrombocytopenic purpura [TTP]) Prosthetic heart valves or severe valvular heart disease Severe burns Snakebite (see p. 733)
"Bite" cells	Hemolysis due to certain drugs with or without glucose-6-PD deficiency
RBC fragmentation (seen on peripheral blood smear [> 10/1000 RBCs] and on histogram of RBC size with automated cell counters)	Cytotoxic chemotherapy for neoplasia Autoimmune hemolytic anemia Severe iron deficiency Megaloblastic anemia Acute leukemia Myelodysplasia Inherited structural abnormality of RBC membrane protein spectrin

SERUM HAPTOGLOBINS

Increased In

One-third of patients witb obstructive biliary disease

Conditions associated with increased erythrocyte sedimentation rate (ESR) and alpha$_2$ globulin (haptoglobin is also an acute-phase reactant) (infection; inflammation; trauma; necrosis of tissue; collagen diseases such as rheumatic fever, rheumatoid arthritis, and dermatomyositis, scurvy, amyloidosis; nephrotic syndrome; disseminated neoplasms such as Hodgkin's disease, lymphosarcoma). *Thus these conditions may mask presence of concomitant hemolysis.*

Therapy with steroids or androgens

Aplastic anemia (normal to very high)

Diabetes mellitus

Decreased Or Absent In

Hemoglobinemia (related to the duration and severity of hemolysis)

- Due To
  - Intravascular hemolysis (e.g., hereditary spherocytosis with marked hemolysis, pyruvate kinase deficiency, autoimmune hemolytic anemia, some transfusion reactions)
  - Extravascular hemolysis (e.g., large retroperitoneal hemorrhage)
  - Intramedullary hemolysis (e.g., thalassemia, megaloblastic anemias, sideroblastic anemias)

Genetically absent in 1% of general population

Parenchymatous liver disease (especially cirrhosis)

Protein loss via kidney, GI tract, skin

Infancy

Haptoglobin Determinations Are Useful

When splenectomy is being considered. Patients with chronic hemolysis (e.g., hereditary spherocytosis, pyruvate kinase deficiency) should not have splenectomy when serum haptoglobin is > 40 mg/dl if infection and inflammation have been ruled out. Increased haptoglobin level following splenectomy for these conditions indicates success of surgery; haptoglobin reappears at 24 hours and becomes normal in 4–6 days in hereditary spherocytosis treated with splenectomy.

In diagnosis of transfusion reaction by comparison of pretransfusion and posttransfusion levels. Posttransfusion reaction serum haptoglobin level decreases in 6–8 hours; at 24 hours it is < 40 mg/dl or < 40% of pretransfusion level.

In paternity studies. May aid by determination of haptoglobin phenotypes.

Hematologic Diseases

Anemias may be classified according to pathogenesis, which is convenient for understanding their pathogenesis (see next section), or according to RBC indices and peripheral blood smear (see Fig. 12-1), which is convenient for workup of a clinical problem.

CLASSIFICATION OF ANEMIAS ACCORDING TO PATHOGENESIS

Marrow hypofunction with decreased RBC production

- Marrow replacement (myelophthisic anemias due to tumor or granulomas [e.g., tuberculosis]). *In absence of severe anemia or leukemoid reaction, nucleated RBCs in blood smear suggest miliary tuberculosis or marrow metastases.*

Marrow injury (hypoplastic and aplastic anemias)
Nutritional deficiency (e.g., megaloblastic anemias due to lack of vitamin B_{12} or folic acid)
Endocrine hypofunction (e.g., pituitary, adrenal, thyroid)
Marrow hypofunction due to decreased hemoglobin production (hypochromic microcytic anemias)
Deficient heme synthesis (iron deficiency anemia, pyridoxine-responsive anemias)
Deficient globin synthesis (thalassemias, hemoglobinopathies)
Excessive loss of RBCs (hemolytic anemias due to genetically defective RBCs)
Abnormal shape (hereditary spherocytosis, hereditary elliptocytosis)
Abnormal hemoglobins (sickle cell anemia, thalassemias, hemoglobin C disease)
Abnormal RBC enzymes (glucose-6-PD deficiency, congenital nonspherocytic hemolytic anemias)
Excessive loss of RBCs
Hemolytic anemias with acquired defects of RBC and positive Coombs' test (autoantibodies, as in SLE, malignant lymphoma; or exogenous allergens, as in penicillin allergy)
Excessive loss of normal RBCs
Hemorrhage
Hypersplenism
Chemical agents (e.g., lead)
Infectious agents (e.g., *Clostridium welchii, Bartonella,* malaria)
Miscellaneous diseases (e.g., uremia, liver disease, cancers)
Physical agents (e.g., burns)
Mechanical trauma (e.g., artificial heart valves, tumor microemboli). *Blood smear shows fragmented bizarre-shaped RBCs in patients with artificial heart valves.*

Anemias are often multifactorial; the resultant characteristics depend on which factor predominates. The diagnosis must be reevaluated after the apparent causes have been treated.

MYELOPHTHISIC ANEMIA

Anemia is usually mild; not more than moderate.
Increased nucleated RBCs and normoblasts in peripheral smear, often without reticulocytosis, are out of proportion to the degree of anemia and may be found even in the absence of anemia. Polychromatophilia, basophilic stippling, and increased reticulocyte count may also occur.
WBC may be normal or decreased; occasionally it is increased up to a leukemoid picture; immature WBC may be found in peripheral smear.
Platelets may be normal or decreased, and abnormal forms may occur.
Abnormalities may occur even when WBC is normal.
Bone marrow demonstrates primary disease.
Metastatic carcinoma of bone marrow (especially breast, lung, prostate, thyroid)
Hodgkin's disease, leukemia
Multiple myeloma (5% of patients)
Gaucher's, Neimann-Pick, and Hand-Schüller-Christian diseases
Osteopetrosis
Myelofibrosis

Mild anemia with normoblastemia should arouse suspicion of infiltrative disease of marrow.

Nonhemolytic normocytic anemias with no obvious cause characterized by marked RBC changes on blood smear should arouse suspicion of malignancy or marrow fibrosis.

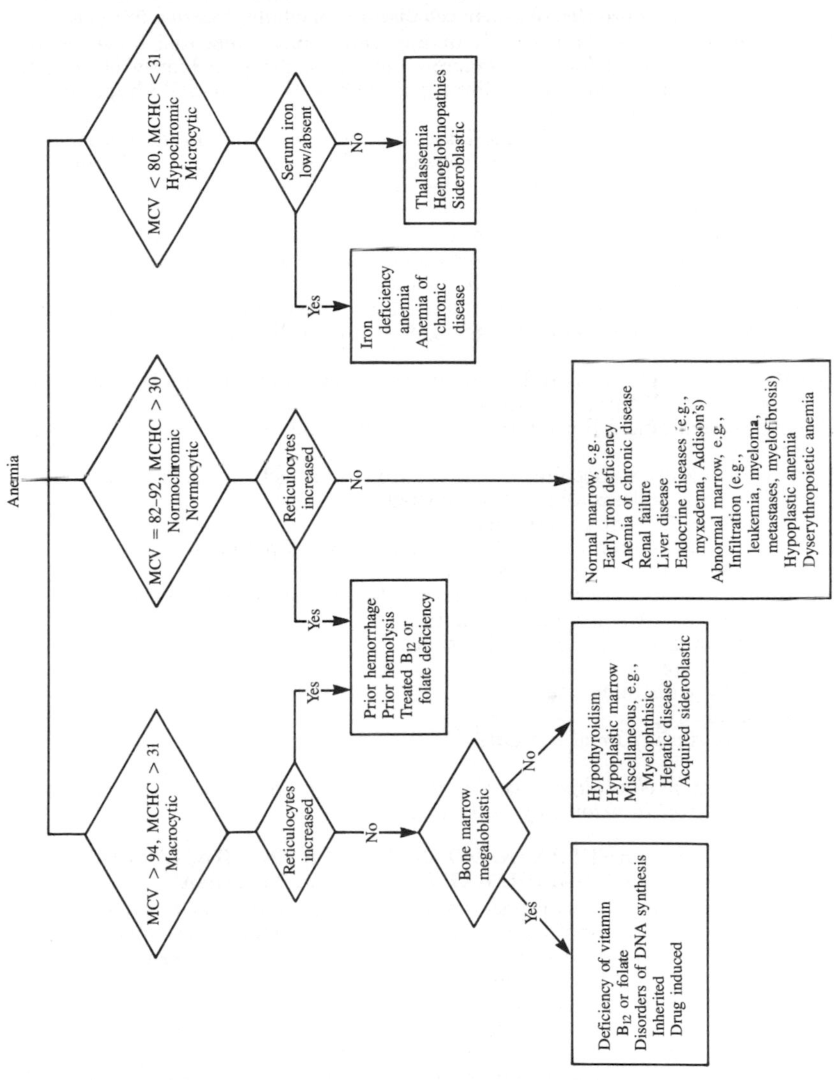

Fig. 12-1. Sequence of laboratory tests in workup of anemia. This algorithm is meant only to illustrate the use of indices for preliminary classification of anemias; many of the subsequent steps in the diagnostic workup are not included. Note also that some conditions may appear in more than one category. (Adapted from M. Wintrobe et al., *Clinical Hematology*. Philadelphia: Lea & Febiger, 1974.)

IDIOPATHIC MYELOFIBROSIS (AGNOGENIC MYELOID METAPLASIA)

(classified as a myeloproliferative stem cell disease stimulating marrow fibroblasts)

Bone marrow shows fibrosis without apparent cause. Repeated bone marrow aspiration often produces no marrow elements. Surgical biopsy of bone for histologic examination shows fibrosis of marrow that is usually hypocellular.

Normocytic anemia is usual.

Peripheral smear shows characteristic anisocytosis, and marked poikilocytosis with teardrop (dacrocytes), polychromatophilia, and occasional nucleated RBCs are found. Rarely seen in other hematologic conditions.

Reticulocyte count is increased ($\leq$ 10%).

WBC may be normal (50% of patients), increased (usually $\leq$ 30,000/cu mm), or decreased, and abnormal forms may occur. Immature cells ($\leq$ 15%) are usual. Basophils and eosinophils may be increased.

Platelets may be normal, increased, or decreased, and abnormal and large forms may occur. Deficient platelet aggregation after collagen or epinephrine may occur.

Needle puncture of spleen and a lymph node shows extramedullary hematopoiesis involving all three cell lines.

Hypersplenism causes thrombocytopenia in 30% and leukopenia in 15% of these patients.

Leukocyte alkaline phosphatase is usually increased (in contrast to chronic myelogenous leukemia); may be marked.

Serum uric acid is often increased.

Prolonged prothrombin time (PT) is found in 75% of patients.

Serum vitamin B_{12} is often increased.

Some patients have trisomies of 8, 9, and 21 (appearance during treatment is a poor prognostic sign), but Ph1 is rare.

Laboratory findings due to complications

- Hemorrhage
- Hemolytic anemia
- Infection
- DIC occurs in 20% of patients.

Rule out other myeloproliferative diseases, especially chronic myelogenous leukemia. May arise in prior polycythemia vera.

PURE RED CELL ANEMIA (AREGENERATIVE ANEMIA; IDIOPATHIC HYPOPLASTIC ANEMIA; PRIMARY RED CELL APLASIA)

Severe normochromic normocytic anemia is present that is refractory to all treatment except transfusion and sometimes adrenocorticotropic hormone (ACTH) or corticosteroids. Reticulocytes are decreased or absent.

WBC and differential blood count are normal.

There is no evidence of hemolysis.

Bone marrow usually shows marked decrease in erythroid series but sometimes is normal. Myeloid cells and megakaryocytes are normal.

Plasma iron (^{59}Fe) clearance is markedly reduced. RBC uptake of ^{59}Fe is markedly decreased.

Increased erythropoietin level

The disease may be related to thymus tumors (see p. 358), leukemia, which develops in 10% of patients, chemicals, bronchogenic carcinoma (rarely), kwashiorkor, etc.

PANCYTOPENIA

Anemia

Leukopenia—absolute myeloid decrease may be associated with relative lymphocytosis or with lymphocytopenia.

Thrombocytopenia

Laboratory findings due to causative disease

Due To

Hypersplenism
- Congestive splenomegaly
- Histiocytoses
- Primary splenic pancytopenia
- Malignant lymphomas
- Infectious diseases (tuberculosis, kala-azar, sarcoidosis)

Diseases of marrow
- Metastatic carcinoma
- Aleukemic leukemia
- Myelosclerosis, myelofibrosis, etc.
- Multiple myeloma
- Osteopetrosis
- Systemic mastocytosis

Aplastic anemias
- Physical and chemical causes (e.g., ionizing irradiation, benzol compounds)
- Idiopathic causes (familial or isolated; "isolated" accounts for 50% of all cases of pancytopenia)

Megaloblastic macrocytic anemias (e.g., pernicious anemia)

Paroxysmal nocturnal hemoglobinuria (rare)

APLASTIC ANEMIA

Peripheral blood pancytopenia associated with variable bone marrow hypocellularity in the absence of underlying myeloproliferative or malignant disease.

Neutropenia (absolute neutrophil count < 1500/cu mm) is always present; often monocytopenia is present.

Lymphocyte count is normal; reduced helper/inducer–cytotoxic/suppressor ratio.

Anemia is usually normochromic, normocytic but may be slightly macrocytic. RDW is normal.

Reticulocyte count corrected for hematocrit is decreased.

No poikilocytes are seen on peripheral blood smear.

Platelet count < 150,000/cu mm; severity varies.

Serum iron is increased.

Both bone marrow aspiration and biopsy should be performed.

Criteria for diagnosis (International Aplastic Anemia Study Group)
- Peripheral blood
  - Neutrophils < 500/cu mm
  - Platelets < 20,000/cu mm
  - Reticulocyte count corrected for hematocrit < 1%
- Marrow
  - Severe hypocellularity
  - Moderate hypocellularity with < 30% of residual cells being hematopoietic
- At least any two peripheral blood criteria plus either of marrow criteria

- Following treatment with marrow transplantation
  - Acute graft-versus-host disease develops in 25–30% of recipients and is fatal in 8%.
  - Chronic graft-versus-host disease develops in 20–30% of patients who survive > 6 months.
  - Most infections occur within 6 months. Interstitial pneumonia occurs in 16% of those conditioned by cyclophosphamide and up to 50% of those conditioned with whole-body irradiation: mortality is 40–50%; one-half of cases are due to cytomegalovirus (CMV) and one-half are of unknown cause.

Laboratory findings represent the whole spectrum, from the most severe condition of the classic type with marked leukopenia, thrombocytopenia, anemia, and acellular bone marrow, to cases with involvement only of erythroid elements. In some cases, the marrow may be cellular or hyperplastic.

Due To

Idiopathic in 50% of cases
Chemicals (e.g., benzene family)
Cytotoxic and antimetabolite drugs
Other drugs (e.g., chloramphenicol, antibiotics, anticonvulsants, phenylbutazone, gold)
Immunologic disorders (graft-versus-host reaction)
Ionizing irradiation (x-ray, radioisotopes)
Malnutrition (e.g., kwashiorkor)
Infections (especially HCV hepatitis)
Constitutional, inherited (e.g., Fanconi's anemia)
Leukemia is the underlying disease in 1–5% of patients who present with aplastic anemia.
Paroxysmal nocturnal hemoglobinuria (PNH) develops in 5–10% of patients with aplastic anemia, and aplastic anemia develops in 25% of patients with PNH.

HEMATOLOGIC EFFECTS OF CHEMICALS THAT INJURE BONE MARROW

(especially benzene; also trinitrotoluene and others)

In order of decreasing frequency
- Anemia
- Macrocytosis
- Thrombocytopenia
- Leukopenia
- Other (e.g., decreased lymphocytes, increased reticulocytes, increased eosinophils)
- Varying degrees of severity up to aplastic anemia
- Hemolytic anemia is sometimes produced.

HEMATOLOGIC EFFECTS OF IRRADIATION

(depends on amount of irradiation received)

Severe
- Severe leukopenia with infection
- Thrombocytopenia and increased vascular fragility, causing hemorrhage; begins in 4–7 days, peak severity in 16–22 days
- Aplastic anemia if patient survives 3–6 weeks; laboratory findings due to complications, such as hemorrhage, infection, dehydration

Mild (< 300 R)
- Increased neutrophils within a few hours with onset of irradiation sickness
- Decreased lymphocytes after 24 hours, causing decrease in total WBC
- No anemia unless dose of radiation is greater; may appear in 4–8 weeks (*Early appearance of anemia with greater irradiation is due to hemorrhage and changes in fluid homeostasis rather than marrow injury.*)
- Platelets slightly decreased (some patients)

Chronic (occupational)
- Decreased granulocytes
- Increased lymphocytes, relative or absolute
- Varying degrees of leukocytosis and leukemoid reactions
- Varying degrees of anemia, normocytic or macrocytic; erythrocytosis
- Thrombocytopenia

Late
- Increased incidence of leukemia (e.g., in survivors of atomic bomb explosions)
- Increased incidence of visceral malignancy (e.g., liver cancer due to Thorotrast, bone cancer due to radium)

PERNICIOUS ANEMIA (PA) (VITAMIN B_{12} DEFICIENCY) AND FOLATE DEFICIENCY

Most Commonly Due To

	Vitamin B_{12} Deficiency	Folate Deficiency
Inadequate intake	Strict vegetarian diet (rare)	Malnutrition, alcoholism
Increased need	Pregnancy, lactation	Pregnancy, lactation, infancy
Defective absorption	Decreased intrinsic factor (e.g., pernicious anemia, congenital deficiency, gastrectomy) Zollinger-Ellison syndrome Pancreatitis Ileal mucosal disease (e.g., sprue, regional enteritis, surgery) Tapeworm infestation, bacterial overgrowth in blind loop Drugs (e.g., colchicine, PAS, alcoholism)	Malabsorption due to drugs (e.g., anticonvulsants, antituberculosis, oral contraceptives), jejunal mucosal disease (e.g., amyloidosis, sprue, lymphoma, surgery)

Normochromic macrocytic anemia is a relatively late event; RBC may be as low as 500,000/cu mm.

MCV is increased (95–110 fl with mild to moderate anemia; 110–150 fl with more severe anemia. MCV increases many months before onset of anemia or clinical symptoms in almost all patients. MCV > 95 fl should prompt further study. MCV > 120 fl is most likely to be due to megaloblastic anemia. MCV may be normal if coexisting iron deficiency, inflammatory disease, renal failure, or thalassemia trait. MCV normal in ~9% of megaloblastic patients.

RDW is usually very increased due to marked anisopoikilocytosis or may be normal.

MCH is increased (33–38 pg with moderate anemia; up to 56 pg with severe anemia).

MCHC is normal.

Large hypersegmented neutrophils (≥ 5 lobes) is the earliest morphologic sign of megaloblastic anemia (rule out congenital hypersegmentation in 1% of white persons and uremia). Occasionally there is moderate eosinophilia. Blood smear may show oval macrocytes, schistocytes, polychromatophilia, stippled RBCs, Howell-Jolly bodies, Cabot's rings, etc. Nucleated RBCs may be found with hematocrit < 20%. Macro-ovalocytes are a good clue, although may also be seen in myelodysplasia.

Poikilocytosis is moderate to marked; is always present in relapse.

Anisocytosis is moderate to marked; is always present in relapse.

Reticulocyte count is usually decreased.

Thrombocytopenia is present in severe cases; abnormal and giant forms may be seen.

Leukopenia is usually < 4000/cu mm in severe cases.

Marrow shows megaloblastic and erythroid hyperplasia and abnormalities of myeloid and megakaryocytic elements. Erythroid megaloblastosis may be masked by concomitant iron deficiency, but granulocytic megaloblastic changes persist.

In PA, serum vitamin B_{12} is very low, usually < 100 pg/ml; 100–150 ng/L usually signifies early vitamin B_{12} deficiency even without neuropathy or macrocytosis. Especially in older persons, vitamin B_{12} deficiency may occur with neurologic symptoms but without anemia. RBC folate is low in many patients with vitamin B_{12} deficiency.

Serum Vitamin B_{12} May Also Be Decreased In

Diet deficient in folic acid (low in 10–30% of patients with simple folate deficiency)

Malabsorption

- Loss of gastric mucosa, e.g., partial or complete gastrectomy, atrophic gastritis, gastric radiation. Annual assay of vitamin B_{12} should be performed, since 100% of patients with total resection and 10% with partial resection will be deficient within 5 years.
- Small-bowel disease (e.g., Crohn's disease, scleroderma, lymphoma, ileal resection, tropical sprue, celiac disease, chronic pancreatic insufficiency)
- Primary hypothyroidism. (Almost 50% of patients have serum achlorhydria with intrinsic factor failure and low vitamin B_{12}; rarely megaloblastic anemia develops.)
- Parasites
    - 5% of persons infested with *Diphyllobothrium latum*
    - Blind loop syndrome diagnosed by positive Schilling test that becomes normal after 2 weeks of tetracycline therapy

Drugs (e.g., chronic PAS or colchicine use, oral contraceptives, aspirin, alcohol)

Pregnancy—progressive decrease during pregnancy (*normal serum B_{12} level in megaloblastic anemia of pregnancy*)

Impaired cell utilization

- Abnormal vitamin B_{12} carrier protein (transcobalamin II deficiency, abnormal protein)
- Enzyme deficiency
- Prolonged nitrous oxide exposure

One-third of patients with multiple myeloma

Others

- Iron deficiency
- Smoking
- Cancer
- Folate deficiency
- Pregnancy
- Vegetarian diet
- Aged persons
- Aplastic anemia
- Hemodialysis
- High doses of vitamin C

Spurious

- Antibiotics (with microbiologic assays)
- Diagnostic radioisotopes for other tests (with radioimmunoassays [RIAs])

Serum Vitamin B_{12} May Be Increased In

Myeloproliferative diseases

- Leukemia—acute and chronic myelogenous; about one-third of the cases of chronic lymphatic; some cases of monocytic. Normal in stem cell leukemia, multiple myeloma, Hodgkin's disease.
- Polycythemia vera

Leukocytosis

Some cases of carcinoma (especially with liver metastases)

Liver disease (acute hepatitis, chronic hepatitis, cirrhosis, hepatic coma)

Ingestion of vitamin A, vitamin C, estrogens, anticonvulsants

Uremia

Serum folate is normal or increased. Decreased serum folate in folate deficiency. Decreased RBC folate in both folate and vitamin B_{12} deficiency. (See Table 12-5, p. 290.)

Serum Folic Acid May Be Decreased In

Nutritional (may fall relatively quickly)
- Alcoholism is most common cause
- Chronic disease
- Anorexia nervosa
- Infancy, prematurity, elderly
- Hemodialysis

Increased requirements due to marked cellular proliferation
- Pregnancy
- Hyperthyroidism
- Neoplasia (e.g., acute leukemia, metastatic carcinoma)
- Hemolytic anemias (e.g., sickle cell, thalassemias, hereditary spherocytosis, paroxysmal nocturnal hemoglobinuria)
- Ineffective erythropoiesis (sideroblastic anemia)

Exfoliative dermatitis

Malabsorption
- Small-bowel disease (e.g., celiac disease, tropical sprue, Crohn's disease, lymphoma, amyloidosis, small-bowel resection)

Defect in utilization
- Drugs—folic acid antagonists (e.g., methotrexate, trimethoprim, primethamine) and anticonvulsants
- Certain enzyme deficiencies

Decreased liver stores

Cirrhosis

Hepatoma

Decreased serum folate is not evidence of tissue deficiency for which RBC folate should be assayed.

Usual normal range for serum folate is 5–15 ng/ml; 3–5 ng/ml is borderline.

Serum folic acid activity < 3 ng/ml is associated with positive hematologic findings.

Serum folic acid activity 3–5 ng/ml is associated with variable hematologic findings.

Serum folic acid activity > 5 ng/ml is associated with normal hematologic findings.

Serum Folic Acid May Be Increased In

Pernicious anemia (or may be normal)

Period following folic acid administration or eating

Vegetarians

Blood transfusion

Some cases of blind loop syndrome (due to folate synthesis by bacteria in gut)

False elevation in hemolyzed specimens (due to folate in RBCs)

Falsely increased to normal in some patients with severe iron deficiency (for unknown reason)

RBC folate reflects folate status at time RBCs were produced; therefore a more reliable indicator of tissue folate deficiency, as it is not subject to daily variation due to diet, etc. Decreased in folate or vitamin B_{12} deficiency. *RBC folate should always be measured in suspected cases of megaloblastic anemia when serum folate and vitamin B_{12} are assayed (see Table 12-5, p. 290).*

Schilling test is diagnostic of PA (shows very decreased absorption of radiolabeled B_{12}, which is corrected only by simultaneous administration of gastric intrinsic factor). Differentiates PA from other causes of vitamin B_{12} deficiency (*commonplace injection of vitamin B_{12} by physicians may make serum level temporarily normal for many weeks*) and can establish the functional absence of intrinsic factor before serum B_{12} deficiency or anemia is present or after patient has received vitamin B_{12} treatment.

Fasting patient is given oral $^{58}Co\ B_{12}$ and $^{57}Co\ B_{12}$ bound to intrinsic factor. In 1–2 hours, a flushing dose of 1 mg of nonradioactive B_{12} is injected IM or subcutaneously, and a 24-hour urine specimen is collected.

In PA, the ^{58}Co in urine is low (usually $< 5\%$ of the administered dose), but the $^{57}Co\ B_{12}$ bound to intrinsic factor is normally absorbed and excreted ($> 10\%$ of the administered dose).

In intestinal malabsorption, ^{57}Co and ^{58}Co in the urine are equally low ($< 5\%$). Both become normal if underlying cause is treated (e.g., antibiotic treatment in patients with bacterial overgrowth, administration of exogenous pancreatic enzyme in patients with pancreatic insufficiency).

For test to be valid, patient must have normal renal function, normal intestinal mucosal absorption, complete 24-hour urine collection.

Some patients cannot absorb dietary vitamin B_{12} but can absorb crystalline vitamin B_{12} used in test, giving false normal result.

Serum antibodies

Intrinsic factor antibody is present in 75% of patients with PA; high serum B_{12} causes false positive results. Positive test strongly supports diagnosis of PA and therefore should be performed in patients with low serum B_{12}; positive test combined with low serum B_{12} is virtually pathognomonic of PA; however, a negative test does not rule out PA, since almost one-fourth of such patients are negative for this antibody. False positive results are rare.

Parietal cell antibodies are more sensitive (90%) for PA but occur frequently in chronic gastritis; found in 2% of normal population; frequency increases with age and presence of insulin-dependent diabetes mellitus. Occurs in 50–100% of cases of PA, but frequency decreases with duration of PA. Intrinsic antibodies are more specific, but sensitivity is only ~50%.

Serum lactic dehydrogenase (LDH) is markedly increased (principally LDH_1 and LDH_2, with $LDH_1 > LDH_2$).

Serum indirect bilirubin is increased (< 4 mg/dl).

Urine urobilinogen and coproporphyrin I are increased.

Stool urobilinogen is increased.

Serum iron, TIBC, ferritin, and marrow iron are almost always increased during relapse unless there is complicating iron deficiency.

Serum methylmalonic acid (MMA) and homocysteine (HCYS) become elevated very early in course of vitamin B_{12} deficiency. Patients with folate deficiency usually increase only HCYS, although some may have mild increase of MMA. These are the most sensitive tests to detect early vitamin B_{12} deficiency and become positive before obvious hematologic evidence of vitamin B_{12} deficiency. Are useful in patients with borderline vitamin B_{12} levels (100 to 300 ng/L). Should be positive in acute neurologic disease due to vitamin B_{12} deficiency, even when hematologic changes are absent. Will remain positive for at least 24 hours after onset of vitamin B_{12} therapy in patients in whom therapy is begun before blood is drawn for vitamin B_{12} levels. Serum is much more sensitive and specific than urine MMA and should be used for testing. Tests should be requested in cases of unexplained hematologic or neuropsychiatric abnormalities with low or borderline serum vitamin B_{12} levels (reference ranges: MMA = 70–279 nmol/L, HCYS = 5–15 μmol/L).

Achlorhydria occurs even after administration of histamine; this is virtually essential for diagnosis of PA. Decreased volume of gastric juice, high pH, and decreased or absent pepsin and renin are also shown. Achlorhydria and gastric changes are rarely found in children.

Increased serum gastrin with low serum vitamin B_{12} suggests PA.

Serum alkaline phosphatase is decreased; increases after treatment.

Serum cholesterol is moderately decreased.

Cholinesterase activity in RBC, plasma, and whole blood is decreased.

There is a characteristic therapeutic response to vitamin B_{12} or folate administration.
RBC survival is decreased.
Recently developed deoxyuridine (dU) suppression test: Patient's marrow cells are cultured with radiolabeled thymidine; in normal marrow, labeled thymidine uptake is suppressed on addition of unlabeled dU because dU can be converted to deoxythymidine, but suppression does not occur when patient is folate or vitamin B_{12} deficient due to inability to convert deoxyuridine; adding folate or vitamin B_{12} to the medium indicates specific cause. May be useful when other test results are masked by recent therapy or are equivocal. Limited availability at present but may become gold standard of megaloblastic states.
50% of PA patients have thyroid antibodies.

Response Of Laboratory Tests To Specific Treatment Of Pernicious Anemia Or Folate Deficiency

RBC count reaches normal between 8th and 12th week regardless of severity of anemia; hemoglobin concentration may rise at a slower rate, producing hypochromia with microcytosis. Peripheral blood is normal in 1–2 months.
Reticulocyte response is proportional to severity of anemia. This response is characteristic: reticulocyte count begins to rise by 4th day after treatment and reaches maximum on 8th to 9th day; returns to normal by 14th day.
Megaloblasts disappear from marrow in 24–48 hours followed by reversal of megaloblastic changes in myeloid cells a few days later.
Serum folate decreases (in PA) at the same time reticulocytosis takes place.
Serum iron decreases to normal or less than normal at the same time reticulocytosis takes place.
Serum uric acid increases; peak precedes maximum reticulocyte count by about 24 hours; remains increased as long as rapid RBC regeneration goes on.
Serum LDH falls but is not yet normal by eighth day.
Serum bilirubin becomes normal.
Serum alkaline phosphatase increases to normal.
Serum cholesterol rises to greater than normal levels; most marked at peak of reticulocyte response.

Table 12-4. Laboratory Tests in Differential Diagnosis of Causes of Vitamin B_{12} Deficiencies

	Gastric Juice		Schilling Test	
Condition	HCl	Intrinsic Factor Assay	Without Intrinsic Factor	With Intrinsic Factor
Lack of intrinsic factor (usually pernicious anemia)	O	O	D	N
Intestinal lesion	P or O	P	D	D
Nutritional	P or O	P	N	N

O = absent; P = present; N = normal; D = decreased.

Presence of free HCl in gastric juice always rules out pernicious anemia (except for very rare cases); absence of HCl is not helpful.

Table 12-5. Laboratory Tests in Differential Diagnosis of Vitamin B_{12} and Folic Acid Deficiencies

	Serum Vitamin B_{12}	Serum Folate	RBC Folate
Normal	N	N or D	N
Vitamin B_{12} deficiency	D	N or I	D
Folic acid deficiency	N	D	D
Vitamin B_{12} and folic acid deficiencies	D	D	D

N = normal; D = decreased; I = increased.

RBC folate does not fall below normal until all body stores are depleted. Low serum folate indicates only negative folate balance, not folate deficiency. Serum folate serves to distinguish combined deficiency from vitamin B_{12} deficiency alone. Thus, all three parameters should be measured simultaneously in suspected cases of megaloblastic anemia.

Iron deficiency is present in one-half of patients with folate deficiency and one-third with vitamin B_{12} deficiency. If iron deficiency is more severe than folate deficiency, results of serum and RBC folate tests are normal, and diagnosis cannot be made from these tests; hypersegmentation of PMNs in blood smear is the only clue.

Increased urinary urobilinogen and coproporphyrin I immediately revert to normal, preceding reticulocyte response.
Achlorhydria persists.
RBC cholinesterase activity increases.

MACROCYTIC ANEMIA OF LIVER DISEASE

Increased MCV (100–125 fl) in one-third to two-thirds of patients. Indices resemble those in other megaloblastic anemias. Low MCHC may indicate associated iron deficiency.
Uniform round macrocytosis is the cardinal finding. Target cells and stomatocytes may be present.
Hemolytic anemia or true folate deficiency is frequent in alcoholic liver disease.
WBC and platelet count may be decreased or normal.

MACROCYTIC ANEMIA OF SPRUE, CELIAC DISEASE, STEATORRHEA

See p. 161.

MEGALOBLASTIC ANEMIA OF PREGNANCY AND PUERPERIUM

Anemia may have been present during previous pregnancy with spontaneous remission after delivery.
Hematologic abnormalities are less marked than in pernicious anemia (see pp. 5–290).
If achlorhydria is present, it often disappears after delivery.
Therapeutic response to folic acid but usually not to vitamin B_{12}.
Urinary excretion of formiminoglutamic acid (FIGLU) is increased.

IRON DEFICIENCY ANEMIA

Due To

(usually a combination of these factors)

Chronic blood loss (e.g., menometrorrhagia, bleeding from GI tract, especially from carcinoma of colon, hiatus hernia, peptic ulcer, parasites in intestine)
Decreased dietary intake (e.g., poverty, emotional factors)

Decreased absorption (e.g., steatorrhea, gastrectomy, achlorhydria)
Increased requirements (e.g., pregnancy, lactation)
The *cause of iron deficiency should always be ascertained* to avoid overlooking *occult carcinoma.*

Laboratory Findings

Hemoglobin is decreased (usually 6–10 gm/dl) out of proportion to decrease in RBC (3.5–5.0 million/cu mm); thus decreased MCV (< 80 fl) is a sensitive indicator; decreased MCHC (25–30 gm/dl) is usually normal until anemia is severe, and MCH is decreased (< 30 pg).

Increased RDW is found more often in iron deficiency than thalassemia; increased RDW may be the first indication of iron deficiency; sensitivity = 89%; negative predictive value of normal RDW = 93%; positive predictive value = 45%; specificity is only 45%.

Hypochromia and microcytosis parallel severity of anemia. Polychromatophilia and nucleated RBCs are less common than in pernicious anemia or thalassemia. Diagnosis from peripheral blood smear is difficult and unreliable. Target cells may be present but are more common in thalassemias; basophilic stippling and polychromasia also favor thalassemia, although absent in 50% of cases. Anisocytosis is less marked in thalassemia.

Serum iron is decreased (usually 40 μg/dl), TIBC increased (usually 350–460 μg/dl), and transferrin saturation decreased (< 15%). TIBC may be normal or moderately increased in many patients with uncomplicated iron deficiency. Serum transferrin may be normal or increased (calculated transferrin = TIBC × 0.7). These have limited value in differential diagnosis, since they are often normal in iron deficiency and abnormal in anemia of chronic disease and may be affected by recent iron therapy.

Decreased serum ferritin is first test to reflect iron deficiency but may be increased when there is coexisting liver disease, inflammation, or other conditions that increase ferritin (see p. 268–269). Thus iron deficiency is suggested by serum ferritin < 25 μg/L in a patient with inflammation, < 50 μg/L in a hemodialysis patient, and < 100 μg/L in liver disease. Ferritin usually distinguishes iron deficiency from thalassemia in uncomplicated cases.

As iron deficiency progresses, decreased serum ferritin is followed in order by anisocytosis, microcytosis, elliptocytosis, hypochromia, fall in hemoglobin, fall in serum iron, fall in transferrin saturation.

Bone marrow shows normoblastic hyperplasia with decreased hemosiderin, later absent, and decreased percentage of sideroblasts. Decreased to absent iron is the "gold standard" test for diagnosis of iron deficiency.

Free erythrocyte protoporphyrin is increased and is a useful screening test, since it is also increased in lead poisoning and normal in thalassemias and can be done on fingerstick sample.

Reticulocytes are normal or decreased, unless there is recent hemorrhage or administration of iron.

WBC is normal or may be slightly decreased in 10% of cases; may be increased with fresh hemorrhage.

Serum bilirubin and LDH are not increased.

Platelet count is usually normal but may be slightly increased or decreased; often increased in children.

Coagulation studies are normal.

RBC fragility is normal or (often) increased to 0.21%.

RBC life span is normal.

Laboratory finding may disclose causative factors (e.g., GI bleeding).

Response to oral iron therapy is the final proof of diagnosis

- Increased reticulocytes with peak of 8–10% on fifth to tenth day; proportional to degree of anemia
- Followed by rising hemoglobin (average 0.25–0.4 gm/dl/day) and rising hematocrit (average = 1%/day) during first 7–10 days; thereafter hemo-

globin increases 0.1 gm/dl/day to level ≥ 11 gm/dl in 3–4 weeks. Should be about half corrected in 3 weeks and fully corrected by 8 weeks. In elderly, increase of 1 gm/dl may take 1 month when younger patients increase hemoglobin 3 gm/dl and hematocrit 10%.

Failure to respond suggests incorrect diagnosis, coexistent deficiencies (folic acid, vitamin B_{12}, thyroid), associated conditions (e.g., lead poisoning, bleeding, malabsorption, liver or kidney disease).

Most difficult differential diagnoses are thalassemias and anemia of chronic disease. See pp. 302 and 292 and Table 12-6, pp. 294–295, for additional laboratory findings.

In U.S., median hemoglobin is about 1 gm/dl lower in blacks without iron deficiency than in whites.

ATRANSFERRINEMIA

(very rare, hereditary isolated absence of transferrin)

Hypochromic, microcytic, iron deficiency anemia is unresponsive to therapy.
TIBC is low (< 85 μg/dl).
Absence of transferrin is demonstrated with immunoelectrophoresis.
Hemosiderosis with involvement of adrenals, heart, etc., is present.
Serum protein electrophoresis shows marked decrease in beta globulins.

ANEMIAS OF CHRONIC DISEASES

Due To

Subacute or chronic infections (especially tuberculosis, bronchiectasis, lung abscess, empyema, bacterial endocarditis, brucellosis)
Neoplasms
Rheumatoid arthritis (anemia parallels activity of arthritis)
Rheumatic fever, SLE
Uremia (serum urea nitrogen [BUN] > 70 mg/dl)
Chronic liver diseases

Laboratory Findings

Anemia is usually mild (hemoglobin > 9 gm/dl) but may be as low as 5 gm/dl in uremia when other factors are present. Is insidious and *not progressive.* May be due to multiple mechanisms, e.g., failure of erythropoiesis, decreased RBC survival, iron deficiency.

Anemia is usually normocytic, normochromic. RDW and indices are usually normal. In one-fourth to one-third of these patients, is hypochromic and/or microcytic, in which case it is always less marked than in iron deficiency anemia.

Moderate anisocytosis and slight poikilocytosis are present.

Reticulocytosis, polychromatophilia, and nucleated RBCs are absent (may be present with severe anemia or uremia).

Serum iron is decreased. TIBC and transferrin saturation are decreased or normal. If TIBC is elevated, presence of iron deficiency must be ruled out, but TIBC is not sufficiently sensitive or specific to distinguish this from iron deficiency anemia. Transferrin saturation is usually normal; < 10% implies iron deficiency.

Serum ferritin is increased or normal in contrast to iron deficiency.

Free erythrocyte protoporphyrin is increased.

WBC and platelets are normal.

Bone marrow cellular elements are generally morphologically normal. Sideroblasts are decreased, and storage iron is substantially increased.

In rheumatoid arthritis, liver disease, or neoplasms, normal serum ferritin does not exclude concomitant iron deficiency.

Marrow hemosiderin is increased or normal; sideroblasts are decreased. Myeloid-erythroid ratio is usually normal.
RBC survival is slightly decreased in patient (80–90 days) but not in normal recipient.
Platelet count is normal.
Increased ESR disproportionate to anemia and increased WBC, CRP, fibrinogen, ceruloplasmin, etc., consistent with inflammation may be found.

See Table 12-6, pp. 294–295.

Hypothyroidism

Occurs in one-third to two-thirds of patients with hypothyroidism; usually mild (hematocrit > 35%)
Normochromic, normocytic or macrocytic. (If hypochromic, rule out associated iron deficiency.)
Serum iron is usually decreased and responds only to treatment of hypothyroidism unless there is concomitant iron deficiency.
No anisocytosis or poikilocytosis
Decreased total blood volume and plasma volume
Normal RBC survival
Concurrent iron deficiency or pernicious anemia may be present.

Chronic Renal Disease

Blood smear frequently shows burr cells or schistocytes.
Usually normochromic, normocytic; hypochromic microcytosis may be due to chronic disease or iron deficiency. Severity of anemia roughly parallels severity of renal disease.
Decreased serum iron and transferrin. Serum iron, TIBC, and ferritin are often not helpful, and bone marrow stained for iron may be necessary for diagnosis of iron deficiency. Concurrent iron deficiency due to GI tract blood loss may be present.
Bone marrow usually shows erythroid hypoplasia.

Chronic Liver Disease

Blood smear often shows round macrocytes and target cells, but presence of hypochromic macrocytes or microcytes may suggest misleading diagnosis of iron deficiency.
Serum iron, TIBC, and ferritin are often not helpful, and bone marrow stained for iron may be necessary for diagnosis of iron deficiency.

SIDEROBLASTIC ANEMIAS

(miscellaneous group of diseases characterized by increased sideroblasts [erythroblasts containing iron inclusions] in marrow) (see Table 12-6, pp. 294–295)

Due To

Drugs (e.g., isoniazid, chloramphenicol, alcohol, lead, cytotoxic drugs such as nitrogen mustard and azathioprine)
Diseases
- Hematologic (e.g., leukemia, polycythemia vera, megaloblastic anemia, hemolytic anemia)
- Neoplastic (e.g., lymphoma, carcinoma)
- Inflammatory (e.g., infection, RA, polyarteritis nodosa)
- Miscellaneous (uremia, myxedema, thyrotoxicosis, porphyria)

Hereditary (pyridoxine-responsive or refractory)
Idiopathic (pyridoxine-responsive or refractory)

Hereditary

Usual onset in young adults but may be in children or infants
Anemia is usually severe, hypochromic, microcytic with anisocytosis, poikilocytosis, target cells, basophilic stippling; dimorphic RBC population.

Table 12-6. Laboratory Tests in Differential Diagnosis of Microcytic (MCV < 80 fl) and Hypochromic (MCHC < 30 gm/dl) Anemias

1. Determine serum iron and TIBC (and also perhaps do iron stain on bone marrow smear—the most reliable index of iron deficiency).
2. If serum iron and TIBC are both normal, hemoglobin electrophoresis will establish the diagnosis of thalassemia.
   If serum iron is abnormal, the cause may be iron deficiency (e.g., blood loss, dietary deficiency) or normochromic microcytic anemia of chronic disease.

Type of Anemia	Serum Iron	TIBC	Transferrin Saturation	Serum Ferritin	FEP*	Marrow Hemosiderin	Sideroblasts	Type of Hemoglobin	Anemia	RBC Count	RDW
Normal values	80–160 μg/dl in men 50–150 μg/dl in women	250–410 μ/dl	20–55%	20–150 ng/dl			30–50%	AA			11.5–14.5
Iron deficiency	D	I	D	D	I	O	D	AA	Hypochromic, normocytic, or microcytic	D	I
Normochromic, normocytic or microcytic, of chronic disease	D	D or N	D or N	N or slightly I	I	N or I	D	AA	Normochromic, normocytic, or microcytic	D	N

Thalessemia											
Major	I	D	I		N	I	I	20–90% F	Hypochromic	I	N
Minor	N or I	N	N or I	I	N	N or I	I	2–8% F, A_2 is 1	Microcytic		
Sideroblastic	N or I	D or N	I	I	D	I	I	AA	Hypochromic and/or microcytic with normocytic or macrocytic changes, dimorphic RBC population	D	I

O = absent; D = decreased; I = increased; N = normal.
*FEP = free erythrocyte protoporphyrin is useful to distinguish between iron deficiency and beta thalassemia.

Iron depletion: Early—serum iron is normal; TIBC may be increased. Later—serum iron decreases; anemia is often normocytic when mild or of rapid onset; anemia first becomes microcytic, then hypochromic.
Iron deficiency may occur without anemia (transferrin saturation < 15%; decreased marrow iron and sideroblasts).

WBC and platelets are usually normal.

Bone marrow shows erythroid hyperplasia with normoblastic maturation; 10–40% of normoblasts are ringed sideroblasts; excessive hemosiderin. Megaloblastic changes indicate complicating folate deficiency.

Transferrin saturation is increased.

< 50% of patients respond to pyridoxine therapy.

Idiopathic Refractory

Usual onset in older adults (rarely < 50 years)

Dimorphic anemia is usually moderate, normocytic, or macrocytic with a small population of hypochromic RBCs on blood smear, some of which show marked stippling.

Reticulocytes are usually not increased.

WBC is variable but usually normal. WBCs may show morphologic changes (hypogranular, Pelger-Huët–like neutrophils). Blasts < 1%.

Platelet counts are variable. Abnormal thrombopoiesis with abnormal morphology (e.g., hypogranular, large platelets or fragments, large nuclei)

Bone marrow shows erythroid hyperplasia; 45–95% of normoblasts are ringed sideroblasts; excessive hemosiderin. Megaloblastic changes due to complicating folate deficiency are found in 20% of patients. Dysgranulopoiesis and dysmegakaryopoiesis may be evident.

Transferrin saturation is increased (> 90% in 33% of patients).

Serum ferritin and iron stores are increased due to ineffective erythropoieses.

Acute leukemia develops in ~10% of patients.

Secondary

Due to drugs and toxic agents (e.g., chloramphenicol, antituberculosis drugs, lead poisoning, alcoholism) or associated with other diseases such as neoplasms (e.g., lymphomas, myeloma), hematologic diseases (e.g., leukemia, polycythemia vera), inflammatory diseases (e.g., SLE, rheumatoid arthritis, polyarteritis nodosa), miscellaneous diseases (e.g., thyroid dysfunction, porphyrias, uremia)

PYRIDOXINE-RESPONSIVE ANEMIA

Severe hypochromic microcytic anemia is present.

Blood smear shows anisocytosis, poikilocytosis with many bizarre forms, target cells, hypochromia. Polychromatophilia and reticulocytosis are not increased.

Serum iron is increased; TIBC is somewhat decreased; transferrin saturation is markedly increased. Marrow sideroblasts and blood siderocytes are increased. Marrow and liver biopsy show increased hemosiderin.

Bone marrow usually shows normoblastic hyperplasia; occasionally it is megaloblastic.

Response to pyridoxine is always incomplete. Even when hemoglobin becomes normal, morphologic changes in RBCs persist.

Tryptophan tolerance test demonstrates pyridoxine deficiency. It may be positive in pyridoxine-responsive anemia, or it may be normal. A positive test produces abnormally large urinary excretion of xanthurenic acid.

CLASSIFICATION OF HEMOLYTIC ANEMIAS*

A useful approach to the diagnosis of hemolytic anemias may be based on

1. Site of RBC destruction (intravascular or extravascular)
2. Site of etiologic defect (intracellular RBC or extracellular)
3. Nature of defect (acquired or hereditary)

*Source: Adapted from M. C. Brain, Hemolytic anemia. *Postgrad. Med.* 64:127, Oct., 1978.

Hemoglobin Disorders

Intrinsic

Autosomal

Sickle cell (SS) disease	Common
Thalassemias	Common
Hemoglobin C, D, E disease	Common
Unstable hemoglobins	Very rare

Membrane Disorders

Intrinsic

Congenital or familial (usually autosomal dominant)

Hereditary spherocytosis	Common (~0.02% North European population)
Hereditary elliptocytosis	Rare
Hereditary stomatocytosis	Very rare
Other	Very rare
Acquired—paroxysmal nocturnal hemoglobinuria	Rare

Extrinsic

Congenital or familial

Abetalipoproteinemia	Very rare

Acquired

Isoimmune (blood transfusion reaction, hemolytic disease of newborn)

Autoimmune (Coombs' test usually positive; spherocytes may be present)	Rare

- Drug induced (e.g., penicillin, methyldopa)
- Diseases (e.g., lymphomas/leukemia, infectious mononucleosis, *Mycoplasma*)
- Idiopathic

Nonimmune (Coombs' test usually negative; morphologic changes in blood smear usually found)

- Physical or mechanical
  - Prosthetic heart valves
  - Microangiopathic hemolytic disease including DIC, thrombotic thrombocytopenic purpura, hemolytic uremic syndrome, etc.
  - Paroxysmal cold hemoglobinuria
  - March hemoglobinuria
  - Severe burns
  - Snakebite (see p. 733)
  - Osmotic—distilled water used in prostate resection
- Infectious
  - Protozoan (e.g., malaria, toxoplasmosis, leishmaniasis)
  - Bacterial (e.g., sepsis, clostridial toxins, bartonellosis)
  - Viral (e.g., echovirus)

Metabolic Disorders

Intrinsic

Glucose-6-PD deficiency	Common
Pyruvate kinase deficiency	Rare
Erythropoietic porphyria	

Extrinsic

Drugs in normal RBCs or in glucose-6-PD deficiency

Others (e.g., lead poisoning, Wilson's disease)

15–20% of acquired immune hemolytic anemias are related to drug therapy.

~3% of patients taking penicillins and cephalosporins develop positive direct Coombs' test; hemolysis is infrequent and usually extravascular.

~10% of patients taking methyldopa develop positive direct Coombs' test but < 1% develop hemolysis.

Hemolytic transfusion reactions occur in ~1 : 12,000 transfusions and are fatal in 1 : 600,000 transfusions, which are almost always due to ABO incompatibility (usually due to clerical error).

Non-ABO antibodies usually cause extravascular hemolysis, producing milder clinical and laboratory findings.

LABORATORY FINDINGS DUE TO INTRAVASCULAR HEMOLYSIS

Anemia varies from mild (Hb = 11.5 gm/dl) to severe (Hb = 2 gm/dl). MCV is usually 80–110 fl; < 70 fl in normochromic anemia suggests hemoglobinopathy or paroxysmal nocturnal hemoglobinuria; > 115 fl suggests macrocytic anemia.

Peripheral smear shows macrocytes, nucleated RBCs, polychromatophilia.

Spherocytes suggest hereditary spherocytosis or autoimmune hemolytic anemia.

Microspherocytes suggest hemoglobin disease, ABO erythroblastosis, burns.

RBC cell fragments suggest DIC, prosthetic valves, hemolytic uremic syndrome.

Target cells suggest hemoglobinopathies, postsplenectomy state.

Plasma haptoglobin level decreases about 100 mg/dl in 6–10 hours and lasts for 2–3 days after lysis of 20–30 ml of blood. Test is relatively reliable and very sensitive.

Urine hemosiderin occurs 3–5 days after hemolysis with positive Prussian blue staining of renal tubular epithelial cells. It may be difficult to detect a single episode. Urine hemosiderin is commonly found in paroxysmal nocturnal hemoglobinuria.

Plasma hemoglobin increases transiently with return to normal in 8 hours; lacks accuracy and precision.

Hemoglobinuria occurs 1–2 hours after severe hemolysis and lasts ≤ 24 hours. It is a transient finding and is relatively insensitive. False positive is due to myoglobinuria or to lysis of RBCs in urine.

Schumm's test for methemalbuminemia becomes positive 1–6 hours after hemolysis of 100 ml of blood and lasts 1–3 days.

Methemalbuminemia also occurs in hemorrhagic pancreatitis.

Serum bilirubin increase depends on liver function and amount of hemolysis. With normal liver function, it is increased 1 mg/dl in 1–6 hours to maximum in 3–12 hours following hemolysis of 100 ml of blood.

Increased serum total LDH; isoenzymes may be useful to confirm RBC source.

Extravascular hemolysis may cause increased serum indirect bilirubin and LDH and decreased serum haptoglobin.

In compensated hemolysis, there is little or no increase in serum LDH, bilirubin, hemoglobin, or urine hemoglobin as in acute hemolytic anemia, but urine hemosiderin may be present.
Increased urine and fecal urobilinogens are insensitive and unreliable as an index of hemolysis.
Bone marrow shows marked normoblastic erythroid hyperplasia. Iron stains show marked increase; absence of iron suggests paroxysmal nocturnal hemoglobinuria.

LABORATORY SCREENING FOR HEMOGLOBINOPATHIES

Normocytic normochromic RBC except in
- Thalassemia syndromes—microcytic hypochromic
- Hemoglobin (Hb) C, D, E diseases—microcytic normochromic

Osmotic fragility—normal or decreased (especially in thalassemia)
- Symmetric shift in Hb C, D, E diseases
- Asymmetric shift in other hemoglobin diseases

Target cells—in many of hemolytic diseases due to hemoglobinopathies; 50% of RBCs in Hb C, D, E diseases
Sickle cell test—proves presence of Hb S
Inclusion bodies—in Hb H and C disorders
Hemoglobin electrophoresis
Alkali denaturation for Hb F

SICKLE CELL DISEASE

Sickle Cell Trait

(heterozygous sickle cell or Hb AS disease; occurs in ~10% of American blacks)

Hemoglobin electrophoresis: Hb S is 20–40%, and Hb A is 60–80%; small amount of Hb F (≤ 2%) may be present.
Sickle cell preparation is positive.
Blood smear shows only a few target cells.
No anemia or hemolysis or jaundice is present.
Anoxia may cause systemic sickling (see next section, Sickle Cell Anemia). *Beware anesthesia, airplane flights, etc.*
Hematuria without any other demonstrable cause may be found.
Hyposthenuria may occur.

Sickle Cell Anemia

(homozygous Hb SS disease; occurs in 1 : 625 American blacks)

Hemoglobin electrophoresis: Hb S is 80–100%, and Hb F comprises the rest (see Fetal Hemoglobin, p. 271); Hb A is absent.
Normocytic normochromic anemia (Hb = 5–10 gm/dl; normal MCV).
Sickle cell preparation is positive; since other Hb variants migrate with Hb S on electrophoresis, it is important to confirm hemoglobin as a sickle type.
Sickle solubility test is positive but does not differentiate anemia from other Hb S genetic variants and may be falsely negative if hemoglobin < 5 gm/dl.
Blood smear shows a variable number of RBCs with target cells (especially in Hb SC disease), abnormal shapes, nucleated RBCs, Howell-Jolly bodies, spherical cells.
Reticulocyte count is increased (5–30%).
WBC is increased (10,000–30,000/cu mm) during a crisis, with normal differential or shift to the left. Infection may be indicated by intracellular bacteria (best seen on buffy coat preparations), Döhle's bodies, toxic granules and vacuoles of WBCs, Westergren ESR > 20 mm/hour.
Platelet count is increased (300,000–500,000/cu mm), with abnormal forms.
Bone marrow shows hyperplasia of all elements.

Decreased ESR becomes normal after blood is aerated. ESR in normal range may indicate intercurrent illness or crisis.
Osmotic fragility is decreased (more resistant RBCs).
Mechanical fragility of RBCs is increased.
RBC survival time is decreased.
Laboratory findings of hemolysis (e.g., increased indirect serum bilirubin [≤ 6 mg/dl], increased urobilinogen in urine and stool but urine is negative for bile).
Hemosiderin appears in urine sediment.
Hematuria is frequent.
Renal concentrating ability is decreased, leading to a fixed specific gravity in virtually all patients after the first few years of life.
Serum uric acid may be increased.
Serum alkaline phosphatase is increased during crisis, representing vaso-occlusive bone injury as well as liver damage.
Leukocyte alkaline phosphatase activity is decreased.
Laboratory findings due to complications

- Vaso-occlusive crisis, e.g., infarction of lungs, spleen, brain, bowel
- Stasis and necrosis of liver—increased direct serum bilirubin ≤ 40 mg/dl, bile in urine, other findings of obstructive type of jaundice
- Infections due to immunocompromised status (functional asplenia)—e.g., *Salmonella* osteomyelitis (see p. 625) occurs almost only in sickle cell syndromes; marked increase in susceptibility to pneumococcal and *Hemophilus influenzae* sepsis and meningitis, *Escherichia coli* and meningococcal infections
- Hyperhemolytic crisis—superimposed further hemolysis due to bacterial or viral infections; hemoglobin falls from usual 6–10 gm/dl to ≤ 5 gm/dl in a few days with increasing reticulocyte count.
- Aplastic crisis—acute, self-limited episode of erythroid aplasia lasting 5–10 days associated with various viral, bacterial, mycoplasmal infections; falling hematocrit and reticulocyte count may require prompt transfusion. Recovery is marked by return of reticulocytosis, usually with resolution of infection.
- Hypoplastic crisis—infection or inflammation causes brief suppression of bone marrow with accentuated brief drop in hematocrit and reticulocyte count.
- Splenic sequestration crisis—seen mostly in children age 5 months to 5 years (before fibrosis of spleen has occurred); enormous enlargement of spleen associated with precipitous drop in hematocrit and hypovolemic shock. Over age 2 years, occurs more often with other Hb S syndromes.
- Megaloblastic crisis—rare occurrence of sudden cessation of erythropoiesis due to folate depletion in persons with inadequate folate (e.g., pregnancy, alcoholism, poor diet).
- Cholelithiasis in 30% of patients by age 18 and 70% by age 30; may cause cholecystitis or biliary obstruction

Anemia and hemolytic jaundice are present throughout life after age 3–6 months; hemolysis and anemia are not increased during crises.

In newborns with SS, anemia is rarely present. May cause unexplained prolonged jaundice. May be difficult to distinguish SS from AS in neonates because of large amount of Hb F, which may obscure the Hb A. Percentage of RBCs that will sickle is much lower in newborn (as low as 0.5%) than in older children. Diagnosis of SS is excluded by Hb A on hemoglobin electrophoresis of infant's blood or if mother has negative sickle cell preparation. *In newborn, cellulose agar electrophoresis is useless to detect Hb S because of the small amount present and acidic citrate agar gel is needed. For exchange transfusion, sickle cell test must be performed on donor blood from blacks, since these*

RBCs may sickle in presence of hypoxia, as in respiratory distress syndrome. Hemoglobin solubility tests (e.g., Sickledex) are usually not suitable on cord blood because a positive result may be easily obscured by a large amount of Hb F. Most children are anemic and symptomatic by age of 1 year; anemia and hemolysis are present throughout life.

Antenatal diagnosis is possible as early as 7–10 weeks gestation using recombinant DNA methodology on amniotic fluid cells or chorionic villi. Diagnosis can also be made by fetal blood sampling.

Hemoglobin SC Disease
(occurs in 1 : 833 of American blacks)

Hemoglobin electrophoresis: Hb A is absent; Hb S predominates (30–60%) with Hb C present; Hb F is 2–15%.
Blood smear shows tetragonal crystals within RBC in 70% of patients.
A valuable diagnostic aid is the presence of target cells with normal MCV.
Other findings are the same as for sickle cell anemia, but there is less marked destruction of RBCs, anemia, etc., and the disease is less severe clinically. *Crises may cause a more marked fall in RBC than occurs in Hb SS disease.*

Sickle Cell–Thalassemia Disease
(occurs in 1 : 1667 American blacks)

Hemoglobin electrophoresis: Hb S is 20–80%; Hb F is 2–20%; Hb A is 0–50%.
Anemia is hypochromic microcytic; target cells are prominent; serum iron is normal.
Other findings resemble those of sickle cell anemia.
A valuable diagnostic aid is the presence of microcytosis and/or splenomegaly with sickle cell syndrome that is mild to moderately severe in a patient with one parent showing microcytosis and increased Hb A_2.

Sickle Cell–Persistent High Fetal Hemoglobin
(occurs in 1 : 25,000 American blacks)

Hemoglobin electrophoresis: Hb F is 20–40%; absent, Hb A and A_2; Hb S is present.
Findings are intermediate between those of sickle cell anemia and of sickle cell trait.

Sickle Cell–Hemoglobin D Disease
(occurs in 1 : 20,000 American blacks)

Findings are intermediate between those of sickle cell anemia and of sickle cell trait.

SICKLING OF RBCs

Occurs In

Sickle cell disease
Sickle cell trait

False Positive In

First 4 months after transfusion with RBCs having sickle cell trait
Mixture on slide with fibrinogen, thrombin, gelatin (glue)
Excessive concentration of sodium metabisulfite (e.g., ≥ 4% instead of 2%)
Drying of wet coverslip preparation
Poikilocytosis

False Negative In

First 4 months after transfusion with normal RBCs
Heating, bacterial contamination, or prolonged washing with saline of RBCs
Newborn because Hb F is high during first months of life

Sickling should be confirmed with hemoglobin electrophoresis and genetic studies.

SICKLE SOLUBILITY TEST

Sodium dithionate is added to lysed RBCs to reduce the hemoglobin.
Solution is turbid when Hb S is present but remains clear with other hemoglobins.
Does not differentiate between sickle cell anemia, trait, and other Hb S genetic variants.
May give false negative results if patient's hemoglobin < 5 gm/dl.
May give false positive results with lipemic specimens.
Unreliable for newborn screening because of high Hb F.
Inadequate for genetic counseling because does not detect carriers of Hb C and beta thalassemia.

THALASSEMIAS

(see Tables 12-6 and 12-8, pp. 294–295, 304)

Beta-chain synthesis is normally low at birth because Hb A becomes predominant only after the first few months. Clinical and laboratory findings correspond to this; thus neonatal anemia occurs only with alpha but not with beta thalassemia.

Thalassemia Minima

Silent carrier of beta thalassemia trait
Normal RBC morphology and hemoglobin electrophoresis
Can only be demonstrated by reduced rate of beta globin synthesis with increased alpha-beta globin chain ratio.

Thalassemia Trait

In uncomplicated cases, hemoglobin is normal or only slightly decreased (11–12 gm/dl), while the RBC is increased (5–7 million/cu mm). Most nonanemic patients with microcytosis have thalassemia minor. Microcytic anemia with anemia < 9.3 gm/dl is unlikely to be thalassemia minor. MCV < 75 fl, may be as low as 55 fl. MCHC > 31%.
Blood smear changes are less than in thalassemia major.
Anisocytosis is less marked than in iron deficiency anemia.
Microcytosis may be difficult to detect morphologically.
Poikilocytosis is mild to moderate; more striking than iron deficiency anemia with hemoglobin = 10–12 gm/dl. Target cells and oval forms may be numerous.
Occasional RBCs show basophilic stippling in beta thalassemia minor (rare in blacks but common in Mediterranean patients).
Reticulocyte count is increased (2–10%).
Serum iron is normal or slightly increased; transferrin saturation may be increased. TIBC is normal.
Cellular marrow contains stainable iron.
Osmotic fragility is decreased.

Beta Thalassemia Minor

(> 50 forms are recognized by gene cloning)

(Most important differential diagnosis is iron deficiency—see pp. 290–292.)
Slight or mild anemia
MCV usually < 75 and hematocrit > 30; RBC is often increased.
Normal iron, TIBC, serum ferritin
Increased Hb A_2 (3–6%) on starch or agar electrophoresis and a slight increase in Hb F (2–10%). Hb A_2 is often decreased in iron deficiency; thus A_2 level may be normal in concomitant iron deficiency and beta thalassemia minor, and the diagnosis of beta thalassemia trait cannot be made until iron defi-

Table 12-7. Representative Laboratory Values of Some Common Hemoglobinopathies

	AS	SS	SC	$S–\beta^+$	$S–\beta^0$
Hb (gm/dl)	N	7.5	11	11	8
Range		(6–9)	(9–14)	(8–13)	(7–10)
Hct (%)	N	22	30	32	25
Range		(18–30)	(26–40)	(25–40)	(20–36)
MCV (fl)	N	93	80	76	69
Reticulocyte count (%)	N	11	3	3	8
Range		(4–30)	(1.5–6)	(1.5–6)	(3–18)
RBC morphology	N				
Sickle cells		Many	Rare	Rare	Varies
Target cells		Many	Many		Many
Microcytosis				Mild	Marked
Hypochromia				Mild	Marked
Nucleated RBC		Many			
Hb electrophoresis (%)	N				
S	38–45	80–90	45–55	55–75	50–85
F		2–20	<8	1–20	2–30
A_2	1–3	<3.6		>3.6	>3.6
A	55–60			15–30	
C			45–55		
Clinical severity	No symptoms	Moderate/severe	Mild/moderate	Mild/moderate	Mild/severe

N = normal.

Table 12-8. Comparison of Sample Values in Iron Deficient States

	Normal	Iron Depletion	Iron Deficiency Erythropoiesis	Iron Deficiency Anemia
RBC morphology	N	N	N	Microcytic hypochromic
Sideroblasts (%)	40–60	40–60	<10	<10
RBC protoporphyrin (μg/dl RBC)	30	30	100	200
Transferrin saturation (%)	20–50	30	<15	<10
Plasma iron (μg/dl)	65–165	115	<60	<40
Plasma ferritin (ng/ml)	40–160	20	10	<10
Transferrin IBC (μg/dl)	300–360	360	390	410
RE marrow iron	2–3+	0–1+	0	0

ciency has been treated. Hb A_2 and F are absent in alpha thalassemia. No specific laboratory identification of alpha thalassemia trait (carrier). Thus, normal hemoglobin electrophoresis and England-Fraser < -6 in the absence of iron deficiency implies alpha thalassemia minor; mild alpha thalassemia is a clinical diagnosis.

Thalassemia Intermedia

(2–10% of thalassemics; may be homozygous delta-beta, beta^0 or beta$^+$, with or without an alpha gene or double heterozygous with an abnormal hemoglobin such as S or E)

Less severe clinical and laboratory findings than major. Same findings occur at later age.

Hemoglobin is usually > 6.5 gm/dl.

Alpha-thalassemias—decreased or absent synthesis of globin chains; very common in African black, Asian, and Mediterranean populations

Alpha Thalassemia 2

One alpha allele is deleted, causing asymptomatic but transmissible trait. Occurs in up to 30% of black populations. Coincident with sickle cell or Hb C trait, it reduces the proportion of Hb S or Hb C below the usual 35–40% (also slightly decreasing the clinical severity); thus < 35% variant hemoglobin is good evidence for coexisting alpha thalassemia in such patients. No clinical or hematologic findings. Definitive diagnosis of older silent carrier depends on special techniques (globin synthesis rates in reticulocytes).

Alpha Thalassemia 1

Two copies of alpha globin gene are deleted from same chromosome.

Minimal hypochromic, microcytic anemia, increased target cells, anisocytosis, resembling beta thalassemia trait but without increased Hb A_2

Table 12-9. Classification of Beta Thalassemia Syndromes

Genotype	Anemia	Microcytosis	Hb Electrophoresis
Normal			
Beta/beta	None	None	Hb $A_2 < 3.5\%$, Hb $F < 1\%$
Thalassemia minima			
Beta/beta$^+$ (mild)	None	None	Hb A_2 = N or slightly I Hb F = I
Thalassemia minor			
Beta/beta$^+$ (severe)	Mild	Mild to moderate	Hb A_2 = 3.5–7.5% Hb F = N or slightly I
Beta/beta^0	Mild	Mild to moderate	Hb A_2 = 3.5–7.5% Hb F = N or slightly I
Beta/delta beta^0	Mild	Mild to moderate	Hb A_2 = N or D Hb F = 5–20%
Beta/beta Lepore	Mild	Mild to moderate	Hb A_2 = N or D Hb F = I Hb Lepore up to 8%
Thalassemia intermedia			
Beta$^+$(mild)/beta$^+$(severe)	Moderate to severe	Moderate to severe	Hb A_2 = 6–8% Hb F = 20–50% Hb A = remainder
Delta beta^0/delta beta^0	Moderate to severe	Moderate to severe	Hb F only
Thalassemia major			
Beta^0/beta^0	Severe	Severe	Hb A_2 = 3–11% Hb F = remainder
Beta$^+$(severe)/beta$^+$(severe)	Severe	Severe	Hb A_2 = 3–11% Hb F = 10–90% Hb A = remainder
Beta^0/beta$^+$(severe)	Severe	Severe	Hb A^2 = 3–11% Hb F = 10–90% Hb A = remainder
Beta^0/beta Lepore	Severe	Severe	Hb F > 80% Hb Lepore = remainder

N = normal; I = increased; D = decreased.

Table 12-10. Classification of Alpha Thalassemia Syndromes

	Gene Deletions	Anemia	Microcytosis	Hb Electrophoresis	
				At birth	Adults
Alpha thalassemia trait 2 (silent carrier)	1	0	0	1–2% Bart's	N
Alpha thalassemia trait 1 (heterozygous)	2	Mild	Present	5–10% Bart's	N
Hg H disease (alpha thalassemia 2 + alpha thalassemia 1)	3	Moderate	Marked	20–40% Bart's	Hb A + Hb H
Hydrops fetalis (homozygous)	4	Fatal at/before birth		>50% Bart's	—

Bart's Hb disappears by age 3–6 months.

Hemoglobin H Disease

Inherited alpha thalassemia 1 from one parent and alpha thalassemia 2 from other, causing absence of 3 of 4 alpha globin alleles and excess of beta globins (Hb H)

Hypochromic, microcytic hemolytic anemia is moderate to severe (Hb = 7–10 gm/dl), accentuated by infection, drugs, etc.

Detected by hemoglobin gel electrophoresis.

Hydrops Fetalis

Deletion of all four alpha globin genes with no normal hemoglobin causes stillbirth or prompt postnatal death due to severe hypoxemia (despite cord hemoglobin up to 10 gm/dl)

Constant Spring hemoglobin

Abnormally elongated alpha chain comprises 0.5–1.0% of total hemoglobin in heterozygote and 5–6% in homozygote. Effects similar to alpha thalassemia 2 or 1 or Hb H disease.

Thalassemia Major

(Cooley's anemia, Mediterranean anemia)

Several hemoglobin electrophoretic patterns are characteristic (see Table 12-9, p. 305).

Classification of beta thalassemia syndromes

- Homozygous beta^0—Hb A is absent; Hb F and Hb A_2 are present.
- Homozygous beta$^+$—Hb A, Hb A_2, and Hb F are all detected.
- Hb F = 10–90%; Hb A is decreased; Hb A_2 may be normal, low, or high.

There is marked hypochromic microcytic regenerative hemolytic anemia. Often Hb = 2.0–6.5 gm/dl, Hct = 10–24%, RBC = 2–3 million, indices are decreased.

Blood smear shows marked anisocytosis, poikilocytosis, target cells, spherocytes, and hypochromic, fragmented, and bizarre RBCs; also many nucleated RBCs—basophilic stippling, Cabot's rings, siderocytes.

Reticulocyte count is increased.

WBCs are often increased, with normal differential or marked shift to the left.

Platelets are normal.

Bone marrow is cellular and shows erythroid hyperplasia and stainable iron.

Serum iron and TIBC are increased. After age 5 years, iron-binding capacity is usually saturated.

Laboratory findings of hemolysis and liver dysfunction (e.g., increased serum LDH, glutamic-oxaloacetic transaminase [SGOT], SGPT, and indirect bilirubin [1–3 mg/dl], urine and stool urobilinogen).

Liver dysfunction causing disturbance of factors V, VII, IX, XI, prothrombin.

Serum haptoglobin and hemopexin are very decreased or absent (due to hemolysis).

RBC survival time is decreased.

Osmotic fragility is decreased.

Mechanical fragility is increased.

Laboratory findings due to complications

- Secondary hypersplenism (usually occurs between age 5–10 years, detected when transfusion requirement > 200–250 mg/kg body weight, at which time splenectomy is indicated)
- Hemosiderosis (hepatic fibrosis and cirrhosis; endocrinopathies with hypofunction of pituitary, thyroid, etc.)

Proteinuria, hyposthenuria, failure to acidify urine, increased urobilin and urobilinogen with dark color may be present.

Prenatal diagnosis is possible at 16 weeks' gestation in 85% of cases by DNA analysis of amniotic cells; the rest can be diagnosed by alpha-beta chain ratios of fetal blood (obtained by fetoscopy).

Hemoglobin E—Beta Thalassemia

Is most common symptomatic thalassemia in Southeast Asia.

Hemolytic anemia varying from moderate to marked severity.

Smear shows severe hypochromia and microcytosis, marked anisopoikilocytosis with many teardrop and target forms. Nucleated RBCs and basophilic stippling may be present.

Hemoglobin E—Alpha Thalassemia

Analogous to alpha thalassemia 1 and 2 and hemoglobin H (see pp. 304, 307)

In American blacks, 28% have mild alpha thalassemia without microcytosis, 3% are homozygous alpha thalassemia with microcytosis, 1% have microcytosis due to beta thalassemia. Median hemoglobin is about 1 gm/dl lower in blacks without iron deficiency than in whites.

Alpha or beta thalassemia or Hb E occurs in ~50% of Southeast Asians and causes microcytosis.

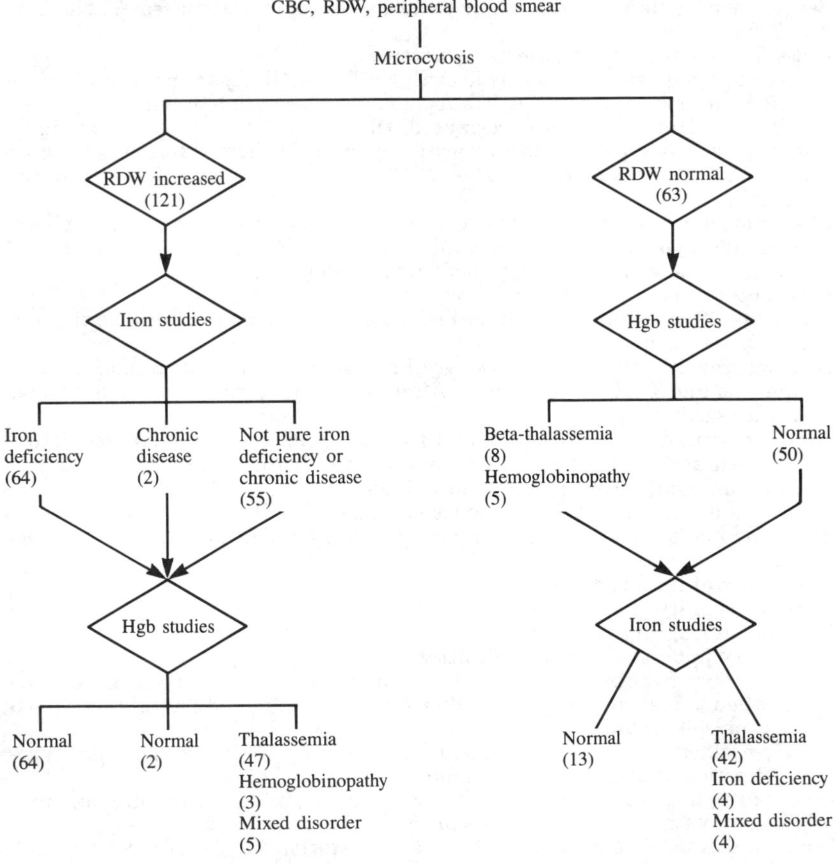

Fig. 12-2. Sequence of diagnostic studies for microcytosis. The classification of 184 cases of microcytosis by this strategy is shown by the numbers in parentheses.

Table 12-11. Comparison of Microcytic Anemias of Iron Deficiency and Thalassemia Minor

	Iron Deficiency	No Differentiation	Thalassemia Minor	Sensitivity (%)[a]	Accuracy (%)[a]
Hb (gm/L)	<9.3 M or F	9.3–13.5 M 9.3–12.5 F	>13.5 M >12.5 F		
MCV (fl)		>68	<68	100	65
MCHC (gm/dl)	<30	>30			
RBC (/cu mm)	<4.2	4.2–5.5	>5.5		
Erythrocytosis				68	90
Mentzer formula[b] (MCV/RBC)	>13		<13	95	65
England-Fraser formula[b] (MCV − (5 × Hgb + RBC + K) if K = 3.4)		Positive number	Negative number	69	77
Shine-Lal formula[b] (MCV squared × MCH)			<1530	100	86
MCV of 1 parent < 79 fl				100	86
Free erythrocyte protoporphyrin = 25 μg/dl				60	67
Hb A_2 >3.5%				85	90

M = males; F = females.

[a]Accuracy in distinguishing anemias of thalassemia minor and iron deficiency (%).

[b]In patients with polycythemia vera who develop iron deficiency with microcytosis, a negative number results. These formulas do not account for the indeterminate zone of no differentiation.

HEMOGLOBIN C DISEASE

Hb C Trait

(occurs in 2% of American blacks, less frequently in other Americans)

Hemoglobin electrophoresis demonstrates the abnormal hemoglobin.
Blood smear shows variable number of target cells.
No other abnormalities are seen.

Hb C Disease

Hemoglobin electrophoresis demonstrates the abnormal hemoglobin.
Significant hypochromic hemolytic anemia is present.
Blood smear shows many target cells, variable number of microspherocytes, occasional nucleated RBCs, a few tetragonal crystals within RBCs that increase following splenectomy.
Reticulocyte count is increased (2–10%).
Osmotic fragility is decreased.
Mechanical fragility is increased.
RBC survival time is decreased.
Hb F is slightly increased.
Increase in serum bilirubin is minimal.
Normoblastic hyperplasia of bone marrow is present.

HEMOGLOBIN D DISEASE

Homozygous Hb D Disease

Hemoglobin electrophoresis demonstrates the abnormal hemoglobin at acid pH.
Mild microcytic anemia
Target cells and spherocytes
Decreased RBC survival time

Heterozygous Hb D Trait

Hemoglobin electrophoresis demonstrates the abnormal hemoglobin at acid pH. There are no other laboratory findings.

Sickle Cell–Hb D Disease

Hemoglobin electrophoresis demonstrates the abnormal hemoglobin at acid pH. Findings are intermediate between those of sickle cell anemia and sickle cell trait.

HEMOGLOBIN E DISEASE

(occurs almost exclusively in Southeast Asia, found in 3% of population in Vietnam up to 35% in Laos; migrates like Hb A_2 on electrophoresis)

Homozygous Hb E Disease

Mild hypochromic hemolytic anemia or no anemia
Marked microcytosis (MCV = 55–70 fl) and erythrocytosis (~5,500,000/cu mm)
Smear shows predominant target cells (25–60%), which differentiates from Hb E trait and microcytes.
Electrophoresis shows 95–97% Hb E and the rest is Hb F.

Heterozygous Hb E Trait

Asymptomatic persons found during family studies or screening programs
Normal hemoglobin
Slight to moderate microcytosis (MCV = 65–80 fl)
Erythrocytosis (RBC = 5,000,000–5,340,000/cu mm)
Electrophoresis shows 30–35% Hb E

Hb E–Beta Thalassemia

See p. 308.

HEREDITARY PERSISTENCE OF HEMOGLOBIN F

Inherited (probably autosomal dominant) persistence of increased Hb F in adult without clinical manifestations. Incidence < 0.2%.

Decreased MCV and MCHC

Increased Hb F on hemoglobin electrophoresis

May be pancellular (Hb F is increased in all RBCs) or heterocellular (Hb F is increased only in some RBCs) as distinguished by Kleihauer-Betke stain of peripheral blood smear.

May be associated with other hemoglobinopathies but is different from the increase of Hb F that is found in some hemoglobinopathies.

UNSTABLE HEMOGLOBINS

(e.g., Hb Koln)

Usually autosomal dominant inheritance

Laboratory evidence of hemolytic anemia

Peripheral blood smear shows hypochromia, anisocytosis, poikilocytosis, increased reticulocytes

Heinz bodies may be few or absent if spleen is present. Supravital stain shows preexistent Heinz bodies.

Excess precipitation at 37°C in 17% isopropanol compared to normal hemoglobin

Hemoglobin electrophoresis is often normal.

HEMOGLOBINS WITH ALTERED OXYGEN AFFINITY

High-oxygen-affinity hemoglobins cause left shift in oxygen dissociation curve, with less oxygen delivered to tissues; autosomal dominance; usually asymptomatic.

- Erythrocytosis without splenomegaly
- Low P_{50} (see Polycythemia, pp. 322–323)

Low-oxygen-affinity hemoglobins cause right shift in oxygen dissociation curve, with more oxygen delivered to tissues; autosomal dominance; cyanosis

- Mild hemolytic anemia in some cases
- High P_{50}
- Identify hemoglobin by gel electrophoresis or measure absorption spectrum at 450–750 nm.

METHEMOGLOBINEMIA

(> 1.5 gm/dl methemoglobin)

Due To

Drugs and chemicals are most common cause, especially aniline derivatives (e.g., acetanilid, phenacetin, certain sulfonamides, various clothing dyes), nitrites, nitrates, local anesthetics (e.g., benzocaine, lidocaine)

Abnormal Hb M (several different Ms)

Inherited enzyme deficiency (methemoglobin reductase)

Laboratory Findings

Normal arterial oxygen saturation in presence of apparent clinical cyanosis

Freshly drawn blood is chocolate-brown; does not become red after exposure to air.

Starch block electrophoresis identifies the Hb M.

Spectroscopic absorption analysis—band at 630 mμ disappears on addition of 5% potassium cyanide.

RBC is slightly increased; no other hematologic abnormalities are found; there is no jaundice.

Patient is cyanotic clinically but in apparent good health. (Clinical cyanosis > 5.0 gm/dl deoxyhemoglobin.)

In newborns with cyanosis, methemoglobin level is usually > 10% and may reach 60–70% in severe cases. Persistent methemoglobinemia in spite of IV methylene blue (1–2 mg/kg) suggests abnormal Hb M.

Recurrence of methemoglobinemia without reexposure to chemicals suggests inherited enzyme deficiency.

Cyanosis without dyspnea in previously pink infant suggests acquired methemoglobinemia due to chemicals, but cyanosis from birth suggests inherited enzyme deficiency or abnormal Hb M.

Hb M causes cyanosis from birth only if it is alpha-chain type; cyanosis of beta-chain type appears at age 2–4 months.

SULFHEMOGLOBINEMIA

(> 0.5 gm/dl sulfhemoglobin)

Due To

Drugs, especially phenacetin (including Bromo-Seltzer) and acetanilid

Laboratory Findings

Spectroscopic absorption analysis—band at 618 mμ does not disappear on addition of 5% potassium cyanide.

Laboratory findings due to associated bromide intoxication.

Bromide intoxication and sulfhemoglobinemia may be due to excessive intake of Bromo-Seltzer.

PAROXYSMAL COLD HEMOGLOBINURIA

Sudden hemoglobinuria follows exposure to cold environment.

Findings are of acute hemolytic anemia.

Cold autohemolysin is present in blood.

Positive direct Coombs' test is present only during the attack.

There may be a biologic false positive test for syphilis, or the attack may be due to congenital syphilis.

ACQUIRED HEMOLYTIC ANEMIA

Laboratory findings due to increased destruction of RBCs

- RBC survival time differentiates intrinsic RBC defect from factor outside RBC.
- Blood smear often shows marked spherocytosis.
- Anisocytosis, poikilocytosis, and polychromasia are seen.
- Slight abnormality of osmotic fragility is shown.
- Increased indirect serum bilirubin (< 6 mg/dl) because of compensatory excretory capacity of liver
- Urine urobilinogen is increased (may vary with liver function; may be obscured by antibiotic therapy altering intestinal flora). Bile is absent.
- Hemoglobinemia and hemoglobinuria are present when hemolysis is very rapid.
- Haptoglobins are decreased or absent in chronic hemolytic diseases (removed following combination with free hemoglobin in serum).
- WBC is usually elevated.

Laboratory findings due to compensatory increased production of RBCs

- Normochromic, normocytic anemia. MCV reflects immaturity of circulating RBCs. Polychromatophilia is present.
- Reticulocyte count is increased.
- Erythroid hyperplasia of bone marrow is evident.

Laboratory findings due to mechanism of RBC destruction

- Positive direct Coombs' test
- Warm antibodies are found.
- Cold agglutinins are found.
- Biologic false positive test for syphilis may occur.

Laboratory findings due to underlying conditions
- Malignant lymphoma
- Collagen diseases (e.g., SLE)
- DIC (see pp. 384, 386, 388)
- Idiopathic pulmonary hemosiderosis
- Infections, especially viral pneumonia, malaria, cholera
- Antibody-induced
  - Drug-induced (e.g., quinidine, quinine, penicillins, cephalothin, alpha methyldopa)
  - Autoantibody (warm, cold)
  - Alloantibody (erythroblastosis fetalis, incompatible transfusion)
  - Paroxysmal cold hemoglobinuria
- Paroxysmal nocturnal hemoglobinuria
- Physical/chemical (e.g., burns, drugs, toxins [e.g., phenylhydrazine, benzene])
- Other

MICROANGIOPATHIC HEMOLYTIC ANEMIA

Peripheral blood smear establishes the diagnosis by characteristic burr cells, schistocytes, helmet cells, microspherocytes.

Nonimmune hemolytic anemia varies in severity depending on underlying condition (see previous section).

Laboratory findings of hemolysis, e.g., increased serum LDH, decreased haptoglobin, hemosiderinuria; hemoglobinemia and hemoglobinuria are less common.

Iron deficiency due to urinary loss of iron.

Direct Coombs' test is usually negative.

Laboratory findings due to causative disease

Due To

Renal disease with uremia

Cardiac valvular disease (e.g., intracardiac valve prostheses, bacterial endocarditis, severe valvular heart disease)

Severe liver disease (e.g., cirrhosis)

DIC (see pp. 384, 386, 388)

Snakebite (see p. 733)

HYPERSPLENISM

Diagnosis is made by exclusion.

Decreased platelet count is moderate to severe (100,000–30,000/cu mm).

Peripheral blood smear may reflect the underlying cause.
- Spherocytes in hereditary spherocytosis
- Target cells in liver disease
- Atypical lymphocytes in infectious mononucleosis or chronic infection
- Leukoerythroblastosis, nucleated RBCs, and immature granulocytes in myeloid metaplasia with extramedullary hematopoiesis
- Teardrop and hand-mirror RBCs in myelofibrosis

Normochromic anemia (Hb = 9.0–11.0 gm/dl) may occur.

WBCs may be decreased with a normal differential count.

Bone marrow is normal or shows increased cellularity of all lines with normal maturation.

Direct Coombs' test is negative.

Laboratory findings due to underlying disease (e.g., portal hypertension, collagen diseases, infections, lymphoma/leukemia, lipid storage disease, Felty's syndrome).

HEREDITARY SPHEROCYTOSIS

(defective RBC membrane due to spectrin deficiency; deficiency ~30% of normal in severe cases to 80% of normal in mildest cases)

Autosomal dominant form in ~75% of cases in which one parent and half the siblings are affected; ~25% appear sporadic and occur without a family history but may be recessive inheritance. Findings vary from only subtle abnormalities with rare spherocytes to marked abnormalities. Abnormal peripheral blood smear is most suggestive finding; numerous microspherocytes and polychromatophilic reticulocytes are present.

Spherocytes are present. Anisocytosis may be marked; poikilocytosis is slight. RBCs show Howell-Jolly bodies, Pappenheimer bodies, Heinz bodies.

Hemolytic anemia is moderate (RBC = 3–4 million/cu mm), microcytic (MCV = 70–80 fl), and hyperchromic (increased MCHC = 36–40 gm/dl). MCHC ≥ 36% means congenital spherocytic anemia if cold agglutinins and hypertriglyceridemia have been excluded.

Osmotic fragility is increased; increase generally reflects clinical severity of disease; when normal in some patients, the incubated fragility test shows increased hemolysis. Diagnosis is not established without abnormal osmotic fragility. Increased osmotic fragility does not distinguish hereditary spherocytosis from autoimmune hemolytic disease with spherocytosis, but latter shows much less increased fragility with incubation.

Autohemolysis (sterile defibrinated blood incubated for 48 hours) is increased (10–20% compared to normal of < 4% of cells); very nonspecific test. May sometimes be found also in nonspherocytic hemolytic anemias.

Abnormal osmotic fragility and autohemolysis are reduced by 10% glucose; false negative test may occur with concomitant diabetes mellitus.

Mechanical fragility is increased.

WBC and platelet counts are usually normal; they may be increased during hemolysis.

Evidence of hemolysis

- Degree of reticulocytosis (usually 5–15%) is greater than in other hemolytic anemias with similar degrees of anemia.
- Bone marrow shows marked erythroid hyperplasia except during aplastic crisis; moderate hemosiderin is present.
- Increased serum LDH and indirect bilirubin.
- Haptoglobins are decreased or absent.
- Direct Coombs' test is negative (in contrast to immune hemolytic conditions in which spherocytosis is common and direct Coombs' test is positive).
- Hemolytic crises usually precipitated by infection cause more profound anemia despite reticulocytosis and increased jaundice and splenomegaly.
- Stool urobilinogen is usually increased.

Laboratory findings due to complications, e.g., gallstones, aplastic crises.

Diagnosis should be questioned if splenectomy does not cause a complete response.

Age at diagnosis is related to severity of hemolysis; more severe forms are diagnosed early in life.

In neonates, is associated with jaundice in about 50% of cases. Serum indirect bilirubin may be > 20 mg/dl. Anemia is usually mild (Hb ≥ 10 gm/dl) during first week of life. Spherocytes are present in infant and one parent and may be present in siblings. Reticulocyte count is usually 5–15%.

HEREDITARY ELLIPTOCYTOSIS (OVALOCYTOSIS)

Autosomal dominant trait affecting 1 : 2500 persons in U.S.

Blood smear shows 20–100% of RBCs are elliptical or oval. In normal individuals, up to 10–15% of RBCs may be oval or elliptical. Also seen frequently in thalassemias, hemoglobinopathies, iron deficiency, myelophthisic anemias; these must be ruled out to establish the diagnosis in a congenital hemolytic anemia with marked elliptocytosis.

Only few ovalocytes are present at birth with gradual increase to stable value at 3–4 months old. Splenectomy does not affect ovalocytosis.

Severity of disease varies. Degree of hemolysis does not correlate with proportion of abnormal RBC.

Moderate to severe in < 5% of patients—a chronic congenital hemolytic anemia (Hb < 9 gm/dl) with decreased RBC survival time, moderate anemia, increased serum bilirubin, and increased reticulocyte count, increased osmotic fragility, and autohemolysis.

Mild normocytic normochromic anemia (Hb = 10–12 gm/dl) in 10–20% of patients.

Elliptocytes are the only hematologic abnormality seen in most patients. Rarely causes hemolysis in newborns. Infants may not show significant numbers of elliptocytes until age 4–6 months. Elliptocytes are found in one parent and may be present in siblings.

Hemoglobin electrophoresis is normal.

Osmotic fragility and autohemolysis are normal in patients without hemolytic anemia.

Mechanical fragility is increased.

Laboratory findings due to complications (e.g., gallstones, hypersplenism)

CONGENITAL STOMATOCYTOSIS

Rare condition of morphologic abnormality of RBCs in which one or more slitlike areas of central pallor produce a mouthlike appearance.

Findings resemble hereditary spherocytosis with variable degree of hemolytic anemia but not cured by splenectomy.

GLUCOSE 6-PHOSPHATE DEHYDROGENASE (GLUCOSE-6-PD) DEFICIENCY IN RBCs

Is the most frequent inherited RBC enzyme disorder

May be associated with several different clinical syndromes

- Class I—Chronic, congenital, nonspherocytic hemolytic anemia not due to drugs or oxidant stress.
- Class II (< 10% of normal RBC activity)—Acute hemolytic crises induced by some oxidant drugs (e.g., primaquine, sulfonamides, acetanilide). Splenectomy is not helpful.
- Class III (RBC glucose-6-PD activity = 10–60% of normal)—Oxidant drugs or infection (e.g., pneumonia, infectious hepatitis) induces acute self-limited (2–3 days) hemolysis in persons without previously recognized hematologic disease. Also reported in hepatic coma, hyperthyroidism, myocardial infarction (first week after), other megaloblastic anemias, and chronic blood loss.
- Many other genetic and clinical variants.

After standard dose of primaquine in adult, intravascular hemolysis is evidenced by the following:

- Falling hematocrit usually begins in 2–4 days; reaches nadir by 8–12 days.
- Heinz bodies and increased serum bilirubin occur during first few days of hemolysis.
- Reticulocytosis begins at about fifth day; reaches maximum in 10–20 days.
  - Hemolysis subsides spontaneously even if primaquine is continued.

In vitro tests of Heinz body formation when patients' RBCs are exposed to acetylphenylhydrazine

Hemoglobin varies from 7 gm/dl to normal; is lower when due to exogenous agent; is usually normochromic, normocytic.

Peripheral smear shows varying degree of nucleated RBCs, spherocytes, poikilocytes, crenated and fragmented RBCs, Heinz bodies but is not distinctive.
WBC is variable.
Diagnosis is established by RBC assay for glucose-6-PD (using fluorescence); heterozygotes have two RBC populations and proportion of each determines degree of deficiency detected.

Decreased In
American black males (13%)
American black females (3%; 20% are carriers)
Some other ethnic groups (e.g., Greeks, Sardinians, Sephardic Jews)
All persons with favism (but not all persons with decreased glucose-6-PD have favism)

Increased In
Pernicious anemia to 3 times normal level; remains elevated for several months, even after administration of vitamin B_{12}
Idiopathic thrombocytopenic purpura (Werlhof's disease); becomes normal soon after splenectomy

HEREDITARY NONSPHEROCYTIC HEMOLYTIC ANEMIAS

This is a heterogeneous group. May be due to pyruvate kinase deficiency, variants of glucose-6-PD deficiency, Hb Zurich, other rare congenital enzyme defects (e.g., glutathione).
Anemia is of the hemolytic type; may be severe; may begin in newborn; may be precipitated by certain drugs.
RBCs show Howell-Jolly bodies, Pappenheimer bodies, Heinz bodies, basophilic stippling; there may be slight macrocytosis.
Increase in reticulocyte count is marked, even with mild anemia.
Bone marrow shows marked erythroid hyperplasia; normal hemosiderin is present.
WBC, platelet count, hemoglobin electrophoresis, osmotic fragility, and mechanical fragility are normal.
Autohemolysis is present in some patients but not in others; reduction by glucose is less than in normal blood.

ERYTHROCYTE PYRUVATE KINASE DEFICIENCY

Congenital autosomal recessive nonspherocytic hemolytic anemia showing wide range of clinical and laboratory findings from severe neonatal anemia requiring transfusion to fully compensated hemolytic process in healthy adults
Laboratory findings due to chronic hemolysis that may be exacerbated by pregnancy or viral infections.
  Beyond early childhood, hemoglobin usually 7–10 gm/dl
  Peripheral smear shows no characteristic changes (i.e., few or no spherocytes, occasional "tailed poikilocytes," macrocytosis, reticulocytosis).
Varying abnormalities of incubated RBC osmotic fragility
Deficiency of pyruvate kinase (10–25% of normal) in RBC assay. If an infant has been transfused, the assay should be performed 3–4 months later. Assay will demonstrate heterozygous carrier state in parents who are hematologically normal.
Diagnosis is difficult to make. May be suggested by increased P_{50} due to elevated 2,3-diphosphoglycerate (DPG).
Laboratory findings due to complications (e.g., cholelithiasis, hemosiderosis)

Other rare deficiencies of RBC enzymes also exist.

PAROXYSMAL NOCTURNAL HEMOGLOBINURIA (MARCHIAFAVA-MICHELI SYNDROME)

(acquired RBC membrane disorder involving increased sensitivity to complement-mediated lysis; a clonal stem cell disorder)

Hemoglobinemia is present; increases during sleep.

Serum haptoglobin is absent during an episode.

Chronic intravascular hemolytic anemia is well developed. Blood smear is not characteristic and often shows hypochromasia and polychromatophilic macrocytes (reticulocytes).

Hemoglobinuria is evident on arising.

Urine contains hemoglobin, hemosiderin (in WBCs and epithelial cells of sediment), and increased urobilinogen.

Sucrose hemolysis test is said to be more sensitive but less specific than Hamm test; if positive, should be confirmed by Hamm test.

Hamm test (RBC fragility is increased in acid medium) and in hydrogen peroxide; amount of change is related to clinical severity. Is most specific test but relatively insensitive.

Autohemolysis is increased.

Negative direct Coombs' test

Osmotic fragility is normal.

Serum iron may be decreased.

Platelet count usually shows mild to moderate decrease.

WBC is usually decreased.

Leukocyte alkaline phosphatase activity is decreased (as in other marrow stem cell disorders, e.g., chronic myelogenous leukemia and myelodysplastic syndromes).

RBC acetylcholinesterase activity is decreased.

Bone marrow most often shows normoblastic hyperplasia with adequate myeloid and megakaryocytic cells, but cellularity may be decreased or aplasia may be present.

Stainable iron is often absent.

Develops in 5–10% of patients with aplastic anemia, and aplastic anemia develops in 25% of patients with paroxysmal nocturnal hemoglobinuria.

Laboratory findings due to recurrent arterial and venous (e.g., hepatic, portal, splenic, cerebral, skin) thromboses that may cause death.

Renal findings very similar to those in sickle cell disease.

Diagnosis should be considered in any patient with Coombs' negative–acquired chronic hemolysis, especially if hemoglobinuria, pancytopenia, or thrombosis is present.

ANEMIA DUE TO ACUTE BLOOD LOSS

RBC, hemoglobin, and hematocrit levels are not reliable initially because of compensatory vasoconstriction and hemodilution. They decrease for several days after hemorrhage ceases. RBCs return to normal in 4–6 weeks. Hemoglobin returns to normal in 6–8 weeks.

Anemia is normochromic, normocytic. (*If hypochromic or microcytic, rule out iron deficiency due to prior hemorrhages.*)

Reticulocyte count is increased after 1–2 days, reaches peak in 4–7 days (≤ 15%). Persistent increase suggests continuing hemorrhage.

Blood smear shows no poikilocytes. Polychromasia and increased number of nucleated RBCs (up to 5 : 100 WBCs) may be found.

Increased WBC (usually ≤ 20,000/cu mm) reaches peak in 2–5 hours, becomes normal in 3–4 days. Persistent increase suggests continuing hemorrhage, bleeding into a body cavity, or infection. Differential count shows shift to the left.

Platelets are increased (≤ 1 million/cu mm) within a few hours; coagulation time is decreased.

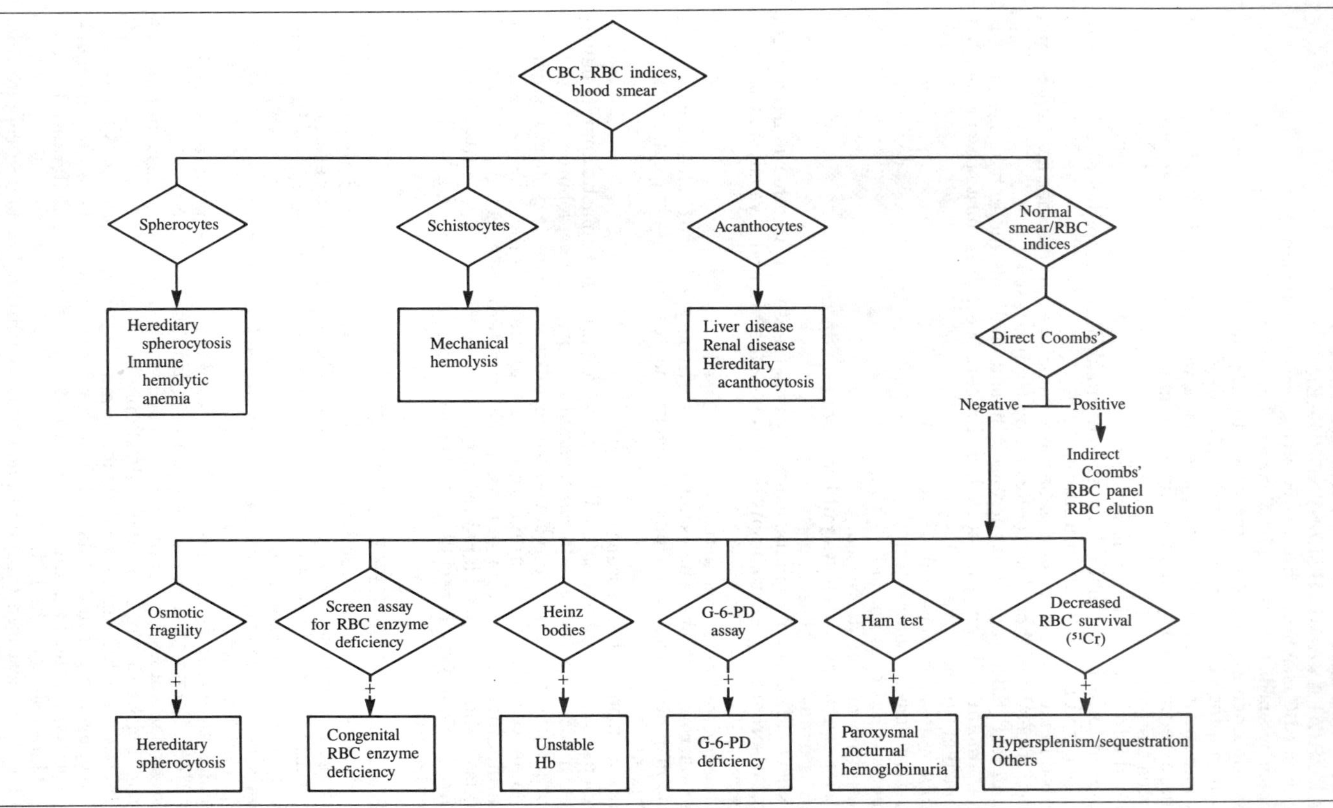

Fig. 12-3. Sequence of laboratory tests for hemolytic anemia with normal hemoglobin electrophoresis.

BUN is increased if hemorrhage into lumen of GI tract occurs.

Serum indirect bilirubin is increased if hemorrhage into a body cavity or cystic structure occurs.

Laboratory findings due to causative disease (e.g., peptic ulcer, esophageal varices, leukemia) are noted.

"ANEMIA" IN PREGNANCY

This is a normal physiologic change due to hemodilution—total blood volume and plasma volume increase more than red cell mass.

Onset is at eighth week; full development by 16–22 weeks; rapid return to normal in puerperium.

Hemoglobin averages 11 gm/dl; hematocrit value averages 33.

RBC morphology is normal.

RBC indices are normal.

If hemoglobin is < 10 gm/dl or there are hypochromic microcytic indices, rule out iron deficiency anemia, which may occur frequently during pregnancy.

ANEMIA IN PARASITIC INFESTATIONS

Anemia due to blood loss, malnutrition, specific organ damage

Malaria
- Hemolytic anemia

Diphyllobothrium latum (fish tapeworm)
- Macrocytic anemia

Hookworm
- Hypochromic microcytic anemia due to chronic blood loss

Schistosoma mansoni

Hypochromic microcytic anemia due to blood loss from intestine

Macrocytic anemia due to cirrhosis of schistosomiasis

Amebiasis
- Due to blood loss and malnutrition

CLASSIFICATION OF ERYTHROCYTOSIS

Polycythemia vera

Hereditary erythrocytosis (rare conditions)
- High-affinity hemoglobinopathies (autosomal dominant)
- Decreased RBC 2,3-DPG (due to high-RBC adenosine triphosphate or autosomal recessive DPG mutase deficiency)
- Increased production of erythropoietin (autosomal recessive)
- Unknown causes

Secondary polycythemia

Relative polycythemia

Neonatal thick blood syndrome

Factitious (due to blood doping or ingestion of steroids by athletes)

POLYCYTHEMIA VERA

RBC is increased; often = 7–12 million; may increase to > 15 million/cu mm.

Increased hemoglobin is 18–24 gm/dl in 71% of cases.

Increased hematocrit > 55% in 83% of cases; > 60% indicates increased RBC mass, but < 60% may be associated with normal RBC mass.

MCV, MCH, and MCHC are normal or decreased.

Increased ^{51}Cr RBC mass is essential for diagnosis; blood volume is increased; plasma volume is variably normal or slightly increased.

Increased platelet count > 400,000/cu mm in 62% of cases; often >1 million.

Increased polymorphonuclear leukocytes (PMNs) > 12,000/cu mm in ~60% of cases; usually >15,000 cu mm; sometimes there is a leukemoid reaction). Mild basophilia in ~60% of cases.

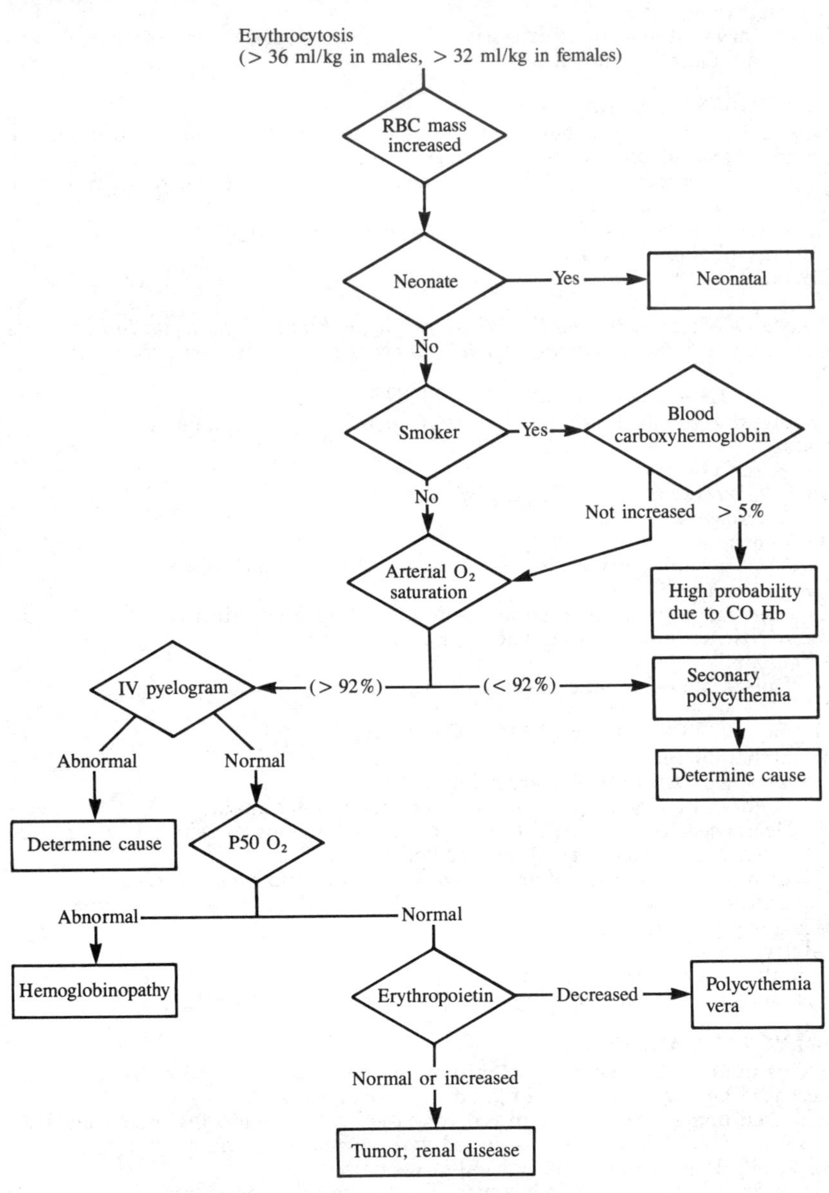

Fig. 12-4. Sequence of laboratory tests in the diagnosis of erythrocytosis.

Oxygen saturation of arterial blood is normal in 84% of cases.
Increased leukocyte alkaline phosphatase score > 100 in 79% of cases.
Increased serum vitamin B_{12} > 900 pg/ml in 13% of cases.
Increased vitamin B_{12}–binding capacity > 2200 pg/ml in 36% of cases.
ESR is decreased.
Blood viscosity is increased.
Osmotic fragility is decreased (increased resistance).
Peripheral blood smear may show macrocytes, microcytes, polychromatophilic RBCs, normoblasts, large masses of platelets, neutrophilic shift to the left.
Reticulocyte count > 1.5% in 44% of cases.
Bone marrow shows general hyperplasia of all elements; mild myelofibrosis may be present. Iron may be decreased or absent.
Increased serum uric acid in ~50% of cases.
Bleeding time and coagulation time are normal, but clot retraction may be poor.
Serum total bilirubin may be slightly increased in ~50% of cases.
Serum iron may be decreased in ~50% of cases.
Urine may contain increased urobilinogen, and occasionally albumin is present.
Laboratory findings of associated diseases
- Gout
- Cirrhosis
- Duodenal ulcer
- Hypertension

Laboratory findings due to complications
- Thromboses (e.g., cerebral, portal vein)
- Intercurrent infection
- Peptic ulcer
- Hemorrhage
- Myelofibrosis
- Myeloid metaplasia
- Chronic myelogenous leukemia (develops in 20% of patients)

Measurement of erythropoietin levels in plasma have become available recently. Suppressed in polycythemia vera and usually normal or increased in secondary polycythemia. Normal level is not helpful, but increased level indicates secondary erythrocytosis. Degree of increase may depend on causative condition. Increases may be intermittent; therefore a single normal level is unreliable.
In vitro culture of erythroid progenitors occurs in polycythemia vera without addition of erythopoietin but not in secondary polycythemia; only available in special labs.

Criteria For Diagnosis*

A1 Increased RBC mass (≥ 36 ml/kg in men; ≥ 32 ml/kg in women)
A2 Splenomegaly (occurs in ~75% of cases)
A3 Normal arterial O_2 saturation (≥ 92%)

If A2 or A3 is absent, then two of four criteria from B must be present.

B1 WBC > 12,000/cu mm
B2 Platelet count > 650,000/cu mm
B3 Increased leukocyte alkaline phosphatase score (occurs in ~70% of cases)
B4 Increased serum vitamin B_{12} (> 900 pg/ml) or vitamin B_{12}–binding capacity (> 2200 pg/ml).

*Data from Polycythemia Vera Study Group, Polycythemia vera. *Semin Hematol* 12(4):13(1), 1976.

Table 12-12. Comparison of Polycythemia Vera, Secondary Polycythemia, and Relative Polycythemia

Test	Polycythemia Vera	Secondary Polycythemia	Relative Polycythemia
Hematocrit	I	I	I
Blood volume	I	I	D or N
Red cell mass	I	I	D or N
Plasma volume	I or N	N or I	D
Platelet count	I	N	N
WBC with shift to left	I	N	N
Nucleated RBC, abnormal RBC	I	N	N
Serum uric acid	I	I	N
Serum vitamin B_{12}	I	N	N
Leukocyte alkaline phosphatase	I	N	N
Oxygen saturation of arterial blood	N	D	N
Bone marrow	Hyperplasia of all elements	Erythroid hyperplasia	N
Erythropoietin level	D	I	N

I = increased; D = decreased; N = normal.

SECONDARY POLYCYTHEMIA

Due To

Hypoxia with decreased arterial oxygen saturation
- Decreased atmospheric pressure (e.g., high altitudes)
- Chronic heart disease
  - Congenital (e.g., pulmonary stenosis, septal defect, patent ductus arteriosus)
  - Acquired (e.g., chronic rheumatic mitral disease)
- Arteriovenous aneurysm
- Impaired pulmonary ventilation
  - Alveolar-capillary block (e.g., Hamman-Rich syndrome, sarcoidosis, lymphangitic cancer)
  - Alveolar hypoventilation (e.g., bronchial asthma, kyphoscoliosis)
  - Restriction of pulmonary vascular bed (e.g., primary pulmonary hypertension, mitral stenosis, chronic pulmonary emboli, emphysema)
- Abnormal hemoglobin pigments (methemoglobinemia or sulfhemoglobinemia due to chemicals, such as aniline and coal tar derivatives) or high oxygen-affinity hemoglobinopathies (50% of hemoglobinopathy cases show an abnormality on standard hemoglobin electrophoresis.) *(Hemoglobin oxygen affinity [P_{50}] is the oxygen tension at which hemoglobin becomes 50% saturated. Normal = 27.5 mmHg. Usually < 20 mmHg in these conditions. Decreased P_{50} indicates increased oxygen affinity, and increased P_{50} indicates decreased oxygen affinity. May be increased by high-affinity hemoglobinopathies, carboxyhemoglobinemia, decreased RBC 2,3-DPG, alkalosis. May be decreased by hemoglobinopathies, increased RBC 2,3-DPG, acidosis.)* Carboxyhemoglobinemia ("smoker's erythrocytosis") can be detected by oximetry but not from PO_2.

Increased erythropoietin secretion
- Associated with tumors and miscellaneous conditions (may be first sign of an occult curable tumor)
- Renal disease (hypernephroma, benign tumors, hydronephrosis, polycystic kidneys; occurs in up to 5% of renal cell carcinomas; occurs in 10–17% of kidney transplant recipients)
- Hemangioblastoma of cerebellum (occurs in 15–20% of cases)
- Uterine fibromyoma
- 5–10% of cases of hepatocellular carcinoma
- Others

Increased androgen
- Pheochromocytoma
- Cushing's syndrome (adrenocortical hyperplasia or tumor)
- Masculinizing ovarian tumor (e.g., arrhenoblastoma)
- Factitious (use of androgens by athletes)

See Table 12-12, p. 322.

RELATIVE POLYCYTHEMIA (STRESS ERYTHROCYTOSIS)

Relative polycythemia is not secondary to hypoxia but results from decreased plasma volume due to unknown mechanism or to decreased fluid intake and/or excess loss of body fluids

Increased RBC (usually < 6,000,000/cu mm), hemoglobin, and hematocrit

RBC mass is normal.

Plasma volume is decreased.

Normal WBC, platelet, and reticulocyte counts

Findings of secondary polycythemia (e.g., decreased O_2 saturation) are not present (see preceding section)

Leukocyte alkaline phosphatase score is normal or mildly increased.

Bone marrow shows normal cellularity and megakaryocyte count; no myelofibrosis; iron may be absent.

Hypercholesterolemia is frequent.

Laboratory findings due to complications (e.g., thromboembolism)

EPSTEIN-BARR VIRUS (EBV) INFECTIONS

Infectious Mononucleosis (IM)

Diagnostic criteria
- Compatible clinical syndrome
- Hematologic findings of absolute (> 4500/cu mm) and relative lymphocytosis (≥ 50%) and ≥ 10% characteristically atypical lymphocytes
- Serologic findings. See Heterophil Agglutination (Paul-Bunnell Test), pp. 324–325.

Leukopenia and granulocytopenia are evident during first week. Later, WBC is increased (usually 10,000–20,000/cu mm) because of increased lymphocytes; peak changes occur in 7–10 days; many persist for 1–2 months. Increased number of bands and > 5% eosinophilia are frequent.

Evidence of mild hepatitis (e.g., increased serum transaminases, increased urine urobilinogen) is very frequent at some stage but may be transient. Clinical jaundice occurs in < 10% of patients. Bilirubin-enzyme dissociation (normal serum bilirubin or < 2 mg/dl with moderate increase of alkaline phosphatase, SGOT, SGPT) occurs in 75% of cases. If no liver function abnormalities can be found, another diagnosis should be sought.

Serologic test for syphilis, rheumatoid arthritis test, and antinuclear antibody (ANA) may show transient false positive results.

Occasional RBCs and albumin are seen in urine.

Mild thrombocytopenia is seen in about 50% of early cases, and platelet dysfunction is frequent.

Hemolytic anemia is rare.

Mononucleosis syndrome is caused by Epstein-Barr virus in > 90% of cases, cytomegalic inclusion disease (see pp. 662–663.) in 5–7%, and *Toxoplasma gondii* in < 1%.

Less common causes include AIDS, herpes simplex II, varicella, viral hepatitis, adenovirus, rubella, certain drugs (e.g., PAS, phenytoin, sulfasalazine, dapsone). Serodiagnostic tests for EBV (see following sections) are required only when the heterophil is negative. When heterophil is negative, primary or recent EBV infection is confirmed by IM-specific heterophil antibody titers: VCA-IgM ≥ 1 : 10, VCA-IgG ≥ 1 : 320, EA-D ≥ 1 : 10, EBNA-Ab ≤ 1 : 2 early after onset.

< 10% atypical lymphocytes are found in other viral diseases (e.g., rubella, roseola, mumps, acute viral hepatitis).

Chronic Mononucleosis Syndrome

(three types are described; many question the existence of this syndrome)

True chronic mononucleosis—typical clinical picture with positive heterophil and serologic evidence of primary EBV infection, but patient does not recover for many months or years; may be related to immunodeficiency.

Severe chronic active EBV infection (very rare) with very high EBV antibody titers and persistent serious disease (e.g., pancytopenia, agranulocytosis, chronic hepatitis, pneumonia); may coexist with true chronic mononucleosis

"Chronic mononucleosis"—no preceding acute mononucleosis, fatigue, fever, lymphadenopathy for > 6 months. Heterophil is positive in ~10% of cases. No definitive diagnostic laboratory tests; usually not more than three of the following are present in a patient:

- Leukopenia (3000–5000/cu mm) with monocytosis (7–15%), relative lymphocytosis (> 40%), atypical lymphocytes (1–20%).
- Low ESR (< 4 mm/hour)
- Mild increase in SGOT and SGPT
- Immunoglobulins may be reduced.
- Low levels of circulating immune complexes may be present.
- Increased CD4/CD8 ratio
- EBV antibodies (sensitivity < 70%; specificity ~20%)
  - IgG–viral capsid antigen (IgG-VCA) > 1 : 64
  - IgM-VCA not detectable
  - Early antigen (EA) > 1 : 40
  - Epstein-Barr nuclear antigen (EBNA) < 1 : 5

Heterophil Agglutination (Paul-Bunnell test)

(agglutination of sheep RBCs by serum of patients with infectious mononucleosis due to EBV)

Titers ≤ 1 : 56 may occur in normal persons and in patients with other illnesses.

A titer of ≥ 1 : 224 is presumptive evidence of IM but may also be caused by recent injection of horse serum or horse immune serum. Therefore a differential absorption test should be performed using guinea pig kidney and beef cell antigens.

Guinea pig absorption will not reduce the titer in IM to < 25% of the original value; most commonly the titer is not reduced by more than 1 or 2 tube dilutions. If > 90% of the agglutination is removed by guinea pig adsorption, the test is considered negative.

Beef red cell absorption takes most (90%) or all of the sheep agglutinations and does reduce the titer in IM; failure to reduce the titer is evidence against a diagnosis of IM.

Heterophil agglutination is positive in 60% of young adults by 2 weeks and 90% by 4 weeks after onset of clinical IM; thus may be negative when positive hematologic and clinical findings are present, and a second heterophil agglutination 1–2 weeks later may be positive. The heterophil agglutination may

Table 12-13. Sample Titers in Heterophil Agglutination

Presumptive Test	After Guinea Pig Kidney Absorption	After Beef RBC Absorption	Interpretation of Diagnosis of Infectious Mononucleosis
1:224	1:112	0	+
1:224	1:56	0	+
1:224	1:28	0	+
1:224	1:14 or less	0	−
1:224	1:56	1:56	−
1:224	0	1:112	−
1:56	1:56–1:7	0	+
1:56	1:56	1:28	−
1:28	1:28–1:7	0	+

have become negative even though some residual hematologic findings are still present.

When horse RBCs are used for the test, results may still be positive up to 12 months after the acute illness in up to 75% of cases.

Heterophil antibodies are found in only 30% of children < 2 years old, 75% of children 2–4 years old, and > 90% of older children with IM.

False positive tests are very rare and occur in relatively low titers. A resurgence of heterophil antibody titer may occur in response to other infections (e.g., viral upper respiratory infection). Occasionally positive in other diseases (e.g., rheumatoid arthritis, rubella).

Titer does not cross react with or correlate with antibodies for EBV; neither correlates with severity of illness.

Heterophil agglutination is almost never positive in Japanese patients with IM for unknown reasons.

Commercial slide agglutination ("spot") tests are now performed as the usual initial test, and tube dilution tests are only done if necessary for confirmation; sensitivity corresponds to tube dilution test (about 98%) except in children < 4 years old when slide test is less sensitive. False positive slide tests may occur in leukemia, malignant lymphoma, malaria, rubella, serum hepatitis, pancreatic carcinoma and have been found for years in some persons with no known explanation. False positive in ~2% and false negative in ~5–7% of adults.

Serologic Tests For Epstein-Barr Virus (EBV)

EBV antibody tests are rarely required, since 90% of cases are heterophil positive and false positive results are rare and because illness is usually mild, self-limited, and relatively mild. May be useful in atypical or very severe cases with negative heterophil tests, especially in young children or immunocompromised patients.

IgG-VCA may be present early in illness, usually before clinical symptoms are present; detected at onset in 100% of cases; has peaked in 80% of patients and only 20% show 4-fold increase in titer after visiting a doctor. Decreases during convalescence but detectable for many years after illness; therefore not helpful in establishing diagnosis of IM. Indicates past infection and immunity.

IgM-VCA is detected at onset in 100% of cases; high titers present in serum 1–6 weeks after onset of illness; starts to fall by third week and usually disappears in 1–6 months; disappears 1–2 months after onset of IM, and sera

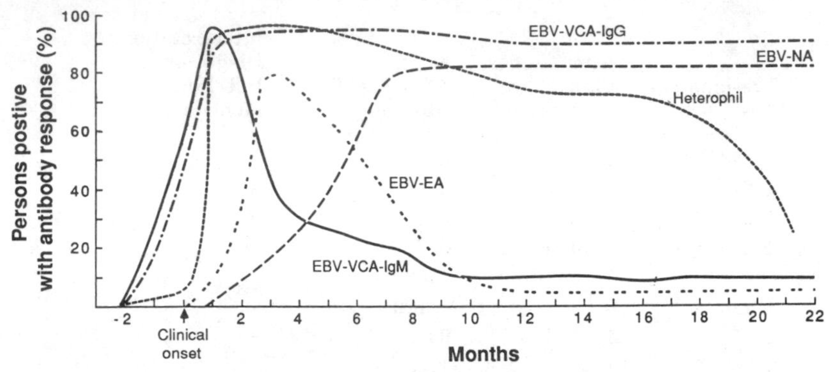

Fig. 12-5. Percent of persons with positive antibody response at specified time intervals. EBV = Epstein-Barr virus; VCA = viral capsid antigen (Ortho Diagnostic Systems, Raritan, NJ); EA = early antigen; NA = nuclear antigen.

are often taken too late to be detected. Is almost always present in active EBV infection and thus most sensitive and specific for acute episode of IM.

Early antigen (anti-D and anti-R): anti-D titers rise later (3–4 weeks after onset; is transient) in course of IM than VCA antibodies and disappear with recovery; combined with IgG-VCA, suggests recent EBV infection; only found in 70% of patients with IM due to EBV.

Early antigen (anti-R) antibodies are only found occasionally, 2 weeks to months after onset; may persist for a year; more often in atypical or protracted cases. Usually found in Burkitt's lymphoma.

EBNA is the last antibody to appear, is rare in acute phase; rises during convalescence (3–12 months) and is found a few weeks after onset of clinical illness; persists for many years after illness. Absence when IgM-VCA and anti-D are present implies recent infection. Appearance after previous negative test evidences recent EBV infection. Recently an ELISA kit (Ortho Diagnostics) detects EBNA IgG and IgM simultaneously; IgM > IgG indicates acute infection, but IgG > IgM indicates previous exposure to EBV. Absent EBNA and presence of VCA indicate acute infection.

Acute primary EBV infection is indicated by ≥ 1 of these serologic findings:

- IgM-VCA that is found early and later declines
- High titer (≥ 1 : 320) or ≥ 4-fold rise in IgG/VCA titer during the illness
- Transient rise in anti-D titer (≥ 1 : 10)
- Early IgG/VCA without EBNA and later appearance of EBNA

Acute or primary EBV infection is excluded when IgG/VCA and EBNA titers are unchanged in acute and convalescent serum samples.

ACUTE INFECTIOUS LYMPHOCYTOSIS

Markedly increased WBC (≥ 40,000/cu mm) is due to lymphocytosis (normal appearing, small-sized lymphocytes).

Heterophil agglutination is negative.

CHRONIC GRANULOMATOUS DISEASE

This is a rare, heterogeneous, genetically determined disorder characterized by chronic recurrent suppurative infections by catalase-positive organisms (e.g., *Staphylococcus aureus, Aspergillus* species; also seen frequently are *Serratia marcescens, Pseudomonas cepacia, Klebsiella species, Escherichia coli, Nocardia, Chromobacterium violaceum*), which usually have low virulence (e.g.,

Table 12-14. Serologic Antibody Patterns in EBV Infection

	Susceptible (no past infection)	Primary EBV (acute infection)	Convalescent (3 months)	Prior (past infection)	Reactivated (chronic infection)
IgM-VCA	–	+	+/–	–	–
IgG-VCA	–	+	+	+	+
EA-D	–	+*	+*	–	+*
EA-R					
EBNA	–	–	+	+	+

VCA = viral capsid antigen; EA-D = early antigen complex, diffuse component; EA-R = early antigen complex, restricted component; EBNA = Epstein-Barr nuclear antigen; + = titer > 1:5.
*Titer <1:5 in 80% of patients.

50% of persons have antibodies to EBV by age 5 years, 90% by age 20, >95% by mid-twenties. EBNA is often absent in immunosuppressed patients. EA-D and EA-R may be increased with no change in VCA.

EBV is associated with Burkitt's lymphoma and with undifferentiated nasopharyngeal carcinoma. Both have anti-VCA titers increased 8–10 times. Anti-EA-R is high and correlated with tumor burden in Burkitt's lymphoma. Anti-EA-D is high and correlated with tumor burden in nasopharyngeal carcinoma.

Salmonella, Candida albicans). Onset in first year of life, causing death by 7 years of age in one-third of patients (PMNs and monocytes ingest normally but fail to kill certain bacteria and fungi).

Due to abnormality of NADPH oxidase system; ~60% are X-linked membrane abnormalities, ~40% due to autosomal recessive inheritance; most are cytosol abnormalities, and 5% are membrane abnormalities, < 1% due to autosomal dominant inheritance.

Failure of these cells to reduce nitroblue tetrazolium to purple formazan on slide test provides a simple rapid diagnosis in patients and in heterozygotes for the X-linked form (carriers).

Other tests include measurement of oxygen consumption, hydrogen peroxide or superoxide production, and chemiluminescence of phagocytes.

WBCs show morphologically normal appearance and granules on routine Wright-Giemsa stained smears.

Prenatal diagnosis has been established using fetal blood obtained before 20 weeks' gestation.

Laboratory findings due to infection (leukocytosis, anemia, increased ESR, elevated gamma globulin levels) are noted.

Laboratory findings due to abscesses of lung, liver, osteomyelitis

Laboratory findings due to granulomas causing obstruction (e.g., GI tract, GU tract)

Serum complement and immunoglobulin levels are normal.

CHÉDIAK-HIGASHI SYNDROME

This is a rare autosomal recessive genetic disease that causes hypopigmentation of skin, hair, and uvea.

Neutrophils contain coarse, deeply staining, peroxidase-positive, large granulations in cytoplasm and are present less frequently in other WBCs.

Pancytopenia appears during the (accelerated) "lymphoma-like" phase.

Laboratory findings due to frequent severe pyogenic infections and hemorrhage (which cause death by age 5) are noted.

Marked deficiency of natural killer (NK) cell function

Heterozygous carriers identified by a granulation anomaly in PMNs.

AGRANULOCYTOSIS

In acute fulminant form, WBC is decreased to ≤ 2000/cu mm, sometimes as low as 50/cu mm. Granulocytes are 0–2%. Granulocytes may show pyknosis or vacuolization.

In chronic or recurrent form, WBC is down to 2000/cu mm with less marked granulocytopenia.

There is relative lymphocytosis and sometimes monocytosis.

Bone marrow shows absence of cells in granulocytic series but normal erythroid and megakaryocytic series.

ESR is increased.

Hemoglobin and RBC count and morphology, platelet count, and coagulation tests are normal.

Laboratory findings due to infection are noted.

Laboratory findings due to underlying causes (see Aplastic Anemia, pp. 283–284) are noted.

PERIODIC (CYCLIC) NEUTROPENIA

Autosomal dominant rare condition with regular periodic occurrence of neutropenia every 10–35 days, lasting 3–4 days.

WBC is 2000–4000/cu mm, and granulocytes are as low as 0%.

Monocytosis may occur.

Eosinophilia may occur during recovery.

Bone marrow during episode may show hypoplasia or maturation arrest at myelocyte stage.

MAY-HEGGLIN ANOMALY

This is an inherited dominant abnormality of WBCs and platelets.

Large, poorly granulated platelets are associated with anomalous area in cytoplasm of all granulocytes (Döhle bodies). Usually no other hematologic abnormalities are present.

The lesion is an asymptomatic familial one. Diagnosis is confirmed by finding Döhle bodies in a parent or sibling.

PELGER-HUËT ANOMALY

This is an autosomal dominant, usually heterozygous, anomaly of WBCs.

Nuclei of granulocytes lack normal segmentation but are shaped like eyeglasses, rods, dumbbells, or peanuts. Coarse chromatin is evident in nuclei of granulocytes, lymphocytes, and monocytes. These cells are present in peripheral blood and bone marrow.

No other hematologic or clinical abnormality is present.

Occasionally cells resembling those in this anomaly are seen following administration of myelotoxic agents in acute and chronic myelogenous leukemia.

ALDER-REILLY ANOMALY

Heavy azurophilic granulation of granulocytes and some lymphocytes and monocytes associated with mucopolysaccharidoses (see pp. 436–437) are seen.

HEREDITARY HYPERSEGMENTATION OF NEUTROPHILS

(simple dominant abnormality found in 1% of whites)

Hypersegmentation of neutrophils resembles that seen in pernicious anemia but is a permanent abnormality. Most neutrophils have four or more lobes.

There is a similar condition that affects only the eosinophilic granulocytes (hereditary constitutional hypersegmentation of the eosinophil).

There is also an inherited giant multilobed abnormality of neutrophilic leukocytes.

Hypersegmentation is also found in almost every patient with chronic renal disease with BUN > 30 mg/dl for more than 3 months.

HYPEREOSINOPHILIC SYNDROME

Diagnosis is based on eosinophilia > 1500/cu mm for > 6 months and no other cause for eosinophilia.

Abnormalities in count and morphology of platelets, WBC, and RBC

Mild anemia is frequent; hypercellular bone marrow with 25–75% eosinophils.

May be asymptomatic or have evidence of organ dysfunction

- Cardiovascular lesions in >80% of patients (e.g., ventricular necrosis, regurgitation due to fibrosis of mitral or tricuspid leaflets; mural thrombi causes systemic embolization in 5% of cases)
- Pulmonary (e.g., pleural effusion, diffuse interstitial infiltrates)
- Neurologic in 30% of patients
- Cutaneous in 25% of patients
- Liver function abnormalities
- Abnormal urine sediment in 20% of patients

CONGENITAL ABSENCE OF SPLEEN

Presence of Heinz bodies in 5–20% of RBCs is the most characteristic finding.

Erythroblastosis (2000–40,000/cu mm) may be present, with increased frequency of Howell-Jolly bodies and target cells.

Decreased osmotic fragility may be found.

Same findings in other causes of functional hyposplenism (e.g., amyloidosis)

POSTSPLENECTOMY STATE

Howell-Jolly bodies (is the most consistent abnormality) and target cells are seen in peripheral blood smears. Heinz bodies can be seen with special stains.

Increased WBC (granulocytosis) for several weeks in 75% of patients and indefinitely in 25%. Lymphocytosis and monocytosis occur for several weeks in 50% of patients; some of these may show increased eosinophils or basophils. Increased platelets occur in postoperative period.

Decreased serum IgM

Increased risk of overwhelming infection (50% are due to *Streptococcus pneumoniae;* another 25% are due to *Hemophilus influenzae, Neisseria meningitidis,* and group A streptococcus; *Staphylococcus, Pseudomonas,* and other gram-negative organisms are rarer), with massive bacteremia, high mortality. Risk of infection is greater in infants less than 2 years old, within 2 years of splenectomy, or if underlying disorder is primary hematologic or splenic disease.

DIC is frequent with septic shock.

HYPERSPLENISM

The disease is either secondary to enlarged spleen or "primary" (with no detectable underlying disease).

There are various combinations of anemia, leukopenia, thrombocytopenia associated with bone marrow showing normal or increased cellularity of affected elements (includes primary splenic pancytopenia and primary splenic neutropenia).

Chromium 51–tagged RBCs from normal person or from patient are rapidly destroyed after transfusion, and radioactivity accumulates in spleen. (Normal spleen-liver ratio = 1.0; in hypersplenism is 1.5–2.0; in hemolysis is >3.0.)

MYELODYSPLASTIC (PRELEUKEMIC) SYNDROMES

(group of clonal proliferative disorders of bone marrow that show peripheral blood cytopenias and dysmyelopoiesis with no detectable cause and progress to acute nonlymphocytic leukemia in >25% or die of complications [e.g., acute infection] or associated diseases)

FAB Classification

Refractory anemia
- Persistent anemia with decreased reticulocytes, variable dyserythropoiesis <1% blasts in peripheral blood, <5% blasts in marrow
- Hypercellular marrow with erythroid hyperplasia and/or dyserythropoiesis
- Normal megakaryocytes and granulocytes
- Dysgranulopoiesis is infrequent.

Refractory anemia with ring sideroblasts (same as acquired idiopathic sideroblastic anemia)

Refractory anemia (see above) with >15% ring sideroblasts
- >10% develop acute myelocytic leukemia

Refractory anemia with excess blasts
- Cytopenia affecting ≥2 cell lines
- <5% blasts in peripheral blood and <20% blasts in marrow
- Granulocytic maturation is present.
- Hypercellular marrow with granulocytic or erythroid hyperplasia
- Dysgranulopoiesis, dyserythropoiesis, and/or dysmegakaryocytopoiesis

Refractory anemia with excess blasts in transformation
- >5% blasts in peripheral blood and/or 20–30% blasts in marrow
- Auer rods may be present.
- 75% develop acute myelocytic leukemia.

Chronic myelomonocytic leukemia
- Same as refractory anemia with excess blasts but with >100 monocytes/μl in peripheral blood
- Mature granulocytes may be increased.
- <5% blasts in peripheral blood and 5–20% blasts in marrow

Abnormal and asynchronous maturation of different cell series is defined as
- Dyserythropoiesis
  - Anisocytosis, poikilocytosis, oval macrocytes, nucleated RBCs, and normochromia are most common changes in RBCs on peripheral smear.
  - Erythroid maturation defects with bizarre (e.g., multinucleated) forms and megaloblastic features unresponsive to folic acid, vitamin B_{12}, and iron.
- Dysgranulomonopoiesis
  - Increased or decreased numbers or abnormal nuclei or granulation in blood
  - Variable increase in mature granulocyte precursors (usually myelocytes) and monocytosis occur frequently in marrow.
- Dysmegakaryocytopoiesis
  - Increased or decreased number
  - Atypical and bizarre platelets are seen in most cases.
  - Marrow megakaryocytes are often atypical or bizarre.

Other clinicopathologic forms include refractory anemias of various types, pure red cell aplasia, paroxysmal nocturnal hemoglobinuria, chronic idiopathic neutropenia, chronic idiopathic thrombocytopenia, etc. For further details on clinical and hematologic classification, see JM Bennett, et al., Proposals for the classification of the myelodysplastic syndromes. *Br J Haematol* 51:189, 1982 and Proposed revised criteria for the classification of acute myeloid leukemia. *Ann Intern Med* 103:460, 1985.

CHROMOSOME ABNORMALITIES IN MALIGNANT HEMATOLOGIC DISORDERS*

At initial diagnosis, routine cytogenetic studies show chromosomal abnormality in >50% of cases

Acute nonlymphocytic leukemia	54%
Acute lymphocytic leukemia	41%
Chronic granulocytic leukemia	94%
Myelodysplastic syndrome	39%
Lymphoma	71%

Structural abnormalities include translocations, deletions, isochromosomes, inversions, duplications, and numeric anomalies (e.g., trisomies, monosomies).

If an abnormal chromosome clone is not observed, the analysis should be considered not diagnostic.

ASSAY (cDNA probe) FOR REARRANGEMENT OF *bcr* GENE

Recently, special procedures using Southern blot techniques following gel electrophoresis for DNA fragment size fractionation can demonstrate reciprocal translocation of DNA from chromosome 9 (including the *abl* locus) to 22 (breakpoint cluster [*bcr*]) giving rise to shorter chromosome 22 (Philadelphia chromosome [Ph^1]). This is found in 95% of patients with chronic granulocytic leukemia (CML), 5–10% of acute lymphoblastic leukemia (ALL), and 1–2% of patients with acute myelogenous leukemia. Presence of Ph^1 affects response to therapy and survival. This rearrangement of *bcr* is typical of Ph^1-positive CML patients and is found in ~30% of Ph^1-positive AML patients. This assay can be done on peripheral blood as well as marrow, does not require dividing cells, and is more sensitive than routine cytogenetic analysis.

*Data from GW Dewald, et al. Chromosome abnormalities in malignant hematologic disorders. *Mayo Clin Proc* 60:675, 1985.

ASSAY FOR REARRANGEMENT OF GENES FOR IMMUNOGLOBULIN HEAVY (IgH) AND LIGHT (IgL-kappa) CHAINS AND FOR REARRANGEMENT OF BETA AND GAMMA T-CELL RECEPTOR GENES (beta-TCR, gamma-TCR)*

Allows classification of almost all cases of ALL as T, B, or pre-B types.

Confirms pathologic-immunologic diagnoses of T- and B-cell lymphomas that are difficult to classify.

Virtually all cases of non-T, non-B leukemias are recognized as pre-B types.

Up to 90% of cases of non-Hodgkin's lymphoma are derived from B cells. Their immunophenotypic abnormalities can be used to distinguish them from benign reactions in lymph nodes.

ACUTE LEUKEMIA

In adults, 20% of acute leukemias are lymphocytic and 80% are nonlymphocytic.

Peripheral blood

- WBC is rarely >100,000/cu mm. It may be normal and is commonly less than normal. Peripheral smear shows many cells that resemble lymphocytes; it may not be possible to differentiate the very young forms as lymphoblasts or myeloblasts, and special cytochemical stains may be used (blast cells are positive for peroxidase, Sudan black B, and nonspecific esterase in AML but negative in ALL; cytoplasmic acid phosphatase may be positive in T-cell ALL). Special immunologic markers distinguish T-cell, B-cell, and non-T, non-B cell types of acute lymphocytic leukemia, which is important because of different prognosis and relapse patterns in the three types. Prognosis is poorer in older children and adults >35 years and those with high initial WBC, with chromosome translocations (e.g., 9 and 22 in Ph^1 chromosome–positive ALL). Favorable response to treatment is more likely if B-cell lymphoblasts are common ALA antigen (CALLA) positive but cytoplasmic μ-chain negative. Presence of leukemic lymphoblasts that express myeloid antigens is associated with an unfavorable prognosis.
- Anemia is almost always present at clinical onset. Usually normocytic and sometimes macrocytic, it is progressive and may become severe. Normoblasts and polychromatophilia are common.

Platelet count is usually decreased at clinical onset and becomes progressively severe. May show poor clot retraction, increased bleeding time, positive tourniquet test, etc.

Bone marrow smear

- Blast cells are present even when none are found in peripheral blood. (This finding is useful to differentiate from other causes of pancytopenia.) There is progressively increasing infiltration with earlier cell types (e.g., blasts, myelocytes).
- The myeloid-erythroid ratio is increased.
- Erythroid and megakaryocyte elements are replaced.
- Histochemical, phenotypical, and cytogenetic studies are often important for classification, prognosis, and therapy.
- Cultures (bacterial, fungal, viral) should be done routinely, as they may be the first clue to occult infection.

DIC may be present (especially with M3; also M4 and M5; less commonly with other forms) at onset.

Serum uric acid is frequently increased.

Tumor lysis syndrome may cause hypokalemia, hypocalcemia, hypomagnesemia, etc.

Increased serum creatinine and BUN reflect infiltration of kidneys, impairing renal function.

*Data from Specialty Laboratories, Inc., San Diego, CA.

In acute myelogenous leukemia, serum LDH and malic dehydrogenase (MDH) are frequently but inconstantly increased; there is normal to slight increase in SGOT, SGPT, aldolase.

Urine lysozyme may be increased in acute nonlymphocytic leukemia (M4 and M5).

Laboratory findings due to complications

- Meningeal leukemia occurs in 25–50% of children and 10–20% of adults with acute leukemia; CSF shows pleocytosis and increased pressure and LDH. CSF should be examined routinely for leukemic cells and to rule out occult infection.
- Urate nephropathy.
- Infection causes 90% of deaths. Most important pathogens are gram-negative rods (especially *Pseudomonas aeruginosa*) and fungi (especially *Candida albicans*).
- Hemolytic anemia

Laboratory findings due to predisposing conditions

- Inherited syndromes (e.g., Down's syndrome, ataxia-telangiectasia, common variable immunodeficiency, severe combined immunodeficiency, Wiskott-Aldrich syndrome, Bloom's syndrome, Fanconi's anemia)
- Ionizing radiation (therapeutic or accidental)
- Chemotherapeutic drugs (e.g., alkylating agents)
- Toxins (e.g., benzene)

Complete remission is possible with drug therapy (e.g., prednisone in acute lymphoblastic leukemia). WBC falls (or rises) to normal in 1–2 weeks with replacement of lymphoblasts by normal PMNs and return of RBC and platelet counts to normal; bone marrow may become normal. Maximum improvement in 6–8 weeks.

Laboratory findings due to toxic effect of therapeutic agents

- Amethopterin toxicity causes a macrocytic type of anemia with megaloblasts in marrow compared to leukemic normocytic anemia with blast cells in marrow.
- Cyclophosphamide can cause hematuria.
- L-Asparaginase can cause coagulopathies, hyperglycemia, etc.
- Daunorubicin can cause cardiac toxicity with fibrosis.

SYNDROMES OF ACUTE NONLYMPHOCYTIC LEUKEMIA*

(French, American, British [FAB] classification)

M1, M2, M3 Leukemias

Predominantly granulocytic

M2 Acute Nonlymphocytic Leukemia with t(8;21)

Incidence: 7–10% of acute nonlymphocytic leukemia patients

Patient age: young (mean = 28 years)

Clinical findings: splenomegaly in 28%; chloromas especially of face area in 20%

Morphology: myeloblasts often with Auer rods (90%) are heterogeneous, hypogranular and frequently show pseudo-Pelger-Huët abnormalities. Sum of types I and II blast cells is 30–89% of nonerythroid cells (differ from M1 in which the sum of types I and II blast cells is >90% of nonerythroid cells and ≥3% of these are peroxidase or Sudan black positive); monocytic cells are <20%; granulocytes from promyelocytes to polymorphonuclear types are >10%. Maturation toward granulocytes is often abnormal; eosinophil precursors are frequently increased and may contain Auer rods.

Histochemistry: cells contain granulocyte but not monocyte enzymes; Sudan black and myeloperoxidase are abnormal (punctate rather than diffuse).

*Data from HP Koeffler, Syndromes of acute nonlymphocytic leukemia. *Ann Intern Med* 107:748, 1987.

Table 12-15. Differential Diagnosis of Chronic Myelogenous Leukemia

	Chronic Myelogenous Leukemia	Acute Myeloblastic Leukemia	Granulocytic Leukemoid Reaction	Myelofibrosis
WBC >100,000/cu mm	Yes	Rare	No	No
Whole spectrum of immature granulocytes	Yes	No (leukemic hiatus)	No	Yes
Myeloblasts and promyelocytes in blood or marrow	>30%	>30%	0	<30%
Leukocyte alkaline phosphatase	Usually <10	30–150	>150	Variable
Bone marrow	Granulocytic hyperplasia	>30% myeloblasts	Granulocytic hyperplasia	Fibrosis
Philadelphia chromosome	Yes	No	No	No

Karyotype: t(8;21)(q22;q22); critical region 21q translocated to 8q; frequent loss of sex chromosome. Increased predilection for this leukemia in Down's syndrome (trisomy 21).
Oncogenes: c-ets-2 translocates from 21q to 8q, but expression data for the gene are unknown; c-mos remains at 8q and c-myc translocates to 21q, but both are probably not important.
Prognosis: 75–85% complete remission rate after chemotherapy, but median survival (9.5 months) is of average duration.

M3 Acute Promyelocytic Leukemia
Incidence: 7% of acute nonlymphocytic leukemia patients
Patient age: median of 31 years
Clinical findings: 50% develop DIC.
Marrow morphology: predominantly neoplastic promyelocytes with coarse azurophilic granules and multiple Auer rods; a variant (M3V) shows microgranular promyelocytes on electron microscopy. Leukemia cells in peripheral blood are usually not high (5000–15,000/cu mm).
Unusual feature: blast cells occasionally can be induced to differentiate into mature granulocytes or macrophages by various agents.
Karyotype: t(15;17)(q22;q21.1) in almost all patients
Oncogene: none known

M4 Acute Myelomonocytic Leukemia With Abnormal Eosinophils
Incidence: 5% of acute nonlymphocytic leukemia patients
Marrow morphology: ≥20% myelomonocytic blasts. 1–30% abnormal eosinophils (precursors). Peripheral blood typically shows myelomonocytic blasts and slight increase in eosinophils (450–1100/cu mm).
Histochemistry: very weak staining for nonspecific esterase; can be distinguished from granulocytic types by monoclonal antibodies demonstrating specific antigens.
Karyotype: almost all patients show inversion of chromosome 16 [inv(16)(p13;q22)]; <10% show balanced translocation between short arm of one chromosome 16 and long arm of other chromosome 16 [t(16;16)(p13.1;q22)].
Oncogene: unknown
Molecular oncology: disruption of metallothionein genes by the chromosomal abnormality
Prognosis: 70–90% complete remission rate probably with prolonged median duration (>18 months). >one-third have relapse in CNS including myeloblastomas (compared to 5% of all acute nonlymphocytic leukemia patients who rarely show CNS myeloblastomas).

M5 Acute Monocytic Leukemia With t(9;11)
Incidence: 10% of acute monoblastic leukemia patients
Patient age: often children and young adults
Clinical findings: leukemia cells may infiltrate skin or gums; increased serum lysozyme.
Morphology: predominantly mature monocytic leukemic cells; can be distinguished from granulocytic types by monoclonal antibodies demonstrating specific antigens.
Karyotype: t(9;11)(p22;q23)
Oncogene: c-ets-1 translocated to 9p22 in region of alpha-interferon gene; expression data not known

M6 Erythroleukemia
Incidence: <5% of acute leukemia
Marrow morphology: ≥30% of nonerythroid cells are blast cells (if <30%, the diagnosis is myelodysplastic syndrome when ≥50% of all nucleated cells are erythroblasts). Erythroid hyperplasia and marked dyserythropoiesis are common. Erythroblasts are PAS positive.

Nucleated RBCs in peripheral blood smear and anemia are common.
Immunologic abnormalities are more frequent in this form, e.g., positive Coombs' test, antinuclear antibodies, positive rheumatoid factor, increased serum gamma globulins, hemolytic anemia.

M7 Acute Megakaryoblastic Leukemia

Incidence: 5% of all acute nonlymphocytic leukemia cases
Marrow morphology: myelofibrosis present in almost all patients; 20–40% present with acute myelofibrosis. Blast cells are highly polymorphic and are often classified as undifferentiated. Leukemic infiltrate ≥30% of all cells. Increased numbers of maturing megakaryocytes may be present.
Histochemistry: no myeloperoxidase or nonspecific esterase reaction. Unlike all other FAB subtypes, diagnosis is based on electron microscope identification of platelet peroxidase or on specific monoclonal antibodies to megakaryocyte antigens.
Karyotype: abnormalities of chromosome 21 have been reported, but specificity is still uncertain.
High serum LDH
Prognosis: preliminary reports of poor response to conventional thracycline-cytarabine based therapy

Acute Nonlymphocytic Leukemia With Normal Or High Platelet Counts And Rearrangement Of 3q21 And q26

Incidence: less than 20 cases known
Clinical findings: platelet count is increased or normal. 40% have a preleukemic phase. Many have prior exposure to a mutagen.
Marrow morphology: increased megakaryocytes that are usually small and dysplastic with 1–3 nuclear lobes. Leukemic cells frequently reported as (M4) myelomonoblasts.
Karyotype: rearrangement of 3q21 and 3q26, especially inv(3), t(3;3), or ins(5;3)
Prognosis: poor response to chemotherapy; often no remission

Therapy-Related Leukemia

Clinical findings: >70% have a preleukemic phase lasting about 11 months; occurs several (median = 4 years) years after chemotherapy (most frequently an alkylating agent, especially melphalan, chlorambucil, or cyclophosphamide) or radiation for another disease (compared to about 20% of all acute nonlymphocytic leukemias that have a preleukemic phase). Risk is 3–10% 10 years after therapy but may be greater after age 40. Risk of 5–20 times following exposure to nontherapeutic compounds (e.g., benzene). Unexplained pancytopenia; infection and hemorrhage.
Karyotype: >75% show deletion of chromosome 5/5q− and/or 7/7q−
Prognosis: short survival; often refractory to therapy

HUMAN T-CELL LEUKEMIA/LYMPHOMA SYNDROME

Recently described syndrome chiefly in black men in U.S. and Caribbean with acute onset, aggressive clinical course, increased antibody titers to human T-lymphotropic virus type I (HTLV-I) that can usually be isolated from malignant lymphoma or leukemia cells.
Leukemic phase with WBC count up to 190,000/cu mm, large or mixed small and large cell immunoblastic types, infrequent anemia, and thrombocytopenia. Bone marrow involvement in 50% of patients correlates poorly with extent of peripheral blood involvement.
Biopsy shows lymphomatous involvement of affected sites (e.g., lymph nodes, liver, spleen, bone, skin).
Laboratory findings due to involvement of various organs (e.g., liver, CNS)
Hypercalcemia in about 75% of patients; may occur without bone involvement.

CHRONIC MYELOGENOUS LEUKEMIA

(20% of all leukemias in U.S.)

Increased WBC due to increase in myeloid series is earliest change. In earlier stages, the more mature forms predominate with sequentially fewer cells of the younger forms and only an occasional blast cell may be seen; in the later, more advanced stages, the younger cells become predominant.

- Eosinophilic, basophilic leukocytes may be slightly increased at first with more marked increases in later stages. Monocytes are normal or only slightly increased.
- Lymphocytes are normal in absolute number but relatively decreased.
- WBC is usually 100,000–500,000/cu mm when disease is discovered.
- Decreased number of leukocytes show positive alkaline phosphatase staining reaction. This leukocyte alkaline phosphatase (LAP) score can rise to normal or high levels with infection, inflammation, secondary malignant disease, remission due to chemotherapy, or onset of blast crisis.

Anemia is usually normocytic; absent in early stage and severe in late stage. Blood smear shows few normoblasts, slight polychromatophilia, occasional stippling. Reticulocyte count is usually $<3\%$. Anemia is due to myelophthisis; also due to bleeding (skin and GI tract), hemolysis (autoimmune hemolytic anemia is rare), and insufficient compensatory hematopoiesis. Degree of anemia is a good index of extent of leukemic process and therefore of prognosis. Anemia improves with appropriate therapy or becomes more marked as the disease progresses.

Platelet count is normal or, commonly, increased; decreased in terminal stages with findings of thrombocytopenic purpura. Low count may increase with therapy. Bleeding manifestations are usually due to thrombocytopenia.

Bone marrow

- Hyperplasia of granulocytic elements occurs, with increase in myeloid-erythroid ratio.
- Granulocytes are more immature than in the peripheral blood.
- The number of eosinophils and basophils is increased.
- Megakaryocytic hyperplasia is often present.
- Hemosiderin deposits are increased.
- Mild fibrosis in 10–15% of cases

Needle aspiration of spleen

- The number of immature leukocytes is increased.
- Normoblastosis is present.
- Megakaryopoiesis is increased.

Serum and urine uric acid are increased, especially with high WBC and antileukemic therapy. Urinary obstruction may develop because of intrarenal and extrarenal uric acid crystallization.

Serum LDH is increased; rises several weeks prior to relapse and falls several weeks prior to remission.

Increased serum LDH, MDH, SGOT, SGPT, and aldolase show less elevation than in acute leukemia. SGOT, SGPT, and aldolase are normal in half the patients. LDH is useful for following course of therapy.

Serum protein electrophoresis shows decreased albumin with increased alpha and gamma globulins.

Thyroid uptake of radioactive iodine is normal.

Coombs' test is positive in one-third of patients.

Serum vitamin B_{12} level is increased (often >1000 μg/ml).

Philadelphia chromosome (reciprocal translocation of material between chromosome 9 and 22) is found in 95% of early chronic phase cases; persists during blast phase and additional abnormalities may appear (e.g., various trisomies, deletion of Y, double Ph^1). Other cytogenic abnormalities occur in one-third of the 5% of patients who are Ph^1-negative. Ph^1 chromosome has also been found in ~20% of adults with ALL, 2% of adults with AML, 5% of children with ALL. Ph^1 chromosome in acute leukemia indicates a poor prognosis.

Laboratory findings due to leukemia infiltration of organs (e.g., kidney [hematuria common; uremia rare], heart, liver). With increasing survival in blast crisis, meningeal leukemia has become more frequent (up to 40%) with leukemic cells in CSF indicative of need for intrathecal chemotherapy.

Chronic stable phase is shorter in men > age 60 with persistent anemia, basophilia, circulating blast cells, increased or decreased platelet count.

Many patients experience an accelerated phase before a blast crisis: progressive anemia, leukocytosis without an increased percentage of blast cells in blood or marrow, basophilia (may be >20%), increased LAP, increased or decreased platelets, new karyotypic abnormalities, and myelofibrosis associated with clinical manifestations of blast crisis (e.g., fever, malaise, increasing splenomegaly) and refractory to therapy.

Approximately one-third of patients with CML in blast crisis have leukemic cells with morphologic, antigenic, enzymatic (TdT), and other lymphoid characteristics. Are increasingly refractory to therapy in blast phase and die of acute leukemia of complications.

Platelet count <15,000 or >1,000,000/cu mm, blasts in peripheral blood, absence of Ph^1, moderate to marked myelofibrosis at time of diagnosis are poor prognostic signs. WBC <25,000/cu ml or hemoglobin >14 gm/dl is good prognostic sign.

Peripheral blood remission due to drugs—decreased WBC to nearly normal levels (decrease in spleen size is usually parallel) with only rare immature cells, correction of anemia, control of thrombocytosis, and LAP may occasionally rise to normal; marrow continues to show granulocytic hyperplasia and Philadelphia chromosome.

CHRONIC LYMPHOCYTIC LEUKEMIA

(30% of all leukemias in U.S.; <5% are T-cell type)

Peripheral blood

- WBC is increased (usually 50,000–250,000/cu mm) with 90% lymphocytes. These are uniformly similar, producing a monotonous blood picture of small mature-looking lymphocytes with minimal cytoplasm indistinguishable from normal. Blast cells are uncommon. Neutropenia is a late occurrence.
- Anemia—see Chronic Myelogenous Leukemia, pp. 337–338. Autoimmune hemolytic anemia occurs in 25% of patients. Anemia and/or thrombocytopenia correlates with marked change in survival time. Progress with rising WBC but may be absent with WBC >50,000/cu mm. Anemia or thrombocytopenia not due to autoimmune factor is poor prognostic sign.
- Platelet count is less likely to increase with therapy than in myelogenous leukemia.

Bone marrow

- Infiltration with earlier cell types is progressively increased.
- There is replacement of erythroid, myeloid, and megakaryocyte series.

Lymph node biopsy shows pattern of diffuse lymphoma with well-differentiated, small, noncleaved cells; aspirate or imprint shows increased number of immature leukocytes, predominantly blast cells.

Serum enzyme levels are less frequently elevated and show a lesser increase than in chronic myelogenous leukemia. Even serum LDH is frequently normal.

Even serum LDH is frequently normal.

Direct Coombs' test is positive in up to one-third of patients.

Hypogammaglobulinemia occurs in two-thirds of patients depending on duration of disease; monoclonal gammopathy (most often IgM) is found in some cases.

Uric acid levels are not increased but may become during therapy.

Table 12-16. Comparison of Chronic Lymphocytic Leukemias

	WBC count × 10^9/L	% Involvement Lymph Nodes	Spleen	Skin	Other
B lymphocytes					
Chronic lymphocytic leukemia	10–200	50	50	5	[a]
Prolymphocytic leukemia	100–>500	25	>90	5	[b]
Waldenström's macroglobulinemia	N–50	30	30	<5	[c]
Leukemic phase of poorly differentiated lymphoma (follicular or diffuse)	N–>100	90	75	5	[d]
Hairy-cell leukemia	<1–100	30	>75	<5	[e]
T lymphocytes					
Chronic lymphocytic leukemia	>20–200	50	50	10	[f]
Adult T-cell leukemia/lymphoma	N–>150	90	>50	>50	[g]
Prolymphocytic leukemia	100–>500	25	>90	<10	[h]
T-gamma-chronic lymphoproliferative disease	N–>300	10	30	<10	[i]
Cutaneous T-cell lymphoma	N–>150	>50	10	100	[j]
Hairy-cell leukemia	Decreased	30	>75	–	[k]

N = normal.

[a]See preceding section. Autoimmune hemolytic anemia, hypogammaglobulinemia.

[b]B-type lymphocytes derived from medullary cords of lymph nodes show less mature forms than in chronic lymphocytic leukemia, extreme leukocytosis with very high blast counts, prominent splenomegaly often without much lymphadenopathy.

[c]Increased serum IgM.

[d]Usually is leukemic phase of lymphoma but up to 50% have marrow involvement when first seen; occasionally may present without node involvement.

[e]Pancytopenia and prominent splenomegaly; usually leukopenia but some patients have increased WBCs with many hairy cells.

[f]Causes <5% of cases of chronic lymphocytic leukemia.

[g]Hypercalcemia, lytic bone lesions; may have HTLV-1 infection; WBC usually >50,000/cu mm.

[h]Morphologically identical to B-cell type, but lymphadenopathy is more frequent in T-cell type.

[i]Decreased WBC with granulocytopenia; recurrent infections are common; usually no lymphadenopathy or skin involvement.

[j]Sézary syndrome refers to both skin and systemic involvement; mycosis fungoides is cutaneous form, which may be present for years before clinical systemic involvement.

[k]Can only be distinguished from B-cell form by immune studies.

Philadelphia chromosome is not found.

Chromosomal abnormalities in ~50% of patients, most often chromosomes 12 (especially trisomy 12) and 14 (especially 14q+).

Minimum requirements for diagnosis are lymphocyte count >15,000/cu mm and marrow infiltration >30% for >6 months.

PROLYMPHOCYTIC LEUKEMIA

Is rare variant of chronic lymphocytic leukemia (CLL). May occur de novo or from CLL. ~80% are B-cell and 20% are T-cell type.

Compared to CLL, has more rapid clinical course, poorer prognosis, slightly older, larger spleen, less frequent lymphadenopathy, higher prolymphocyte count (>55%), and immunologic differences (mouse erythrocytes, rosettes, surface immunoglobulin staining).

SÉZARY SYNDROME

Syndrome of skin lesion due to infiltration of Sézary cells associated with presence of these cells in peripheral blood.

Increased peripheral blood lymphocyte count, >15% of which are atypical lymphocytes (Sézary cells)

Total WBC often increased

ESR, hemoglobin, and platelet counts usually normal

Bone marrow, lymph nodes, and liver biopsy usually normal

LEUKEMIC RETICULOENDOTHELIOSIS

This is a rare condition of splenomegaly and absence of lymphadenopathy with characteristic pathologic changes in marrow and spleen that often respond to splenectomy but not to chemotherapy.

Diagnosis is established by finding the characteristic cells in the peripheral blood or bone marrow. These cells show a characteristic histochemical reaction of tartrate-resistant acid phosphatase (isoenzyme 5) activity. This isoenzyme 5 may also be increased in the serum.

Hypersplenism causing thrombocytopenia, anemia, and leukopenia of varying degrees is present.

Increased ESR may be present.

Abnormal platelet function may be found.

Leukocyte alkaline phosphatase activity is markedly increased in some patients.

HODGKIN'S DISEASE AND OTHER MALIGNANT LYMPHOMAS

Diagnosis is established by histologic findings of biopsied lymph node.

Blood findings may vary from completely normal to markedly abnormal.

Moderate normochromic normocytic anemia occurs, occasionally of the hemolytic type; may become severe.

Peripheral blood changes in Hodgkin's disease are common (~25% of cases at time of diagnosis) but not specific. WBC may be normal, decreased, or slightly or markedly increased (25,000/cu mm). Leukopenia, marked leukocytosis, anemia are bad prognostic signs. Eosinophilia occurs in ~20% of patients. Relative and absolute lymphopenia may occur. If lymphocytosis is present, look for another disease. Neutrophilia may be found. Monocytosis may be found. These changes may all be absent or may even be present simultaneously or in various combinations. Rarely, Reed-Sternberg cells are found in marrow or peripheral blood smears in advanced disease.

Small lymphocytic and follicular lymphomas often have malignant lymphocytes in peripheral blood; leukemic phase in 5–15% of patients. Cytopenias occur commonly due to hypersplenism, immune effect, or lymphoma effect on marrow.

Bone marrow involvement at time of diagnosis in <10% of patients with Hodgkin's disease; 50% of patients with diffuse, small cleaved lymphoma and mixed cell type; 70–80% of patients with follicular, small cleaved cell lymphoma; less frequent in large cell lymphomas.

Increased serum LDH, uric acid, and abnormal liver function tests are common in non-Hodgkin's lymphomas.

Serum protein electrophoresis: Albumin is frequently decreased. Increased $alpha_1$ and $alpha_2$ globulins suggest disease activity. Decreased gamma globulin is less frequent in Hodgkin's disease than in lymphosarcoma. Gamma globulins may be increased, with macroglobulins present and evidence of autoimmune process (e.g., hemolytic anemia, cold agglutinins, positive LE test).

ESR and CRP are increased during active stages in ~50% of patients; may be normal during remission.

Hodgkin's disease patients commonly have deficiencies of cell-mediated immunity with increased susceptibility to bacterial, fungal, and viral (especially herpes zoster and varicella) infections; these persist even after cure. Serum immunoglobulins are usually normal.

Laboratory findings due to involvement of other organ systems (e.g., liver, kidney) are noted.

Laboratory findings due to effects of treatment (e.g., radiation, chemotherapy, splenectomy) including acute and long-term toxicity and second neoplasms.

Non-Hodgkin's lymphoma occurs frequently in AIDS patients and shows rapid course, poor prognosis, frequent extranodal and CNS involvement.

MYCOSIS FUNGOIDES

Biopsy of lesion (usually skin) shows microscopic findings that parallel clinical findings.

Laboratory findings are generally not helpful.

Bone marrow may show increase in reticuloendothelial cells, monoblasts, lymphocytes, plasma cells.

Peripheral blood may occasionally show increased eosinophils, monocytes, and lymphocytes.

Mycosis fungoides cells in peripheral blood or marrow suggest extensive disease.

ANGIOIMMUNOBLASTIC LYMPHADENOPATHY

(rare lymphoproliferative disorder with sudden onset of constitutional symptoms and lymphadenopathy; very poor prognosis)

Diagnosis requires a lymph node biopsy that shows characteristic changes (loss of architecture and germinal centers, arborization of postcapillary venules, proliferation of immunoblasts, B- and T-lymphocytes and plasma cells), but these alone do not permit diagnosis, and the clinical findings are required.

Anemia is often hemolytic, Coombs' positive.

Leukocytosis with lymphopenia

Thrombocytopenia

Nonspecific hypergammaglobulinemia

High frequency of autoantibodies and often associated with other autoimmune syndromes, especially SLE.

Death usually due to infection associated with T-cell immune deficiency (e.g., CMV, EBV, herpes simplex, *Pneumocystis carinii,* mycobacteria, opportunistic fungi).

Lymphomas (B- or T-cell type or rarely Hodgkin's disease) develop in 5–20% of patients.

Serologic tests for HIV are negative.

CLASSIFICATION OF MONOCLONAL GAMMOPATHIES

- Malignant
  - Multiple myeloma
    - Symptomatic
    - Asymptomatic and indolent (smoldering)

Table 12-17. Comparison of Diseases with Monoclonal Immunoglobulins

	Multiple Myeloma	Macroglobulinemia	Benign Monoclonal Gammopathy	Heavy-Chain Diseases		
				Gamma	Alpha	Mu
Clinical	Bone lesions Anemia Infections	Enlarged LNN, L, S	None	Enlarged LNN, L, S	Intestinal malabsorption	Enlarged LNN, L, S
Bone marrow	Sheets of plasma cells	Lymphocytosis or lymphocytoid plasma cells	Up to 10% plasma cells	Plasma cells or lymphocytoid plasma cells	—	Lymphocytosis or lymphocytoid plasma cells with vacuoles
Monoclonal Ig in serum (electrophoresis)	80%	Present	Present	Present	Present	Present

Bence Jones protein in urine (electrophoresis)	70–80%	80–95%	Rare	Common	Rare	Common
Serum (immunoelectrophoresis)	1 type of M chain[a] 1 type of L chain[b]	Mu chain 1 type of L chain[b]	1 type of M chain[a] 1 type of L chain[b]	Gamma chain No L	Alpha chain No L	Mu chain Free kappa or lambda in two-thirds
Urine (immunoelectrophoresis)	Kappa or lambda	Kappa or lambda	Rare kappa or lambda	Gamma chain	—	Kappa or lambda in two-thirds

LNN = lymph nodes; L = liver; S = spleen.

[a] M chain is gamma, alpha, mu, delta, or epsilon.

[b] L chain is kappa or lambda.

Monoclonal proteins (paraproteins, M proteins) are immunoglobulins synthesized by atypical cells of reticuloendothelial system. Each is a homogeneous product of a single clone of proliferating cells and is expressed as a monoclonal gammopathy. Monoclonal proteins consist of two heavy polypeptide chains of the same class (e.g., gamma, alpha, mu) and subclass and two light polypeptide chains of the same type (either kappa or lambda); may be present in serum, urine, and CSF. Heavy-chain disease is production of only heavy chains without accompanying light chains; light-chain disease is the reverse. They are detected by conventional protein electrophoresis and identified by immunoelectrophoresis.

Table 12-18. Immunochemical Frequency (%) of Monoclonal Gammopathies

IgG (with/without BJ)	60
IgA (with/without BJ)	15
IgM (with/without BJ)	10–15
Light chain (BJ only)	15
Rare	
IgD (with/without BJ)	1
Heavy chain	1
Gamma heavy-chain disease	
Alpha heavy-chain disease	
Mu heavy-chain disease	
IgE (with/without BJ)	0.1
Biclonal (IgG + IgM)	
Triclonal	

BJ = Bence Jones proteins.

- Plasma cell leukemia
- Nonsecretory
- Osteosclerotic

Plasmacytoma
- Solitary of bone
- Extramedullary

Malignant lymphoproliferative diseases
- Waldenström's macroglobulinemia
- Malignant lymphoma

Heavy-chain diseases
- Gamma
- Alpha
- Mu
- Delta (very rare)

Amyloidosis
- Secondary to multiple myeloma
- Primary

Unknown significance
- Idiopathic
- Others

IDIOPATHIC ("BENIGN," "ASYMPTOMATIC") MONOCLONAL GAMMOPATHY (PLASMA CELL DYSCRASIA OF UNKNOWN SIGNIFICANCE) (MGUS)

(found in 0.5% of normal persons > age 30, 3% > age 70, and ≤10% age 80)

The following changes are present for a period of >5 years.

- Monoclonal serum protein concentration < 3 gm/dl; IgG type in 90% of patients; normal immunoglobulins may be depressed. In contrast, multiple myeloma always shows depression of background immunoglobulins and higher monoclonal serum protein (>3 gm/dl).
- Normal serum albumin
- <5% plasma cells in bone marrow
- Absence of Bence Jones protein, anemia, myeloma bone lesions
- Monoclonal light-chain proteinuria may occur (up to 1 gm/24 hours).
- May be associated with aging, cholecystitis, neoplasms, many chronic diseases (most often rheumatoid arthritis).

Periodic reexamination is essential because approximately 10% of these patients will develop myeloma, macroglobulinemia, lymphoma, or amyloidosis

Table 12-19. Comparison of Multiple Myeloma and MGUS

	Multiple Myeloma	MGUS
Paraprotein level	Higher	Lower (rarely >3 gm/dl)
Nonparaprotein immunoglobulins suppressed	96% of cases	12% of cases
Bence Jones proteinuria	57% of cases	17% of cases
Bone marrow plasmacytosis >20%	100% of cases	4% of cases

within 5 years and 20% at 10 years; no definite predictive factors permit recognition of this group but more likely to become malignant if these criteria are present and converse if these criteria are absent:

IgG > 200 mg/dl, or either IgA or IgM > 100 mg/dl or IgD or IgE paraprotein is found at any concentration.
Ig fragments in urine (usually Bence Jones protein) or serum
Progressive increase in paraprotein concentration
Low levels of polyclonal Ig

One study (Malacrida V, DeFrancesco D, Banf G, et al. Laboratory investigation of monoclonal gammopathy during 10 years of screening in a general hospital. *J Clin Pathol* 40:793, 1987) showed the following:

Paraproteinemia by electrophoresis was found in 730 of 102,000 samples (0.7%) in a general hospital. 375 had paraprotein ≥200 mg/dl (2 gm/L).
114 of these were B lymphocytic malignancy:
- 96—multiple myeloma
- 4—Waldenström's macroglobulinemia
- 8—chronic lymphatic leukemia
- 6—non-Hodgkin's lymphoma

261 were monoclonal gammopathy of undefined significance (MGUS).

MULTIPLE MYELOMA

Essential Diagnostic Criteria

Bone marrow shows sheets or >20% plasma cells and
Abnormality of immunoglobulin formation (monoclonal spike >4 gm/dl or Bence Jones (BJ) proteinuria >0.5 gm/24 hours)
If monoclonal spike is <4 gm/dl, then substitute criteria:
Reciprocal depression of normal immunoglobulins or panhypogammaglobulinemia and osteolytic bone lesions or plasmacytosis not due to other causes (see Plasma Cells, p. 264)

Very elevated serum total protein is due to increase in globulins (with decreased albumin-globulin [A/G] ratio) in one-half to two-thirds of the patients.
Serum protein immunoelectrophoresis characterizes protein as monoclonal (i.e., one light-chain type) and classifies disease by identifying specific heavy chain. It reveals abnormal immunoglobulins in 80% of patients. An immunoelectrophoretic serum or urine monoclonal paraprotein can be identified in >98% of patients with multiple myeloma.

% of Patients	Show
60%	Serum monoclonal spike
20%	Both serum and urine monoclonal protein
20%	Monoclonal light chains in urine only
<2%	Hypogammaglobulinemia only without serum or urine paraprotein

60%	IgG myeloma protein
20%	IgA myeloma protein
Very rare	IgE myeloma protein
<1%	IgD myeloma protein*

BJ proteinuria occurs in 35–50% of patients. >50% of IgG or IgA myeloma and 100% of light-chain myelomas have BJ proteinuria. (Dipstick tests for urine protein will miss BJ protein, and heat precipitation is not a reliable test; see pp. 87, 89, 91.)

Electrophoresis of both serum and urine is abnormal in almost all patients. If only serum electrophoresis is performed, kappa and some lambda light-chain myelomas will be missed. 15% of patients have hypogammaglobulinemia (<0.6 gm/dl).

Bone marrow aspiration usually shows 20–50% plasma cells or myeloma cells, usually in sheets; abnormal plasma cells may be found (flaming cells, morular cells, Mott cells, thesaurocytes); multiple sites may be required.

Hematologic findings

- Anemia (normocytic, normochromic; rarely macrocytic) in 60% of patients
- Usually normal WBC and platelet count; 40–55% lymphocytes frequently present on differential count, with variable number of immature lymphocytic and plasmacytic forms.
- Decreased WBC and platelet counts are seen in about 20% of patients, usually with extensive marrow replacement.
- Eosinophilia may be found.
- Rouleaux formation (due to serum protein changes) in 85% of patients, occasionally causing difficulty in cross matching blood
- Increased ESR in 90% of patients and other abnormalities due to serum protein changes. May be normal in light-chain myeloma. >100 is rare in any condition other than myeloma.
- Cold agglutinins or cryoglobulins

Hyperviscosity syndrome is characteristic of IgM and occurs in 4% of IgG and 10% of IgA myeloma and may be the presenting feature. Symptoms are usually present when relative serum viscosity = 6–7 centipoises (normal <1.8).

Clinical amyloidosis occurs in 15% of cases of multiple myeloma, but monoclonal spikes are present in urine in most, if not all, cases of primary amyloidosis. IgD myeloma and light-chain disease are associated with amyloidosis and early renal failure more frequently than other types of myeloma.

Serum beta$_2$ microglobulin is increased in proliferative disorders where there is rapid cell multiplication or increased tumor burden. >6 μg/ml indicates poor prognosis (normal <2 μg/ml); may also be increased by renal failure.

Chromosome analysis frequently shows translocation t(11;14)(q13;q32).

Laboratory findings of repeated bacterial infections, especially those due to *Diplococcus pneumoniae, Staphylococcus aureus,* and *Escherichia coli.*

See bone diseases of calcium and phosphorus, Table 14-6, pp. 472–473.

- Serum calcium is markedly increased in 25–50% of patients.†
- Serum phosphorus is usually normal.
- Serum alkaline phosphatase is usually normal or slightly increased. Increase may reflect amyloidosis of liver rather than bone disease.
- Hypercalciuria causing dehydration and tubular dysfunction

See Kidney in Multiple Myeloma, p. 589.

- BUN and creatinine are increased in about 50% of patients.

*IgD myeloma is difficult to recognize because serum levels are relatively low, specific antiserum is required to demonstrate IgD; on electrophoresis, IgD is often included in beta globulin peak, and clinical features are the same as in other types of myeloma. *Bence Jones proteinuria is almost always present, and total protein is often normal.*

†Corrected calcium (mg/dl) = serum calcium (mg/dl) − serum albumin (gm/dl) + 4.0

Uric acid is increased in 60% of patients, but uric acid stones and gout are rare.
Renal function is decreased in <50% of patients.
Urinalysis abnormalities appear—e.g., albumin, casts.
Renal failure is usually present when there is a marked increase of BJ protein in blood.

Presymptomatic phase (may last many years) may show only
Unexplained persistent proteinuria
Increased ESR
Myeloma protein in serum or urine
Repeated bacterial infections, especially pneumonias (6 times greater incidence)
Amyloidosis (see pp. 702–704)

High tumor mass (clinical stage III) is present when any of the following are present:
Hemoglobin <8.5 gm/dl
Corrected calcium >12 mg/dl
Serum IgG >7 gm/dl
Serum IgA >5 gm/dl
BJ proteinuria >12 gm/day
Advanced lytic bone lesions
Low tumor mass (stage I) is present when all of the following are present:
Hemoglobin >10 gm/dl
Normal corrected calcium
Serum IgG <5 gm/dl
Serum IgA <3 gm/dl
BJ proteinuria <4 gm/day
Generalized lytic bone lesions are absent.
Stage II has intermediate values.
Subclassified as A if serum creatinine <2 mg/dl or B if >2 mg/dl
Survival varies from 61 months for stage IA patients to 15 months for stage IIIB patients.
Serial measurement of serum globulins and/or BJ proteinuria is excellent indication of efficacy of chemotherapy; decrease in BJ proteinuria occurs before decrease in abnormal serum globulin peak

Lowered anion gap in IgG myeloma only (due to cationic IgG paraproteins causing retention of excess chloride ion)
Increased incidence of other neoplasms (not known if related to chemotherapy)
Acute myelomonocytic leukemia, often preceded by sideroblastic refractory anemia, is increasingly seen.
20% of patients develop adenocarcinoma of GI tract, biliary tree, or breast.

LOCALIZED PLASMACYTOMA

Diagnosis is based on histologic finding of tumor of plasma cells, which are identical to those of multiple myeloma.
Bone marrow shows no evidence of plasmacytosis.
X-rays and bone scans are negative for other myeloma bone lesions.
Myeloma proteins are low or normal concentration in serum or concentrated urine.
Nonmyeloma immunoglobulin concentration in serum is generally normal.
Paraprotein is detectable in 80–90% of cases of solitary plasmacytoma of bone, often at very low concentrations. IgG kappa is most common; IgA and Bence Jones have been described.
Following local radiotherapy, level of any myeloma protein is reduced and level of nonmyeloma immunoglobulins may be increased above normal.

Table 12-20. Comparison of Immunoproliferative Disorders

Disease	Relative Frequency (%)	Ig		Urine BJ (%)	Complications/ Associated Conditions
		Heavy Chain	Light Chain		
Myelomas					
IgG	75	γ	κ or λ	60	Infection
IgA	15	α	κ or λ	70	Infection
IgD	<2	δ	Usually λ	100	Amyloidosis
IgE	Very rare	ϵ	κ or λ	?	Plasma cell leukemia
Light-chain myeloma	10	None	κ or λ	100	Amyloid kidney Hypercalcemia
Macroglobulinemia		μ	κ or λ	30–40	Hyperviscosity Hemolytic anemia (cold agglutinin) Bleeding
Heavy-chain disease					
Gamma			None	γ chain	
Alpha			None	None	GI tract lymphoma Malabsorption
Mu			None	κ chain BJ	Amyloidosis Chronic lymphocytic leukemia

Solitary plasmacytoma of bone is considered to represent the earliest stage of multiple myeloma and 50–60% of cases progress to multiple myeloma within 5 years. 15% remain solitary; 12% develop local recurrence; 15% develop new distant lesions.

CSF total protein, albumin, and IgG may be increased if a vertebral lesion extends into the spinal canal.

In addition to solitary plasmacytoma of bone, extramedullary plasmacytoma may occur, chiefly in upper respiratory tract. Diagnosis is based on histologic examination of tumor and same criteria as above. Development of multiple myeloma is infrequent.

PLASMA CELL LEUKEMIA

WBC usually >15,000, with >20% plasma cells in peripheral blood varying from typical plasmacytes to immature and atypical forms; absolute plasma cell count > 2000/cu mm. Occasionally, special studies (cytochemical stains, cell surface and cytoplasmic markers, electron microscopy) are needed to confirm identity of plasma cells.

Plasma cell monoclonality

- ~60% of cases are primary, and the rest occur in 2% of previously diagnosed cases of multiple myeloma. Primary cases have smaller M-protein peak in serum, higher platelet count, younger age and longer survival. Other findings (see under Multiple Myeloma, pp. 345–347)

SMOLDERING MULTIPLE MYELOMA

Serum M protein > 3 gm/dl; uninvolved immunoglobulins are decreased.

Bone marrow shows >10% atypical plasma cells.

Urine frequently contains a small amount of M protein.

No anemia, renal insufficiency, or bone lesions

OSTEOSCLEROTIC MYELOMA

Diagnosis based on biopsy from single or multiple osteosclerotic bone lesion

Bone marrow aspiration shows <5% plasma cells.

Lambda M protein is usually present.

Absence of anemia, hypercalcemia, renal insufficiency

Erythrocytosis and thrombocytosis may occur.

CNS protein is increased.

CRYOGLOBULINEMIA

Type I—cryoglobulins (monoclonal immunoglobulin, especially IgM)

- Causes 25% of cases, most commonly multiple myeloma and Waldenström's macroglobulinemia; may be idiopathic
- Often present in large amounts (>5 mg/dl serum)

Type II (monoclonal immunoglobulin mixed with at least one other type of polyclonal immunoglobulin, most commonly IgM and polyclonal IgG; often has rheumatoid factor)

- Causes up to 25% of cases

Type III (mixed polyclonal immunoglobulin, most commonly IgM-IgG combinations)

- Causes ~50% of cases
- Usually present in small amounts (<1 mg/dl serum)

May Be Associated With

Infections

- Viral (e.g., EBV, CMV, hepatitis B)
- Bacterial (e.g., endocarditis, leprosy, lymphogranuloma venereum)
- Spirochetal (e.g., syphilis, Lyme disease)
- Fungal (e.g., coccidioidomycosis)
- Parasitic (e.g., malaria, toxoplasmosis, schistosomiasis)

Autoimmune
- SLE
- Polyarthritis nodosa
- Rheumatoid arthritis
- Sjögren's syndrome
- Scleroderma
- Sarcoidosis
- Behçet's syndrome
- Thyroiditis
- Schönlein-Henoch purpura
- Idiopathic thrombocytopenic purpura
- Autoimmune hemolytic anemia

Lymphoproliferative diseases
- Multiple myeloma
- Waldenström's macroglobulinemia
- Lymphoma, chronic lymphocytic leukemia

Idiopathic (essential) mixed cryoglobulinemia
- No other major disease is present.
- Predominantly mixed type

Recurrent purpura may occur.
Cryoprecipitate may be seen in serum.
Rheumatoid factor is present in cryoglobulins.
Serum protein electrophoresis is unremarkable or shows diffuse hyperglobulinemia.
May cause erroneous WBC when performed on electronic cell counter
Rouleaux formation may occur.
ESR may be increased at 37°C but is normal at room temperature.
Components of complement system (especially C2) are decreased.
Laboratory findings of other associated conditions may occur
- Liver disease—e.g., serologic evidence of hepatitis B virus in 60%
- Renal disease—e.g., nephrosis, immune glomerular disease. Renal failure develops in ~50%, and marked proteinuria occurs in ~25%.
- Skin biopsy shows cutaneous vasculitis, often with immune reactants in vessel walls.

CRYOFIBRINOGENEMIA

Plasma precipitates when oxalated blood is refrigerated at 4°C overnight.
May cause erroneous WBC when performed on electronic cell counter
May be associated with increased $alpha_1$ antitrypsin, haptoglobin, $alpha_2$ macroglobulin (by immunodiffusion technique), and with increased plasma fibrinogen; not associated with cryoglobulins
Has been reported in association with many conditions, especially
- Neoplasms
- Thromboembolic conditions

MACROGLOBULINEMIA (PRIMARY; WALDENSTRÖM'S)

Electrophoresis of serum shows an intense sharp peak in globulin fraction, usually in the gamma zone, identified typically as IgM by immunoelectrophoresis. The pattern may be indistinguishable from that in multiple myeloma.
Total serum protein and globulin are markedly increased.
ESR is very high.
Rouleaux formation is marked; positive Coombs' reaction; difficulty in cross matching blood.
Severe anemia, usually normochromic normocytic, occasionally hemolytic
WBC is decreased, with relative lymphocytosis; monocytes or eosinophils may be increased.
Bone marrow sections are always hypercellular and show extensive infiltration

with atypical "lymphocytes" and also plasma cells; increased number of mast cells

Lymph node shows malignant lymphoma, usually well-differentiated lymphocytic lymphoma with plasmacytoid features.

Flow cytometry shows ≤50% of patients have circulating monoclonal B-lymphocyte population.

Spleen and liver involvement occurs in ~50% of patients.

Persistent oronasal hemorrhage occurs in ~75% of patients.

Coagulation abnormalities: may be decreased platelets, abnormal bleeding time, coagulation time, PT, prothrombin consumption, etc.

50% of patients with Waldenström's macroglobulinemia have hyperviscosity syndrome due to large IgM molecule causing coagulation abnormalities (see previous sentence). (Normal serum viscosity ≤1.8 centipoises.)

IgM may also cause cryoglobulinemia.

Bence Jones proteinuria is found in 10% of patients.

Impaired renal function is much less common than in myeloma.

Amyloidosis is rare.

Lytic bone lesions are absent.

Macroglobulinemia may also be associated with neoplasms, collagen diseases, cirrhosis, chronic infections.

GAMMA HEAVY-CHAIN DISEASE

(a lymphoma-like disease with excessive production of heavy-chain proteins)

Serum protein electrophoresis
- Abnormal protein related to heavy chain (Fc fragment) and unrelated to light chain and Bence Jones; similar in serum and urine
- Gamma globulin almost absent
- Localized spikes or bands may be absent.

Serum tests
- Reversed A/G ratio
- Increased uric acid (>8.5 mg/dl)
- Increased BUN (30–50 mg/dl)

Hematologic findings
- Autoimmune hemolytic anemia almost always present; leukopenia and thrombocytopenia common (probably due to hypersplenism)
- Eosinophilia sometimes marked; relative lymphocytosis
- Vacuolated mononuclear cells sometimes seen
- Bone marrow and lymph nodes show many atypical plasmacytic and lymphocytic cells.

Urine tests
- Trace to 1+ protein
- Negative for Bence Jones protein
- Identical to abnormal serum protein on electrophoresis

Marked susceptibility to bacterial infection

Histologic findings of associated lymphoma, e.g., extranodal non-Hodgkins's lymphoma

ALPHA HEAVY-CHAIN DISEASE

(Mediterranean-type abdominal lymphoma)

Chronic diarrhea and malabsorption due to diffuse lymphoma-like proliferation in small intestine and mesentery

Laboratory findings of malabsorption

Biopsy of small intestine shows marked infiltration with abnormal plasma cells.

Serum protein electrophoresis shows distinctive increase in monoclonal IgA heavy chains (alpha chains) causing an elevated broad peak in half the cases and is normal in half the cases. Relatively low concentration of alpha chains in urine (compared to gamma heavy-chain disease)

Bence Jones proteinuria is absent.

Mu HEAVY-CHAIN DISEASE

(usually associated with chronic lymphocytic leukemia or a lymphoma)

Serum electrophoresis shows hypogammaglobulinemia, usually without a localized peak or band
Bence Jones proteinuria in two-thirds of patients
Bone marrow shows vacuolated plasma cells.

CONGENITAL X-LINKED AGAMMAGLOBULINEMIA (BRUTON'S DISEASE)

Probably represents a heterogeneous group of defects
Male patients suffer severe pyogenic infections (commonly due to *Streptococcus pneumoniae, Hemophilus influenzae, Neisseria meningitidis*) after age 4–6 months.
- Often have persistent viral (e.g., chronic, progressive, fatal CNS infection with echoviruses) or parasitic infections

Inability to make functional antibody is the distinguishing feature; antibody responses to immunization are usually absent. Live virus vaccination may cause severe disease (e.g., paralytic polio).
Serum levels of immunoglobulins (IgG, IgA, IgM) are very low (total <100 mg/dl).
B cells in peripheral blood detected by surface immunoglobulin techniques are absent or found in very low numbers; however, cells bearing complement receptor (EAC rosettes determination) may be normal.
Plasma cells in lymph nodes and GI tract are absent or found in very low numbers.
T cell numbers and function are intact.
There are no markers for detection of heterozygotes.
Hypoplasia of tonsils, adenoids, lymph nodes. Thymus appears normal with Hassall's corpuscles and abundant lymphoid cells.
Increased frequency of lymphoreticular malignancy (up to 6%).

IMMUNODEFICIENCY WITH INCREASED IgM

Normal or increased number of IgM-producing B cells and plasma cells
Normal or more frequently markedly increased serum IgM with very low serum IgG and IgA
B cells with IgG or IgA are virtually absent.
Normal titers of isohemagglutinins and opsonic antibodies to many polysaccharide-coated bacteria
No IgG antibody response following immunization or infection
Increased frequency of autoimmune disorders
Autoimmune hemolytic anemia and thrombocytopenia are commonly associated findings.
Neutropenia is common.
Lymphoid hyperplasia is frequently present.

SELECTIVE IgM DEFICIENCY

(few cases are well-documented)

Decreased serum IgM
Decreased to absent isohemagglutinins
Low levels of opsonins to gram-negative and polysaccharide-coated bacteria
In children and adults who often have serious infections, e.g., sepsis, meningitis

SELECTIVE IgA DEFICIENCY

(a more common immunodeficiency syndrome; lack of IgA-producing cells in intestinal lamina propria)

Secretory and serum IgA is very low (<10 mg/dl) or absent.
Serum IgM and IgG are usually normal.

Table 12-21. Tests for Immune Deficiency

Arm of the Immune System Deficient	Screening Tests	Definitive Tests[a]	Type of Infection[b]	Suggestive Organism	Example of Immunodeficiency Disease
Antibody	Quantitative IgM, IgG, IgA Rubella titer Isohemagglutinins	Diphtheria-tetanus titer Pneumococcal titer B-lymphocytes Plasma cells	Sinusitis, diarrhea, failure to thrive	*S. pneumoniae*, nontypeable *H. influenzae*, *Giardia lamblia* from gut	Bruton's disease, selective IgA deficiency, hypogammaglobulinemia with normal or increased IgM
Complement	Total hemolytic C3, C4, C5 Factor B	Chemotactic factors Opsonins Immunoelectrophoretic analysis	Sinusitis	*S. pneumoniae*, *Neisseria* species	Deficiency of C3, C3b inactivator, Factor B, C6, C7, C8
Phagocytes	WBC and differential count Nitroblue tetrazolium test (NBT) IgE	Chemotaxis Adhesion Aggregation Chemiluminescence Phagocytosis and killing	Osteomyelitis, eczema, stomatitis, furunculosis, liver abscess, draining lymphadenitis	*S. aureus*, *S. epidermidis*, *C. albicans*, *S. marcescens*	Primary or secondary neutropenia, chronic granulomatous disease, Chédiak-Higashi syndrome
Cell-mediated immunity	Skin tests (e.g., *C. albicans*)	T-cell rosette Mitogen responses Suppressor or helper cells	Failure to thrive, autoimmune disease, eczema, diarrhea, candidiasis (perineal/oral)	Lungs—CMV, *Pneumocystis carinii*, varicella-zoster virus, *Cryptococcus*, *Nocardia*, recurrent *Candida*	Wiskott-Aldrich syndrome, ataxia-telangiectasia, thymic hypoplasia, severe combined immunodeficiency disease

[a] At special immunologic centers.
[b] Severe or recurrent pneumonia, acute otitis media in all groups.

Table 12-22. Classification of Primary Immunologic Defects

Syndrome	Number of Circulating Lymphocytes	Number of Plasma Cells	Immunoglobulin Changes	Thymus	Lymph Node: Germinal Center	Lymph Node: Paracortical Zone	Other Laboratory Findings
Infantile sex-linked agammaglobulinemia (Bruton's disease)	N	O	Markedly D in all	N	O	N	X; increased frequency of malignant lymphoma
Selective inability to produce IgA	N	IgA-producing plasma cells, especially in lamina propria	IgA is O; others are usually N	N	N	N	May have malabsorption syndrome, steatorrhea, bronchitis
Transient hypogammaglobulinemia of infancy	N	D	IgG is D		O or rare		X
Non-sex-linked primary immunoglobulin deficiencies (e.g., dysgammaglobulinemias—acquired, congenital)	N	V (usually D)	Present, but type and amount are V	N	Usually O; Reticulum hyperplasia	Often D; Reticulum hyperplasia	X, Z; increased frequency of malignant lymphoma and autoimmune diseases
Agammaglobulinemia with thymoma (Good's syndrome)	Progressively D, often to very low levels	D or O	Markedly D in all	Enlarged (stromal epithelial spindle-cell type)	D or O	May be D	X, Z; thymoma (see p. 358); pure red cell aplasia may occur; eosinophils O or markedly D
Wiskott-Aldrich syndrome (X-linked, recessive immune deficiency with thrombopenia and eczema)	Usually progressively D	N	Usually present, but type and amount are V (frequently IgM is D and IgA is I); IgG usually N	N	May be D	Progressively D in lymphocytes	X, Z; eczema and thrombocytopenia; increased frequency of malignant lymphoma; serum lacks isohemagglutinins; platelets ½ normal size

Ataxia-telangiectasia (Louis-Bar syndrome), autosomal recessive	V (usually slightly D)	V (usually present)	Usually present, but type and amount are V (frequently IgA and IgE are D or O, and D IgG)	Embryonic type (no Hassall's corpuscles or cortical medullary organization)	May be D	Lymphocytes D	Progressive cerebellar ataxia; telangiectasia in tissues; ovarian dysgenesis; increased frequency of malignant lymphoma; frequent pulmonary infections when IgA is D
Primary lymphopenic immunologic deficiency (Gitlin's syndrome)	V–D	V	Always present, but type and amount are V	Hypoplastic (Hassall's corpuscles and lymphoid cells D)	Marked D in tissue lymphocytes; foci of lymphocytes may be present in spleen and lymph nodes		Z
Autosomal recessive alymphocytic agammaglobulinemia (Swiss type agammaglobulinemia; Glanzmann and Riniker's lymphocytophthisis)	Markedly D	O	Markedly D in all	Hypoplastic (Hassall's corpuscles and lymphoid cells O)	Lymphocytes O or markedly D		X, Z; increased frequency of malignant lymphoma
Autosomal recessive lymphopenia with normal immunoglobulins (Nezelof's syndrome)	D	Present	N	Hypoplastic (Hassall's corpuscles and lymphoid cells O)	May be present	Lymphocytes markedly D	Z
DiGeorge's syndrome (thymic aplasia)	V (usually N)	Present	N	Absent	Present	Rare paracortical lymphocytes present	Z; absent parathyroids (tetany of the newborn); frequent cardiovascular malformations

N = normal; O = absent; D = decreased; V = variable; X = recurrent infections with pyogenic organisms; Z = frequent virus, fungus, or *Pneumocystis* infection.
Source: Adapted from M Seligmann, HH Fudenberg, and RA Good, A proposed classification of primary immunologic deficiencies. *Am. J. Med.* 45:818, 1968.

Serum antibodies to IgA in >40% of patients; therefore IV or IM blood products that contain IgA (e.g., immune serum globulin) are contraindicated.
Peripheral blood lymphocytes bearing IgA, IgM, and IgG are normal.
Plasma cells producing IgA are absent in GI and respiratory epithelium.
Clinical—asymptomatic or recurrent pyogenic respiratory infections; increased incidence of atopic disease, rheumatoid arthritis, lymphonodular hyperplasia of small intestine. Found in 1:333 blood donors.

COMMON VARIABLE (OR "ACQUIRED") HYPOGAMMAGLOBULINEMIA

(a more common immunodeficiency syndrome in children and adults)

Can result from three different immunologic causes: intrinsic B-cell defects, immunoregulatory T-cell imbalances, or autoantibodies to T or B cells.
Clinically, may resemble X-linked agammaglobulinemia, but infections are less severe, have equal sex distribution, and may have normal or enlarged tonsils and lymph nodes and enlarged spleen.
Serum IgG is decreased (<250 μg/μl).
Other immunoglobulin abnormalities are variable.
Severe infections due to *S. pneumoniae, H. influenzae* causing sepsis, pneumonia, meningitis are common. Usually present with chronic progressive bronchiectasis. Many have sprue-like syndrome due to *Giardia lamblia.* Sterile noncaseating granulomas can occur in liver, spleen, lung, skin.
Associated with autoimmune diseases, e.g., pernicious anemia occurs in about one-third of patients, SLE, rheumatoid arthritis.
T-lymphocyte function may be impaired.
Number of peripheral blood B cells may be low or high but fail to differentiate into antibody-secreting cells.
Alternative complement pathway defects
- Special studies show contribution of alternative pathway to opsonization.
- Decreased levels of specific factors (e.g., Factor B) may be found.
- Impaired generation of chemotactic factors or decreased hemolytic activity may occur.
- Due to
  - Sickle cell disease with splenic infarction
  - Postsplenectomy
  - Nephrotic syndrome

IMMUNODEFICIENCY WITH THYMOMA

Adults develop recurrent infection, panhypogammaglobulinemia, defective cell-mediated immunity, benign thymoma (usually spindle cell type).
Poor antibody formation with decreased or absent B-lymphocytes.
May show pancytopenia or agranulocytosis, increased or decreased eosinophils, hemolytic or aregenerative anemia.

HYPERIMMUNOGLOBULINEMIA E SYNDROME

Very rare condition shows recurrent severe staphylococcal abscesses.
Increased eosinophils in blood, sputum, and sections of tissues
Very high serum IgE, increased serum IgD, other Ig are usually normal.
Normal count of lymphocytes and subsets

COMPLEMENT DEFICIENCIES

See Serum Complement, p. 78–81.

HEREDITARY ANGIOEDEMA

CBC and ESR are usually normal when the manifestation is peripheral or facial angioedema, but they may be abnormal when the manifestation is diarrhea and abdominal pain.

Serum C-1-esterase inhibitor is either decreased (5–30% of normal) or is functionally inactive. (Test is performed only at reference laboratories.)

BISALBUMINEMIA

Two albumin bands are present on serum protein electrophoresis in clinically healthy homozygotes or carriers.

ALPHA$_1$ ANTITRYPSIN (AAT) DEFICIENCY

This is an autosomal recessive deficiency associated with familial pulmonary emphysema and liver disease. The heterozygous state occurs in 10–15% of general population who have serum levels of alpha$_1$ antitrypsin ~60% of normal; homozygous state occurs in 1:2000 persons who have serum levels ~10% of normal.

There are many alleles of AAT gene.

	Serum AAT	AAT Function	Phenotype
Normal	Normal (20–48 μM) (150–350 mg/dl)	Normal	Pi MM
Deficient severe	(2.5–7.0 μM)	Normal	Pi ZZ (>95% of cases)
			Pi SZ (rare)
	(15–33 μM)		Pi SS
	(12–35 μM)		Pi MZ
Null	Undetectable		Pi null-null
			Pi Z-null
Dysfunctional	Normal	Abnormal	

Z alleles are rare in Orientals and blacks.

Threshold protection levels for emphysema = 11 μM (80 mg/dl).

Pulmonary emphysema occurs in family of 25% of patients; occurs in heterozygotes and homozygotes. Causes 2% of cases of emphysema. Secondary bronchitis and bronchiectasis may occur.

Liver disease occurs in 10–20% of children with this deficiency. Clinical picture may be neonatal hepatitis (in 15% of those with ZZ phenotype), 25% of whom develop prolonged obstructive jaundice during infancy, juvenile cirrhosis, and die by age 8; or abnormal liver functions tests (e.g., SGPT) in 50% of apparently healthy asymptomatic patients. Liver biopsy (in both heterozygotes and homozygotes) shows characteristic intracytoplasmic inclusions; these may be found in patients with emphysema without liver disease and in asymptomatic heterozygous relatives, but these inclusions must be searched for and stained specifically, since the rest of the pathology in the liver is not specific. ~9% of adults with nonalcoholic cirrhosis are MZ phenotype. Hepatoma may occur in cirrhotic livers.

Decreased serum alpha$_1$ antitrypsin is typically <50 mg/dl. May also be decreased in prematurity, severe liver disease, malnutrition, renal losses (e.g., nephrosis), GI losses (e.g., pancreatitis, protein-losing diseases), exudative dermopathies. Serum alpha$_1$ antitrypsin may be increased in infections, neoplasia (especially cervical cancer and lymphomas), pregnancy, and use of birth control pills.

Purified AAT is now available for augmentation therapy.

- Indicated when AAT <11 μM, abnormal lung function tests show deterioration.
- Not indicated when lung function is normal, even if AAT deficiency with liver disease, or pulmonary emphysema is associated with normal or heterozygous phenotypes.

TUMORS OF THYMUS

(>40% have parathymic syndromes noted below, which are multiple in one-third)

Associated With

Myasthenia gravis in about 35% of patients. May appear up to 6 years after excision of thymoma in 5% of patients. Thymoma develops in 15% of patients with myasthenia gravis. See p. 243.

Acquired hypogammaglobulinemia. 7–13% of adults with this condition have an associated thymoma; does not respond to thymectomy.

Pure red cell aplasia (PRCA) is found in approximately 5% of thymoma patients. 50% of patients with PRCA have thymoma, 25% of whom benefit from thymectomy; onset followed thymectomy in 10% of patients. May be accompanied or followed, but not preceded, by granulocytopenia or thrombocytopenia or both in one-third of cases; thymectomy is not useful therapy. PRCA occurs in one-third of patients with hypogammaglobulinemia and thymoma.

Autoimmune hemolytic anemia with positive Coombs' test and increased reticulocyte count

Cushing's syndrome

Multiple endocrine neoplasia (usually Type I)

SLE

Miscellaneous disorders (e.g., giant cell myocarditis, nephrotic syndrome)

Cutaneous disorders (e.g., mucocutaneous candidiasis, pemphigus)

ACQUIRED IMMUNE DEFICIENCY SYNDROME (AIDS)

See pp. 653–657.

HYPOANABOLIC HYPOALBUMINEMIA

(an inherited disorder present from birth, without kidney or liver disease)

Growth and development are normal. The patient is unaffected except for periodic peripheral edema.)

Serum albumin is <0.3 gm/dl.

Total globulins are 4.5–5.5 gm/dl.

Serum cholesterol is increased.

Albumin synthesis is decreased, with decreased catabolism of IV injected albumin.

Coagulation Tests

(See Table 12-26, pp. 372–373, for specific diseases and test results.)

PLATELET COUNT

(see also Tables 12-27, p. 378, and Table 12-28, p. 379)

May Be Increased (>500,000/cu mm) In

Malignancy, especially disseminated, advanced, or inoperable

Myeloproliferative disease (e.g., polycythemia vera, chronic myelogenous leukemia, agnogenic myeloid metaplasia, essential thrombocytosis)

Patients recently having surgery, especially splenectomy

Collagen disorders, e.g., rheumatoid arthritis

Iron deficiency anemia

Pseudothrombocytosis

- Cryoglobulinemia
- Malaria parasites
- Fragments of RBCs or WBCs
- Microspherocytes
- Howell-Jolly bodies, nucleated RBCs, Heinz bodies, clumped Pappenheimer bodies

Miscellaneous disease states (e.g., acute infection, cardiac disease, cirrhosis of the liver, chronic pancreatitis)

Approximately 50% of patients with "unexpected" increase of platelet count are found to have a malignancy.

Decreased In

Thrombocytopenia

Acquired

Drugs (e.g., quinidine, quinine, sulfonamides, trimethoprim-sulfamethoxazole, gold, thiazides, alcohol, chemotherapeutic agents, aspirin, nonsteroidal anti-inflammatory agents, dipyridamole, aminophylline, penicillins, dextran, beta-blocking agents, calcium-channel blocking agents, halothane anesthetics, phenothiazines. Heparin causes thrombocytopenia in ≤10% of patients, usually in 5–10 days.)

Aplastic anemia

Myelophthisis

Viral infections

Renal deficiency

Paroxysmal nocturnal hemoglobinuria

Nutritional deficiencies

Ionizing radiation

Inherited

Alport's syndrome

Bernard-Soulier syndrome

Chédiak-Higashi syndrome

Ehlers-Danlos syndrome

May-Hegglin anomaly

Wiskott-Aldrich syndrome

Glanzmann's thrombasthenia

Hermansky-Pudiak syndrome

Thrombocytopenia–absent radius (TAR) syndrome

When associated with anemia and microangiopathy on peripheral smear, rule out DIC, thrombotic thrombocytopenic purpura, prosthetic valve dysfunction, malignant hypertension, eclampsia, vasculitis, leaking aortic aneurysm, disseminated metastatic cancer, hemolytic-uremic syndromes.

Pseudothrombocytopenia (laboratory artifact; diagnosis by examination of stained peripheral blood smear)

Platelet clumping induced by EDTA blood collection tubes is the most common cause.

Platelet satellitosis

Platelet cold agglutinins

Giant platelets

RBC count >6,500,000/cu mm

PLATELET AGGREGATION STUDIES

(platelet aggregation stimulated by certain agonistic drugs is measured in vitro by turbidimeter shown graphically by wave patterns)

Useful to study qualitative platelet functional abnormalities of adhesion, release, or aggregation

Adenosine diphosphate (ADP) and epinephrine produce primary and secondary waves of aggregation; collagen, arachidonic acid, and ristocetin produce only primary waves.

Thrombasthenia causes absent primary and secondary aggregation with all agents except ristocetin.

Storage pool disease and release defect cause absent secondary aggregation.

Defective arachidonic acid aggregation: release defects due to abnormal thromboxane A2 synthesis.

Release defects: decreased secondary waves with ADP and epinephrine and decreased primary wave with collagen

Aspirin may produce characteristic abnormalities of release defects with decreased thromboxane A_2 synthesis

Decreased ristocetin aggregation: Bernard-Soulier syndrome, some cases of von Willebrand's disease

Myeloproliferative diseases and uremia: abnormal aggregation to epinephrine, ADP, and collagen

MEAN PLATELET VOLUME (MPV)

(limited value when measured by routine automated hematology instruments)

Usually requested for thrombocytopenic patients

- Increased MPV with thrombocytopenia indicates that thrombopoiesis is stimulated and platelet production is increased.
- Normal MPV with thrombocytopenia indicates impaired thrombopoiesis.

Increased In

Immune thrombocytopenic purpura
Thrombocytopenia due to sepsis (recovery phase)
Myeloproliferative disorders
Massive hemorrhage
Prosthetic heart valve
Splenectomy
Vasculitis

Decreased In

Wiskott-Aldrich syndrome

BLEEDING TIME (BT)*

Mielke modification of Ivy method: should use a standardized technique—blood pressure cuff on upper arm inflated to 40 mm Hg; two small standardized skin incisions are made on volar surface of forearm using a specially calibrated template.

Normal = 4–7 minutes. Longer in women than men.

Usually Prolonged In

Thrombocytopenia

- Plate count <100,000/cu mm and usually <80,000/cu mm before BT becomes abnormal and <40,000/cu mm before abnormality becomes pronounced. BT is almost always abnormal when platelet count <60,000/cu mm except in conditions that have young supereffective platelets. BT may be normal in some patients with immune thrombocytopenic purpura with marked decrease in platelet count. Platelet count = 80,000/cu mm should have BT ~10 minutes and platelet count = 40,000/cu mm should have BT ~20 minutes if platelet function is normal; beyond these values the patient may also have a qualitative platelet abnormality. No value in performing BT if platelet count <10,000/cu mm, as BT will always be >30 minutes.

Platelet function disorders

- Hereditary
  - Defect in plasma proteins
    - von Willebrand's disease (especially 2 hours after ingestion of 300 mg of aspirin)

*Data from ER Burns and C Lawrence, Bleeding time: A guide to its diagnostic and clinical utility. *Arch Pathol Lab Med* 113:1219, 1989.

Deficient release platelet glycoproteins
Glanzmann's thrombasthenia
Bernard-Soulier syndrome
Defective release mechanisms
Gray platelet syndrome
Aspirin-like defect
Storage pool deficiency
Others
Wiskott-Aldrich syndrome
Chédiak-Higashi syndrome
Oculocutaneous albinism (Hermansky-Pudlak syndrome)
Hereditary hemorrhagic telangiectasia
Ehlers-Danlos syndrome
Acquired—abnormal plasma factors
Drugs
Aspirin, nonsteroidal anti-inflammatory agents (e.g., indomethacin, ibuprofen, phenylbutazone). Recent (up to 7 days) ingestion is the most common cause of prolonged BT. Aspirin may double the baseline BT, which may still be within normal range. 325 mg of aspirin will increase BT of most persons.
Antimicrobials (e.g., penicillins, cephalosporins, nitrofurantoin, hydroxychloroquine)
Tricyclic antidepressants (e.g., imipramine, amitriptyline, nortriptyline)
Phenothiazines (e.g., chlorpromazine, promethazine, trifluoperazine)
Anesthetic (e.g., halothane, local)
Methylxanthines (e.g., caffeine, theophylline, aminophylline)
Others (e.g., dextrans, calcium channel-blocking agents, x-ray contrast agents, beta-adrenergic blockers, alcohol)
Uremic (may be corrected with vasopressin or cryoprecipitate)
Fibrin degradation products (e.g., DIC, liver disease, fibrinolytic therapy)
Macromolecules (e.g., dextran, paraproteins [e.g., myelomas, Waldenström's macroglobulinemia])
Other immune thrombocytopenias
Myeloproliferative diseases, including myelodysplastic syndrome, preleukemia, acute leukemia, hairy-cell leukemia)
Vasculitis
Others (e.g., amyloidosis, viral infections, scurvy, after circulating through an oxygenator during cardiac bypass surgery)
Increased BT or BT increased out of proportion to platelet count suggests von Willebrand's disease or qualitative platelet defect.
BT is best single screening test for platelet functional disorders. A normal test without suggestive history usually excludes platelet dysfunction.

Usually Normal In
Hemophilia
Severe hereditary hypoprothrombinemia
Severe hereditary hypofibrinogenemia
Other

Sensitivity, specificity, and predictive value of BT in perioperative hemorrhage are not known.
Not recommended for routine preoperative screening because
General surgery patients without obvious risk factors for bleeding rarely have clinically significant increase in BT.

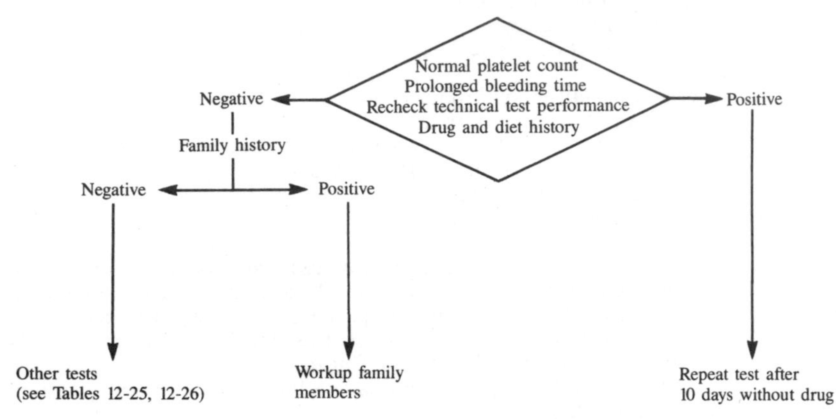

Fig. 12-6. Flow chart for prolonged bleeding time.

Even with a prolonged BT, blood loss does not exceed that of patients with normal BT.

Prolonged BT does not necessarily cause increased bleeding.

Therapeutic decisions are not likely to be changed by results of BT.

Clinical history is the best preoperative screening.

Not recommended for preoperative evaluation of patients receiving aspirin or nonsteroidal anti-inflammatory drugs, with liver disease, for coronary bypass

Not recommended for prediction of bleeding in myeloproliferative diseases or neonates receiving nonsteroidal anti-inflammatory drugs

BT may be useful in preoperative screening of patients for eye, middle ear, brain, or knee surgery. May also be useful to monitor treatment of active hemorrhage in patients with prolonged BT due to uremia, von Willebrand's disease, congenital platelet function abnormalities, or severe anemia

BT is useful as part of workup for coagulation disorders in patients with history of excess bleeding (e.g., associated with dental extraction, childbirth, circumcision, tonsillectomy) even with a normal platelet count.

COAGULATION (CLOTTING) TIME (CT) ("LEE-WHITE CLOTTING TIME")

Prolonged In

Severe deficiency (<6%) of any known plasma clotting factors except Factors XIII (fibrin-stabilizing factor) and VII

Afibrinogenemia

Presence of a circulating anticoagulant (including heparin)

Normal In

Thrombocytopenia
Deficiency of Factor VII
von Willebrand's disease
Mild coagulation defects due to any cause

This was the routine method for control of heparin therapy but now replaced by activated partial thromboplastin time (aPTT). It is not a reliable screening test for bleeding conditions because it is not sensitive enough to detect mild conditions but will only detect severe ones. Normal CT does not rule out a coagulation defect. There are many variables in the technique of performing the test.

Routine preoperative bleeding and coagulation times are of little value for routine preoperative screening.

TOURNIQUET TEST

Positive In

Thrombocytopenic purpuras
Nonthrombocytopenic purpuras
Thrombocytopathies
Scurvy

PROTHROMBIN TIME (PT)

Prolonged By Defect In

Factor I (fibrinogen)
Factor II (prothrombin)
Factor V (labile factor)
Factor VII (stable factor)
Factor X (Stuart-Prower factor)

Prolonged In

Inadequate vitamin K in diet
Premature infants
Newborn infants of vitamin K–deficient mothers (hemorrhagic disease of the newborn)
Poor fat absorption (e.g., obstructive jaundice, fistulas, sprue, steatorrhea, celiac disease, colitis, chronic diarrhea)
Severe liver damage (e.g., poisoning, hepatitis, cirrhosis)
Drugs (e.g., coumarin-type drugs for anticoagulant therapy, salicylates)
Factitious ingestion of warfarin
Idiopathic familial hypoprothrombinemia
Circulating anticoagulants
Hypofibrinogenemia (acquired or inherited)

The PT is primarily used for three purposes:

- Control of long-term oral anticoagulant therapy with coumarins and indanedione derivatives.
- Evaluation of liver function—PT is the most useful test of impaired liver synthesis of prothrombin complex factors (Factors II, VII, X, Proteins C and S).
- Evaluation of coagulation disorders—screens for abnormality of factors involved in extrinsic pathway (factors V, VII, X, prothrombin, fibrinogen); should be used with aPTT

PT should be reported as ratio of patient to control rather than as a percentage.

ACTIVATED PARTIAL THROMBOPLASTIN TIME (aPTT)

Prolonged By

Defect in Factors
- I (fibrinogen)
- II (prothrombin)
- V (labile factor)
- VIII
- IX
- X (Stuart-Prower factor)
- XI
- XII (Hageman factor)

Presence of specific inhibitors of clotting factors (most frequently antibody against factor VIII, which occurs in ~15% of multitransfused patients with severe hemophilia A and less frequently in mild/moderate hemophilia A; and circulating lupus anticoagulant). *Mixing equal parts of patient and normal plasma corrects PTT if due to coagulation factor deficiency but not if due to an inhibitor.*

Values may be falsely very high if plasma is very turbid or icteric when photoelectric machines are used.

Normal In

Thrombocytopenia
Platelet dysfunction
von Willebrand's disease (may be prolonged in some patients)
Isolated defects of Factor VII

Used To

Monitor heparin therapy
Screen for hemophilia A and B
Detect clotting inhibitors

aPTT is the *best single screening test* for disorders of coagulation; it is abnormal in 90% of patients with coagulation disorders when properly performed. Screens for all coagulation factors that contribute to thrombin formation except VII and XIII.

The test may not detect mild clotting defects (25–40% of normal levels), which seldom cause significant bleeding.

Is not recommended for preoperative screening of asymptomatic adult unless patient has specific clinical indication (e.g., active bleeding, known or suspected bleeding disorders [including anticoagulant use], liver disease, malabsorption, malnutrition, other conditions associated with acquired coagulopathies, where procedure may interefere with normal coagulation)

PROTHROMBIN CONSUMPTION

Impaired By

Any defect in phase I or phase II of blood coagulation
- Thrombocytopathies
- Thrombocytopenia
- Hypoprothrombinemia
- Hemophilias
- Circulating anticoagulants
- Other

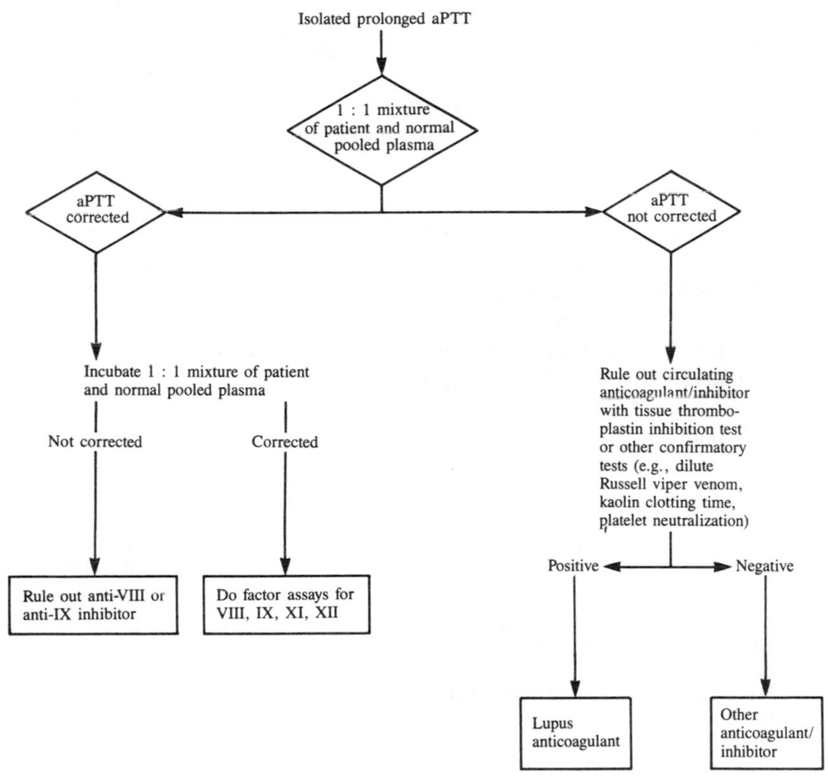

Fig. 12-7. Algorithm for isolated prolonged aPTT.

THROMBIN TIME

Increased In

Very low fibrinogen level (<80 mg/dl)
Interference with polymerization of fibrin
- Fibrin degradation products, especially DIC
- Paraproteinemias
- Uremia

Dysfibrinogenemia (abnormal fibrinogen present)
Heparin contamination of specimen is common cause in hospital patients, but a reptilase test is normal in presence of heparin but prolonged by other causes listed above.

THROMBOPLASTIN GENERATION TEST (TGT)

This test uses three components ($BaSO_4$-adsorbed plasma, serum, washed platelets) that are individually substituted in turn to mixtures of patient's blood

Table 12-23. Thrombоplastin Generation Test

Components	Mixtures
$BaSO_4$-adsorbed plasma (Factors V, VIII present; VII, IX, X absent) from	P P N N
Serum (VII, IX, X present; V, VII absent) from	P N P N
Washed platelets from	N N N P
Abnormality	
Normal	+ + + +
Thrombocytopenia, thrombasthenia	+ + + 0
von Willebrand's disease	0 0 + +
Factor V deficiency (severe)	0 0 + +
Factor VII deficiency	+ + + +
Factor VIII deficiency (hemophilia)	0 0 + +
Factor IX deficiency (Christmas disease)	0 + 0 +
Factor X deficiency	0 + 0 +
Factor XI (PTA) deficiency	0 + + +
Factor XII deficiency	0 + + +
Circulating anticoagulant	0 0 0 +

P = patient; N = normal control; + = thromboplastin is generated (i.e., fibrin clot forms); 0 = thromboplastin is not generated (i.e., fibrin clot does not form).

to localize the defect in thromboplastin generation. It can be used to localize coagulation defects due to

- Factor VIII
- Factor IX (may not detect mild deficiencies)
- Factor X
- Factor V
- Factor VII
- Thrombasthenia
- Circulating anticoagulant (equal mixture of normal and patient's plasma causes normalization of coagulation tests in coagulation factor deficiency states but does not correct in presence of anticoagulant)

It may not detect disease after recent blood or plasma transfusion.

POOR CLOT RETRACTION

May Occur In

Various thrombocytopenias
Thrombasthenia
Poor test of clotting function; little value for detection of mild-to-moderate bleeding disorders

FIBRINOGEN DEGRADATION PRODUCTS (FDP)

(rapid latex agglutination test kit detects 10 μg/ml in serum and parallels results with hemagglutination inhibition [HAI] method; detects major breakdown products of fibrin or fibrinogen; does not distinguish between fibrinolysis and fibrinogenolysis)

Chief use is to aid in diagnosis of DIC

Increased In Serum

Acute myocardial infarction during first 24–48 hours
Pulmonary embolism—peak values may be transient.

Postoperative deep vein thrombosis
Certain disorders of pregnancy
Small increases with exercises, anxiety, stress

Increased In Urine

Kidney disease
- Urinary tract infection—increased in infection of upper tract but not of bladder
- Proliferative glomerulonephritis—level falls during response to drug therapy
- Rejection of renal transplant

Conditions causing increased serum level (see above)

ANTITHROMBIN III

To detect hypercoagulable state associated with episodes of venous thrombosis; decreased in ~4.5% of patients with idiopathic venous thrombosis

Functional test is preferred to immunologic, since the antigen level may be normal in ~10% of cases of hereditary deficiency.

Decreased In

Chronic liver disease (>80% of cases of cirrhosis)
Nephrotic syndrome
Protein-wasting diseases
Heparin therapy for >3 days
L-Asparaginase therapy
Active thrombotic disease (e.g., thrombophlebitis, deep venous thrombosis) (not diagnostically useful)
Hereditary familial deficiency (typically 40–60% of normal)
DIC (not diagnostically useful)
Oral contraceptives (slightly)
Last trimester of pregnancy (rarely <75% of normal)
Newborns (~50% of adult level, which is attained by age 6 months)
Others (e.g., acute leukemia, carcinoma, burns, postsurgical trauma)

PLASMINOGEN

(normal adults = 76–124% males; 65–153% females; infants = 27–59%)

Used to monitor fibrinolytic therapy with streptokinase or urokinase

May Be Decreased In

Some familial or isolated cases of idiopathic deep venous thrombosis
Diabetics with thrombosis
DIC and systemic fibrinolysis
Behçet's disease
Cirrhosis of the liver

PLASMA PROTEIN C

(normal range = 70–130%; to detect hypercoagulable states associated with episodes of venous thrombosis. *Purpura fulminans is seen in homozygous infants. Warfarin-induced skin necrosis is almost pathognomonic for protein C deficiency.*)

Decreased In

Hereditary (autosomal recessive) deficiency (heterozygote levels are usually 30–65%; thrombosis is not usual if level >50%)
Chronic liver disease
DIC
Postoperatively
Malignancy
Acute respiratory distress syndrome

Protein S should be assayed whenever protein C is assayed; performed in special laboratories. Heterozygotes with levels of 30–60% may have episodes of recurrent thrombosis.

Hemorrhagic Disorders

CLASSIFICATION OF HEMORRHAGIC DISORDERS

Vascular abnormalities
- Congenital (e.g., hereditary hemorrhagic telangiectasia [Osler-Weber-Rendu disease])
- Acquired (see Nonthrombocytopenic Purpura, p. 377)
  - Infection (e.g., bacterial endocarditis, rickettsial infection)
  - Immunologic (e.g., Schönlein-Henoch, allergic purpura, drug sensitivity)
  - Metabolic (e.g., scurvy, uremia, diabetes mellitus)
  - Miscellaneous (e.g., neoplasms, amyloidosis, angioma serpiginosum)

Connective tissue abnormalities
- Congenital (e.g., Ehlers-Danlos syndrome)
- Acquired (e.g., Cushing's syndrome)

Platelet abnormalities (see sections on thrombocytopenic purpura, thrombocythemia, thrombocytopathies)

Plasma coagulation defects
- Causing defective thromboplastin formation
  - Hemophilia (Factor VIII deficiency)
  - Plasma thromboplastin components (PTC) (Factor IX) deficiency (Christmas disease)
  - Plasma thromboplastin antecedent (PTA) (Factor XI) deficiency
  - von Willebrand's disease
- Causing defective rate or amount of thrombin formation
  - Vitamin K deficiency (due to liver disease, prolonged bile duct obstruction, malabsorption syndrome, hemorrhagic disease of the newborn, anticoagulant therapy)
  - Congenital deficiency of Factor II (prothrombin), Factor V (proaccelerin, labile factor), Factor VII (proconvertin, stable factor), Factor X (Stuart factor)
- Decreased fibrinogen due to intravascular clotting and/or fibrinolysis
  - Obstetric abnormalities (e.g., amniotic fluid embolism, premature separation of placenta, retention of dead fetus)
  - Congenital deficiency of Factor XIII (fibrin-stabilizing factor), congenital afibrinogenemia, hypofibrinogenemia, etc.
  - Neoplasms (e.g., leukemia, carcinoma of prostate)
  - Transfusion reactions
  - Gram-negative septicemia, meningococcemia
- Circulating anticoagulants
  - Heparin therapy
- Dysproteinemias, SLE, postpartum state, some cases of hemophilia, etc.

THROMBOCYTOPENIC PURPURA

Due To

Idiopathic thrombocytopenic purpura

Hematologic disorders
- Myelophthisic diseases (e.g., leukemia, lymphoma, metastatic carcinoma)
- Anemias (aplastic, vitamin B_{12} or folic acid deficiency, acquired hemolytic)
- Hypersplenism (e.g., Gaucher's disease, Felty's syndrome, sarcoidosis, congestive splenomegaly)

Table 12-24. Comparison of Coagulation Disorders with Platelet or Vascular Disorders

	Coagulation Disorder	Platelet or Vascular Disorder
Hemarthroses and deep hematomas in muscle	Characteristic	Rare
Delayed bleeding	Characteristic	Rare
Bleeding from superficial cuts	Uncommon	Persistent; may be profuse
Petechiae	Rare	Characteristic
Ecchymoses	Common, usually single and large	Characteristic, usually multiple and large
Epistaxis, melena	Seldom predominant	Often causes significant bleeding
Hematuria	Common	Uncommon

- Thrombotic thrombocytopenic purpura
- DIC
- Post-transfusion and massive blood transfusions

Hereditary
- May-Hegglin anomaly
- Bernard-Soulier syndrome
- Wiskott-Aldrich syndrome

Infections (e.g., AIDS, subacute bacterial endocarditis, septicemia, typhus)
Other diseases (e.g., SLE, alcohol binges)
Marrow suppressive agents (e.g., ionizing radiation, benzol, nitrogen mustards and other antitumor drugs)
Drug sensitivity reactions (e.g., sulfonamides, chloramphenicol and other antibacterial drugs, tranquilizers, antipyretic drugs, heparin, gold)

Antiplatelet antibodies (IgG and IgM) may be found in plasma and by flow cytometry may be detected on platelets in most patients with drug-induced thrombocytopenia (e.g., heparin, quinidine, procainamide, quinine) (sensitivity = 90%). 15–29% of patients with autoimmune thrombocytopenia have only platelet-associated IgM. Negative results in plasma and on platelets strongly oppose or contradict an immune etiology of thrombocytopenia.

IDIOPATHIC THROMBOCYTOPENIC PURPURA (WERLHOF'S DISEASE)

Laboratory Findings

Decreased platelet count (<100,000/cu mm); no bleeding until <50,000/cu mm; postoperative and minor spontaneous bleeding may occur at 20,000–50,000/cu mm. Serious bleeding may occur at <20,000/cu mm.
Positive tourniquet test
Increased bleeding time
Poor clot retraction
Normal PT, PTT, and coagulation time
Bone marrow is normal or may show only increased number of megakaryocytes but without marginal platelets.
Normal blood count and blood smear except for decreased number of platelets; platelets may appear abnormal (small or giant or deeply stained).
Laboratory findings due to hemorrhage
- Increased WBC with shift to left
- Anemia proportional to hemorrhage, with compensatory increase in reticulocytes, polychromatophilia, etc.

Table 12-25. Screening Tests for Presumptive Diagnosis of Common Bleeding Disorders[a]

Platelet Count	Bleeding Time	Prothrombin Time[b]	Activated Partial Thromboplastin Time[b]	Location of Defect	Most Frequent Causes	
					Acquired	Hereditary
N	N	I	N	Extrinsic pathway[c]	Liver disease, coumarin therapy, vitamin K deficiency, DIC (very rare)	Deficiency of Factor VII (very rare)
N	N	N	I	Intrinsic pathway[d]	Heparin therapy, inhibitors	Hemophilia A or B deficiency of XI, XII, prekallikrein, high-molecular-weight kininogen, Passavoy factor
N[e]	N	I	I	Common or multiple pathways	Heparin therapy, liver disease, vitamin K deficiency, DIC, fibrinogenolysis (very common)	Deficiency of V, X, prothrombin; dysfibrinogenemias (very rare)

D	I	N	N	Thrombocytopenia	ITP, secondary (e.g., drugs)	Aldrich's syndrome, etc.
N or I	I	N	N	Disorder of platelet function	Thrombocythemia, drugs, uremia, dysproteinemias	Thrombasthenia, deficient release reaction
N	I	N	I	Von Willebrand's disease		
N	N	N	N	Vascular abnormality	Allergic purpura, drugs, scurvy, etc.	Deficiency of XIII, telangiectasia

N = normal; I = increased; D = decreased.

[a]Screening tests may be normal in mild von Willebrand's disease that has borderline or intermittent normal bleeding time, in mild hemophilia, and in Factor XIII deficiency.

[b]Concentration of factors must be decreased to ≦ 30% of normal for these tests to be abnormal.

[c]Extrinsic pathway function depends on Factors VII, X, V, II (prothrombin), I (fibrinogen); is assessed by prothrombin time.

[d]Intrinsic pathway depends on Factors XII, XI, IX, VIII, X, V, II, I; is assessed by partial thromboplastin time.

[e]May be I in acquired disorders that produce abnormalities of platelets and multiple coagulation factors.

Table 12-26. Summary of Coagulation Studies in Hemorrhagic Conditions

	Screening Tests				Accessory Tests			Tests to Identify Deficiency	
Condition	Platelet Count	Bleeding Time	Prothrombin Time	Partial Thromboplastin Time (PTT)	Capillary Fragility (Rumpel-Leede tourniquet test)	Coagulation Time	Clot Retraction	Prothrombin Consumption Time	Thromboplastin Generation Test (TGT)
Thrombocytopenic purpura	D	I	N	N	+	N	Poor	I	I
Nonthrombocytopenic purpura	N	N	N	N	V	N	N	N	N
Glanzmann's thrombasthenia	N[a]	N or I	N		+ or N	N	Poor	I Corrected by platelet substitute	I
von Willebrand's disease	N	I or N	N	N or I	N + in severe	V	N	I	V[b]
AHG (Factor VIII) deficiency (hemophilia)	N	N	N	I	N	I N in mild	N	I	I[b]

PTC (Factor IX) deficiency (hemophilia B; Christmas disease)	N	N	N	I[c]	N	I N in mild	N	I	I[c]
Factor X (Stuart) deficiency	N	N	I[c]	I[c]	N	N or slightly I	N	I	I
PTA (Factor XI) deficiency	N	N I in severe	N	I[d]	N	I	N	I	I[d]
Factor XII (Hageman) deficiency	N	N	N	I[d]	N	I	N	I	I[d]
Factor XIII deficiency	N	N	N	N	N	N	N	N	N
Fibrinogen deficiency	N	N I in severe	I	I	N	I	N	N	N
Hypoprothrombinemia	N	N or I	I	I	N	I	N	N	N
Excess dicumarol therapy	N	N I in severe	I	I	N + in severe	I N in mild	N	N	N
Heparin therapy	N	N to I	May be I	I	N	I	N		

Table 12-26 (continued)

Condition	Screening Tests				Accessory Tests			Tests to Identify Deficiency	
	Platelet Count	Bleeding Time	Pro-thrombin Time	Partial Thrombo-plastin Time (PTT)	Capillary Fragility (Rumpel-Leede tourni-quet test)	Coagula-tion Time	Clot Retrac-tion	Prothrom-bin Con-sumption Time	Thrombo-plastin Generation Test (TGT)
Vascular purpura (e.g., Schönlein-Henoch, hereditary hemorrhagic telangiectasia)	N	N	N	N	N	N	N	N	N
Increased antithrom-boplastin	N		I			I		I	May be I and not corrected by absorbed plasma or aged serum
Increased anti-thrombin	N	N	I		N	N May be I in severe	N	N[e]	
Increased fibrinolysin	N	N or I	N		N	N or I	Lysis of clot	N[e]	N

D = decreased; I = increased; N = normal; V = variable.
[a]Platelets appear abnormal.
[b]Corrected by absorbed plasma.
[c]Corrected by serum.
[d]Corrected by serum or plasma.
[e]Not useful; may be difficult to do.

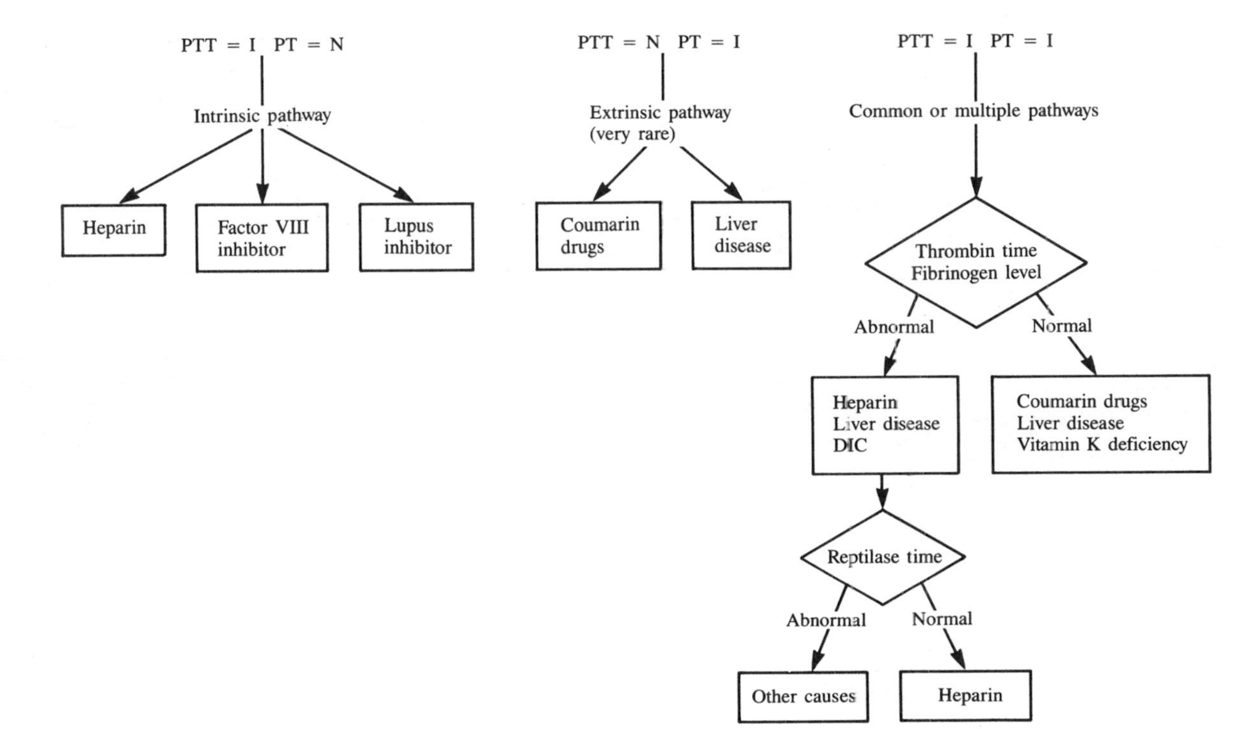

Fig. 12-8. Algorithm for acquired coagulation disorders.

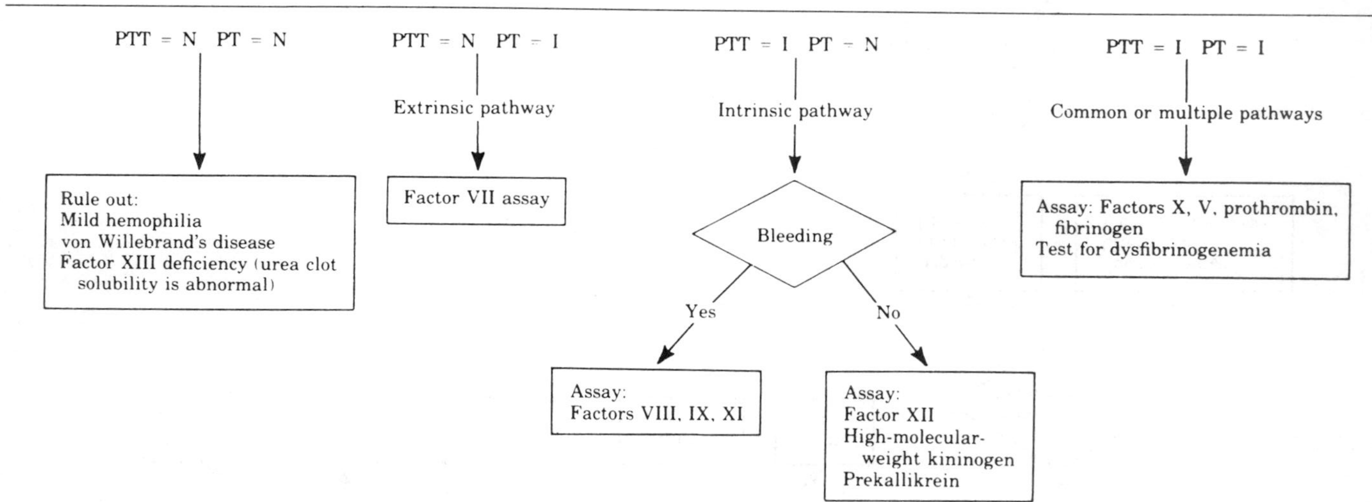

Fig. 12-9. Algorithm for hereditary coagulation disorders.

One unit of platelet concentrate will raise the platelet count by 15,000/cu mm in the average 70-kg adult; therefore minimal dose to administer is 6 units. No increment in 60 minutes suggests alloimmunization has occurred (should use single-donor platelets); >5000/cu mm increment suggests that alloimmunization has not occurred.

NONTHROMBOCYTOPENIC PURPURA

Abnormal platelets (e.g., thrombocytopathies, thrombasthenia, thrombocythemia)
Abnormal serum globulins (e.g., multiple myeloma, macroglobulinemia, cryoglobulinemia, hyperglobulinemia)
Infections (e.g., meningococcemia, subacute bacterial endocarditis, typhoid, Rocky Mountain spotted fever)
Other diseases (e.g., amyloidosis, Cushing's syndrome, polycythemia vera, hemochromatosis, diabetes mellitus, uremia)
Drugs and chemicals (e.g., mercury, phenacetin, salicylic acid, chloral hydrate)
Allergic reaction (e.g., Schönlein-Henoch purpura, serum sickness)
Diseases of the skin (e.g., Osler-Weber-Rendu disease, Ehlers-Danlos syndrome)
von Willebrand's disease
Avitaminosis (e.g., scurvy)
Miscellaneous (e.g., mechanical, orthostatic)
Blood coagulation factors (e.g., hemophilia)

THROMBOTIC THROMBOCYTOPENIC PURPURA

Diagnostic criteria are thrombocytopenia, microangiopathic hemolytic anemia, neurologic involvement, frequently with renal involvement and fever.
Severe thrombocytopenic purpura with normal or increased megakaryocytes in bone marrow. Platelet count usually <50,000/cu mm.
Microangiopathic hemolytic anemia (normochromic, normocytic) with
- Hemoglobin usually <10 gm/dl.
- Numerous fragmented and misshapen RBCs (burr cells, schistocytes) on blood smear are virtually required for this diagnosis.
- Increased serum indirect bilirubin, LDH, and serum hemoglobin and decreased serum haptoglobin
- Increased reticulocytes, nucleated RBCs, basophilic stippling and polychromatophilia
- Negative Coombs' test

Increased or normal WBCs and neutrophils
PT and PTT are usually normal (in contrast to DIC) or may be mildly increased.
Fibrin split products are usually present in low levels.
Abnormal urine findings (e.g., RBCs, protein), increased BUN and creatinine occur frequently. Oliguria and acute renal failure are uncommon.
SGOT and SGPT may be slightly increased.
High initial BUN and creatinine, falling hemoglobin, and failure of platelet count to rise are poor prognostic signs.
Arteriolar thrombi in various organ systems result in clinical manifestations, especially neurologic in ~90% and hemorrhagic in up to 70% of cases. Presence in gingival biopsy supports the diagnosis but present in <50%. Other sites (skin, liver, lymph nodes, kidney) are rarely useful.

PRIMARY THROMBOCYTOSIS

(classified as a myeloproliferative disorder involving the thrombocytes)

Platelets >600,000/cu mm; normal aggregation
No cause for reactive thrombocytosis
No evidence of leukemia (and absent Philadelphia chromosome) or polycythemia (hemoglobin <13 gm/dl or normal RBC mass) in peripheral blood or marrow. Not due to iron deficiency (marrow contains stainable iron or <1 gm hemoglobin increase after 1 month of iron therapy)

Table 12-27. Some Congenital Hemorrhagic Diseases Due to Disorders of Platelet-Vessel Wall

Platelet Defects	
Bernard-Soulier syndrome	Moderate thrombocytopenia Bleeding time markedly increased Large platelets Decreased ristocetin-induced agglutination not corrected by vWF
Glanzmann's thrombasthenia	Normal platelet count and morphology Increased bleeding time Clot retraction absent or much decreased No platelet aggregation with any agonists
Pseudo–von Willebrand's disease	Variable mild thrombocytopenia Increased bleeding time Increased ristocetin-induced agglutination Variable plasma immunoreactive vWF
Gray-platelet syndrome	Moderate thrombocytopenia Large platelets Bleeding time slightly increased Platelets agranular on blood smear Abnormal platelet aggregation with collagen or thrombin
Dense-granule deficiency syndrome	Normal platelet count Normal platelet morphology on blood smear Bleeding time variably increased Abnormal aggregation with ADP and collagen
Deficiency of platelet enzyme (cyclooxygenase or thromboxane synthetase)	Normal platelet count and morphology Abnormal aggregation with ADP, collagen, and arachidonic acid
May-Hegglin anomaly	Autosomal dominant trait Moderate thrombocytopenia with huge platelets; normal platelet function Doehle bodies in granulocytes
Plasma Defects	
von Willebrand's disease	Normal platelet count and morphology Increased bleeding time Abnormal ristocetin-induced agglutination Abnormal plasma vWF
Afibrinogenemia	Normal platelet morphology Mild thrombocytopenia occasionally Bleeding time variably increased Plasma coagulation abnormalities
Vessel Wall Defects	
Genetic disorders of connective tissue	Platelets may be large Collagen-induced aggregation may be abnormal

vWF = von Willebrand factor; ADP = adenosine diphosphate.

Table 12-28. Congenital Functional Platelet Disorders

	Platelet Retention in Glass Bead	Platelet Aggregation: ADP or Epinephrine 1st Phase	Platelet Aggregation: ADP or Epinephrine 2nd Phase	Platelet Aggregation: Ristocetin	Platelet Aggregation: Collagen
Bernard-Soulier syndrome	D	N	N	D	N
Glanzmann's thrombasthenia	D	D	D	N	D
Release defect	N or D	N	D	N	D
Storage pool disease	N or D	N	D	N	D
von Willebrand's disease	D	N	N	D	N

ADP = adenosine diphosphate; D = depressed; N = normal.
Source: Data from DJW Bowie, Recognition of easily missed bleeding diseases. *Mayo Clin Proc* 57:263, 1982.

Bone marrow—fibrosis is minimal or absent; hyperplasia of all elements, with predominance of megakaryocytes and platelet masses, eosinophilia, basophilia

Thrombohemorrhagic disease (bleeding—skin, GI tract, nose, gums in 35% of patients)

Mild anemia (10–13 gm/dl) in one-third of patients

WBC usually >12,000/cu mm without cells earlier than myelocyte forms; leukocyte alkaline phosphatase is usually normal.

GLANZMANN'S THROMBASTHENIA

Probably represents a heterogeneous group of conditions incompletely studied and delineated

Normal platelet count with abnormal platelet morphology (e.g., variation in platelet size, increased platelet size, abnormal clumping and spreading)

Poor clot retraction and increased bleeding time may be present.

Normal coagulation time

TGT and prothrombin consumption tests abnormal but corrected by adding platelet substitute

Capillary fragility sometimes abnormal

ALLERGIC PURPURA

This is called Henoch's purpura when abdominal symptoms are predominant and Schönlein's purpura when joint symptoms are predominant.

Platelet count, bleeding time, coagulation time, and clot retraction are normal.

Tourniquet test may be negative or positive.

WBC and neutrophils may be increased; eosinophils may be increased.

Stool may show blood.

Urine usually contains RBCs and slight to marked protein.

Renal biopsy shows positive immunohistologic findings and typical glomerular histologic changes.

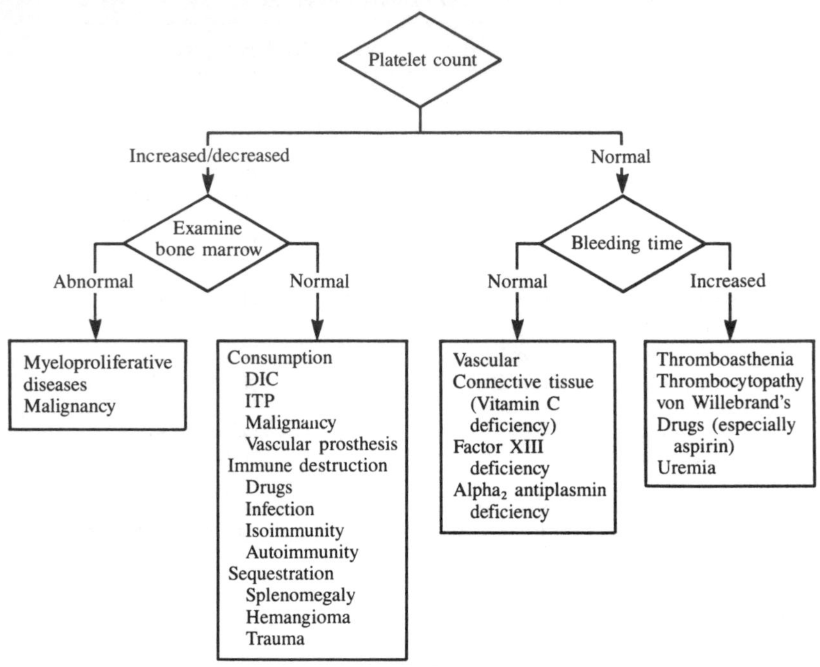

Fig. 12-10. Evaluation of hemostatic abnormalities. (PT and aPTT—see Figs. 12-8 and 12-9.)

VON WILLEBRAND'S DISEASE

Autosomal dominant heterozygous hereditary deficiency of a high-molecular-weight plasma protein (von Willebrand factor [vWF]) that mediates adherence of platelets to injured endothelium (various types are recognized). There is also a rare recessive homozygous with complete (or almost complete) absence of vWF and severe hemorrhage. Acquired form due to inhibitors to vWF in patients with autoimmune or lymphoproliferative disorders.

Difficulty in diagnosis arises from temporal variation in clinical and laboratory findings in an individual patient as well as from patient to patient; since many patients do not have the classic laboratory findings, five clinical variants have been described.

Bleeding time is prolonged using a calibrated template; in a few patients, may only be prolonged after administration of 300 mg of aspirin.

aPTT is prolonged.

Platelet adhesiveness to glass beads is decreased. Ristocetin-induced aggregation of platelets is deficient.

PT, platelet count, and clot retraction are normal.

Tourniquet test may be positive.

Factor VIII coagulant activity may range from normal to severely reduced (indicated by direct assay, PTT, or TGT tests).

Factor VIII-related antigen measured by special electroimmunoassay is decreased.

Table 12-29. Types of von Willebrand's Disease

	Autosomal Dominant Type			Autosomal Recessive
	I	IIa	IIb	
Bleeding time	I	I	I	I
Factor VIII procoagulant activity	D	D or N	D or N	D
Factor VIII–related antigen	D	D or N	D or N	D
Factor VIII von Willebrand's protein	D	D	D or N	D
Ristocetin-induced platelet aggregation	D or N	D	I	D

I = increased; D = decreased; N = normal.

Transfusion of normal plasma (or of hemophiliac plasma, cryoprecipitate, serum) causes a rise in Factor VIII activity greater than the amount of Factor VIII infused, which does not peak until 8–10 hours and slowly declines for days; in contrast, hemophilia shows rapid peak and fall after infusion of normal plasma or cryoprecipitate. This response to transfusion is a good diagnostic test in patients in whom diagnosis is equivocal. Factor VIII levels may increase to normal during pregnancy or use of oral contraceptives with subsidence of hemorrhagic episodes, although bleeding time is often unaffected. Therefore diagnostic evaluation should not be done in the presence of these two circumstances.

Screening of family members may be useful in difficult diagnostic cases even if they are asymptomatic and have no history of unusual bleeding.

Pseudo–von Willebrand's disease is a rare platelet disorder in which platelets have marked avidity for vWF that depletes the plasma of factor and may cause mild to moderate thrombocytopenia.

HEMOPHILIA

(Factor VIII deficiency; antihemophilic globulin [AHG] deficiency)

Classic hemophilia (assay of Factor VIII <1%) shows increased bleeding time, coagulation time, prothrombin consumption time, and aPTT (see Table 12-26).

Moderate hemophilia (assay of Factor VIII 1–5%) shows normal coagulation time and normal prothrombin consumption time but increased aPTT.

In mild hemophilia (assay of Factor VIII <16%) and "subhemophilia" (assay of Factor VIII 20–30%), these laboratory tests may be normal.

Abnormal TGT is corrected by absorbed plasma.

Laboratory findings due to hemorrhage and anemia are noted.

Acquired deficiency may occur in DIC and when an inhibitor is present (e.g., some cases of SLE, multiple myeloma, rheumatoid arthritis).

Screening tests for Factor VIII deficiency: PT, aPTT, thrombin time, bleeding time, platelet count

Secondary tests: Factor VIII:C, Factor VIIIR:Ag, platelet aggregation, platelet agglutination, ristocetin cofactor

COMPARISON OF LABORATORY TESTS IN HEMOPHILIA A AND VON WILLEBRAND'S DISEASE

	Hemophilia A	von Willebrand's Disease
Bleeding time	Normal	Prolonged
Factor VIIIR:Ag	Normal	Low
Factor VIII:C	Low	Prolonged-normal
Platelet adhesion	Normal	Retarded
Platelet aggregation (RIPA)	Normal	Decreased
Ristocetin cofactor	Normal	Deficient
aPTT	Prolonged	Prolonged-normal

FACTOR V DEFICIENCY (PARAHEMOPHILIA)

Inherited autosomal recessive deficiency syndrome or acquired in association with severe liver disease or DIC.

PT and aPTT are increased but corrected by addition of absorbed plasma.

FACTOR VII DEFICIENCY

Inherited form is autosomal recessive trait and is rare.

Acquired type may be due to liver disease, vitamin K deficiency, or dicumarol therapy.

PT is increased but corrected by aged serum.

aPTT is normal.

CONGENITAL FACTOR VII DEFICIENCY

With this infrequent autosomal trait, bleeding occurs when the gene is homozygous; heterozygotes have little or no manifestations.

Increased PT (normal when viper venom is used as thromboplastin; this does not correct PT in Factor X deficiency) is not corrected by administration of vitamin K.

Bleeding time, coagulation time, clot retraction, prothrombin consumption, and TGT are normal.

CONGENITAL FACTOR V DEFICIENCY (PARAHEMOPHILIA)

This is an infrequent autosomal recessive defect in which bleeding occurs only in the homozygote.

Variable increase in PT, prothrombin consumption, and coagulation time is not corrected by administration of vitamin K.

FACTOR IX (PLASMA THROMBOPLASTIN COMPONENTS [PTC]) DEFICIENCY (CHRISTMAS DISEASE; HEMOPHILIA B)

Inherited recessive sex-linked deficiency

In mild deficiency, only the TGT may be abnormal.

In more severe cases, increased coagulation time, bleeding time, prothrombin consumption time, and aPTT are found.

Defect is corrected by frozen plasma just as well as by bank blood.

FACTOR X (STUART-PROWER) DEFICIENCY

This rare autosomal recessive defect resembles Factor VII deficiency; heterozygotes show mild or no clinical manifestations.

Increased PT (not corrected by use of viper venom as thromboplastin) is not corrected by administration of vitamin K. Heterozygotes may have only slight increase in PT.

Acquired form may be associated with amyloidosis, coumarin anticoagulant therapy, vitamin K deficiency, liver trauma.

FACTOR XI (PLASMA THROMBOPLASTIN ANTECEDENT [PTA]) DEFICIENCY

Inherited autosomal recessive deficiency is usually mild; acquired forms are recognized.
In mild form, coagulation may be normal, prothrombin consumption time is slightly increased, and TGT is abnormal.
In severe cases, increased coagulation time, increased prothrombin consumption time, and abnormal TGT are found.

Postoperative bleeding may not begin until several days after surgery.

FACTOR XII (HAGEMAN FACTOR) DEFICIENCY

Coagulation time and prothrombin consumption time are increased.
TGT is abnormal.
Specific factor assay is needed to distinguish from Factor XI deficiency.

No hemorrhagic symptoms occur.

CONGENITAL DEFICIENCY OF FACTOR XIII (FIBRIN-STABILIZING FACTOR)

This is an inherited autosomal recessive deficiency with severe coagulation defect.
All standard clotting tests appear normal.
Patient's fibrin clot is soluble in 5M urea.
Whole blood clot is qualitatively friable.
Acquired type may occur in

- Acute myelogenous leukemia
- Liver disease
- Association with hypofibrinogenemia in obstetric complications
- Presence of circulating inhibitors

CONGENITAL AFIBRINOGENEMIA

This is a rare inherited autosomal recessive congenital condition.
Plasma fibrinogen is absent.
Bleeding time is often increased (one-third of patients).
PT, aPTT, and thrombin time are abnormal.
Platelet-to-glass adhesiveness is abnormal unless fibrinogen is added.

CONGENITAL HYPOFIBRINOGENEMIA

Inherited autosomal dominant
Plasma fibrinogen is moderately decreased (usually <80 mg/dl).
Bleeding and coagulation times are normal.
Blood clots are soft and small.

DYSFIBRINOGENEMIA

Fibrin formation is abnormally slow with prolonged plasma thrombin time.
Dysfibrinogenemia is present if immunologic fibrinogen is >2 times functional fibrinogen.
Other coagulation factors are normal.

Due To

Liver disease
Cancer
Fibrinolysis
DIC

Congenital, inherited autosomal dominant rare condition; may have no bleeding diathesis.

DISSEMINATED INTRAVASCULAR COAGULATION (DIC)*

(see Tables 12-30, p. 385, and 12-31, p. 386)

Not only is the clinical picture very variable, but the laboratory findings in a particular patient differ from the textbook composite, depending on the underlying disease, duration (acute or chronic), and compensatory or over-reactive coagulation mechanisms.

Many of the laboratory abnormalities may be present in patients with predisposing conditions (e.g., carcinoma of prostate, lung carcinoma) in whom DIC is latent; these abnormalities may predict development of DIC precipitated by surgery. These preexisting laboratory abnormalities may obscure changes due to DIC, e.g., increased fibrinogen in neoplasia, infection, and pregnancy may produce an apparently "normal" level in a case of DIC.

Criteria for specific diagnosis are not well defined. No single test is diagnostic, and diagnosis usually depends on combination of findings. Single normal level does not rule out DIC, and a repeat test screen should be done a few hours later for changes in platelet count and fibrinogen.

Repeated PTs (if initially prolonged) and fibrinogen levels are particularly useful. Normal PT rules out significant consumption coagulopathy.

Most sensitive and specific tests
- Protamine sulfate or ethanol gelation. A negative protamine is against ongoing DIC; ethanol test is less sensitive and may produce false negatives.
- Test for fibrin degradation products (FDP) in serum may be >100 μg/ml (normal = 0–10 μg/ml).
- Tests for fibrinopeptide A
- Serial fibrinogen levels (normal = 200–400 μg/dl)
- D-dimer assay (uses monoclonal antibodies to detect only cross-linked D-dimer fragments) is specific for fibrin and is more reliable indicator of DIC than FDP assay, since D-dimer is negative in cases of primary fibrinolysis.

Less sensitive and specific tests
- PT (done serially if prolonged)
- aPTT
- Thrombin time
- Serial platelet counts

Least sensitive and specific tests
- Euglobulin clot lysis measures fibrinolytic activity in plasma
- Factor assays
- Peripheral blood smear examination

In addition to the findings listed in Table 12-31 (p. 386), the following abnormalities often occur.
- Schistocytes in the peripheral blood smear and other evidence of microangiopathic hemolytic anemia may be present (e.g., increased serum LDH, decreased serum haptoglobin).
- Ethanol gelation and protamine gelation tests (that reflect fibrinogen degradation products but are less specific)
- Cryofibrinogen may be present.
- Observation of the blood clot may show the clot that forms to be small, friable, and wispy because of the hypofibrinogenemia.
- Plasma Factors V, VIII, and XIII are usually significantly decreased but are not used for primary diagnosis because of time and technical complexity.

*Data from M Sirridge, Laboratory evaluation of the bleeding patient. *Clin Lab Med* 4:285, 1984.

Table 12-30. Effect of Anticoagulant Drugs on Coagulation Tests

Test	Heparin	Warfarin	Aspirin	Dipyridamole/ sulfinpyrazone	Urokinase/ streptokinase
Platelet count	N[a]	N	N	N	N
Inhibition of platelet aggregation	N or I	N	I	N	I
Bleeding time	N or I	N[b]	I	N	I
Clotting time	I	N[b]	N	N	I
Thrombin time	I	N	N	N	I
Prothrombin time	I	I	N[b]	N	I
PTT	I	N[b]	N	N	I
Fibrinogen	N	N	N	N	D

N = no change; I = increased; D = decreased.
[a]Decreased in 25% of cases.
[b]Increased with high drug dosage.

Table 12-31. Disseminated Intravascular Coagulation (Consumption Coagulopathy)

Determination	% of Cases Abnormal	Abnormal Level for DIC	Mean Values for DIC	Response to Heparin Therapy	Tests
Decreased platelet count (per cu mm)	93	<150,000	52,000	None or may take weeks*	Platelet count, prothrombin time, fibrinogen level are performed first as screening tests; if all three are positive, diagnosis is considered established. If only two of these are positive, diagnosis should be confirmed by at least one of the tests for fibrinolysis.
Increased prothrombin time (seconds)	90	>15	18.0	Becomes normal or falls > 5 sec in few hours to 1 day	
Decreased fibrinogen level (mg/dl)	71	<160	137	Rises significantly (>40 mg) in 1–3 days	
Latex test for fibrinogen degradation products (titer)	92	>1:16	1:52	Begins to fall in 1 day; if very high, may take > 1 week to become normal	Tests for fibrinolysis
Prolonged thrombin time (seconds)	59	>25	27		
Euglobulin clot lysis time (minutes)	42	<120		Returns to normal	

*Platelet count is not a satisfactory indicator of response to heparin therapy.

Source: Adapted from RW Colman, SJ Robboy, and JD Minna, Disseminated intravascular coagulation (DIC): An approach. *Am J Med* 52:679, 1972.

Table 12-32. Comparison of Acute and Chronic DIC

	Acute DIC	Chronic DIC
Platelet count	D—moderate/marked	D—mild/marked
PT	I	N or slight I
aPTT	I	N or D
Thrombin time	I	N or moderate I
Fibrinogen	D	I, N, or moderate D
Fibrin degradation products	Present	Present
Protamine sulfate test	Positive	Positive
Factors V & VIII	D	N

D = decreased; I = increased; N = normal.

Table 12-33. Comparison of Acute DIC and Primary Fibrinogenolysis

	Acute DIC	Fibrinogenolysis
Platelet count	D	Usually N
Fibrinogen	D	D
Fibrin degradation products	0 to very marked I	Very marked I
Protamine sulfate test	Positive	Negative
Euglobulin clot lysis time	N	D
Factor V	D	D
Factor VIII	D	N to moderate D

D = decreased; I = increased; N = normal.

Survival time of radioiodine-labeled fibrinogen and rate of incorporation of ^{14}C-labeled glycine ethyl ester into soluble "circulating fibrin" are sensitive indicators of DIC.

Clotting time determinations are used to monitor heparin therapy.

Underlying conditions

- Sepsis (especially due to gram-negative bacteria) is most common cause.
- Tissue injury—pregnancy and obstetric complications (e.g., abruptio placentae, intrauterine fetal death, amniotic fluid embolism), extensive surgery, neoplasms (especially prostate), leukemias, chemotherapy of neoplasia, large traumatic injuries and burns
- Endothelial injury—infections, prolonged hypotension
- Injury of platelets or RBCs—immunologic hemolytic anemias
- Reticuloendothelial system injury—liver disease (cirrhosis, hepatitis), postsplenectomy
- Vascular malformations—giant hemangiomas, aortic aneurysm

Suspect clinically in patients with underlying conditions who show bleeding (frequently acute and dramatic), purpura or petechiae, acrocyanosis, arterial or venous thrombosis.

CIRCULATING ANTICOAGULANTS

Various types of endogenous anticoagulants may interfere with coagulation at different stages, especially Factor VIII, heparin-like activity, antithromboplastins.

May be acquired (antibodies) due to multiple transfusion for congenital deficiency of a coagulation factor or spontaneous.

Table 12-34. Differential Diagnosis of DIC

	DIC	Chronic Liver Disease	Primary Fibrinolysis	TTP	Hemolytic Uremic Syndrome	Multiple Transfusion
Platelet count	D	D	N	N–D	D	D
PT	I	I	I	N	N	I
aPTT	I	N–I	I	N	N	I
FDP	I	N–I	I	N–I	N–I	N
D-dimer assay	I	N	I	N	N	N
Fibrinogen	D	V	D	N	N	I
Schistocytes	+	0	+	+	+	0
BUN	I	N	N	I	I	N
Liver function tests	N	I	N	N	N	N
Protamine sulfate	I	N–I	I	N–I	N	N
Euglobulin clot lysis	N	N	D	N	N	N

D = decreased; I = increased; N = normal; V = variable; + = present; 0 = absent

Abnormal PTT or aPTT screening is not corrected by equal mixtures of patient and normal plasma but is corrected if due to deficient coagulation factor.

Circulating Anticoagulants Associated with Clinical Disorders

Various types of anticoagulants may interfere with coagulation at different stages, especially Factor VIII, heparin-like activity, antithromboplastins.

Inhibitors of specific coagulation factors are often associated with a bleeding tendency, but lupus anticoagulant predisposes to arterial and venous thrombosis.

Factor	Disorder
VIII and IX	Following replacement therapy for hereditary deficiency
XI	SLE—very rare
IX	SLE—rare
VIII	SLE, rheumatoid arthritis, drug reaction, asthma, pemphigus, inflammatory bowel disease, postpartum period, advanced age
X	Amyloidosis (tissue binding rather than circulating)
V	Associated with streptomycin administration, idiopathic
X, V	SLE—common
II	Myeloma, SLE
XIII	Associated with isoniazid administration, idiopathic

SYSTEMIC LUPUS ERYTHEMATOSUS (SLE)

Criteria for diagnosis of lupus anticoagulant
- Increased aPTT
- 1:1 mixture with normal plasma is >4 seconds longer than control aPTT
- Decrease in ≥2 factors (VIII, IX, XI, or XII) by one-stage assay but normal by two-stage assay
- Activity increases with dilution

Other findings
- Increased PT in 10%
- Tissue thromboplastin inhibition test and dilute Russell viper venom times (RVVT) are abnormal in almost all cases.
- Platelet neutralization procedure (addition of platelets will shorten the prolonged aPTT and RVVT due to lupus anticoagulants but not due to Factor VIII inhibitors)

Arterial and venous thrombi occur in up to 30% of patients; therefore this inhibitor may be a marker for predisposition to thrombosis.

Lupus anticoagulant may occur in patients with
- Autoimmune diseases
- Infectious diseases (e.g., AIDS)
- Due to drugs
- SLE is associated wtih <50% of cases of lupus anticoagulant

LIVER DISEASE

Screening tests may include any combination of abnormal PTT, aPTT, thrombin time, euglobulin or whole-blood clot lysis times, increased fibrin degradation products. These will be corrected by equal mixture of patient and normal plasma except thrombin time in presence of large amounts of fibrin degradation products due to hyperplasminemia or if fibrin polymerization is faulty.

Special tests may show decreased antithrombin-III, decrease in any coagulation factor (except VIII:C, which is normal or increased in liver disease but decreased in DIC), decreased $alpha_2$ antiplasmin.

SOME INDICATIONS FOR TRANSFUSION OF BLOOD PRODUCTS

Red Cell Transfusion

Hgb < 8 gm/dl (Hct < 26%) and MCV within normal limits (81–100 fl; 70–125 fl if age 14 years or less)

Hb < 8 gm/dl (Hct < 26%) in patients with acute bleed or high risk*
Hb < 11 gm/dl (Hct < 36%) and clinically symptomatic†
Hb < 11 gm/dl (Hct <36%) or bleeding >1 unit/24 hours
Any Hb level in high-risk* patients with acute bleed
Any Hb level in symptomatic† patients with acute bleed
Any Hb level in patients bleeding >2 units/24 hours or >15% of blood volume/24 hours

Cryoprecipitate Transfusion

Received massive transfusions >8 units/24 hours
Received transfusion >6 RBC units/case (e.g., open heart surgery)
Bleeding or invasive procedure in patients with hypofibrinogenemia or DIC
Deficient Factor VIII or von Willebrand's disease or abnormal fibrinogen in presurgical or bleeding patients

Platelet Transfusion

- Platelet count <20,000 in patients without
  - Thrombotic thrombocytopenic purpura
  - Idiopathic thrombocytopenic purpura
  - Posttransfusion purpura
  - Hemolytic uremic syndrome
- Platelet count <50,000 in patients with
  - Minor bleeding
  - Pre-op for a minor procedure
  - Prematurity
- Platelet count <90,000 in patients with
  - Bleed requiring RBC transfusion
  - Pre-op for a major procedure
- Received massive RBC transfusion (>8 units/24 hours)
- Bleeding time >10 minutes
- Received transfusion >6 RBC units/case (e.g., open heart surgery)

Fresh Frozen Plasma Transfusion

Massive transfusion >8 units RBC/24 hours (>1 blood volume in infants/children)
Abnormal coagulation test result(s) (e.g., PT >15 or PTT >45 seconds) during prior 24 hours
Known congenital coagulation factor disorder (e.g., Factor II, V, VII, IX, X, XI, XII) and bleeding or prophylaxis for major procedures
Clinical evidence of abnormal bleeding (e.g., bleeding from venipuncture sites or generalized oozing)
Patients with diagnosis of thrombotic thrombocytopenic purpura
Received transfusion >6 RBC units/case (e.g., open heart surgery)

*High risk: for example, patients with coronary artery disease, chronic pulmonary disease, cerebrovascular disease, or known anemia.
†Symptomatic: for example, patients with signs or symptoms of anemia (e.g., tachycardia, angina, ECG changes); or of respiratory distress; known hemoglobinopathy, etc.

Metabolic and Hereditary Diseases

BLOOD VITAMIN LEVELS

Vitamin A (retinol)	360–1200 μg/L
Carotene	
0–6 months	0–40 mg/dl
6 months to adult	40–180 mg/dl
Vitamin C (ascorbic acid)	0.2–2.0 mg/dl
Vitamin D	Indirect estimate by measuring serum alkaline phosphatase, calcium, and phosphorus
Total 25-hydroxyvitamin D	14–42 ng/ml (winter)
	15–80 ng/ml (summer)
1,25-Dihydroxyvitamin D	15–60 pg/ml
Vitamin E (alpha-tocopherol)	
Children	3.0–15.0 μg/ml
Adults	5.5–17.0 μg/ml
Deficiency	<3.0 μg/ml
Excess	>40 μg/ml
Vitamin B_1 (thiamine)	5.3–7.9 μg/dl
Vitamin B_2 (riboflavin)	3.7–13.7 μg/dl
Vitamin B_{12} (cobalamin)	
Low	<100 pg/ml
Indeterminate	100–200 pg/ml
Normal	
Males	
0–50 years	200–1079 pg/ml
50–59 years	191–770 pg/ml
60–69 years	168–687 pg/ml
70–79 years	152–630 pg/ml
Females	190–765 pg/ml
Elevated	>1100 pg/ml
Unsaturated vitamin B_{12}–binding capacity	870–1800 pg/ml
Folate (serum)	
Low	<2.0 ng/ml
Normal	2.0–20 ng/ml
Increased	>20 ng/ml
Folate (RBC)	>140 ng/ml

ACID-BASE DISORDERS

In analyzing acid-base disorders, several precautions should be kept in mind:

Determination of pH and blood gases should be performed on *arterial* blood.

Venous blood is useless for judging oxygenation but may offer a crude estimate of acid-base status.

The blood specimen should be packed in ice immediately; delay of even a few minutes will cause erroneous results, especially if WBC is high.

Determination of electrolytes, pH, and blood gases ideally should be performed on blood specimens obtained simultaneously, since the acid-base situation is very labile.

Repeated determinations may often be indicated because of the development of complications, the effect of therapy, and other factors.

Table 13-1. Metabolic and Respiratory Acid-Base Changes in Blood

	pH	PCO_2	HCO_3^-
Acidosis			
Acute metabolic	D	N	D
Compensated metabolic	N	D	D
Acute respiratory	D	I	N
Compensated respiratory	N	I	I
Alkalosis			
Acute metabolic	I	N	I
Chronic metabolic	I	I	I
Acute respiratory	I	D	N
Compensated respiratory	N	D	D

D = decreased; N = normal; I = increased.

Acid-base disorders are often mixed rather than in the pure form usually described in textbooks. These mixed disorders may represent simultaneously occurring diseases, complications superimposed on the primary condition, or the effect of treatment.

Changes in chronic forms may be notably different from those in the acute forms.

For judging hypoxemia, it is also necessary to know the patient's hemoglobin or hematocrit and whether the patient was breathing room air or oxygen when the specimen was drawn.

Arterial blood gases cannot be interpreted without clinical information about the patient.

Most laboratories measure pH and PCO_2 directly and calculate HCO_3^- using the Henderson-Hasselbalch equation:

$$\text{Arterial pH} = 6.1 + \log \frac{HCO_3}{0.03 \times PCO_2}$$

where 6.1 is the dissociation constant for CO_2 in aqueous solution and 0.03 is a constant for the solubility of CO_2 in plasma at 37°C.

A normal pH does not ensure the absence of an acid-base disturbance if the PCO_2 is not known.

An abnormal HCO_3^- means a metabolic rather than a respiratory problem; decreased HCO_3^- indicates metabolic acidosis, and increased HCO_3^- indicates metabolic alkalosis. Respiratory acidosis is associated with a $PCO_2 >$ 45 mmHg, and respiratory alkalosis is associated with a $PCO_2 <$ 35 mmHg. Thus mixed metabolic and respiratory acidosis is characterized by low pH, low HCO_3^-, and high PCO_2. Mixed metabolic and respiratory alkalosis is characterized by high pH, high HCO_3^-, and low PCO_2. (See Table 13-1, Metabolic and Respiratory Acid-Base Changes in Blood.)

In severe metabolic acidosis, respiratory compensation is limited by inability to hyperventilate PCO_2 to <20 mmHg. In metabolic alkalosis, respiratory compensation is limited by CO_2 retention, which rarely causes PCO_2 >50–60 mmHg (because CO_2 stimulates respiration very strongly); thus pH is not returned to normal.

Pearls

Pulmonary embolus: Mild to moderate respiratory alkalosis is present unless sudden death occurs. The degree of hypoxia often correlates with the size and extent of the pulmonary embolus.

$PO_2 > 90$ mmHg when breathing room air virtually excludes a lung problem.

Acute pulmonary edema: Hypoxemia is usual. CO_2 is not increased unless the situation is grave.

Asthma: Hypoxia occurs even during a mild episode and increases as the attack becomes worse. As hyperventilation occurs, the PCO_2 falls (usually <35 mmHg); a normal PCO_2 (>40 mmHg) implies impending respiratory failure; increased PCO_2 in a true asthmatic (not bronchitis or emphysema) indicates impending disaster and the need to consider intubation and ventilation assistance.

Chronic obstructive pulmonary disease (bronchitis and emphysema) may show two patterns—"pink puffers" with mild hypoxia and normal pH and PCO_2 and "blue bloaters" with hypoxia and increased PCO_2; normal pH suggests compensation, and decreased pH suggests decompensation.

Neurologic and neuromuscular disorders (e.g., drug overdose, Guillain-Barré syndrome, myasthenia gravis, trauma, succinylcholine): Acute alveolar hypoventilation causes uncompensated respiratory acidosis with high PCO_2, low pH, and normal HCO_3^-. Acidosis appears before significant hypoxemia, and rising CO_2 indicates rapid deterioration and need for mechanical assistance.

Sepsis: Unexplained respiratory alkalosis may be the earliest sign of sepsis. It may progress to cause metabolic acidosis, and the mixed picture may produce a normal pH; low HCO_3^- is useful to recognize this. With deterioration and worsening of metabolic acidosis, the pH falls.

Salicylate poisoning characteristically shows poor correlation between serum salicylate level and presence or degree of acidemia (because as pH drops from 7.4 to 7.2, the proportion of nonionized to ionized salicylate doubles and the nonionized form leaves the serum and is sequestered in the brain and other organs, where it interferes with function at a cellular level without changing blood levels of glucose, etc.). Salicylate poisoning in adults typically causes respiratory alkalosis, but in children this progresses rapidly to mixed respiratory alkalosis-metabolic acidosis and then to metabolic acidosis (in adults, metabolic acidosis is said to be rare and a near-terminal event).

Isopropyl (rubbing) alcohol poisoning produces enough circulating acetone to produce a positive nitroprusside test (and therefore may be mistaken for diabetic ketoacidosis; thus insulin should not be given until the blood glucose is known). In the absence of a history, positive serum ketone test associated with normal anion gap, normal serum HCO_3^-, and normal blood glucose suggest rubbing alcohol intoxication.

Acid-base maps (see Fig. 13-1) are a graphic solution of the Henderson-Hasselbalch equation that predicts the HCO_3^- value for each set of pH/PCO_2 coordinates. They also allow a check of the consistency of arterial blood gas and SMA-6 determinations, since the SMA-6 determines the total CO_2 content, of which 95% is HCO_3^-. These maps contain bands that show the 95% probability range of values for each disorder. If the pH/PCO_2 coordinate is outside the 95% confidence band, then the patient has at least two acid-base disturbances. These maps are of particular use when one of the acid-base disturbances is not suspected clinically. If the coordinates lie within a band, it is not a guarantee of a simple acid-base disturbance.

METABOLIC ACIDOSIS

With Increased Anion Gap (AG > 15 mEq/L)

Lactic acidosis—commonest cause of metabolic acidosis with increased AG (frequently > 25 mEq/L) (see following section)

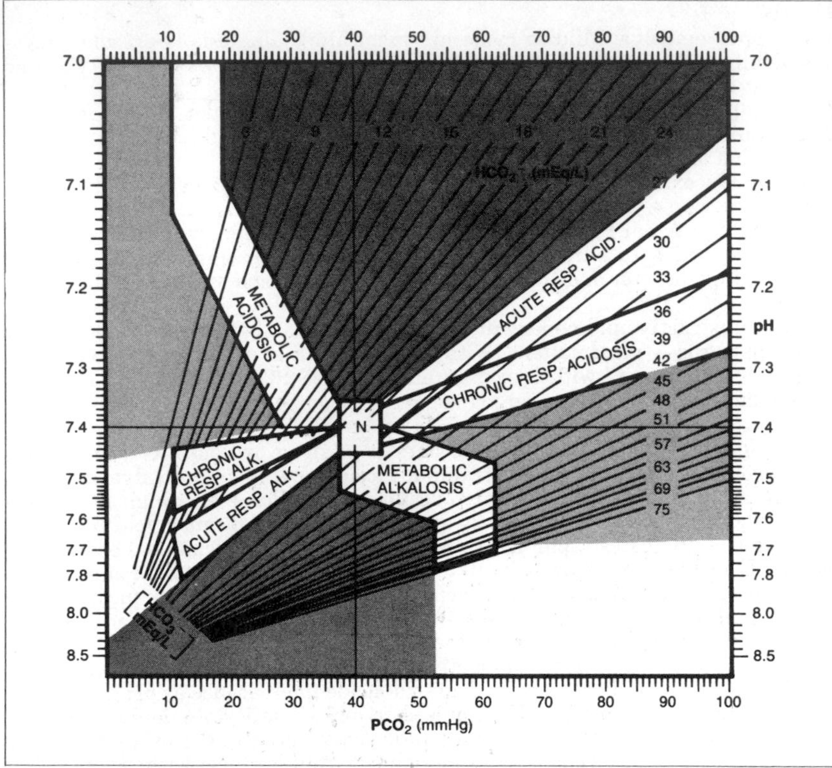

Fig. 13-1. Acid-base map. The values demarcated for each disorder represent a 95% probability range for each *pure* disorder (N = normal). Coordinates lying outside these zones suggest mixed acid-base disorders. (Adapted from M Goldberg, SB Green, ML Moss, et al., Computer-based instruction and diagnosis of acid-base disorders. *JAMA* 223:269, 1973. Copyright 1973 American Medical Association.)

Renal failure (AG < 25 mEq/L)
Ketoacidosis
- Diabetes mellitus (AG frequently > 25 mEq/L)
- Associated with alcohol abuse (AG frequently 20–25 mEq/L)
- Starvation (AG usually 5–10 mEq/L)

Drugs
- Salicylate poisoning (AG frequently 5–10 mEq/L; higher in children)
- Methanol poisoning (AG frequently > 20 mEq/L)
- Ethylene glycol poisoning (AG frequently > 20 mEq/L)
- Paraldehyde (AG frequently > 20 mEq/L)

With Normal Anion Gap
(hyperchloremic acidosis)

Decreased serum potassium
- Renal tubular acidosis
- Acquired (e.g., drugs, hypercalcemia)
- Inherited (e.g., cystinosis, Wilson's disease)
- Carbonic anhydrase inhibitors (e.g., acetazolamide, mafenide)

Table 13-2. Illustrative Serum Electrolyte Values in Various Conditions

Condition	pH	Bicarbonate	Potassium	Sodium	Chloride
Normal	7.35–7.45	24–26	3.5–5.0	136–145	100–106
Metabolic acidosis					
Diabetic acidosis	7.2	10	5.6	122	80
Fasting	7.2	16	5.2	142	100
Severe diarrhea	7.2	12	3.2	128	96
Hyperchloremic acidosis	7.2	12	5.2	142	116
Addison's disease	7.2	22	6.5	111	72
Nephritis	7.2	8	4	129	90
Nephrosis	7.2	20	5.5	138	113
Metabolic alkalosis					
Vomiting	7.6	38	3.2	150	94
Pyloric obstruction	7.6	58	3.2	132	42
Duodenal obstruction	7.6	42	3.2	138	49
Respiratory acidosis	7.1	30	5.5	142	80
Respiratory alkalosis	7.6	14	5.5	136	112

Increased loss of alkaline body fluids (e.g., diarrhea, loss of pancreatic or biliary fluids)
Ureteral diversion (e.g., ileal bladder or ureter, ureterosigmoidostomy)
Normal or increased serum potassium
Hydronephrosis
Early renal failure
Administration of HCl (e.g., ammonium chloride)
Hypoadrenalism (diffuse, zona glomerulosa, or hyporeninemia)
Renal aldosterone resistance
Sulfur toxicity

In lactic acidosis the increase in AG is usually greater than the decrease in HCO_3^-, in contrast to diabetic ketoacidosis in which the increase in AG is identical to the decrease in HCO_3^-.

Laboratory Findings

Serum pH is decreased (<7.3).
Total plasma CO_2 content is decreased; <15 mEq/L almost certainly rules out respiratory alkalosis.
Serum potassium is frequently increased; it is decreased in renal tubular acidosis, diarrhea, or carbonic anhydrase inhibition.
Azotemia suggests metabolic acidosis due to renal failure.
Urine is strongly acid (pH = 4.5–5.2) if renal function is normal.
In evaluating acid-base disorders, calculate the anion gap (see the following section).

ANION GAP (AG) CLASSIFICATION

(calculated as Na − [Cl + HCO_3]; normal = 8–16 mEq/L; if K is included, normal = 10–20 mEq/L)

Increased In

Increased "unmeasured" anions
Organic (e.g., lactic acidosis, ketoacidosis)
Inorganic (e.g., administration of phosphate, sulfate)
Protein (e.g., hyperalbuminemia, transient)
Exogenous (e.g., salicylate, formate, nitrate, penicillin, carbenicillin)
Not completely identified (e.g., hyperosmolar hyperglycemic nonketotic coma, uremia, poisoning by ethylene glycol, methanol, salicylates)
Laboratory error
Falsely increased serum sodium
Falsely decreased serum chloride or bicarbonate
Decreased unmeasured cations (e.g., hypokalemia, hypocalcemia, hypomagnesemia)

When AG >12–14 mEq/L, diabetic ketoacidosis is the most common cause, uremic acidosis is the second most common cause, and drug ingestion (e.g., salicylates, methyl alcohol, ethylene glycol, ethyl alcohol) is the third most common cause; lactic acidosis should always be considered when these three causes are ruled out.

Decreased In

Decreased unmeasured anion (e.g., hypoalbuminemia is probably commonest cause of decreased anion gap)
Laboratory error
"Hyperchloremia" in bromide intoxication (if chloride determination by colorimetric method)
Hyponatremia due to viscous serum
False decrease in serum sodium; false increase in serum chloride or HCO_3^-

Increased unmeasured cations
- Hyperkalemia, hypercalcemia, hypermagnesemia
- Increased proteins in multiple myeloma, paraproteinemias, polyclonal gammopathies (these abnormal proteins are positively charged and lower the AG)
- Increased lithium, TRIS buffer (tromethamine)

AG > 30 mEq/L almost always indicates organic acidosis even in presence of uremia. AG = 20–29 mEq/L occurs in absence of identified organic acidosis in 25% of patients.

AG is rarely >23 mEq/L in chronic renal failure.

Simultaneous changes in ions may cancel each other out, leaving anion gap unchanged (e.g., increased Cl and decreased HCO_3^-).
AG may provide a clue to the presence of a mixed rather than simple acid-base disturbance.

LACTIC ACIDOSIS

Should be considered in any metabolic acidosis with increased AG (>15 mEq/L).
Diagnosis is confirmed by exclusion of other causes of metabolic acidosis and serum lactate ≥ 5 mEq/L (upper limit of normal = 1.6 for plasma and 1.4 for whole blood). Considerable variation in literature in limits of serum lactate and pH to define lactic acidosis.
Exclusion of other causes by
- Normal serum creatinine and BUN *(Increased acetoacetic acid [but not beta-hydroxybutyric acid] will cause false increase of creatinine by colorimetric assay.)*
- Osmolar gap < 10 mOsm/L
- Negative nitroprusside reaction *(Nitroprusside test for ketoacidosis measures acetoacetic acid but not beta-hydroxybutyric acid; thus blood ketone test may be negative in diabetic ketoacidosis.)*
- Urine negative for calcium oxalate crystals
- No known ingestion of toxic substances

Laboratory findings due to underlying diseases (e.g., diabetes mellitus, renal insufficiency)
Laboratory tests for monitoring therapy
- Arterial pH, PCO_2, HCO_3, serum electrolytes every 1–2 hours until patient is stable
- Urine electrolytes every 6 hours

Associated or compensatory metabolic or respiratory disturbances (e.g., hyperventilation or respiratory alkalosis may result in normal pH)

Due To

Type A due to clinically apparent tissue hypoxia (e.g., acute hemorrhage, severe anemia, shock, asphyxia)
Type B without clinically apparent tissue hypoxia
- Common disorders (e.g., diabetes mellitus, uremia, liver disease, infections, malignancies, alkaloses)
- Drugs and toxins (e.g., ethanol, methanol, ethylene glycol, salicylates)
- Hereditary enzyme defects (e.g., methylmalonic aciduria, glucose-6-PD deficiency)

Laboratory Findings

With a typical clinical picture (acute onset following nausea and vomiting, altered state of consciousness, hyperventilation, high mortality)

Decreased serum bicarbonate
Low serum pH, usually 6.98–7.25
Increased serum potassium, often 6–7 mEq/L
Serum chloride normal or low with increased AG
WBC is increased (occasionally to leukemoid levels).
Increased serum uric acid is frequent (up to 25 mg/dl in lactic acidosis).
Increased serum phosphorus. Phosphorus-creatinine ratio > 3 indicates lactic acidosis either alone or as a component of other metabolic acidosis.
Increased SGOT, LDH, and phosphorus in serum

METABOLIC ALKALOSIS

Due To

Loss of acid
- Vomiting, gastric suction, gastrocolic fistula
- Diarrhea in mucoviscidosis (rarely)
- Aciduria secondary to potassium depletion

Excess of base due to administration of
- Absorbable antacids (e.g., sodium bicarbonate)
- Salts of weak acids (e.g., sodium lactate, sodium or potassium citrate)

Some vegetable diets

Potassium depletion (causing sodium and H^+ to enter the cells)
- Gastrointestinal loss (e.g., chronic diarrhea)
- Lack of potassium intake (e.g., anorexia nervosa, IV fluids without potassium supplements for treatment of vomiting or postoperatively)
- Diuresis (e.g., mercurials, thiazides, osmotic diuresis)
- Extracellular volume depletion and chloride depletion
- All forms of mineralocorticoid excess (e.g., primary aldosteronism, Cushing's syndrome, administration of steroids, large amounts of licorice)
- Glycogen deposition
- Chronic alkalosis
- Potassium-losing nephropathy

Hypoproteinemia per se may cause a nonrespiratory alkalosis. Decreased albumin of 1 gm/dl causes an average increase in standard bicarbonate of 3.4 mM/L, an apparent base excess of +3.7 mEq/L and a decrease in AG of ~3 mEq/L.*

Laboratory Findings

Serum pH is increased.
Total plasma CO_2 is increased (bicarbonate > 30 mEq/L).
PCO_2 is normal or slightly increased.
Serum pH and bicarbonate above those predicted by the PCO_2 (by nomogram or Table 13-3)
Serum potassium is usually decreased, which is the chief danger in metabolic alkalosis.
Decreased serum chloride is relatively lower than sodium.
BUN may be increased.
Urine pH is >7.0 (≤7.9) if potassium depletion is not severe and concomitant sodium deficiency (e.g., vomiting) is not present. With severe hypokalemia (<2.0 mEq/L), urine may be acid in presence of systemic alkalosis.
When the urine chloride is low (<10 mEq/L) and the patient responds to chloride treatment, the cause is more likely loss of gastric juice, diuretic therapy, or rapid relief of chronic hypercapnia. Chloride replacement is completed when urine chloride remains >40 mEq/L. When the urine chloride is high

*Data from JJ McAuliffe, et al., Hypoproteinemic alkalosis. *Am J Med* 81:86, 1986.

Table 13-3. Upper Limits of Arterial Blood pH and Bicarbonate Concentrations (expected for blood PCO_2 values)

Arterial Blood		
PCO_2 (mmHg)	pH	Bicarbonate (mEq/L)
20	7.66	22.8
30	7.53	25.6
40	7.47	27.3
60	7.29	27.9
80	7.18	28.9

Values shown are the upper limits of the 95% confidence bands.
Source: Data from FL Coe, Metabolic alkalosis. *JAMA* 238:2288, 1977.

(>20 mEq/L) and the patient does not respond to NaCl treatment, the cause is more likely hyperadrenalism or severe potassium deficiency.

RESPIRATORY ACIDOSIS

Laboratory findings differ in acute and chronic conditions.

Acute

Due to decreased alveolar ventilation impairing CO_2 excretion
- Pneumonia
- Pulmonary edema
- Laryngospasm, bronchospasm
- General anesthesia
- Pneumothorax
- Foreign body aspiration
- Mechanical ventilation
- Oversedation

Acidosis is severe (pH 7.05–7.10), but HCO_3^- concentration is only 29–30 mEq/L.

Severe mixed acidosis is common in cardiac arrest when respiratory and circulatory failure cause marked respiratory acidosis and severe lactic acidosis.

Chronic

Due to chronic obstructive or restrictive disease
- Nerve disease (e.g., poliomyelitis)
- Muscle disease (e.g., myopathy)
- Central neurologic disorder (e.g., brain tumor)
- Restriction of thorax (e.g., musculoskeletal, scleroderma)
- Pulmonary disease (e.g., prolonged pneumonia, primary alveolar hypoventilation)

Acidosis is not usually severe.

Beware of commonly occurring mixed acid-base disturbances (e.g., chronic respiratory acidosis with superimposed acute hypercapnia resulting from acute infection, such as bronchitis or pneumonia).

Superimposed metabolic alkalosis (e.g., due to diuretics or vomiting) may exacerbate the hypercapnia.

RESPIRATORY ALKALOSIS

(decreased $PCO_2 < 38$ mmHg)

Due To

Hyperventilation

- CNS disorders (e.g., infection, tumor, trauma, cerebrovascular accident
- Salicylate intoxication
- Fever
- Gram-negative bacteremia
- Liver disease
- Pulmonary disease (e.g., pneumonia, pulmonary emboli, asthma)
- Mechanical overventilation
- Congestive heart failure
- Hypoxia (e.g., decreased barometric pressure, ventilation-perfusion imbalance)

Laboratory Findings

Acute hypocapnia—usually only a modest decrease in plasma HCO_3^- concentrations and marked alkalosis

Chronic hypocapnia—usually only a slight alkaline pH

MIXED ACID-BASE DISTURBANCES

(must always be interpreted with clinical data and other laboratory findings)

Respiratory Acidosis With Metabolic Acidosis

Examples: Acute pulmonary edema, cardiopulmonary arrest (lactic acidosis due to tissue anoxia and CO_2 retention due to alveolar hypoventilation)

Acidemia may be extreme with pH < 7.0 ($H^+ > 100$ mEq/L)

$HCO_3^- < 26$ mEq/L. Failure of HCO_3^- to increase ≥ 3 mEq/L for each 10 mmHg rise in $PaCO_2$ suggests metabolic acidosis with respiratory acidosis.

Mild metabolic acidosis superimposed on chronic hypercapnia causing partial suppression of HCO_3^- may be indistinguishable from adaptation to hypercapnia alone.

Metabolic Acidosis With Respiratory Alkalosis

Examples: Rapid correction of severe metabolic acidosis, salicylate intoxication, gram-negative septicemia, initial respiratory alkalosis with subsequent development of metabolic acidosis

pH may be normal or decreased.

Hypocapnia remains inappropriate to decreased HCO_3^- for several hours or more.

Respiratory Acidosis With Metabolic Alkalosis

Examples: Chronic pulmonary disease with CO_2 retention developing metabolic alkalosis due to administration of diuretics, severe vomiting, or sudden improvement in ventilation ("posthypercapnic" metabolic alkalosis)

Decreased or absent urine chloride indicates that chloride-responsive metabolic alkalosis is a part of the picture.

In clinical setting of respiratory acidosis but with normal blood pH and/or HCO_3^- higher than predicted, complicating metabolic alkalosis may be present.

Respiratory Alkalosis With Metabolic Alkalosis

Examples: Hepatic insufficiency with hyperventilation plus administration of diuretics or severe vomiting; metabolic alkalosis with stimulation of ventilation (e.g., sepsis, pulmonary embolism, mechanical ventilation) that causes respiratory alkalosis

Marked alkalemia with decreased PCO_2 and increased HCO_3^- is diagnostic.

Acute and Chronic Respiratory Acidosis

Examples: Chronic hypercapnia with acute deterioration of pulmonary function causing further rise of PCO_2

HCO_3^- in intermediate range between acute and chronic respiratory acidosis (similar findings in chronic respiratory acidosis with superimposed metabolic acidosis or acute respiratory acidosis with superimposed metabolic alkalosis)

Coexistence of Metabolic Acidoses of Hyperchloremic Type and Increased AG Type

May be suspected by plasma HCO_3^- that is lower than is explained by the increase in anions (e.g., AG = 16 mEq/L and HCO_3^- = 5 mEq/L)

Examples are uremia and proximal renal tubular acidosis (RTA), lactic acidosis with diarrhea, excessive administration of NaCl to patient with organic acidosis

Coexistence of Metabolic Alkalosis and Metabolic Acidosis

Examples: vomiting causing alkalosis plus bicarbonate-losing diarrhea causing acidosis

May be suspected by acid-base values that are too normal for clinical picture

PROTEIN-CALORIE MALNUTRITION

Adult Malnutrition and Kwashiorkor

Occurs in patients with inadequate protein intake in presence of low or normal caloric intake and increased catabolism (e.g., trauma, severe burns, respiratory or renal failure, nonmalignant GI tract disease); may develop quickly. Major loss of protein from visceral compartments may impair organ function.

Decreased serum albumin (2.1–3.0 mg/dl in moderate; <2.1 mg/dl in severe) is a poor marker; uncertain significance of level 2.9–3.5 mg/dl.

Decreased serum prealbumin (transthyretin) is more sensitive than albumin due to shorter half-life; (normal range = 16–40 mg/dl: severe malnutrition <10.7 mg/dl; moderate malnutrition = 10.7–16.0 mg/dl; is likely to benefit from early therapy). With therapy, increases >1 mg/dl daily. Other protein markers with short half-lives that have been suggested are retinol-binding protein and fibronectin.

Decreased total iron-binding capacity (TIBC) or serum transferrin (moderate = 100–150 mg/dl; severe <100 mg/dl); increase in transferrin due to inflammation decreases diagnostic utility. Direct measurement is preferred because calculation is affected by iron metabolism and laboratory variability. Poor sensitivity in this condition.

All serum complement components except C4 and sometimes C5 are decreased. Decreased total lymphocyte count evidencing diminished immunologic resistance (normal = 2000–3500/cu mm; <1500/cu mm is indication for further assessment; moderate = 800–1200/cu mm; severe < 800;) (should always be interpreted with total WBC count).

Diminished delayed hypersensitivity reaction (measured by skin testing).

Normal anthropometric measurements (e.g., creatinine-height index, triceps skinfold, arm circumference measurements).

Clinically, may show pitting edema, ascites, enlarged liver, diarrhea.

Table 13-4. Summary of Pure and Mixed Acid-Base Disorders

	Decreased pH	Normal pH	Increased pH
Increased PCO_2	Respiratory acidosis with or without incompletely compensated metabolic alkalosis or coexisting metabolic acidosis	Respiratory acidosis and compensated metabolic alkalosis	Metabolic alkalosis with incompletely compensated respiratory acidosis or coexisting respiratory acidosis
Normal PCO_2	Metabolic acidosis	Normal	Metabolic alkalosis
Decreased PCO_2	Metabolic acidosis with incompletely compensated respiratory alkalosis or coexisting respiratory alkalosis	Respiratory alkalosis and compensated metabolic acidosis	Respiratory alkalosis with or without incompletely compensated metabolic acidosis or coexisting metabolic alkalosis

Source: Adapted from HH Friedman, *Problem-Oriented Medical Diagnosis* (3rd ed.). Boston: Little, Brown, 1983.

These laboratory tests all have low sensitivity and specificity or are not easily available.

Marasmus

Chronic deficiency in total energy intake as in wasting illnesses (e.g., cancer) with protein loss from somatic compartment without necessary losses in visceral component

Normal serum protein levels

Impaired immune function

Clinically, show severe wasting of skeletal muscle and fat; edema is distinctively absent. May progress to marasmic kwashiorkor.

Laboratory findings due to underlying diseases (e.g., cancer) or complications (e.g., infection)

Monitor Nutritional Therapy

Weekly 24-hour urine nitrogen excretion reflects degree of hypermetabolism and correction of deficits.

Increase of serum prealbumin and retinol-binding proteins by 1 mg/dl/day indicates good response. Measure 2–3 times/week. May precede improvement in albumin levels by 7–10 days.

Somatomedin C has also been suggested for monitoring.

Fluid and electrolyte levels should be corrected.

VITAMIN A DEFICIENCY

Decreased plasma level of vitamin A. <25 IU/ml is significantly low.

Elevated carotenoids may cause false low values for vitamin A.

Laboratory findings due to preceding conditions (e.g., malabsorption, alcoholism, restricted diet).

Table 13-5. Illustrative Values in Acid-Base Disturbances

Condition	Sodium	Chloride	HCO_3^-	PCO_2	pH
Normal	140	105	25	40	7.40
Metabolic acidosis	140	115	15	31	7.30
Chronic respiratory alkalosis	136	102	25	40	7.44
Mixed metabolic acidosis and chronic respiratory alkalosis	136	108	14	24	7.39
e.g., Sepsis: addition of respiratory alkalosis to metabolic acidosis further decreases HCO_3^- but pH may remain normal. Lactic acidosis plus respiratory alkalosis due to severe liver disease, pulmonary emboli, or sepsis					
Metabolic alkalosis	140	92	36	48	7.49
Chronic respiratory acidosis	140	102	28	50	7.37
Mixed metabolic alkalosis and chronic respiratory acidosis	140	90	40	67	7.40
e.g., COPD patient receiving glucocorticoids or diuretics. PCO_2 and HCO_3^- are increased by both conditions but pH is neutralized.					
Metabolic alkalosis	139	89	35	47	7.49
Respiratory alkalosis	136	102	20	30	7.44
Mixed alkalosis, mild	139	92	32	39	7.53
Mixed alkalosis, severe	139	92	32	30	7.63
e.g., Postoperative patient with severe hemorrhage stimulating hyperventilation (respiratory alkalosis) plus massive transfusion and nasogastric drainage (metabolic alkalosis)					
Chronic respiratory acidosis	140	100	30	55	7.36
Mixed chronic respiratory acidosis and acute metabolic acidosis	136	102	22	55	7.22
e.g., COPD (chronic respiratory acidosis) with severe diarrhea (metabolic acidosis). pH is too low for PCO_2 of 55 in chronic respiratory acidosis indicating low pH due to mixed acidosis, but HCO_3^- effect is offset					
Metabolic acidosis	140	105	25	40	7.40
Metabolic alkalosis	138	90	36	48	7.49
Mixed metabolic acidosis and metabolic alkalosis	140	103	25	40	7.40
e.g., Gastroenteritis with vomiting (metabolic alkalosis) and diarrhea (metabolic acidosis due to loss of HCO_3^-). Surprisingly normal findings with marked volume depletion					

SCURVY (VITAMIN C DEFICIENCY)

Plasma level of ascorbic acid is decreased—usually 0 in frank scurvy. (Normal = 0.5–1.5 mg/dl, but lower level does not prove diagnosis.) Ascorbic acid in buffy coat (WBC) is decreased—usually absent in clinical scurvy. (Normal = 30 mg/dl.)

Tyrosyl compounds are present in urine (detected by Millon's reagent) in patients with scurvy but are absent in normal persons after protein meal or administration of tyrosine.

Serum alkaline phosphatase is decreased; serum calcium and phosphorus are normal.

Rumpel-Leede test is positive.

Microscopic hematuria is present in one-third of patients.
Stool may be positive for occult blood.
Laboratory findings due to associated deficiencies (e.g., anemia due to folic acid deficiency) are present.

BERIBERI (THIAMINE DEFICIENCY)

Increased blood pyruvic acid level
Decreased thiamine level in blood and urine; becomes normal within 24 hours after therapy begins (thus baseline levels should be established first)
RBC transketolase < 8 IU (baseline) and addition of thiamine pyrophosphate causes >20% increase
Laboratory findings due to complications (e.g., heart failure)
Laboratory findings due to underlying conditions (e.g., chronic diarrhea, inadequate intake, alcoholism)

RIBOFLAVIN DEFICIENCY

Decreased riboflavin level in plasma, RBCs, WBCs
RBC glutathione reductase activity coefficient ≥ 1.20

PELLAGRA (NIACIN DEFICIENCY)

Whole blood niacin level < 24 μmol/L
Decreased excretion of niacin metabolites (nicotinamide) in 6- or 24-hour urine sample
Plasma tryptophan level markedly decreased

PYRIDOXINE (VITAMIN B_6) DEFICIENCY

Decreased pyridoxic acid in urine
Decreased serum levels of vitamin B_6

VITAMIN B_{12} AND FOLIC ACID DEFICIENCY

See pp. 285–290 and Table 12-5, p. 290.

VITAMIN D DEFICIENCY OR EXCESS

See p. 290.

VITAMIN E DEFICIENCY

Plasma tocopherol < 0.4 mg/dl in adults; < 0.15 mg/dl in infants age 1 month
Laboratory findings due to underlying conditions (e.g., malabsorption in adults; diet high in polyunsaturated fatty acids in premature infants)

VITAMIN K DEFICIENCY

See p. 368.

COPPER DEFICIENCY

Nutritional Copper Deficiency

Found in patients on parenteral nutrition and in children recovering from severe protein-calorie malnutrition fed iron-fortified milk formula with cane sugar and cottonseed oil
Anemia not responsive to iron and vitamins
Leukopenia with WBC < 5000/cu mm and neutropenia (<1500/cu mm)
Copper administration corrects neutropenia in 3 weeks, and anemia responds with reticulocytosis.
Decreased copper and ceruloplasmin in plasma and decreased hepatic copper confirm diagnosis.

"Kinky Hair" Syndrome

Syndrome of neonatal hypothermia, feeding difficulties, and sometimes prolonged jaundice; at 2–3 months, seizures and progressive change of hair from

normal to steel-wool light color; striking facial appearance, increasing mental deterioration, infections, failure to thrive, death in early infancy; changes in elastica interna of arteries
Decreased copper in serum and liver; normal in RBCs
Increased copper in amniotic fluid, cultured fibroblasts, and amniotic cells

Serum Copper Also Decreased In
Nephrosis (ceruloplasmin lost in urine)
Wilson's disease
Acute leukemia in remission
Some iron deficiency anemias of childhood (that require copper as well as iron therapy)
Kwashiorkor

Serum Copper Increased In
Anemias
- Pernicious anemia
- Megaloblastic anemia of pregnancy
- Iron deficiency anemia
- Aplastic anemia

Leukemia, acute and chronic
Infection, acute and chronic
Malignant lymphoma
Biliary cirrhosis
Hemochromatosis
Collagen diseases (including systemic lupus erythematosus [SLE], rheumatoid arthritis, acute rheumatic fever, glomerulonephritis)
Hypothyroidism
Hyperthyroidism
Frequently associated with increased C-reactive protein (CRP)
Ingestion of oral contraceptives and estrogens

ZINC DEFICIENCY

Occurs In
Acrodermatitis enteropathica (rare autosomal recessive disease of infancy)
Inadequate nutrition (e.g., parenteral alimentation)
Excessive requirements
Decreased absorption or availability
Increased losses
Iatrogenic
Plasma zinc levels do not always reflect nutritional status.
Measurement of zinc in hair may be helpful.
Decreased or very excessive urinary zinc excretion may be helpful.

CLASSIFICATION OF SOME INHERITED METABOLIC CONDITIONS

Disorders of carbohydrate metabolism
- Diabetes mellitus
- Pentosuria
- Fructosuria
- Familial lactose intolerance
- Galactosemia
- Glycogen storage diseases
- Mucopolysaccharidoses

Disorders of amino acid metabolism
- Phenylketonuria
- Tyrosinosis
- Maple syrup urine disease
- Alkaptonuria

Disorders of purine and pyrimidine metabolism
- Gout
- Orotic aciduria
- Beta-aminoisobutyric aciduria

Disorders of lipid metabolism
- Essential familial hypercholesterolemia
- Inherited deficiency of lipoprotein lipase
- Disorders of porphyrin metabolism

Disorders of metabolism involving metals
- Wilson's disease
- Hemochromatosis
- Periodic paralysis
- Adynamia episodica hereditaria

Disorders of renal tubular function
- Fanconi's syndrome of cystinosis
- Vitamin D–resistant rickets of primary hypophosphatemia
- Cystinuria
- Renal glycosuria

Disorders of serum enzymes
- Hypophosphatasia

Disorders of plasma proteins
- Analbuminemia
- Agammaglobulinemia
- Atransferrinemia

Disorders of blood
- Coagulation diseases (e.g., hemophilias)
- RBC glucose-6-PD deficiency
- Hemoglobinopathies and thalassemias
- Hereditary spherocytosis
- Hereditary nonspherocytic hemolytic anemia

Disorders of Lipid Metabolism

SERUM CHOLESTEROL

(Note effect of illness, intra-individual variation, position, season, drugs, etc. when these values are used to diagnose and treat hyperlipidemias.)

Increased In

Idiopathic hypercholesterolemia

Hyperlipoproteinemias

Biliary obstruction
- Stone, carcinoma, etc., of duct
- Cholangiolitic cirrhosis
- Biliary cirrhosis
- Cholestasis

von Gierke's disease

Hypothyroidism

Nephrosis (due to chronic nephritis, renal vein thrombosis, amyloidosis, SLE, periarteritis, diabetic glomerulosclerosis)

Pancreatic disease
- Diabetes mellitus
- Total pancreatectomy
- Chronic pancreatitis (some patients)

Pregnancy

Certain drugs (e.g., progestins, anabolic steroids)

Decreased In

Severe liver cell damage (due to chemicals, drugs, hepatitis)
Hyperthyroidism
Malnutrition (e.g., starvation, terminal neoplasm, uremia, malabsorption in steatorrhea)
Chronic anemia
- Pernicious anemia in relapse
- Hemolytic anemias
- Marked hypochromic anemia

Cortisone and adrenocorticotropic hormone (ACTH) therapy
Hypobeta- and abetalipoproteinemia
Tangier disease

SERUM HIGH-DENSITY LIPOPROTEIN (HDL) CHOLESTEROL

Increased In

Vigorous exercise
Increased clearance of triglyceride very low-density lipoprotein (VLDL)
Moderate consumption of alcohol
Insulin treatment
Estrogen

Decreased In (<32 mg/dl in men, <38 mg/dl in women)

Stress and recent illness (e.g., acute myocardial infarction, stroke, surgery, trauma) *(Thus tests for hyperlipidemia should not be performed on hospitalized patients until 2–3 months after illness.)*
Starvation
Obesity
Lack of exercise
Cigarette smoking
Diabetes mellitus
Hypothyroidism
Liver disease
Nephrosis
Uremia
Elevated serum triglyceride
Certain drugs (e.g., anabolic steroids, progesterone, antihypertensive beta blockers)
Familial hypoalphalipoproteinemia
Rare genetic disorders
- Homozygous Tangier disease
- Familial lecithin-cholesterol acyltransferase deficiency (LCAT) and fish eye disease
- HDL deficiency with planar xanthomas
- Apolipoprotein A-I and apolipoprotein C-III deficiency variant I and variant II

SERUM LOW-DENSITY LIPOPROTEIN (LDL) CHOLESTEROL

Increased In (>190 mg/dl)

Familial hypercholesterolemia
Familial combined hyperlipidemia
Diabetes mellitus
Hypothyroidism
Nephrotic syndrome
Chronic renal failure
Diet high in cholesterol, total and saturated fat
Pregnancy

Multiple myeloma, dysgammaglobulinemia
Porphyria
Pregnancy
Anorexia nervosa
Certain drugs (e.g., estrogens, anabolic steroids, antihypertensive beta blockers, progestins, carbamazepine)

Can estimate LDL if fasting triglycerides < 400 mg/dl by this formula:

LDL = total cholesterol − ([triglycerides/5] + HDL cholesterol)

VLDL = triglycerides/5

LDL cholesterol is directly related to risk of coronary heart disease.

Desirable level	<130 mg/dl
Borderline elevation	130–159 mg/dl
Elevated level	≥160 mg/dl

HDL cholesterol is inversely related to risk of coronary heart disease.

Low risk (desirable level)	>60 mg/dl
Moderate risk	35–60 mg/dl
High risk	<35 mg/dl

Some laboratories also report various ratios, e.g.,

LDL/HDL ratio

Low risk	0.5–3.0
Moderate risk	3.0–6.0
High risk	>6.0

Cholesterol/HDL ratio

Low risk	3.3–4.4
Average risk	4.4–7.1
Moderate risk	7.1–11.0
High risk	>11.0

TRIGLYCERIDES

Increased In

Familial hyperlipidemia
Liver diseases
Nephrotic syndrome
Hypothyroidism
Diabetes mellitus (higher values correlate with hyperglycemia and poorer control of diabetes; reduced by insulin therapy)
Alcoholism
Gout
Pancreatitis
von Gierke's disease
Acute myocardial infarction (rise to peak in 3 weeks; increase may persist for 1 year)
Certain drugs (e.g., oral contraceptives, high-dose estrogens, beta blockers, hydrochlorothiazide)

Mild elevation of serum triglycerides (up to 250 mg/dl) probably does not represent increased risk for any disease. Range of 250–500 mg/dl may be a marker for patients with genetic forms of hyperlipoproteinemias who need specific therapy because of increased cardiovascular risk. >500 mg/dl should be labeled "hypertriglyceridemia" with danger of pancreatitis; >1000 mg/dl carries substantial risk of pancreatitis.

Decreased In

Congenital abetalipoproteinemia
Malnutrition

Total and HDL cholesterol levels are similar in fasting and nonfasting, but triglycerides should be measured after 12–14 hours fasting. Serum levels are about 5% higher than plasma levels.

Triglyceride levels are not a strong predictor of atherosclerosis or coronary heart disease and are not an independent risk factor.

SERUM LIPOPROTEINS

Decreased In

Abetalipoproteinemia (Bassen-Kornzweig syndrome)
Tangier disease
Hypobetalipoproteinemia

Increased In

Hyperbetalipoproteinemia
Hyperalphalipoproteinemia

APOLIPOPROTEINS

(are protein component of lipoprotein and regulate their metabolism; each of four major groups consists of a family of 2 or more immunologically distinct proteins)

Apolipoprotein (Apo) A is the major protein of HDL; Apo A-I and A-II constitute 90% of total HDL protein in ratio of 3:1.

Apo B is the major protein in LDL; important in regulating cholesterol synthesis and metabolism.

Apo C-I, C-II, and C-III are associated with all lipoproteins except LDL; C-II is important in triglyceride metabolism.

Serum Apo A-I and B levels are more highly correlated with severity and extent of coronary artery stenosis than total cholesterol and triglycerides.

Apo A-I/B ratio showed greater sensitivity and specificity for coronary artery disease than LDL/HDL cholesterol ratio or HDL cholesterol-triglyceride ratio or any of the individual components.*

HYPERLIPIDEMIAS

Independent risk factors for coronary artery disease (CAD) are increased LDL cholesterol or decreased HDL cholesterol. Tests should not be performed during stress or acute illness, recent myocardial infarction, stroke, pregnancy, trauma, weight loss, or use of drugs that affect blood lipids; severe illness lowers LDL cholesterol and LDL Apo B, and one should allow 3 months after such illness to do these tests. Intra-individual variation in serum triglycerides

*Data from *J Clin Immunoassay* 9:11, 1986.

Table 13-6. Comparison of Classic Types of Hyperlipoproteinemia

Point of Comparison	Type I (rarest)	Type IIa (relatively common)	Type IIb (relatively common)	Type III (relatively uncommon)	Type IV (most common)	Type V (uncommon)
Origin	Exogenous hyperlipidemia due to deficient lipoprotein lipase		Overindulgence lipidemia		Endogenous hyperlipidemia	Mixed endogenous and exogenous hyperlipidemia (combined Types I and IV)
Definition	Familial fat-induced hyperglycidemia	Hyperbetalipoproteinemia (hypercholesterolemia)	Combined hyperlipidemia (mixed hyperlipidemia)	Carbohydrate-induced hyperglyceridemia with hypercholesterolemia	Carbohydrate-induced hyperglyceridemia without hypercholesterolemia	Combined fat and carbohydrate-induced hyperglyceridemia
Age	Usually under age 10			Not known under age 25	Only occasionally seen in children	
Gross appearance of plasma	On standing: supernatant creamy, infranatant clear	Clear (no cream layer on top)	No cream layer on top; clear to turbid infranatant	Clear, cloudy, or milky	Slightly turbid to cloudy Unchanged on standing	Markedly turbid On standing: supernatant creamy, infranatant milky
Serum cholesterol	N or slightly I	Markedly I (300–600 mg/dl)	Markedly I (300–600 mg/dl)	Markedly I (300–1000 mg/dl)	N or slightly I	I (250–500 mg/dl)
LDL-cholesterol	N	I	I	I	N	N
HDL-cholesterol	N to D	N to D	N to D	N to D	N to D	N to D

Apolipoprotein	I (B-48) I (A-IV) V (CII)	I (B-100)	I (B-100)	I (E-II) D (E-III) D (E-IV)	V (CII) I (B-100)	V (CII) I (B-48) I (B-100)
Increased lipoprotein	Chylomicrons	LDL	LDL, VLDL	IDL	VLDL	VLDL Chylomicrons
Serum triglycerides	Markedly I (usually >2000 mg/dl)	N	I ≤400 mg/dl	Markedly I (200–1000 mg/dl)	Markedly I (500–1500 mg/dl)	Markedly I (500–1500 mg/dl)
Appearance of lipoprotein components visualized by electrophoresis						
Chylomicron[a]	Marked I	0	0	0	0	I
Beta-lipoprotein[b]	N or D	I	I	I Floating beta	N or I	N or I
Prebetalipoprotein[c]	N or D	N	I	I	I	I
Alpha-lipoprotein[d]						
Other laboratory abnormalities	Glucose tolerance usually N			Hyperglycemia; glucose tolerance often abnormal; serum uric acid I	Glucose tolerance often abnormal; serum uric acid often I	Glucose tolerance usually abnormal; serum uric acid usually I
Triglyceride-cholesterol ratio	8	1	Variable	<2	1–5	> 5

(Continued)

Table 13-6. (continued)

Point of Comparison	Type I (rarest)	Type IIa (relatively common)	Type IIb (relatively common)	Type III (relatively uncommon)	Type IV (most common)	Type V (uncommon)
Lipid changes resembling primary hyperlipidemias						
Diet		Very high cholesterol diet	Same as Type IIa		Caffeine or alcohol before testing	
Drugs		Triglyceride-lowering drugs in Types III and IV	Same as Type IIa	Triglyceride-lowering drugs in Type IV	Cholesterol-lowering drugs Chlorothiazide Birth control pills or estrogens	
Primary disease		Myxedema Nephrosis Obstructive liver disease Stress Porphyria Anorexia nervosa Idiopathic hypercalcemia	Same as Type IIa	Myxedema Dysgammaglobulinemia Liver disease	Nephrotic syndrome Hypothyroidism Pregnancy Glycogen storage disease	Myeloma Macroglobulinemia Nephrosis

0 = absent; N = normal; I = increased; D = decreased.

	[a]Chylomicrons	[c]VLDL (pre-beta-lipoprotein)	[b]LDL (beta-lipoprotein)	[d]HDL (alpha-lipoprotein)
Triglycerides	90%	60%	5%	5%
Cholesterol	5%	15%	50%	20%
Phospholipids	4%	15%	25%	25%
Protein	1%	10%	20%	50% (Apo A-1, II)

Since Apo B is the only protein in LDL and Apo A-I is the major protein constituent of HDL and VLDL, the ratio Apo-B/Apo A-I reflects the ratio LDL/HDL and may be a better discriminator of coronary artery disease than the individual components, but data on apoliproproteins are still limited.

Obtain blood only after at least 12–14 hours' fasting and when patient has been on usual diet for at least 2 weeks.
Rule out diabetes and pancreatitis in all groups.
Increased susceptibility to coronary artery disease occurs in Types II, III, IV; accelerated peripheral vascular disease in Type III.
Xanthomas appear in Types I, II, III.
Abdominal pain occurs in Types I, V.
If dietary or drug treatment has begun, it may not be possible to classify the lipoproteinemia or the classification may be erroneous.

Type IIb is overindulgence hyperlipemia; shows increased cholesterol and triglycerides, with increased beta and prebeta; can only be distinguished from Type III by detecting abnormal beta-migrating lipoprotein in serum fraction with density > 1.006.

Source: Data from Office of Medical Application of Research, NIH. Treatment of hypertriglyceridemia. *JAMA* 251:1196, 1984.

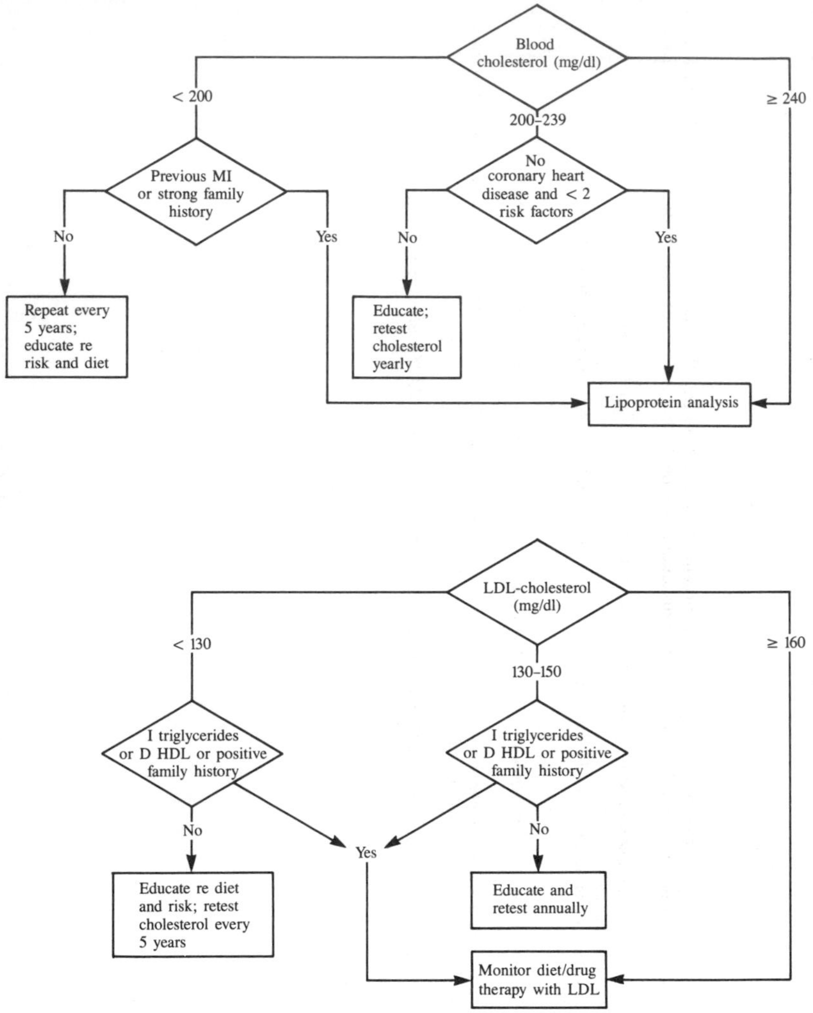

Blood cholesterol (mg/dl)

< 200

200–239

≥ 240

Previous MI or strong family history

No

Yes

Repeat every 5 years; educate re risk and diet

No coronary heart disease and < 2 risk factors

No

Yes

Educate; retest cholesterol yearly

Lipoprotein analysis

LDL-cholesterol (mg/dl)

< 130

130–150

≥ 160

I triglycerides or D HDL or positive family history

No

Educate re diet and risk; retest cholesterol every 5 years

Yes

I triglycerides or D HDL or positive family history

No

Educate and retest annually

Monitor diet/drug therapy with LDL

Fig. 13-2. Flow chart of recommended testing and treatment of increased serum cholesterol. Measure serum total cholesterol, HDL cholesterol, and triglycerides after 12- to 14-hour fast. Average of 2–3 tests, 1–8 weeks apart.

$$\textbf{Estimate LDL} = \textbf{total cholesterol} - \textbf{HDL cholesterol} - \frac{\textbf{triglycerides}}{\textbf{5}}$$

D = decreased; I = increased.
(Adapted from Report of the Expert Panel on Detection, Evaluation and Treatment of High Blood Cholesterol in Adults. National Cholesterol Education Program Coordinated by the National Heart, Lung, and Blood Institute, US Department of Health and Human Services, PHS, NIH. NIH Publication No. 88-2025, Jan 1988.)

is 12–40%; analytical variation is 5–10%. Intra-individual variation may be about 4–10% for serum total cholesterol and 3.6–12.4% for HDL. Anabolic steroids increase total and LDL cholesterol and decrease HDL. Contraceptive agents and some beta-blocking antihypertensive drugs tend to increase triglycerides and decrease HDL. Some diuretics increase total cholesterol. Cholesterol values are up to 8% higher in winter than summer, 5% lower if bled when sitting compared to when standing, and 10–15% different when recumbent compared to when standing. Tourniquet in place longer than 3 minutes may cause 5% variation in lipid values. Diurnal variation causes triglycerides to be lowest in the morning and highest around noon. Cholesterol values of EDTA plasma can be multiplied by 1.03 to be comparable to serum values. Serum cholesterol and HDL can be nonfasting, but serum for triglycerides and for calculating LDL should follow a 12-hour fast. Nonfasting cholesterol >200 mg/dl indicates need for further study; if confirmed by repeat study, perform fasting total and HDL cholesterol and triglycerides. For all of the above reasons, abnormal lipid test results should always be confirmed with a new specimen before beginning or changing therapy. Repeat cholesterol values should be within 30 mg/dl.

Fasting level LDL cholesterol > 160 mg/dl, HDL cholesterol < 35 mg/dl, or triglycerides > 250 mg/dl indicate lipoprotein disorder. Should first rule out secondary causes.

Definite coronary heart disease: definite myocardial infarction or definite angina pectoris

Other coronary heart disease risk factors

- HDL cholesterol < 35 mg/dl (not part of initial screen)
- Diabetes mellitus
- Family history of premature coronary heart disease
- Hypertension
- Cigarette smoking
- Male
- Extreme obesity (>30% above ideal body weight)
- History of stroke or peripheral vascular disease

Notes

- Use total cholesterol for initial case finding and classification.
- Use LDL cholesterol to decide about treatment.
- Use total cholesterol to monitor diet therapy.
- Repeat initial cholesterol within 2 months for confirmation before performing lipoprotein screening. Repeat LDL before treatment. If the repeat values are within 30 mg/dl, use the average; if not, repeat and average the three values.
- Do not use age- or sex-specific cholesterol values as decision levels.
- Always rule out secondary and familial causes of hypercholesterolemia.

Step I diet (also appropriate for all Americans)

- Total fat < 30% of total calories
- Saturated fat < 10% of total calories
- Cholesterol intake < 300 mg/day

Step II diet

- Total fat < 30% of total calories
- Saturated fat < 7% of total calories
- Cholesterol intake < 200 mg/day

Primary Hyperlipidemias (see Table 13-6, pp. 410–413)

Lipoprotein electrophoresis shows a specific abnormal pattern in <2% of Americans (usually Type II, IV). Chief purpose of test now is to identify rare familial disorders (e.g., I, III, V) to anticipate problems in children.

Lipoprotein electrophoresis may be indicated if
- Serum triglycerides > 300 mg/dl
- Fasting serum is lipemic.
- Hyperglycemia is significant.
- Glycosuria
- Impaired glucose tolerance
- Increased serum uric acid
- Strong family history of premature coronary heart disease
- Clinical evidence of coronary heart disease or atherosclerosis in patient <age 40

If lipoprotein electrophoresis is abnormal, tests should be performed to rule out diabetes mellitus, liver disease, nephrotic syndrome, dysproteinemias, hypothyroidism

Familial Hypercholesterolemia (Type II)

LDL receptors in fibroblasts or mononuclear blood cells are absent in homozygous patients and 50% of normal levels in heterozygous patients (performed at specialized laboratories).

Homozygous—very rare condition in which serum cholesterol is very high (e.g., 600–1000 mg/dl) with corresponding increase (6–8 times normal) in LDL. Both parents are heterozygous. Clinical manifestations of increased cholesterol (xanthomata, corneal arcus, CAD that causes death usually before age 30 years). Neonatal diagnosis requires finding increased LDL cholesterol in cord blood; serum cholesterol is unreliable. Because of marked variation in serum cholesterol levels during first year of life, diagnosis should be deferred until infant is 1 year old. Prenatal diagnosis of homozygous fetus can be made by estimation of binding sites on fibroblasts cultured from amniotic fluids; useful when both parents are heterozygous. Occurs 1 per million in the population.

Heterozygous—increased serum cholesterol (300–500 mg/dl) and LDL (2–3 times normal) with similar change in a parent or first-degree relative; serum triglycerides and VLDL are normal in 90% and slightly increased in 10% of these patients. Gene frequency occurs 1 in 500 in general population, but 5% in survivors of acute myocardial infarction < age 60 years. Premature CAD, tendinous xanthomas, and corneal arcus are often present.

Familial Combined Hyperlipidemia (IIa, IIb, IV, V)

Occurs in 0.5% of general population and 15% of survivors of acute myocardial infarction < 60 years old.

There may be any combination of increased LDL and VLDL and chylomicrons; HDL is often low; different family members may have increased serum cholesterol or triglycerides or both.

Premature CAD occurs later in life (after age 30 years) than with familial hypercholesterolemia.

Xanthomas are rare. Patient is often overweight.

Polygenic Hypercholesterolemia (Type IIa)

Persistent cholesterol elevation (>240 mg/dl) and increased LDL without familial hypercholesterolemia or familial combined hypercholesterolemia

Premature CAD occurs later in life than with familial combined hyperlipidemia.

Xanthomas are rare.

Familial Dysbetalipoproteinemia (Type III)

Excess of abnormal lipoprotein (beta mobility–VLDL) is present; cholesterol > 300 mg/dl plus triglycerides > 400 mg/dl should suggest this diagnosis. VLDL cholesterol–plasma triglyceride ratio = 0.3.

Tuberous and tendinous xanthomas and palmar and plantar xanthomatous streaks are present.

Atherosclerosis is more common in peripheral than coronary arteries.

Familial Hypertriglyceridemia (Type IV)

Elevated triglycerides (usually 200–500 mg/dl and VLDL with normal LDL and decreased HDL.

Distinction from familial combined hyperlipidemia is made only by extensive family screening.

Autosomal dominant condition present in 1% of general population and 5% of survivors of acute myocardial infarction < age 60 years.

Severe Hypertriglyceridemia (Type I)

Persistent high triglycerides (>1000 mg/dl) with marked increase in VLDL and chylomicrons.

Associated with recurrent pancreatitis rather than CAD.

Usually in middle-aged with diabetes mellitus, increased uric acid, obesity; may be precipitated by alcohol, estrogens, renal insufficiency. Less often in young nonobese, nondiabetic adults due to familial lipoprotein lipase deficiency.

Abetalipoproteinemia (Bassen-Kornzweig syndrome)

Chylomicrons, LDL, and VLDL are absent; HDL are normal.

Marked decrease in plasma triglycerides (<30 mg/dl) and cholesterol (<100 mg/dl).

Patients also have acanthotic RBCs and low serum carotene levels.

Arteriosclerosis is absent.

The condition is an autosomal recessive trait. A variant is normotriglyceridemic abetalipoproteinemia in which patient can secrete Apo B-48 but not Apo B-100, resulting in normal postprandial triglyceride values but marked hypocholesterolemia; associated with mental retardation and vitamin E deficiency.

Hypobetalipoproteinemia

Familial disorder with increased longevity and lower incidence of atherosclerosis. Marked decrease in LDL and LDL/HDL ratio.

Homozygous patients have decreased plasma cholesterol (<60 mg/dl) and triglycerides and undetectable or trace amounts of chylomicrons, VLDL, and LDL.

Heterozygotes have plasma cholesterol, LDL, and Apo B values 50% of normal (consistent with codominant disorder). May also be caused by malabsorption of fats, infection, anemia, hepatic necrosis, hyperthyroidism, acute myocardial infarction (AMI), acute trauma.

Tangier Disease

There is a marked decrease (heterozygous) or absence (homozygous) of HDL.

Pre-beta-lipoprotein is absent.

Serum cholesterol (<100 mg/dl), LDL cholesterol, and phospholipid are decreased; triglycerides are normal or increased (100–250 mg/dl).

Premature coronary artery disease is present.

Deposits in reticuloendothelial cells cause enlarged liver, spleen, lymph nodes, enlarged orange tonsils; may have CAD, mild corneal opacification, and neuropathy in homozygous type.

Increased In

Hyperbetalipoproteinemia: See Table 13-6, pp. 410–413.

Hyperalphalipoproteinemia: See next paragraph.

Familial lipid disorders with protection against atherosclerosis (illustrates importance of measuring HDL to evaluate hypercholesterolemia)

- Hyperalphalipoproteinemia (HDL excess): 1 in 20 adults with mild increased cholesterol levels (240–300 mg/dl) secondary to increased HDL (>70 mg/dl); LDL not increased; triglycerides are normal. Inherited as simple autosomal dominant trait in families with longevity or may be caused by alcoholism, extensive exposure to chlorinated hydrocarbon pesticides, exogenous estrogen supplementation.

Hypobetalipoproteinemia (see Table 13-6, pp. 410–413)

Conditions With HDL Deficiency

Associated with men, obesity, sedentary life, smoking, diabetes mellitus, use of androgenic substances, hypertriglyceridemia

Homozygous Tangier disease

Familial lecithin-cholesterol acyltransferase deficiency (LCAT) and fish-eye disease

HDL deficiency with planar xanthomas

Apo A-I and Apo C-III deficiencies are rare genetic conditions associated with premature CAD and marked HDL deficiency.

Familial hypoalphalipoproteinemia

Common autosomal dominant condition, with premature CAD and stroke

HDL < 10th percentile (<30 mg/dl in men and <38 mg/dl in women of middle age)

One-third of patients with premature CAD may have this disorder.

Secondary Hyperlipidemias

Poorly controlled diabetes mellitus

Most common findings—increase in VLDL with increased serum triglycerides and less marked increase in cholesterol

Less common findings—as above with chylomicrons also increased

Least common—normal pattern despite poor control

Hypothyroidism

Most common pattern is Type II with increased LDL and total cholesterol.

Less common pattern is Type III.

Serum cholesterol is not always increased.

Rapidly becomes normal with treatment.

Nephrotic syndrome

Increased serum cholesterol is usual.

Increased LDL is common.

Increased VLDL and therefore increased serum triglyceride may also occur.

Hepatic glycogenoses

Increased serum lipoprotein is common in any of the forms, but the pattern cannot be used to differentiate the type of GSD.

Predominant increase in VLDL in glucose-6-phosphatase deficiency

Predominant increase in LDL in debrancher and phosphorylase deficiencies

Obstructive liver disease

Increased serum cholesterol is common until liver failure develops.

The type of lipoproteinemia is variable.

In intrahepatic biliary atresia, there is often increase in lipoprotein X with marked increase in serum cholesterol and even more marked increase in serum phospholipids.

Chronic alcoholism

Marked increase in VLDL producing Type IV or V pattern

Hyperlipoproteinemia of “affluence” (dietary)

Disorders of Amino Acid Metabolism

HOMOCYSTINURIA

Autosomal recessive error of methionine metabolism with deficient cystathionine synthetase in liver and brain with inability to change homocystine to cystathionine.

Urine excretion of homocystine is increased (positive nitroprusside screening test). May also contain increased methionine and other amino acids.

Table 13-7. Summary of Primary Overflow Aminoacidurias (increased blood concentration with overflow into urine)

Disease	Increased Blood Amino Acids	Urine Abnormalities*	Other Laboratory Findings
Phenylketonuria	Phenylalanine	*o*-Hydroxyphenylacetic acid; phenylpyruvic, acetic, and lactic acids	Blood tyrosine does not rise after phenylalanine load
Maple syrup urine disease			
Severe infantile form	Valine, leucine, isoleucine, alloisoleucine	Branched-chain ketoacids in great excess; urine has odor of maple syrup	
Intermittent form	Same	Ketoaciduria and urine odor present only during attacks	
Hypervalinemia	Valine		
Homocystinuria	Methionine; homocystine slightly increased	Homocystine in great excess in urine	Blood cystine low; vascular accidents, Marfan-like syndrome, osteoporosis
Tryptophanemia	Tryptophan	Decreased excretion of kynurenin after tryptophan load	
Hyperlysinemia	Lysine	Ornithine, gamma-aminobutyric acid, and ethanolamine in excess	
Congenital lysine intolerance	Lysine, arginine		Ammonia intoxication
Tyrosinosis	Tyrosine; methionine may be markedly increased	*p*-Hydroxyphenylpyruvic, acetic, and lactic acids; methionine may be prominent	Generalized aminoaciduria, renal glycosuria, renal rickets, cirrhosis; Fanconi's syndrome

Table 13-7. (continued)

Disease	Increased Blood Amino Acids	Urine Abnormalities*	Other Laboratory Findings
Cystathioninuria	Cystathionine slightly increased	Cystathionine (may be > 1 gm/day)	Congenital acidosis, thrombocytopenia, pituitary gland abnormalities
Hyperglycinemia			
Severe infantile	Glycine (other amino acids may be elevated)	Acetone	May have ammonia intoxication, ketosis, neutropenia, and osteoporosis
With hypo-oxaluria	Glycine	Decreased oxalate excretion	
Argininosuccinic aciduria	Argininosuccinic acid (≅4 mg/dl)	Argininosuccinic acid (2.5–9.0 gm/day)	Ammonia intoxication
Citrullinemia	Citrulline		Liver disease, ammonia intoxication; may have low BUN
Ornithinemia	Ornithine	Ornithine may be normal	Ammonia intoxication
Histidinemia	Histidine (alanine may also be increased)	Alanine may be increased; imidazolepyruvic, acetic, and lactic acids	Urocanic acid absent in sweat and urine after oral histidine load
Carnosinuria		Carnosine (20–100 mg/day)	
Hyper-beta-alaninemia	Beta-alanine, gamma-aminobutyric acid (GABA)	Beta-aminoisobutyric acid, GABA and taurine in excess	Beta-alanine and GABA increased in CSF
Hyperprolinemia			
Type I	Proline	Hydroxyproline, glycine elevated	May have hereditary nephritis
Type II	Proline	Δ^1-Pyrroline-5-carboxylate, hydroxyproline, glycine elevated	No nephritis

Hydroxyprolinemia	Hydroxyproline	No excretion of Δ^1-pyrroline-3-hydroxy-5-carboxylate or gamma-hydroxyglutamic acid after hydroxyproline load	
Hypophosphatasia	Phosphoethanolamine slightly elevated ($\cong$ 0.4 mg/dl)	Phosphoethanolamine ($\geqq$150 mg/day)	Bone disease

*In addition to overflow aminoaciduria:

Mental retardation is often present in these patients.

For proper interpretation of aminoaciduria, avoid all drugs and medications for 3–4 days (unless immediate diagnosis is required), since they may cause renal tubular damage with aminoaciduria or may produce confusing spots on chromatograms. Use fresh urine specimens without urinary tract infection or else amino acid pattern may be abnormal. Since aminoaciduria may occur with various acute illnesses, repeat amino acid chromatogram after recovery from acute illness to avoid misdiagnosis.

Some aminoacidurias may not be clinically significant (e.g., newborn aminoaciduria, glycinuria, beta-aminoisobutyric aciduria).

Source: Data from MD Efron and MG Ampola, The aminoacidurias. *Pediatr Clin North Am* 14:881, 1967.

Increased homocystine (up to 250 mg/day; normal = trace or not detected) and methionine (up to 2000 mg/day; normal up to 30 mg/day) in serum; also increased in CSF.
Laboratory findings due to associated clinical conditions (e.g., mental retardation, Marfan's syndrome, osteoporosis, arterial and venous thromboembolic accidents [due to increased platelet stickiness], mild variable hepatocellular dysfunction) are noted.
Serum methionine levels should be kept at 20–150 μmol/L by low-methionine diet and pyridoxine therapy.
Patients have enzyme activity levels of 0–10% in fibroblasts and lymphocytes; heterozygotes (their parents) have levels < 50% of normal.
Neonatal detection is possible; incidence = 1:200,000 live births.

CYSTATHIONINURIA

(rare disorder of intermediate metabolism of methionine)

Increased cystathionine in urine

HYPERGLYCINEMIA

Long-chain ketosis (without hypoglycemia) and ketonuria accentuated by leucine ingestion
Same clinical picture (neutropenia, thrombocytopenia, hypogammaglobulinemia, increased glycine in blood and urine, osteoporosis, hypoglycemia) may occur in propionic acidemia, methylmalonic acidemia, isovaleric acidemia, 3-keto-thiolase deficiency.

PROPIONIC ACIDEMIA

Autosomal recessive defect in enzyme activity of propionyl-CoA carboxylase preventing degradation and therefore intolerance of isoleucine, valine, threonine, methionine
Recurrent episodes (often following infections) of massive ketosis, acidosis, vomiting, dehydration progressing to coma
Same picture as hyperglycinemia (see preceding section)
Urine is tested (daily in infants) for ketones (e.g., Acetest reagent strips or tablets) and blood for propionic acid to monitor treatment.
Laboratory findings of complications (e.g., sepsis, ventricular hemorrhage)
Prenatal diagnosis is available.
Positive assay of enzyme in cultured fibroblasts can indicate heterozygosity but negative assay may not be reliable to indicate absence.

ARGININOSUCCINIC ACIDURIA

Autosomal recessive deficiency of argininosuccinase
Fasting blood ammonia is normal but may be markedly increased after eating.
Argininosuccinic acid is increased in urine; may also be increased in blood and CSF.
Serum alkaline phosphatase may be increased.
Heterozygous carriers show increased argininosuccinic acid in urine and decreased argininosuccinase in RBCs.
Prenatal diagnosis by assay of enzyme in cultured amniocytes (*Mycoplasma* contamination may cause a false negative result) or assay of amniotic fluid for argininosuccinic acid

CITRULLINEMIA

(rare autosomal recessive deficiency of argininosuccinate synthetase of metabolic block in citrulline utilization and associated mental retardation)

Genetically heterogeneous (like other disorders of urea cycle) with various different clinical pictures and onset from neonatal to adult period
Massive hyperammonemia in neonatal form
Markedly increased citrulline levels in blood, CSF, and urine

Table 13-8. Summary of Renal Transport Aminoacidurias (blood amino acids are normal or low)

Disease	Amino Acids Increased in Urine
Oasthouse urine disease	Methionine (may not be much increased on normal diet but is on high-methionine diet); smaller amounts of valine, leucine, isoleucine, tyrosine, and phenylalanine
Hartnup disease	Neutral (monoamine, monocarboxylic) amino acids; basic amino acids, methionine, proline, hydroxyproline, and glycine normal or only slightly increased
Glycinuria (may be harmless; may be heterozygous for benign prolinuria; may be associated with many conditions)	Glycine
Severe prolinuria (Joseph's syndrome)	Proline, hydroxyproline, and glycine in great excess (≤3 gm/day of proline)
Benign prolinuria	Proline, hydroxyproline, and glycine (≤600 mg/day of proline)
Cystine-lysinuria Type I (renal calculi) Type II Type III	Cystine and dibasic amino acids
Isolated cystinuria (familial hypoparathyroidism, ? incidental)	Cystine

Source: Data from MD Efron and MG Ampola, The aminoacidurias. *Pediatr Clin North Am* 14:881, 1967.

Serum levels of glutamine, alanine, and aspartic acid are usually increased; arginine is usually decreased.
Laboratory findings due to liver disease
Deficient enzyme activity can be demonstrated in liver cells and cultured fibroblasts.
Prenatal diagnosis by assay of citrulline in amniotic fluid or of enzyme in cultured amniocytes

HISTIDINEMIA

(rare autosomal recessive deficiency of histidase in liver and skin converts histidine to urocanic acid)

Blood histidine is increased to 500–1000 μmol/L (normal = 85–120 μmol/L).
Urine histidine is increased to 0.5–4.0 gm/day (normal < 0.5 gm/day). Histidine metabolites (imidazole acetic, imidazole lactic, and imidazole pyruvic acids) are also increased in urine; alanine may be increased.
Urine may show positive Phenistix test because of imidazole pyruvic acid.
With oral histidine load, no formiminoglutamic acid (FIGLU) appears in urine.
Incidence = 1:14,000–1:20,000 live births in U.S. and 1:8000 in Japan
Most children show no sequelae; therefore neonatal screening is not performed. Heterozygote detection is not established yet.

HYPERPROLINEMIA

Increased proline in blood
Increased glycine and hydroxyproline in urine

HYDROXYPROLINEMIA

Increased hydroxyproline in blood

OASTHOUSE URINE DISEASE

(distinctive odor of urine)

Increase of various amino acids in blood and also in urine (e.g., phenylalanine, tyrosine, methionine, valine, leucine, isoleucine)

HARTNUP DISEASE

(hereditary abnormality of tryptophan metabolism)

Urine chromatography shows greatly increased amounts of indoleacetic acid, alpha-*N* (indole-3-acetyl) glutamine, and tryptophan.

JOSEPH'S SYNDROME (SEVERE PROLINURIA)

Urine shows marked increase in proline, hydroxyproline, and glycine.
Heterozygotes may show mild prolinuria.

BENIGN PROLINURIA

Increased proline, hydroxyproline, and glycine appear in urine.
Heterozygotes may show glycinuria but not prolinuria.
Prolinuria may occur in association with various diseases; may be harmless.

CYSTINURIA

(failure of renal tubular reabsorption and of intestinal uptake of cystine and dibasic amino acids)

Increased cystine in urine (20–30 times normal)
Increased urinary arginine, lysine, and ornithine
Cystine renal stones

BETA-AMINOISOBUTYRIC ACIDURIA

(familial recessive disorder of thymine metabolism)

Increased beta-aminoisobutyric acid in urine (50–200 mg/24 hours)

May also occur in leukemia due to increased breakdown of nucleic acids.

FAMILIAL IMINOGLYCINURIA

(inherited autosomal defect of renal transport; may be associated with mental retardation)

Increased urine glycine
Increased urine imino acids (proline, hydroxyproline)

METHYLMALONIC ACIDURIA

(very rare autosomal recessive error of metabolism with neonatal metabolic acidosis and mental and somatic retardation; at least 4 distinct forms)

Metabolic acidosis
Increased methylmalonic acid in urine and blood
Long-chain ketonuria
Intermittent hyperglycinemia
All findings accentuated by high-protein diet or supplemental ingestion of valine or isoleucine
Neutropenia
Possibly, thrombocytopenia
Heterozygote detection is not reliable.
Prenatal diagnosis by assay of methylmalonyl-CoA mutase in cultured amniocytes, increased methylcitric or methylmalonic acids in amniotic fluid, or (late in pregnancy) increased methylmalonic acid in maternal urine
Screening incidence = 1:48,000 in infants 3–4 weeks old

Methylmalonic aciduria also occurs in vitamin B_{12} deficiency.
Organic acidemias (e.g., methylmalonic, propionic, isovaleric) show
- *Metabolic acidosis and ketoacidosis*
- *Ketonuria*
- *Hyperammonemia*
- *Hypoglycemia*
- *Sweat and urine with odor of sweaty feet*

FAMILIAL LECITHIN-CHOLESTEROL ACYLTRANSFERASE DEFICIENCY

(rare genctic disorder of adults)

Anemia with large RBCs that are frequently target cells
Proteinuria
Serum cholesterol level normal but cholesterol esters virtually absent

PRIMARY OXALOSIS

(rarc familial disease)

Increased serum and urinary oxalic acid
Incrcased urinary glycolic and glyoxylic acid
Calcium oxalate renal calculi and nephrocalcinosis with extrarenal deposition of calcium oxalate
Uremia causes death.
Manifestations of hyperoxaluria are the same, but extrarenal calcium oxalate deposits are absent.

L-GLYCERIC ACIDURIA

(genetic variant of primary hyperoxaluria; autosomal trait that causes disease only when homozygous)

Renal calculi composed of calcium oxalate
Increased urinary oxalic acid (3–5 times normal)
L-Glyceric acid in urine (not found in normal urine)

CYSTINOSIS

(lysosomal storage disease due to impaired transport of cystine out of lysosomes; only this one amino acid is accumulated)

Adults (benign disease)
- Urinary tract calculi
- Cystinuria (cystine crystals in urine; >200 mg of cystine in 24-hour urine)

SECONDARY AMINOACIDURIA

Severe liver disease
Renal tubular damage due to
- Lysol
- Heavy metals
- Maleic acid
- Burns
- Galactosemia
- Wilson's disease
- Scurvy
- Rickets
- Fanconi's syndrome (e.g., outdated tetracycline, multiple myeloma, inherited)

Neoplasm
- Cystathionine excretion in neuroblastoma of adrenal gland; ethanolamine excretion in primary hepatoma

Disorders of Carbohydrate Metabolism

GALACTOSEMIA

(inherited defect in liver and in RBCs of galactose-1-phosphate uridyl transferase that converts galactose to glucose causing accumulation of galactose-1-phosphate)

Increased blood galactose up to 300 mg/dl (normal < 5 mg/dl)

Increased urine galactose of 500–2000 mg/dl (normal < 5 mg/dl)

Serum glucose may appear to be elevated in fasting state but falls as galactose increases; hypoglycemia is usual.

Galactose tolerance test is positive but not necessary for diagnosis and may be hazardous because of induced hypoglycemia and hypokalemia.

- Use an oral dose of 35 gm of galactose/sq m body area.
- Normal: Serum galactose increases to 30–50 mg/dl; returns to normal within 3 hours.
- Galactosemia: Serum increase is greater, and return to baseline level is delayed.
- Heterozygous carrier: Response is intermediate.
- The test is not specific or sensitive enough for genetic studies.

Lack of RBC galactose-1-phosphate uridyl transferase establishes the diagnosis.

General ammoaciduria is identified by chromatography.

Proteinuria

Laboratory findings due to complications

- Jaundice (onset at age 4–10 days)
- Liver biopsy—dilated canaliculus filled with bile pigment with surrounding rosette of liver cells
- Coagulation abnormalities
- Cataracts
- Mental and physical retardation
- Decreased immunity (infants often die of *Escherichia coli* sepsis)

Findings disappear (but are not reversed) when galactose is eliminated from diet (e.g., milk).

Screening incidence = 1:62,000 live births. Cord blood is preferred, but this prevents also screening for phenylketonuria (PKU), which is normal in neonatal cord blood. Filter paper blood may show false positive test for PKU, tyrosinemia, and homocystinuria. Test is invalidated by exchange transfusion.

Prenatal diagnosis by measurement of galactose-1-phosphate uridyl transferase in cell culture from amniotic fluid. Parents show <50% enzyme activity in RBCs.

CONGENITAL FRUCTOSE INTOLERANCE

This is a severe familial genetic disease of infancy due to defect involving fructose 1-phosphoaldolase and fructose 1,6-diphosphoaldolase; it resembles galactosemia.

Fructose in urine of 100–300 mg/dl gives a positive test for reducing substances (Benedict's reagent, Clinitest) but not with glucose-oxidase methods (Clinistix, Tes-Tape). Identify fructose by paper chromatography.

Aminoaciduria and proteinuria may be present.

Fructose tolerance test shows prolonged elevation of blood fructose and marked decrease in serum glucose. Serum phosphorus shows rapid prolonged decrease. Hypoglycemia with convulsions and coma follows ingestion of fructose.

Increased serum bilirubin and cirrhosis may occur.

BENIGN FRUCTOSURIA

This is a benign asymptomatic disorder due to fructokinase deficiency.

Large amount of fructose in urine gives a positive test for reducing substances (Benedict's reagent, Clinitest) but not with glucose-oxidase methods (Clinistix, Tes-Tape).

Identify fructose by paper chromatography.

Fructose tolerance test shows that blood fructose increases to 4 times more than in normal persons, blood glucose increases only slightly, and serum phosphorus does not change.

ALKAPTONURIA

Recessive inherited absence of liver homogentisic acid oxidase causes excretion of homogentisic acid in urine.

Cardinal features are urine changes, scleral pigmentation, lumbosacral spondylitis (see Ochronosis, p. 259). May also cause deformity of aortic valve cusps.

Presumptive diagnosis by urine that becomes brown-black on standing and reduces Benedict's solution (urine turns brown) and Fehling's solution, but glucose-oxidase methods are negative. Ferric chloride test is positive (urine turns purple-black).

Thin-layer chromatography and spectrophotometric assay identify urinary homogentisic acid but are not generally necessary for diagnosis.

An oral dose of homogentisic acid is largely recovered in the urine of affected patients but not in normal persons.

SUCROSURIA

Urine specific gravity is very high (≤1.07).

Urine tests for reducing substances are negative.

Sucrosuria may follow IV administration of sucrose or the purposeful addition of cane sugar to urine.

PENTOSURIA

Pentosuria is due to a block in oxidation of glucuronic acid; the patient can metabolize only the sixth carbon, excreting the 5-carbon fraction as pentose.

Urinary excretion of L-xylulose is increased (1–4 gm/day), and the increase is accentuated by administration of glucuronic acid and glucuronogenic drugs (e.g., aminopyrine, antipyrine, menthol).

Differential Diagnosis

Alimentary pentosuria—arabinose or xylose excreted after ingestion of large amount of certain fruits (e.g., plums, cherries, grapes)

Healthy normal persons—small amounts of D-ribose in urine

Healthy normal persons—trace amounts of ribulose in urine

Muscular dystrophy—small amounts of D-ribose in urine (some patients)

MANNOHEPTULOSURIA

Mannoheptulose in urine after the eating of avocados occurs in some persons; not clinically important.

INTESTINAL DEFICIENCY OF SUGAR-SPLITTING ENZYMES (MILK ALLERGY; MILK INTOLERANCE; CONGENITAL FAMILIAL LACTOSE INTOLERANCE; LACTASE DEFICIENCY; DISACCHARIDASE DEFICIENCY)

Familial disease that often begins in infancy with diarrhea, vomiting, failure to thrive, malabsorption, etc.; patient becomes asymptomatic when lactose is removed from diet.

Oral lactose tolerance test shows a rise in blood sugar <20 mg/dl in blood drawn at 15, 30, 60, 90 minutes (usual dose = 50 gm).

In diabetics, blood sugar may increase >20 mg/dl despite impaired lactose absorption. Test may also be influenced by impaired gastric emptying or small bowel transit.

If test is positive, repeat using glucose and galactose (usually 25 gm each) instead of lactose; subnormal rise indicates a mucosal absorptive defect; normal increase (>25 gm/dl) indicates lactase deficiency only.
Biopsy of small intestine mucosa shows low level of lactase in homogenized tissue. Is used to assess other diagnostic tests but is seldom required except to exclude secondary lactase deficiency with histologic studies.
Hydrogen breath test (measured by gas chromatography) is noninvasive, rapid, simple, sensitive, quantitative. Patient expires into a breath-collecting apparatus; complete absorption causes no increase of H_2 formed in colon to be excreted in breath. Malabsorption causes H_2 production by fermentation in colon that is proportional to amount of test dose not absorbed. False negative test in ~20% of patients due to absence of H_2-producing bacteria in colon or prior antibiotic therapy.
Lactose in urine amounts to 100–2000 mg/dl. It produces a positive test for reducing sugars (Benedict's reagent, Clinitest) but a negative test with glucose-oxidase methods (Tes-Tape, Clinistix).
After ingestion of milk or 50–100 gm of lactose, stools have a pH of 4.5–6.0 (normal pH is >7.0) and are sour and frothy.
Fecal studies are of limited value in adults.

CLASSIFICATION OF PORPHYRIAS

(1) Congenital Erythropoietic Porphyria (CEP)

Very rare, autosomal recessive, probably due to decreased activity of uroporphyrinogen III cosynthetase in RBCs. Usual onset in infancy, extreme cutaneous photosensitivity with mutilation, red urine and teeth with ultraviolet fluorescence of urine, teeth, and bones.
Normocytic, normochromic, anicteric hemolytic anemia that tends to be mild; may be associated with hypersplenism.
Urine—marked increase of uroporphyrin is characteristic; coproporphyrin shows lesser increase. Excretion of porphobilinogen (PBG) and delta-aminolevulinic acid (ALA) is normal. Watson-Schwartz test is negative.
Stool—marked increase of porphyrins, especially coproporphyrins
RBCs and plasma—marked increase of uroporphyrins; increased coproporphyrin

(2) Porphyria Cutanea Tarda (PCT)

Most common porphyrin disorder. Autosomal dominant deficiency of hepatic and RBC uroporphyrinogen decarboxylase. Associated with alcoholic liver disease and hepatic siderosis. Skin changes and photosensitivity are present. Acquired form may be due to hepatoma, cirrhosis, chemicals (an epidemic in Turkey was caused by contamination of wheat by hexachlorobenzene).
Laboratory findings of underlying liver disease
Liver biopsy shows morphologic changes of underlying disease and fluorescence under ultraviolet light.
Serum iron and transferrin saturation are increased in ~50% of patients, but liver usually shows iron overload.
Urine—marked increase of uroporphyrin (frequently up to 1000–3000 μg/24 hours (normal < 300 μg) with only slight increase of coproporphyrin and ratio of uroporphyrin-coproporphyrin > 7.5 (ratio < 1 in variegate porphyria). In biochemical remission, 24-hour uroporphyrin < 400 μg.
Stool—slight increase of coproporphyrin
Plasma—increased protoporphyrin

(3) Erythropoietic Protoporphyria

Relatively common type of porphyria due to autosomal dominant deficiency of heme synthetase activity in bone marrow, reticulocytes, liver, and other cells
Mild anemia with slight hypochromia is common.

Laboratory findings due to liver disease (in 5–10% of cases) with increased direct bilirubin, serum glutamic-oxaloacetic transaminase (SGOT), alkaline phosphatase (due to intrahepatic cholestasis) and gallstones containing porphyrins may be found.
Urine—porphyrins within normal limits
RBCs—marked increase of free protoporphyrin in symptomatic patients (may also be increased in iron deficiency anemia and lead poisoning in zinc chelate form but nonchelated in protoporphyria). May be normal or slightly increased in asymptomatic carriers. Examination of dilute blood by fluorescent microscopy may show rapidly fading fluorescence in variable part of RBCs.
Stool—protoporphyrin is usually increased in symptomatic patients and in some carriers even when carrier RBC porphyrins are normal.

(4) Acute Intermittent Porphyria (AIP)

Most frequent and severe form of porphyria in U.S. Is autosomal dominant deficiency of uroporphyrinogen I synthetase in RBCs, liver, and other cells. Adult onset with episodes of abdominal pain, neurologic, and mental symptoms that may be precipitated by certain drugs (especially barbiturates, alcohol, and sulfonamides; also diphenylhydantoin, chlordiazepoxide, ergots, etc.), infection, starvation, and certain steroids; no photosensitivity.
Definitive test is decreased (~50% of normal). PBG deaminase in RBCs (performed in special laboratories); normal in other porphyrias.
Urine—marked increase of PBG and, to a lesser extent, of delta-ALA; these decrease during remission but are rarely normal; also increased in plasma. Coproporphyrin and uroporphyrin may be increased.
Stool—protoporphyrin and coproporphyrin are usually normal.
Urine may be of normal color when fresh and become brown, red, or black on standing.
During acute attack, there may be slight leukocytosis, decreased serum sodium, chloride, and magnesium, and increased serum urea nitrogen (BUN).
Liver function tests are normal except for sulfobromophthalein (BSP) retention.
Other frequent laboratory abnormalities are increased serum cholesterol, hyperbetalipoproteinemia (Type IIa), increased serum iron, abnormal glucose tolerance, increased T-4, and thyroxine-binding globulin without hyperthyroidism.

(5) Variegate Porphyria (VP)

Autosomal dominant condition probably due to deficiency of protoporphyrinogen oxidase causes episodes of abdominal pain and neuropsychiatric symptoms that cannot be distinguished from acute intermittent porphyria but are almost always precipitated by a drug. Skin changes of excessive mechanical fragility of sun-exposed areas.
Stool—characteristic change is marked increase of protoporphyrin and coproporphyrin, which is found during attack, remission, or only with skin manifestations.
Urine—marked increase of delta-ALA and PBG during an acute attack, which are usually normal after acute episode or with only skin manifestations (in contrast to acute intermittent porphyria).
Blood—porphyrin levels are not increased.

(6) Hereditary Coproporphyria (HC)

Autosomal dominant deficiency of coproporphyrinogen oxidase in WBC, liver, and other cells. Two-thirds of patients are latent. Acute attacks resemble acute intermittent and variegate porphyrias and may be precipitated by same factors, i.e., drugs (e.g., barbiturates, sedatives, anticonvulsants, alcohol), starvation, infection; skin photosensitivity may occur.

Stool—coproporphyrin is always increased; very markedly during an acute attack; also increased in plasma. Protoporphyrin is normal or only slightly increased.

Urine—coproporphyrin is markedly increased and is usually normal during remission.

RBC, but not plasma, protoporphyrins are also increased in iron deficiency anemia and lead intoxication. Screening tests using fluorescence microscopy of RBCs or Wood's lamp viewing of treated whole blood may also be positive in iron deficiency anemia, lead intoxication, and other dyserythropoietic states. In congenital erythropoietic porphyria, 5–20% of RBCs show fluorescence that lasts up to a minute or more in contrast to erythropoietic protoporphyria where fluorescence is half that and lasts about 30 seconds and in lead poisoning where almost all RBCs fluoresce for only a few seconds. Fluorescence of hepatocytes occurs in erythropoietic protoporphyria, porphyria cutanea tarda, porphyria variegata, hereditary coproporphyria.

Laboratory evaluation for porphyrias may include 24-hour urine for quantitative aminolevulinic acid, porphobilinogen, uroporphyrin, and coproporphyrin (urine should be kept refrigerated as porphyrins quickly deteriorate, especially at room temperature); plasma porphyrin; free RBC protoporphyrin; spot stool quantitative coproporphyrin and protoporphyrin; Watson-Schwartz test to demonstrate porphyrin precursors in urine (Ehrlich's reagent and sodium acetate added to urine; positive turns cherry red with chloroform); evidence of hemolytic anemia, liver disease; fluorescence of appropriate tissues; enzyme activity assay of RBCs, liver tissue, or cultured fibroblasts.

I-CELL DISEASE (MUCOLIPIDOSIS II)

Autosomal recessive transmission of fundamental defect in recognition and uptake of certain lysosomal enzymes due to deficient activity of *N*-acetylglucosaminylphosphotransferase.

Vacuolation (cytoplasmic inclusions) in lymphocytes, fibroblasts, liver, and kidney cells is positive for Sudan and acid phosphatase. Lysosomal enzyme activity (hexosaminidase A and B and alpha-galactosidase) is low in these cells but high in serum or culture medium. Urine mucopolysaccharides are not increased.

Prenatal diagnosis by high levels of multiple acid hydrolases in amniotic fluid or deficiency of them in cultured amniocytes.

Some heterozygotes have abnormal inclusions in fibroblasts.

Some heterozygotes may have intermediate enzyme levels in leukocytes and cultured fibroblasts.

Clinical features resemble Hurler's syndrome but without corneal changes or increased mucopolysaccharides in urine.

MUCOLIPIDOSIS III (*N*-ACETYLGLUCOSAMINYLPHOSPHOTRANSFERASE DEFICIENCY; PSEUDO-HURLER DYSTROPHY)

Clinical features resemble Hurler's syndrome but without increased mucopolysaccharides in urine.

Autosomal recessive transmission of fundamental defect in recognition or catylsis and uptake of certain lysosomal enzymes due to deficient activity of *N*-acetylglucosaminylphosphotransferase.

Prenatal diagnosis has not been reported yet.

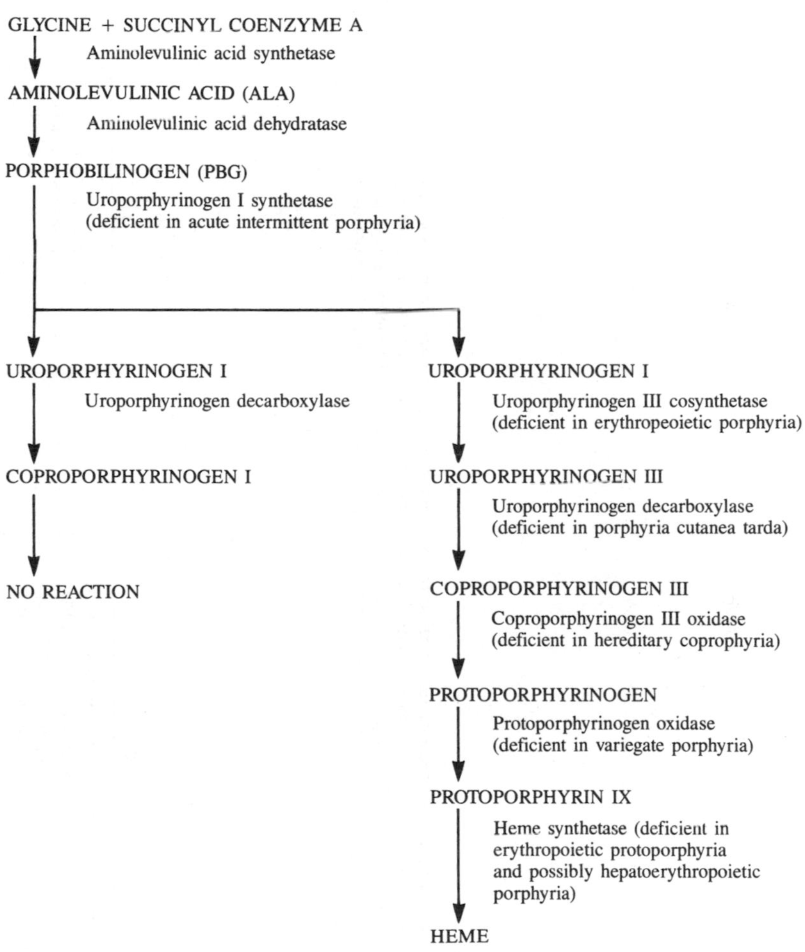

Fig. 13-3. Heme biosynthesis pathway showing effect of enzyme defect. Accumulation of porphyrins and their precursors preceding the enzyme block are responsible for the clinical and laboratory findings in each syndrome. PBG and ALA cause abdominal pain and neuropsychiatric symptoms. Increased formation of porphyrins (with or without increased PBG or ALA) causes photosensitivity. Thus deficiencies near end of metabolic path cause more photosensitivity and less neuropsychiatric findings.

Fig. 13-4. Diagnostic strategy (algorithm) for suspected porphyria according to symptoms. Excess production of porphyrins is associated with cutaneous photosensitivity. Excess production of only porphyrin precursors is associated with neurologic symptoms. Excess production of both is associated with both types of clinical symptoms.

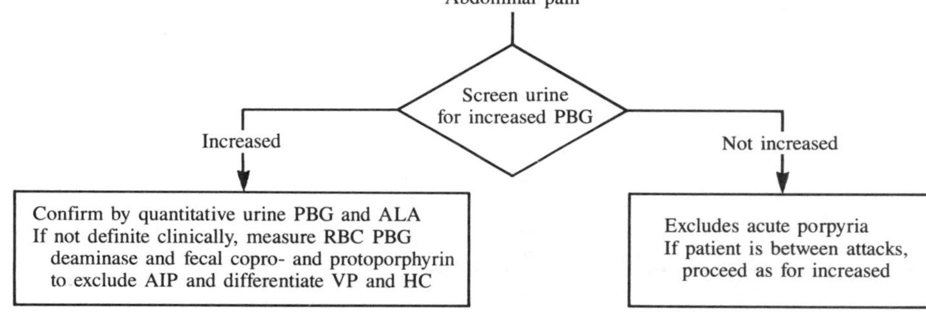

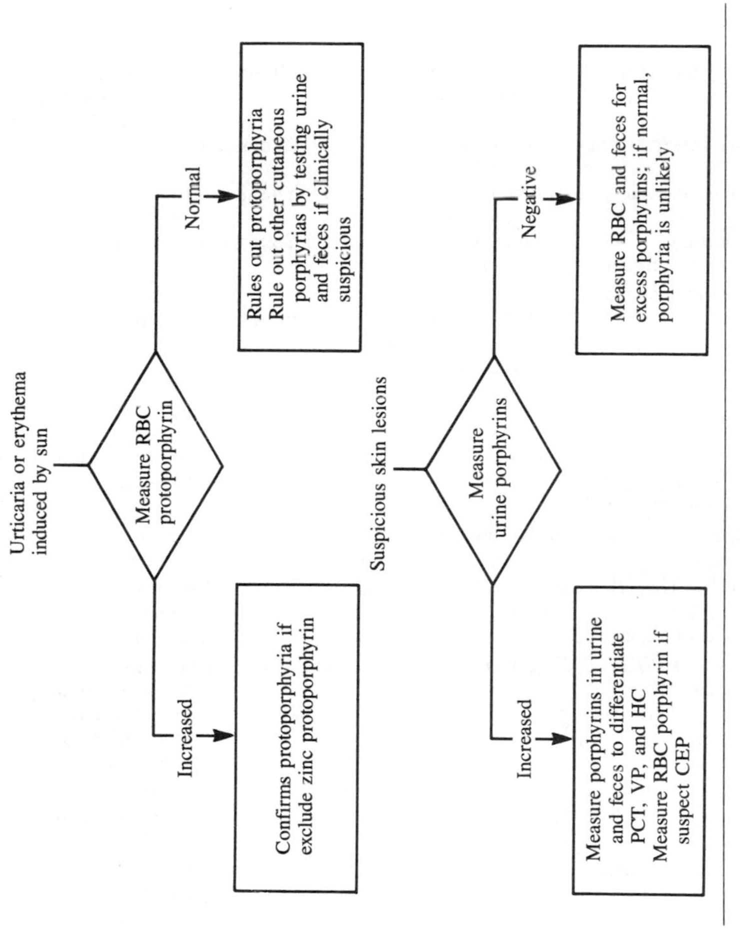
Urticaria or erythema induced by sun
Measure RBC protoporphyrin
Increased
Confirms protoporphyria if exclude zinc protoporphyrin
Normal
Rules out protoporphyria
Rule out other cutaneous porphyrias by testing urine and feces if clinically suspicious
Suspicious skin lesions
Measure urine porphyrins
Increased
Measure porphyrins in urine and feces to differentiate PCT, VP, and HC
Measure RBC porphyrin if suspect CEP
Negative
Measure RBC and feces for excess porphyrins; if normal, porphyria is unlikely

Table 13-9. Comparison of Porphyrias

Type	Enzyme Defect	Age at Onset	Frequency
Erythropoietic			
(1) Erythropoietic porphyria	Uroporphyrinogen III cosynthetase	Infancy	
(2) Erythropoietic protoporphyria	Heme synthetase	Childhood	
Hepatic			
(3) Porphyria cutanea tarda	Uroporphyrinogen decarboxylase	Middle age	Commonest type in U.S. and Europe
(4) Acute intermittent	Uroporphyrinogen I synthetase	Adolescence	
(5) Variegate porphyria	Protoporphyrinogen oxidase	Young adult	
(6) Hereditary coproporphyria	Coproporphyrinogen oxidase	Young adult	Rarest
Hepatic, erythropoietic			
(7) Hepatoerythropoietic porphyria	Heme synthetase Uroporphyrinogen decarboxylase	Infancy	Rarest

Type	Urine	Feces	RBCs	Comment
(1)	Uro I, Copro I Watson-Schwartz negative*	Copro I	Uro I, stable fluor	Hemolytic anemia Red teeth
(2)	Negative	Proto constant	Proto transient fluor	Liver disease Gallstones
(3)	Uro I > Uro III constant Constant fluor	Isocopro > Copro	Negative	Decreased liver function Siderosis
(4)	ALA and PBG constant* Watson-Schwartz positive	Negative	Negative	Abdominal pain, psychosis neuropathy SIADH with low sodium and osmolarity
(5)	ALA and PBG during attack* Copro > Uro	Proto constant Some Copro X-porphyrin	Negative	Abdominal pain, psychosis, neuropathy
(6)	Copro, ALA, and PBG during attack*	Copro III constant	Negative	Abdominal pain, psychosis, neuropathy
(7)	Uro I, Uro III	Copro I, Copro III Isocopro	Proto	Decreased liver function

Skin manifestations in all except acute intermittent porphyria.
Autosomal dominant except erythropoietic porphyria and hepatoerythropoietic porphyria.

Uro = uroporphyrin; Copro = coproporphyrin; Proto = protoporphyrin; Iso = isocoproporphyrin; PBG = porphobilinogen; ALA = aminolevulinic acid; fluor = fluorescence.
*Present during acute attack; may be absent during remission.

Heterozygotes may have intermediate enzyme levels in leukocytes and cultured fibroblasts.

LYSOSOMAL STORAGE DISORDERS*

	Deficient Enzyme	Major Organ Involved
Disorders of glycoprotein degradation		
Fucosidosis	Alpha-fucosidase	CNS
Mannosidosis	Alpha-mannosidase	CNS, bone, liver, spleen
Sialidosis (mucolipidosis I)	Oligosaccharide neuraminidase	CNS, bone, liver, spleen
Glycogen storage disease	Alpha-glucosidase	Muscle, heart
Aspartylglycosaminuria	Amidase	CNS, bone marrow, connective tissue
Disorders of enzyme Localization		
Mucolipidosis II (I-cell disease) (formerly MPS VII)	*N*-Acetylglucosaminylphosphotransferase	CNS, bone, connective tissue
Mucolipidosis III (pseudo-Hurler polydystrophy)	*N*-Acetylglucosaminylphosphotransferase tissue	Predominantly joint and connective
Disorders of lysosomal efflux		
Cystinosis	?	Kidney
Salla's disease	?	CNS
Mucopolysaccharidoses (see Table 13-10, pp. 436–437)		
Sphingolipidoses (see Table 13-12, p. 443)		
Lipidoses		

GENETIC MUCOPOLYSACCHARIDOSES (MPS)
See Table 13-10, pp. 436–437, for a classification of MPS.

Glycogen Storage Diseases (GSD)

VON GIERKE'S DISEASE (TYPE I GSD; GLUCOSE-6-PHOSPHATASE DEFICIENCY)

May appear in first days or weeks of life. Autosomal recessive trait with incidence of 1:200,000 births.

After overnight fast, marked hypoglycemia, increased blood lactate, and occasionally pyruvate with severe metabolic acidosis, ketonemia, and ketonuria. *(Recurrent acidosis is commonest cause for hospital admission.)*

Blood glucose is markedly decreased.

Blood triglycerides are very high; cholesterol is moderately increased, and serum free fatty acids are increased. Results in xanthomas and lipid-laden cells in bone marrow.

*Classification from S Kornfeld and WS Sly, Lysosomal storage defects. *Hosp Pract*, pp. 71–82, Aug. 15, 1985.

Table 13-10. Classification of Mucopolysaccharidoses (MPS)

MPS Type (Clinical Name)	Deficient Enzyme	Mucopolysaccharide Excreted in Urine	Signs/Symptoms
Ih (Hurler's syndrome)	Alpha-L-iduronidase	Dermatan sulfate & heparan sulfate	Progressive mental/physical disability from age 1 year; corneal opacity; hyperplastic gums; coarse face; stiff joints (clawhands); organomegaly; dwarfing; dysostosis multiplex
Ia (Scheie's syndrome)	Alpha-L-iduronidase	Dermatan sulfate & heparan sulfate	Mild form of MPS I; mild or no mental retardation; corneal opacity; clawhands; aortic stenosis
II (Hunter's syndrome)	Iduronate sulfatase	Dermatan sulfate & heparan sulfate	Dysostosis multiplex; mild to severe mental retardation; no corneal opacity and longer life compared to MPS I
IIIa (Sanfilippo's syndrome, Type A)	Heparan *N*-sulfatase (sulfamidase)	Heparan sulfate	Mild or no connective tissue abnormalities; marked hirsutism; behaviorism progresses to severe mental retardation
IIIb (Sanfilippo's syndrome, Type B)	Alpha-*N*-acetylglucosaminidase	Heparan sulfate	Same as MPS IIIa
IIIc (Sanfilippo's syndrome, Type C)	Acetyl CoA–alpha-glucosaminide-*N*-acetyltransferase	Heparan sulfate	Same as MPS IIIa
IIId (Sanfilippo's syndrome, Type D)	*N*-Acetylglucosamine-6-sulfate sulfatase	Heparan sulfate	Same as MPS IIIa
IVa (Morquio A)	Galactosamine-6-sulfatase	Keratan sulfate	Marked skeletal abnormalities, small stature, short neck, prominent lower ribs, normal intellect; coma
IVb (Morquio B)	Beta-galactosidase	Keratan sulfate, heparan sulfate	
VI (Maroteaux-Lamy syndrome)	*N*-Acetylgalactosamine-4-sulfatase (arylsulfatase B)	Dermatan sulfate	Severe dysostosis multiplex and corneal opacity, retarded growth, normal intellect; cardiac abnormalities

VII (beta-glucuronidase deficiency)	Beta-glucuronidase	Dermatan sulfate, heparan sulfate, chondroitin 4,6-sulfate	Mild mental retardation, organomegaly, corneal opacity may occur; coarse facies; gingivitis

All MPS show metachromatically staining inclusions of mucopolysaccharides in circulating polymorphonuclear leukocytes (PMNs) (Reilly granulations) or lymphocytes, cells of inflammatory exudate, and bone marrow cells (most consistently in clasmatocytes). Mucopolysaccharide is also deposited in various parenchymal cells. Diagnosis of deficient lysosomal enzyme in cultured fibroblasts makes prenatal diagnosis possible. Serum can be used for diagnosis in MPS II, IIIb, and VI. Leukocytes can be used for diagnosis in MPS I, Ia, IIIa, and IIIc. RBCs can be used for diagnosis in III, IV, VI. Enzyme deficiency is demonstrable in liver in all except V, VII; demonstrable in muscle in all except I, II. Increased glycogen in affected organs except in IV; glycogen structure is normal except in III, IV.

Inheritance in Hunter's syndrome is X-linked recessive; others are autosomal recessive.
Cloudy cornea in Ih, Is, IVa, IVb, VI, VII.
Mental retardation in Ih, II, IIIa, IIIb, IIIc, IIId, VII.
Hepatosplenomegaly in Ih, II, IIIa, IIIb, IIIc, IIId, IVb, VI, VII.
Skeletal defects in all.

Hurler's syndrome (MPS Ih)—Initial diagnosis by quantitative increase of MPS in urine; followed by assay of alpha-L-iduronidase on leukocytes or cultured fibroblasts. Similar enzyme assay detects carriers who have ~50% activity, but the wide range with overlap between normal and carriers may make the diagnosis difficult in individual cases. Prenatal diagnosis by assay of enzyme or MPS in amniocytes. Most die by age 10 years.
Hunter's syndrome (MPS II)—Clinically similar to Hurler's syndrome but milder and no corneal opacity. Initial diagnosis by quantitation of total glucosaminoglycans in urine and confirmed by enzyme assay on serum, cells, or tissues. Heterozygous female carriers recognized by MPS in fibroblasts or enzyme assay in individual hair roots. Diagnosis by accumulation of keratan sulfate in tissues is verified by enzyme assay in fibroblasts or leukocytes. Prenatal diagnosis by enzyme assay or amniotic fluid, which should be confirmed by assay of cultured cells.
Sanfilippo's Type A syndrome (MPS III)—Is only MPS that shows only heparan sulfate in urine, which confirms diagnosis. Assay of fibroblasts and leukocytes shows deficiency of enzyme in patient and decrease of normal activity in carrier who also shows MPS accumulation. Metachromatic inclusion bodies in lymphocytes are coarser and sparser than in Hurler's syndrome and may be seen in bone marrow cells. Severe cerebral changes with relatively mild changes in other body tissues. Four types of Sanfilippo's syndrome cannot be distinguished clinically.
Morquio syndrome—Keratan sulfate is increased in urine (often 2–3 times normal). Metachromatic granules may be seen in PMNs. Prenatal diagnosis by assay of enzymes in cultured amniocytes.
Maroteaux-Lamy syndrome (MPS VI)—Metachromatic cytoplasmic inclusions (Alder granules) may be seen in 50% of lymphocytes and 100% of granulocytes and more marked than in other MPSs. Large amount of dermatan sulfate occurs in urine. Diagnosis is established by deficiency of specific enzyme in cultured fibroblasts. Enzyme assay also allows diagnosis of heterozygotes and prenatal diagnosis.
I-cell diseases (mucolipidosis II)—Clinically resembles severe Hurler's syndrome. Classified as a mucolipidosis; due to defect in *N*-acetylglucosaminylphosphotransferase, whose deficiency in cultured fibroblasts establishes the diagnosis. Urine MPS is not increased. Heterozygotes can be diagnosed, and prenatal diagnosis is possible.
Other rare diseases due to enzyme deficiencies that resemble these conditions include mucolipidosis III and related disorders.

Mild anemia is present.
Impaired platelet function may cause bleeding tendency.
Increased serum uric acid, which may cause clinical gout.
Serum phosphorus and alkaline phosphatase are decreased.
Urinary nonspecific amino acids are increased, without increase in blood amino acids.
Other renal function tests are relatively normal despite kidney enlargement; Fanconi's syndrome can occur.
Liver function tests (other than related to carbohydrate metabolism) are relatively normal but SGOT and serum glutamic-pyruvic transaminase (SGPT) may be increased.
Glucose tolerance may be normal or diabetic type; diabetic type is more frequent in older children and adults.
Functional tests
- Administer 1 mg of glucagon IV or IM after 8-hour fast.
- Blood glucose increases 50–60% in 10–20 minutes in the normal person. Little or no increase occurs in infants or young children with von Gierke's disease; delayed response may occur in older children and adults.
- Administration of glucose precursors (e.g., galactose or fructose IV) causes no rise in blood glucose in von Gierke's disease (demonstrating block in gluconeogenesis), but normal rise occurs in limit dextrinosis (Type III GSD).

Biopsy of liver
- Biochemical studies
  - Absent or markedly decreased glucose-6-phosphatase on assay of frozen liver provides definitive diagnosis.
  - Increased glycogen content (>4% by weight) but normal biochemically and structurally.
  - Other enzymes (other GSD) are present in normal amounts.
- Histology is not diagnostic; shows vacuolization of hepatic cells and abundant glycogen granules. Confirm with Best's stain.

Biopsy of jejunum
- Intestinal glucose-6-phosphatase is decreased or absent.

Biopsy of muscle shows no abnormality of enzyme activity or glycogen content.
Can be cured by liver transplant.

Type IB
- Shows all the clinical and biochemical features of von Gierke's disease except that liver biopsy does not show deficiency of glucose-6-phosphatase.
- May have maturation-arrest neutropenia; varies from mild to agranulocytosis; usually constant but may be cyclic. Associated increased frequency of staphylococcal and *Candida* infection.
- Establish diagnosis by impaired function of glucose 6-phosphate activity in granulocytes.

POMPE'S DISEASE (TYPE II GSD; GENERALIZED GLYCOGENOSIS; ALPHA-1,4-GLUCOSIDASE DEFICIENCY GLYCOGENOSIS)

Features of this autosomal recessive disease are imbecility, varying neurologic defects, muscle hypotonia, cardiac enlargement, and frequent liver enlargement.
May occur in classic infantile form (Type IIA) with neurologic, cardiac, and muscle involvement; juvenile form (Type IIB) with muscle disease resembling pseudohypertrophic dystrophy; adult form (Type IIC) as progressive myopathy.
Fasting blood sugar, glucose tolerance test (GTT), glucagon responses, and rises in blood glucose after fructose infusion are normal. No acetonuria is present.
General hematologic findings are normal.

Table 13-11. Classification of Glycogen Storage Diseases

Type	% Frequency	Clinical Name	Deficient Enzyme
I	20	von Gierke's disease	Liver glucose-6-phosphatase
II	20	Pompe's disease	Lysosomal alpha-1,4-glucosidase
III	30	Forbes' disease	Amylo-1,6-glucosidase (debranching enzyme)
IV	<1	Andersen's disease	Amylo-(1,4 → 1,6)-transglucosidase (branching enzyme)
V	5	McArdle's disease	Muscle phosphorylase
VI	25% for VI + VII	Hers' disease	Liver phosphorylase
VII		Tarui's disease	Muscle phosphofructokinase
VIII	Very rare	Hug, Huijing	Phosphorylase kinase

All are autosomal recessive except Type VIII, which is X-linked recessive.

Staining of circulating leukocytes for glycogen shows massive deposition.

Confirm diagnosis by absence of alpha-1,4-glucosidase in muscle and liver biopsy or cultured fibroblasts from skin biopsy, and perhaps WBCs. Assay in amniotic cell culture allows prenatal diagnosis. Special assay of peripheral blood cells for diagnosis of heterozygotes.

TYPE III GLYCOGEN DEPOSITION DISEASE (FORBES' DISEASE; DEBRANCHER DEFICIENCY; LIMIT DEXTRINOSIS)

This is a familial disease with enlarged liver, retarded growth, chemical changes, and benign course.

Mild increase in cholesterol and triglycerides is less marked than in Type I.

Marked fasting acetonuria (as in starvation)

Fasting hypoglycemia is less severe than in Type I.

Normal blood lactate; uric acid is usually normal.

SGOT and SGPT are increased in children but normal in adults.

There is a diabetic type of glucose tolerance curve with associated glucosuria.

Infusions of gluconeogenic precursors (e.g., galactose, fructose) cause a normal hyperglycemic response in contrast to Type I.

Low fasting blood sugar does not show expected rise after administration of subcutaneous glucagon or epinephrine but does increase 2 hours after high-carbohydrate meal.

Confirm diagnosis by liver and muscle biopsy that show biochemical findings of increased glycogen, abnormal glycogen structure, absence of specific enzyme activity. Normal phosphorylase and glucose-6-phosphatase activity.

TYPE IV GLYCOGEN DEPOSITION DISEASE (ANDERSEN'S DISEASE; BRANCHER DEFICIENCY; AMYLOPECTINOSIS)

This extremely rare fatal condition is due to absence of amylo-(1,4 → 1.6)-transglucosidase.

Hypoglycemia is not present.

Liver function tests may be altered as in other types of cirrhosis (e.g., slight increase in bilirubin, reversed albumin-globulin [A/G] ratio, increased SGOT, decreased serum cholesterol). There may be a flat blood glucose response to epinephrine and glucagon. There may be increased WBC and decreased hemoglobin.

Biopsy of liver may show a cirrhotic reaction to the presence of polysaccharide of abnormal structure, which stains with Best's carmine and periodic acid–Schiff stain but has a very low glycogen content.

TYPE V GLYCOGEN DEPOSITION DISEASE (MCARDLE'S DISEASE; MYOPHOSPHORYLASE DEFICIENCY)

This is a familial autosomal recessive disease showing very limited ischemic muscle exercise tolerance in the presence of normal appearance of muscle.

Epinephrine or glucagon causes a normal hyperglycemic response.

Biopsy of muscle is microscopically normal in young; vacuolation and necrosis are seen in later years. Increased glycogen is present. Definitive diagnosis is made by absence of phosphorylase. Following exercise that quickly causes muscle cramping and weakness, the regional blood lactate and pyruvate do not increase (in a normal person it increases 2–5 times). Similar abnormal response occurs in Type III involving muscle and in Types VII, VIII, X.

Myoglobulinuria may occur after strenuous exercise.

Increased muscle enzymes (e.g., lactic dehydrogenase [LDH], creatine kinase [CK], aldolase) for several hours after strenuous exercise.

TYPE VI GSD (HEPATIC PHOSPHORYLASE DEFICIENCY)

Enlarged liver present from birth is associated with hypoglycemia.

Hypoglycemia (mild to moderate) is unusual.

Serum cholesterol and triglycerides are mildly increased.

Serum uric acid and lactic acid are normal.

Liver function tests are normal.

Fructose tolerance is normal.

Response to glucagon and epinephrine is variable but tends to be poor.

Diagnosis is based on decreased phosphorylase activity in liver, leukocytes, and RBC hemolysate, but muscle phosphorylase is normal.

TYPE VII GSD (MUSCLE PHOSPHOFRUCTOKINASE DEFICIENCY; TARUI'S DISEASE)

Fasting hypoglycemia is marked.

Other members of family may have reduced tolerance to glucose.

RBCs show 50% decrease in phosphofructokinase activity.

Biopsy of muscle shows marked decrease (1–3% of normal) in phosphofructokinase activity.

Clinically identical to Type V

TYPE VIII GSD

This is a very rare X-linked recessive deficiency of phosphorylase kinase enzyme.

Blood glucose is markedly decreased, causing hypoglycemic seizures and mental retardation.

Glucagon administration causes no increase in blood glucose (see von Gierke's disease, pp. 435–438), but ingestion of food causes a rise in 2–3 hours.

Biopsy of liver shows marked decrease in glycogen synthetase.

LESCH-NYHAN SYNDROME

(X-linked recessive trait of complete absence of hypoxanthine-guanine phosphoribosyl transferase [HGPRT] that catalyzes hypoxanthine and guanine to their nucleotides causing accumulation of purines)

The syndrome appears in male children, with choreoathetosis, mental retardation, tendency to self-mutilating, biting, and scratching.

Increased serum uric acid levels (9–12 mg/dl).

Hyperuricuria

- 3–4 mg of uric acid/mg creatinine
- 40–70 mg of uric acid/kg body weight

600–1000 mg/24 hours in patients weighing ≥ 15 kg
Marked variation in purine diet causes very little change.
Orange crystals or sand in infants' diapers

Laboratory findings due to secondary gout (tophi after 10 years, crystalluria, hematuria, urinary calculi, urinary tract infection, gouty arthritis, response to colchicine); patients die of renal failure by age 10 years unless treated.

Deficiency of HGPRT activity can be detected in cultured fibroblasts (< 1.2% of normal), RBC hemolysates (0%) establish the diagnosis; in amniotic cells allows diagnosis in utero. DNA probes allow prenatal diagnosis.

Heterozygotes can be detected by study of individual hair follicles.

Variants with partial deficiency of HGPRT show 0–50% of normal activity in RBC hemolysates and > 1.2% in fibroblasts; accumulate purines but no orange sand in diapers; no abnormality of CNS or behavior

XANTHINURIA

(rare autosomal recessive deficiency of xanthine oxidase in tissues that catalyzes conversion of hypoxanthine to xanthine and xanthine to uric acid)

Decreased serum uric acid; < 1 mg/dl strongly suggests this diagnosis (see pp. 36–37).

Decreased urine uric acid (usually < 30 mg/24 hours; normal up to 500 mg/24 hours)

Increased urine and serum levels of xanthine and hypoxanthine

Laboratory findings due to urinary calculi

Enzyme activity < 10% of normal in biopsy of liver and jejunal mucosa

FAMILIAL DYSAUTONOMIA (RILEY-DAY SYNDROME)

This condition is due to an autosomal recessive trait occurring in Ashkenazi Jews, who show difficulty in swallowing, corneal ulcerations, insensitivity to pain, motor incoordination, excessive sweating, diminished gag reflex, lack of tongue papillae, progressive kyphoscoliosis, pulmonary infections

Urine vanillylmandelic acid (VMA) (3-methoxy-4-hydroxymandelic acid) may be low, and homovanillic acid (HVA) increased.

In asymptomatic carriers, urine VMA may be lower than in healthy adults.

BATTEN'S DISEASE (BATTEN-SPIELMEYER-VOGT DISEASE)

(autosomal recessive type of juvenile amaurotic idiocy)

Azurophilic hypergranulation of leukocytes occurs in patients and in heterozygous and homozygous members of their families. In Giemsa- and Wright-stained smears, it resembles toxic granulation but differs by the absence of supravital staining in Batten's disease and by normal leukocyte alkaline phosphatase activity (markedly increased in toxic granulation). This granulation occurs in ≥ 15% of neutrophils.

GAUCHER'S DISEASE

Gaucher's cells appear in bone marrow aspiration, needle biopsy, or aspiration of spleen, liver, or lymph nodes.

Serum acid phosphatase is increased (if substrate for test is different from that for prostatic acid phosphatase; i.e., use phenyl phosphate or *p*-nitrophenylphosphate instead of glycerophosphate). It may return to normal following splenectomy.

Serum cholesterol and total fats are normal.

Laboratory findings due to involvement of specific organs

Spleen—hypersplenism occurs with anemia (normocytic normochromic), leukopenia (with relative lymphocytosis; monocytes may be increased), and/or thrombocytopenia.
Bone—serum alkaline phosphatase may be increased.
Liver—serum SGOT may be increased.
CSF—GOT may be increased.

Table 13-12. Classification of Gangliosidoses

Clinical Name	Enzyme Defect	Major Lipid Accumulation	Signs/Symptoms
Gaucher's disease	Beta-glucosidase	Glucocerebroside	Enlarged spleen and liver; erosion of long bones and pelvis; mental retardation only in infantile form
Niemann-Pick disease	Sphingomyelinase	Sphingomyelin	Enlarged liver and spleen; mental retardation; ~30% with red spot in retina
Krabbe's disease (globoid leukodystrophy)	Galactosylceramide beta-galactosidase	Galactosylceramide	X-linked; mental retardation; almost total absence of myelin; globoid bodies in brain white matter; CSF protein may be abnormal
Metachromatic leukodystrophy	Arylsulfatase A	Sulfatide	Mental retardation; psychological disturbances in adult form; nerves stain yellow-brown with cresyl violet dye; CSF protein normal or increased ($\leq$200 mg/dl)
Ceramide lactoside lipidosis	Beta-galactosidase	Ceramide lactoside	Slowly progressing brain damage; enlarged liver and spleen
Fabry's disease (angiokeratoma corporis diffusum universale)	Alpha-galactosidase A	Ceramide	Skin lesions; loss of renal function; involvement of heart and brain vessels; pain in lower limbs; red spot in retina
Tay-Sachs disease	Hexosaminidase A	Ganglioside GM_2	Mental retardation; red spot in retina; blindness; muscle weakness
Sandhoff's disease	Hexosaminidase A and B	Ganglioside GM_2 and globoside	Clinical picture same as Tay-Sachs
Landing's disease	Acid beta-galactosidase	Ganglioside GM_1	Psychomotor deterioration; red spot in retina; enlarged liver & spleen; x-ray findings resemble Hunter's and Hurler's syndromes
Fucosidosis	Alpha-fucosidase	H-isoantigen	Cerebral degeneration; muscle spasticity; thick skin

NIEMANN-PICK DISEASE

Foamy histiocytes may be found in bone marrow aspiration and may appear in peripheral blood terminally.

Peripheral blood lymphocytes and monocytes may be vacuolated (2–20% of cells).

WBC is variable.

Rectal biopsy may show changes in ganglion cells of myenteric plexus.

Laboratory findings due to involvement of specific organs

- Anemia is due to hypersplenism or microcytic anemia associated with anisocytosis, poikilocytosis, and elliptocytosis.
- SGOT may be increased in serum and spinal fluid.
- Enzyme changes in CSF are same as in Tay-Sachs disease, except that LDH is normal.

Acid phosphatase is increased (same as in Gaucher's disease—see preceding section).

Serum aldolase is increased.

LDH is normal in serum and CSF.

HISTIOCYTOSIS X

Letterer-Siwe Disease

Bone marrow aspiration or biopsy of lymph node may show characteristic histiocytes and histologic changes.

Progressive normocytic normochromic anemia is present.

Hemorrhagic manifestations (thrombocytopenia) occur.

Hand-Schüller-Christian Disease

Histologic examination of skin, bone, etc., is diagnostic.

Anemia, leukopenia, thrombocytopenia may or may not be present.

Diabetes insipidus may occur.

Eosinophilic Granuloma

Biopsy of bone is diagnostic.

Blood is normal; eosinophilia is unusual.

Development of leukopenia and thrombocytopenia suggests poorest prognosis.

DOWN'S SYNDROME (TRISOMY 21; MONGOLISM)

Karyotyping shows 47 chromosomes with trisomy 21 in most patients; due to translocation, usually to chromosome 14 or other D group chromosome in <5% of cases. 2% have mosaicism with one cell population trisomic.

Increased leukocyte alkaline phosphatase staining reaction.

Leukocytes show decreased incidence of drumsticks (see p. 108) and mean lobe counts.

Serum acid phosphatase may be decreased.

Incidence of leukemia is increased (~1%).

Increased susceptibility to infection (e.g., hepatitis is common in institutionalized patients where Australia antigen was first noted).

Laboratory findings due to associated congenital abnormalities (e.g., GI, GU, cardiovascular systems).

Prenatal Screening and Diagnosis

Increased maternal serum human chorionic gonadotropin (HCG) ≥ 2.5 times multiple of the median (MOM) at 18–25 weeks of gestation will detect ~56% of cases. One study that detected 73% of cases had a 4% false positive rate at that serum level.

Decreased maternal serum unconjugated estriol level (reflects fetal adrenal, liver, and placental function) detects 45% of cases with a 5.2% false positive rate.

≤0.6 MOM in 5% of unaffected pregnancies and 26% of Down's syndrome

Decreased maternal serum alpha-fetoprotein (AFP)

<0.5 MOM in 5% of unaffected pregnancies and ~20% of Down's syndrome

Optimum screening combines maternal age > 35 years with HCG, AFP, and unconjugated estriol levels in maternal serum; detects 60% of cases with 5% false-positive rate.*

Chromosomal analysis of amniotic fluid detects ~20% of cases, since 80% of Down's syndrome patients are born to women < 35 years old.

D_1 TRISOMY (TRISOMY 13; PATAU'S SYNDROME)

In peripheral blood smears, up to 80% of PMNs (neutrophils and eosinophils) show an increased number of anomalous nuclear projections (tags, threads, drumsticks, clubs); the nuclear lobulation may appear abnormal (e.g., nucleus may look twisted without clear separation of individual lobes, coarse lumpy chromatin). Present in almost all complete trisomic cases. Nuclear coils of chromatin by electron microscopy.

Fetal hemoglobins may persist longer than normal (i.e., be increased); these include Hb F, Bart's, Gower 2.

Decreased AFP in maternal serum and AFP

Laboratory findings due to multiple congenital abnormalities (including almost pathognomonic tetrad of narrow palpebral fissures, microphthalmos, cleft palate, parieto-occipital scalp defect, polydactyly).

Karyotyping shows numerical abnormality in 80% of cases 47 XX, +13 or 47 XY, +13. 20% are due to translocations.

TRISOMY 18

Usually sporadic; due to nondisjunction; increased maternal age.

Laboratory findings due to congenital abnormalities (e.g., cardiovascular, GU, GI systems).

FAMILIAL PAROXYSMAL PERITONITIS (FAMILIAL MEDITERRANEAN FEVER; "PERIODIC DISEASE")

WBC is increased (10,000–20,000/cu mm), and there may be increased eosinophils during an attack but a return to normal between attacks. Erythrocyte sedimentation rate (ESR) is increased during an attack but normal between attacks.

Mild normocytic normochromic anemia is occasionally seen.

Serum glycoprotein is increased in patients and their relatives.

Increased alpha-2 globulin and fibrinogen are common.

Amyloidosis develops in 10–40% of patients; it is not related to frequency or severity of clinical attacks.

Etiocholanolone is increased in urine and blood during attacks in a few patients.

*Data from NJ Wald, HS Cuckle, JW Densem, et al., Maternal serum screening for Down's syndrome in early pregnancy. *Br Med J* 297(6653):883, 1988.

Endocrine Diseases

GENERAL PRINCIPLES IN DIAGNOSIS OF ENDOCRINE DISEASES

Perform stimulatory tests if hypofunction is suspected and suppression tests if hyperfunction is suspected.

Suppression tests will suppress normal glands but not autonomous secretion (e.g., functioning neoplasm).

Multiple or pooled samples of baseline specimens and drawing specimens from indwelling lines are often required to obtain optimal specimens.

Patient preparation is particularly important for hormone studies, results of which may be markedly affected by many factors such as stress, position, fasting state, time of day, preceding diet, and drug therapy, all of which should be recorded on the laboratory test requisition form and discussed with the laboratory prior to test ordering.

Appropriate (e.g., frozen) and timely transportation to laboratory and preparation of specimen (e.g., separation of serum may be vital for some tests)

No single test adequately reflects the endocrine status in all conditions.

Tests of Thyroid Function

SERUM TOTAL THYROXINE ASSAY (T-4)

Increased In

Hyperthyroidism

Pregnancy

Certain drugs (estrogens, birth control pills, D-thyroxine, thyroid extract, thyroid-stimulating hormone (TSH), amiodarone, heroin, methadone, amphetamines, some radiopaque substances for x-ray studies [ipodate, iopanoic acid])

"Euthyroid sick" syndrome

Increase in thyroxine-binding globulin (TBG) or abnormal thyroxine-binding prealbumin (TBPA)

- Familial dysalbuminemic hyperthyroxinemia—albumin binds T-4 but not T-3 more avidly than normal, causing changes similar to thyrotoxicosis (total T-4 $\sim$ 20 μg/dl, normal thyroid hormone–binding ratio, increased free T-4 index), but patient is not clinically thyrotoxic.

Decreased In

Hypothyroidism

Hypoproteinemia (e.g., nephrosis, cirrhosis)

Certain drugs (phenytoin, triiodothyronine, testosterone, adrenocorticotropic hormone [ACTH], corticosteroids)

"Euthyroid sick" syndrome

Decrease in TBG

Not Affected By

Mercurial diuretics

Nonthyroidal iodine

FREE THYROXINE (T-4) ASSAY (NORMALIZED THYROXINE)

This determination gives corrected values in patients in whom the total thyroxine (T-4) is altered on account of changes in serum proteins or in binding sites, e.g.,

- Pregnancy
- Drugs (e.g., androgens, estrogens, birth control pills, phenytoin [Dilantin])
- Altered levels of serum proteins (e.g., nephrosis)

Increased In

Hyperthyroidism
Hypothyroidism treated with thyroxine
"Euthyroid sick" syndrome

Decreased In

Hypothyroidism
Hypothyroidism treated with triiodothyronine
"Euthyroid sick" syndrome

SERUM TRIIODOTHYRONINE (T-3) ASSAY

T-4 and free thyroxine index (FTI) are the usual initial tests for thyroid disease.
Serum T-3 parallels T-4 and may be helpful
- When serum free T-4 is borderline elevated
- When serum T-4 is normal in presence of symptoms of hyperthyroidism
- When overlooking diagnosis of hyperthyroidism is very undesirable (e.g., unexplained atrial fibrillation)
- Monitoring the course of hyperthyroidism

May decrease by up to 25% in healthy older persons while T-4 remains normal

SERUM REVERSE T-3 (rT-3)

(hormonally inactive isomer of T-3)

Usually increased in hyperthyroidism and increased serum TBG; often decreased in hypothyroidism but overlap with normal range. Usually normal in euthyroid patients; has been suggested to distinguish "sick thyroid" patients who are euthyroid from true hypothyroid cases, but serum TSH is probably more reliable.

SERUM TRIIODOTHYRONINE (T-3) RESIN UPTAKE

This test should be used only with a simultaneous measurement of serum T-4 to exclude the possibility that an increased T-4 is due to an increase in T-4–binding globulin. American Thyroid Association now recommends term *thyroid hormone–binding ratio* (THBR) for this value reported as ratio of patient to normal plasma pool; = 1 ± 10%). *Measurement of serum T-3 concentration should be done by radioimmunoassay (RIA) for diagnosis of hyperthyroidism.*

Increased In

See causes of *decreased* serum thyroxine-binding globulin, p. 447.

Decreased In

See causes of *increased* serum thyroxine-binding globulin, p. 447.

Normal In

Pregnancy with hyperthyroidism
Nontoxic goiter
Carcinoma of thyroid
Diabetes mellitus
Addison's disease
Anxiety
Certain drugs (mercurials, iodine)

Variable In

Liver disease

FREE THYROXINE INDEX (T-7)

American Thyroid Association now recommends the term *thyroid hormone–binding ratios* (THBR).

Table 14-1. Free Thyroxine Index in Various Conditions

Condition	T-3	T-4	Free Thyroxine Factor (T-7) (T-3 Uptake × T-4)
Normal			
Range	24–36	4–11	96–396
Mean	31	7	217
Hypothyroid	22	3	66
Hyperthyroid	38	12	456
Pregnancy, estrogens (especially birth control pills)	20	12	240*

*Normal even though T-3 and T-4 alone are abnormal.

Table 14-2. Sensitivity and Specificity of Thyroid Function Tests

	Sensitivity			Specificity	
Patients	All	Hyperthyroid	Hypothyroid	All	Nonthyroid Illness
T-4	76	89	61	90	83
Free T-4	82	96	65	94	94
T-3	80	85	74	87	72
Free T-3	73	93	48	90	80
TSH	89–95	86–95	92–94	92–95	85–90

Source: Data from ET de los Santos, GH Starich, and EL Mazzaferri, Sensitivity, specificity, and cost-effectiveness of the sensitive thyrotropin assay in the diagnosis of thyroid disease in ambulatory patients. *Arch Intern Med* 149:526, 1989.

This is the calculated product of T-3 resin uptake and serum total thyroxine (T-4).

It permits correction of misleading results of T-3 and T-4 determinations caused by conditions that alter the thyroxine-binding protein concentration (e.g., pregnancy, estrogens, birth control pills).

SERUM THYROXINE-BINDING GLOBULIN (TBG)

Increased In

Pregnancy
Excess TBG, genetic or idiopathic
Certain drugs (estrogens, birth control pills, perphenazine [Trilafon], clofibrate, heroin, methadone)
Estrogen-producing tumors
Acute intermittent porphyria
Acute or chronic active hepatitis
Sometimes used to detect recurrent or metastatic differentiated thyroid carcinoma, especially follicular type and where patient has had an increased level due to carcinoma.
Lymphocytic painless subacute thyroiditis
Neonates

Decreased In

Nephrosis and other causes of marked hypoproteinemia such as liver disease, severe illness, stress (thyroxine-binding prealbumin [TBPA] also decreased)
Deficiency of TBG, genetic or idiopathic
Acromegaly (TBPA also decreased)
Severe acidosis
Certain drugs
- Androgens, anabolic steroids
- Glucocorticoids (TBPA is increased)

Testosterone-producing tumors
Factitious hyperthyroidism (useful to distinguish this from lymphocytic painless thyroiditis)

Decreased Binding Of T-3 And T-4 Due To Drugs

Salicylates
Phenytoin
Orinase, Diabinase
Penicillin, heparin, barbital

An increased TBG is associated with increased serum T-4 and decreased T-3 resin uptake; a converse association exists for decreased TBG.

SERUM THYROGLOBULIN

Increased in most patients with differentiated thyroid carcinoma but not with undifferentiated or medullary thyroid carcinomas
May be useful to assess the presence and possibly the extent of residual or recurrent or metastatic carcinoma
In differentiated thyroid carcinoma treated with total thyroidectomy or radioiodine and taking thyroid hormone therapy, thyroglobulin levels are undetectable if functional metastases are absent but elevated if functional metastases are present.
Is not useful for screening high-risk groups (e.g., neck radiation in childhood) because
- May not be increased in patients with small occult thyroid carcinomas
- Increased levels may also be found in patients with nontoxic nodular goiter.
- Presence of autoantibodies interferes with the test procedure for which the patients' serum must first be screened.

In differential diagnosis of hyperthyroidism, level is very low or not detectable in factitious hyperthyroidism and high in all other types of hyperthyroidism (e.g., thyroiditis).

SERUM THYROID-STIMULATING HORMONE (TSH; THYROTROPIN)

(hormone secreted by anterior pituitary; newest test technology uses immunoradiometric assay [IRMA], which can measure much lower levels than RIA. Since all of these assays are not equivalent, the clinician must know which technique is being used and what the various ranges are for that laboratory.)

Reference range (mIU/L) IRMA (*values differ from C10 as different reference laboratory*)
- Euthyroid: 0.4–6.0
- Possible hypothyroid: >6.0
- Possible hyperthyroid: <0.10
- Borderline: 0.10–0.39

Recommended Uses Include

Diagnosis of hypothyroidism
Therapy of hypothyroidism (treatment should bring TSH into normal range)
Differentiation of primary (increased levels) from central [pituitary or hypothalamic] hypothyroidism (decreased levels)

Establish adequate thyroid hormone replacement therapy in primary hypothyroidism although T-4 may be mildly increased
Establish adequate thyroid hormone therapy to suppress thyroid carcinoma (should suppress to undetectable levels) or goiter or nodules (should suppress to subnormal levels)
Help differentiate euthyroid sick syndrome from primary hypothyroid patients
Initial screening test for hyperthyroidism (decreased to undetectable levels)
Replace thyrotropin-releasing hormone (TRH) stimulation test in hyperthyroidism, since most patients with euthyroid TSH level will have a normal TSH response and patients with undetectable TSH level almost never respond to TRH stimulation
Screening for euthyroidism—normal level in stable ambulatory patient not on interfering drugs excludes thyroid hormone excess or deficiency. Has been recommended as the initial test of thyroid function rather than T-4
Diagnosis of hyperthyroidism by IRMA method

Increased In

Primary untreated hypothyroidism. Increase is proportionate to the degree of hypofunction, varying from 3 times normal in mild cases to 100 times normal in severe myxedema. A single determination is usually sufficient to establish the diagnosis. Useful to distinguish from pituitary or hypothalamic hypothyroidism. Especially useful in early or subclinical hypothyroidism before the patient develops clinical findings, goiter, or abnormalities of routine laboratory thyroid tests. In very early cases with only marginal elevation, the TRH stimulation test may be preferred. Serum TSH suppressed to normal level is the best monitor of dosage of thyroid hormone for treatment of hypothyroidism, but it does not indicate overtreatment.
Hashimoto's thyroiditis, including those with clinical hypothyroidism and about one-third of those patients who are clinically euthyroid
Various drugs (e.g., amphetamine abuse)
- Iodine-containing (e.g., iopanoic acid, ipodate, amiodarone)
- Dopamine antagonists (e.g., metochlopramide, domperidone, chlorpromazine, haloperidol)

Other conditions (test is not clinically useful)
- Iodide deficiency goiter
- Iodide-induced goiter or lithium treatment
- External neck irradiation
- Post-subtotal thyroidectomy
- Neonatal period

Thyrotoxicosis due to pituitary tumor or pituitary resistance to thyroid hormone
Some patients with euthyroid sick syndrome
TSH antibodies

Decreased In

Newer IRMA method measures much lower levels, making serum TSH useful for primary screening or confirmation of hyperthyroidism. Older RIA method does not extend to very low levels found in hyperthyroidism, and it may not be possible to differentiate low range of normal from an abnormally decreased value. A TRH stimulation test used to be required to establish the diagnosis.
Thyrotoxicosis due to thyroiditis or extrathyroidal thyroid hormone source
Secondary pituitary or hypothalamic hypothyroidism
Euthyroid sick patients
- Acute psychiatric illness
- Acute medical illness
- Hyperemesis gravidarum
- Hepatic disease
- Malnutrition
- Hyponatremia

Addison's disease
Acromegaly
Drug effect, especially large doses
Glucocorticoids, dopamine, dopamine agonists (bromocriptine), levodopa, T-4 replacement therapy, apomorphine, pyridoxine; T-4 may be normal or low.
Antithyroid drug for thyrotoxicosis, especially early in treatment; T-4 may be normal or low.
Assay interference, e.g., antibodies to mouse IgG, autoimmune disease
First trimester of pregnancy.

May Be Normal By IRMA In
Central hypothyroidism
Recent rapid correction of hyperthyroidism or hypothyroidism
Pregnancy
Phenytoin therapy

Normal By RIA In Some Patients With
Cushing's syndrome
Acromegaly
Pregnancy at term

THYROID-RELEASING HORMONE (TRH) STIMULATION TEST*

Now being replaced by new serum TSH (IRMA)

Serum TSH is measured before and 20 minutes after IV administration of TRH (usually 500 or 200 μg).

The TSH response to TRH is modified by thyroxine, antithyroid drugs, corticosteroids, estrogens, and levodopa. Response is increased during pregnancy. Absent response may also occur in exophthalmic Graves' disease and nodular goiter. Response may also be suppressed in nonthyroidal conditions (e.g., starvation, renal failure, elevated levels of glucocorticoids, depression, some elderly patients). Blunted response may occur in uremia, Cushing's syndrome, acromegaly, administration of certain drugs (corticosteroids, levodopa, large amounts of salicylates).

Normal response—a significant rise from a basal level of about 1 μU/ml to 8 μU/ml at 20 minutes and return to normal by 120 minutes. Response is usually greater in women than in men.

Hyperthyroidism—shows no rise in the depressed TSH level. A normal rise virtually excludes hyperthyroidism. This test may be particularly useful in T-3 toxicosis in which the other tests are normal or in patients clinically suspicious for hyperthyroidism with borderline serum T-3 levels. TRH stimulation test is superior to the T-3 suppression test of thyroid uptake of radioactive iodine (RAIU).

Primary hypothyroidism—an exaggerated rise of an already increased TSH level

Secondary (pituitary) hypothyroidism—no rise in the decreased TSH level

Hypothalamic hypothyroidism—low serum T-3 and T-4 and TSH levels, with a TRH response that may be exaggerated or normal or (most characteristically) with a peak delay of 45–60 minutes

Diagnosis must be based on clinical studies that exclude the pituitary gland as the site of the disease.

Test is useful for the following evaluations:
Confirm hyperthyroidism when other test results are equivocal

*Data from RN Kolesnick and MC Gershengorn, Thyrotropin-releasing hormone and the pituitary. *Am J Med* 79:729, 1985.

Lack of response shows adequate therapy in patients receiving thyroid hormones to shrink thyroid nodules and goiters and during long-term treatment of thyroid carcinoma.
Differentiate two forms (whether or not due to tumor) of thyrotropin-induced hyperthyroidism
May help differentiate hypothalamic from pituitary hypothyroidism (see above)
Help differentiate euthyroid sick syndrome

	Baseline TSH (μU/ml)	**Change in TSH 30 Minutes After TRH Administration (μU/ml)**
Euthyroidism	<10	>2 (95% of cases)
Hyperthyroidism	<10	<2
Primary hypothyroidism	>10	>2 (exaggerated)
Secondary hypothyroidism	<10	<2
Tertiary hypothyroidism	<10	>2 (delayed or exaggerated or normal)

TRH test may remain abnormal even after successful therapy of Graves' disease.
Abnormal TSH response to TRH administration does not definitely establish the diagnosis of hyperthyroidism (because autonomous production of normal or slightly increased amounts of thyroid hormones causes pituitary suppression).

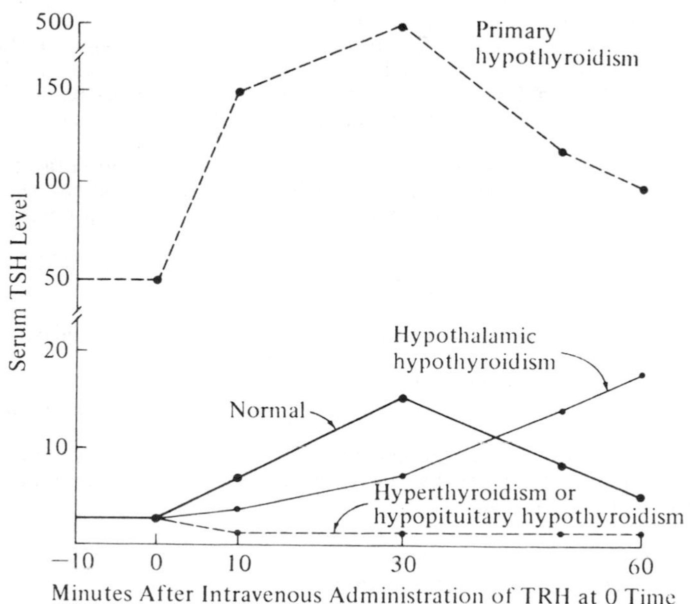

Fig. 14-1. Sample curves of serum TSH response to administration of TRH in various conditions.

THYROID AUTOANTIBODY TESTS

(antithyroglobulin and antimicrosomal antibodies)

Positive in >85% of Hashimoto's disease and ~80% of Graves' disease. Very high titer is pathognomonic of Hashimoto's thyroiditis, but absence does not exclude Hashimoto's thyroiditis. >1:1000 occurs virtually only in Graves' disease or Hashimoto's thyroiditis. Significant titer of microsome antibodies indicates Hashimoto's thyroiditis or postpartum thyroid dysfunction.

Occasionally positive in papillary-follicular carcinoma of thyroid, subacute thyroiditis (briefly), lymphocytic (painless) thyroiditis (in ~60% of patients)

Primary thyroid lymphoma often shows very high titers; should suggest need for biopsy in elderly patient with a firm enlarging thyroid.

Positive in 7% of normal population, reaching peak of 15% in females in sixth decade

Useful to distinguish subacute thyroiditis from Hashimoto's thyroiditis, as antibodies are more common in the latter

Hashimoto's thyroiditis is very unlikely cause of hypothyroidism in the absence of thyroglobulin and microsome antibodies.

Significant titer of thyroglobulin and microsome antibodies in euthyroid patient with unilateral exophthalmos suggests the diagnosis of euthyroid Graves' disease.

Occasionally useful to distinguish Graves' disease from toxic multinodular goiter when physical findings are not diagnostic.

Graves' disease with elevated titers of antimicrosomal antibodies should direct surgeon to perform a more limited thyroidectomy to avoid late postthyroidectomy hypothyroidism.

THYROID UPTAKE OF RADIOACTIVE IODINE (RAIU)

A tracer dose of radioactive iodine (^{131}I or ^{123}I) is administered orally, and the radioactivity over the thyroid is measured at specific time intervals (e.g., 2–6 hours and again at 24 hours). The percent of administered iodine in the thyroid is an index of thyroid trapping and organification of iodide. (Normal uptake is 9–19% in 1 hour; 7–25% in 6 hours; 5–30% in 24 hours. Varies with local iodine intake. 40–70% of administered dose is excreted in urine in 24 hours.)

Contraindicated in pregnancy, lactation, childhood. It is invalidated for 2–4 weeks after administration of antithyroid drugs, thyroid, or iodides; the effect of organic iodine (e.g., x-ray contrast media) may persist for a much longer time.

Because of widespread dietary use of iodine in the United States, RAIU should not be used to evaluate euthyroid state.

Indications for test

- Detection of hyperthyroidism associated with low RAIU, e.g., factitious hyperthyroidism, subacute thyroiditis, struma ovarii
- Evaluate use of radioiodine therapy
- Determine presence of an organification defect in thyroid hormone production

T-3 suppression test. Administration of triiodothyronine causes less suppression in the hyperthyroid patient than in the normal person; has been replaced by the TRH stimulation test.

Increased In

Hyperthyroidism (Graves' disease, toxic nodule)

Thyroiditis (early Hashimoto's; recovery stage of subacute thyroiditis)

TSH excess (TSH administration, TSH production by neoplasm, defective thyroid hormone synthesis)

Withdrawal rebound (thyroid hormones, propylthiouracil)

Increased iodine excretion (e.g., diuretics, nephrotic syndrome, chronic diarrhea)
Decreased iodine intake (salt restriction, iodine deficiency)

Decreased In

Hypothyroidism (tertiary, secondary, late primary)
Thyroiditis (late Hashimoto's; active stage of subacute thyroiditis; RAIU does not usually respond to TSH administration in subacute thyroiditis)
Thyroid hormone administration (T-3 or T-4) (therapeutic, factitious [RAIU is augmented after TSH administration in factitious thyrotoxicosis])
Antithyroid medication
Increased iodine intake (e.g., x-ray contrast media, iodine-containing drugs, iodized salt)
Drugs (e.g., calcitonin, thyroglobulin, corticosteroids, dopamine)

PERCHLORATE WASHOUT TEST

Perchlorate is given 2–4 hours after administration of ^{131}I, and RAIU is calculated before and at intervals after perchlorate.
Decreased uptake >10% from peak value is positive test, indicating an organification defect as the cause of hypothyroidism. Free iodide is present within the thyroid in such patients. Perchlorate blocks the trapping mechanism, causing rapid discharge of iodine so that RAIU within the thyroid diminishes. Normal thyroid gland contains very little inorganic iodine.

SERUM CALCITONIN

Basal fasting level may be increased in patients with medullary carcinoma of the thyroid even when there is no palpable mass in the thyroid. Circadian rhythm with rise to peak after lunchtime
Calcium infusion and/or pentagastrin injection are used as provocative tests in patients with normal basal levels who have a family history of thyroid carcinoma, a calcified thyroid mass, pheochromocytoma, hyperparathyroidism, hypercalcemia, amyloid-containing metastatic carcinoma of unknown origin, or facial characteristics of the mucosal neuroma syndrome.
Serum calcitonin levels are also useful to detect recurrence of medullary carcinoma or metastases after the primary tumor has been removed or to confirm complete removal of the tumor.
Increased levels have also been reported in some patients with
- Carcinoma of lung, breast, islet cell, or ovary and carcinoid due to ectopic production
- Hypercalcemia of any etiology stimulating calcitonin production
- Zollinger-Ellison syndrome (hypergastrinemia)
- Pernicious anemia
- Acute or chronic thyroiditis
- Chronic renal failure

Basal calcitonin levels
- >2000 pg/ml is almost always associated with medullary carcinoma of thyroid with rare cases due to obvious renal failure or ectopic production of calcitonin.
- 500–2000 pg/ml generally indicates medullary carcinoma, renal failure, or ectopic production of calcitonin.
- 100–500 pg/ml should be interpreted cautiously, with repeat assays and provocative tests; if these and repeat tests in 1–2 months are still abnormal, some authors recommend total thyroidectomy.
- Normal basal levels
  - Males ≤19 pg/ml
  - Females ≤14 pg/ml

IODINE TOLERANCE TEST

A fasting patient who has received no iodine for 1 week is given 0.3–0.5 ml of strong iodine solution in milk. Blood iodine determinations are made every half hour for 2½ hours.

Normal: Blood iodine increases from 10 to ≤160 or 170 μg/dl in one-half hour; by 2½ hours it decreases to only 150 μg.

Hyperthyroidism: Blood iodine increases from 15 μg to only 40 μg after 1 hour.

Indications for thyroid function tests

- Not indicated for community screening programs (overall yield ~0.5% and varies from 0% in young men to 1% in women >40 years old).
- Not indicated for hospital patients with acute medical or psychiatric illness
- Not indicated for screening of healthy asymptomatic patients
- May be useful in some women >40 years old with nonspecific complaints

T-4, T-7, free thyroxine, and sensitive TSH are all effective initial tests for screening; interpretation and follow-up of abnormal tests are most important.

Diseases of the Thyroid

HYPERTHYROIDISM

Causes of Hyperthyroidism

Diffuse toxic goiter (Graves' disease)
Toxic adenoma
Toxic multinodular goiter
Thyroiditis
- Hashimoto's
- Lymphocytic (painless)
- Subacute granulomatous

Iodide-induced (Jod-Basedow)
Metastatic functioning thyroid carcinoma
Factitious
Struma ovarii with hyperthyroidism
Thyrotropin-induced (TRH) hyperthyroidism
- With pituitary tumor
- Without pituitary tumor

Neoplasms that secrete thyroid stimulators
- Choriocarcinoma, hydatidiform mole
- Embryonal carcinoma of testis
- Others

Severity of hyperthyroidism does not correlate with thyroid hormone levels.

Serum total and free thyroxine (T-4) are increased. With a typical clinical picture of hyperthyroidism, serum T-4 >16 μg/dl confirms the diagnosis.

Serum triiodothyronine (T-3) concentration on RIA and T-3 resin uptake are increased in up to 85% of patients. T-3 is usually elevated to a greater degree than T-4. Ratio T-3/T-4 > 20:1 in T-3 dependent type of Graves' disease.

Free thyroxine index (FTI) (serum T-4 concentration × T-3 resin uptake) is the best initial screening test, since it is not affected by alterations in thyroxine-binding protein sites. Is increased in about 90% of hyperthyroid patients.

Serum TSH is decreased in all forms of thyrotoxicosis except the very rare cases of pituitary neoplasms that secrete TSH; routine measurement of TSH by sensitive IRMA method has been suggested by some authors as initial screening test for thyrotoxicosis since it will detect virtually all hyperthyroid patients, but a number of euthyroid patients are also included. TRH administration does not cause a significant rise in serum TSH in hyperthyroid patients as it does in normal persons; a normal rise (>2 μU/ml) virtually excludes hyperthyroidism. This test may be indicated in the following situations:

Hyperthyroid patients in whom associated nonthyroid conditions result in only slight elevation of serum T-4 and T-3

Euthyroid Graves' disease presenting with only exophthalmos (unilateral or bilateral). *TRH stimulation test may sometimes be normal in these patients, and T-3 suppression test may be required.*

Elderly patients with or without symptoms of hyperthyroidism may have serum T-4 and T-3 in upper normal range.

Euthyroid sick syndrome (see pp. 461–462)—generally serum TSH is normal with a relatively normal TSH response to TRH.

Serum thyroxine-binding globulin (TBG) is normal.

Radioactive iodine uptake (RAIU) is increased. It is relatively more affected at 1, 2, or 6 hours than at 24 hours. It may be normal with recent iodine ingestion. RAIU is no longer useful for diagnosis of hyperthyroidism but should be performed prior to administration of therapeutic dose of ^{131}I.

Microsomal antibodies are found in moderate to high titers in most patients with Graves' disease; may be helpful in confirming diagnosis in a hyperthyroid patient without ocular findings or a euthyroid patient with eye findings.

Other thyroid autoantibodies are thyroid-stimulating immunoglobulins (TSI) and TSH-binding inhibitory immunoglobulins (TBII) found only with Graves' disease; these are sometimes helpful in diagnosis and management.

Thyroid suppression test: T-3 administration decreases RAIU in normal persons but not in hyperthyroid persons. Now replaced by TRH stimulation test.

Salivary excretion and urinary excretion of RAI are increased.

Iodine tolerance test shows increased utilization of iodine.

Serum cholesterol is decreased, and total lipids are usually decreased.

Glucose tolerance is decreased with early high peak and early fall.

Hyperglycemia and glycosuria are present.

Liver function tests show impairment.

Creatinine excretion in urine and creatine tolerance are increased.

Normal serum creatine almost excludes hyperthyroidism.

Serum total and ionized calcium are increased in >10% of patients. Serum phosphorus is high normal or increased. Parathormone level is decreased. Serum 1,25-dihydroxyvitamin D is decreased. Urinary and fecal excretion of calcium are increased.

Unusual laboratory manifestations of hyperthyroidism include increased alkaline phosphatase, hypoproteinemia, malabsorption, anemia.

T-3 Toxicosis

Causes 5% of cases of hyperthyroidism

Should be suspected in patients with clinical thyrotoxicosis in whom usual laboratory tests are normal (serum T-4, FTI, 24-hour RAI, TBG, and thyroxine-binding albumin [TBPA]), but serum T-3 is increased.

RAIU is autonomous (not suppressed by T-3 administration).

TSH may be increased.

Abnormal TRH test (lack of TSH response to TRH)

Factitious Hyperthyroidism

Self-induced hyperthyroidism by ingestion of thyroxine (T-4) or Cytomel (T-3)

Increased total and free serum T-4 or T-3, depending on which drug is ingested. T-4 may be absent when T-3 is ingested.

RAIU is low when all other thyroid function tests indicate hyperthyroidism

Augmented RAIU after TSH administration, whereas patients with subacute and painless thyroiditis usually do not have any response to TSH administration

Serum thyroglobulin is depressed to low-normal level or undetectable unless patient is taking desiccated thyroid extract of thyroglobulin; therefore may be useful to distinguish from early or recovery phases of subacute thyroiditis and most causes of hyperthyroidism, in which it is increased.

Normal Serum T-4 Levels May Be Found In Hyperthyroid Patients With

T-3 thyrotoxicosis
Factitious hyperthyroidism due to T-3 (Cytomel)
Decreased binding capacity due to hypoproteinemia or ingestion of certain drugs (e.g., phenytoin, salicylates)

Increased Serum T-4 Levels May Be Found In Euthyroid Patients With

Increased serum TBG

Thyroid Storm

Thyroid function test values may be somewhat higher than in uncomplicated thyrotoxicosis but are useless for differentiation.
Transient hyperglycemia is common.
Abnormal liver function tests are common.
Abnormal serum electrolytes (especially decreased potassium, mild to moderate hypercalcemia) and decreased arterial PCO_2 are common.
Laboratory findings due to associated conditions, especially bacterial infection (increased WBC, shift to left; bacteria in urine, sputum, etc.), pulmonary or arterial embolism.

Hyperthyroidism With Decreased RAIU (<3%)

Factitious thyrotoxicosis*
Iodine-induced hyperthyroidism (Jodbasedow)†,‡
Graves' disease with iodine excess
Subacute thyroiditis
Lymphocytic (painless) thyroiditis†
Ectopic hypersecreting thyroid tissue
Metastatic functioning thyroid carcinoma*
Struma ovarii*

Hyperthyroidism With Increased RAIU (>12%)

Graves' disease (diffuse toxic goiter)
Plummer's disease (toxic multinodular goiter)
Toxic adenoma (uninodular goiter)
TSH-producing pituitary tumor (TSH >4 μU/ml)
Hyperthyroidism and lymphocytic thyroiditis (see p. 463)
Trophoblastic tumor
Thyrotropin-producing neoplasms (e.g., choriocarcinoma, hydatidiform mole, embryonal carcinoma of testis)

HYPOTHYROIDISM

Causes Of Hypothyroidism

Treatment of preceding hyperthyroidism
Autoimmune disease
Pituitary/hypothalamic disease
Radiation (e.g., treatment of head and neck cancer)
Iodine deficiency
Organification defect (diagnosis by perchlorate washout test)

*TSH injection causes increase ≥50% of RAIU in normal persons.
†TSH injection does not cause a normal increase ≥ 50% of RAIU.
‡Urinary iodine > 2000 μg/24 hours.

Serum TSH is increased in proportion to degree of hypofunction; is at least 2 times and often 10 times normal value. A single determination is usually sufficient to establish the diagnosis. Since increased serum TSH is earliest evidence of hypothyroidism, it should be measured to document subclinical hypothyroidism and begin early therapy in patients with Graves' disease treated with RAI or surgery or with chronic thyroiditis. TSH is especially useful in cases where T-4 and FTI are not diagnostic and is essential when the diagnosis of hypothyroidism must be confirmed. Serum TSH should always be measured prior to treatment of all patients with hypothyroidism to distinguish primary from secondary (pituitary) or tertiary (hypothalamic) types, since the latter two are often associated with secondary adrenal insufficiency, which could be lethal if unrecognized. Serum TSH is increased in primary hypothyroidism but undetectable or inappropriately low in relationship to degree of thyroid hormone deficiency in secondary or tertiary hypothyroidism. A TRH-provocative test shows a normal or delayed response in tertiary, no response in secondary and exaggerated, and prolonged response in primary hypothyroidism. (See Fig. 14-1, p. 451, and Table 14-3, p. 459.)

Increased TSH and decreased free T-4 establish diagnosis of primary hypothyroidism.

Increased TSH and normal free T-4 indicate early stage of primary hypothyroidism.

Normal or decreased TSH and decreased free T-4 suggest hypothyroidism secondary to decreased TSH secretion (hypopituitarism).

Serum T-4 and free thyroxine concentration are decreased; T-4 >7 μg/dl almost certainly excludes hypothyroidism. Serum free T-4 and TSH together is diagnostic method of choice.

Serum T-3 concentration (RIA) is decreased (may be normal in 20–30% of hypothyroid patients), and serum T-3 resin uptake is decreased (may be normal in $\leq 50\%$ of hypothyroid patients). Thus serum T-4 is a better test than T-3 for hypothyroidism, and T-3 has little role in this diagnosis.

Free thyroxine index is decreased.

Serum T-3/T-4 ratio is increased.

TSH stimulation (20 units/day for 3 days) increases RAIU to ~normal (20%) in secondary but not in primary hypothyroidism. Diagnosis of primary hypothyroidism is unlikely if RAIU increases substantially after administration of TSH. Replaced by serum TSH.

Laboratory findings indicative of other autoimmune diseases (e.g., pernicious anemia and primary adrenocortical insufficiency occur with increased frequency in primary hypothyroidism)

Serum TBG is normal.

RAIU is usually decreased and is not helpful in diagnosis.

Salivary excretion and urinary excretion of RAI are decreased.

Iodine tolerance test shows decreased utilization of iodine.

Serum cholesterol is increased (may be useful to follow effect of therapy, especially in children).

Glucose tolerance is increased (oral glucose tolerance test [GTT] is flat; IV GTT is normal); fasting blood sugar is decreased.

Serum calcium is sometimes increased.

Serum alkaline phosphatase is decreased.

Serum lactic dehydrogenase (LDH), glutamic-oxaloacetic transaminase (SGOT), and creatine kinase (CK) are increased in 40–90% of cases.

Serum carotene is increased.

Normocytic normochromic anemia is present.

Serum iron and total iron-binding capacity (TIBC) may be decreased.

Serum sodium is decreased in approximately 50% of cases.

CSF protein is elevated (100–340 mg/dl) in 25% of cases of myxedema.

Serum luteinizing hormone (LH) may be decreased, and urine 17-ketosteroids and 17-hydroxyketosteroids may be increased.

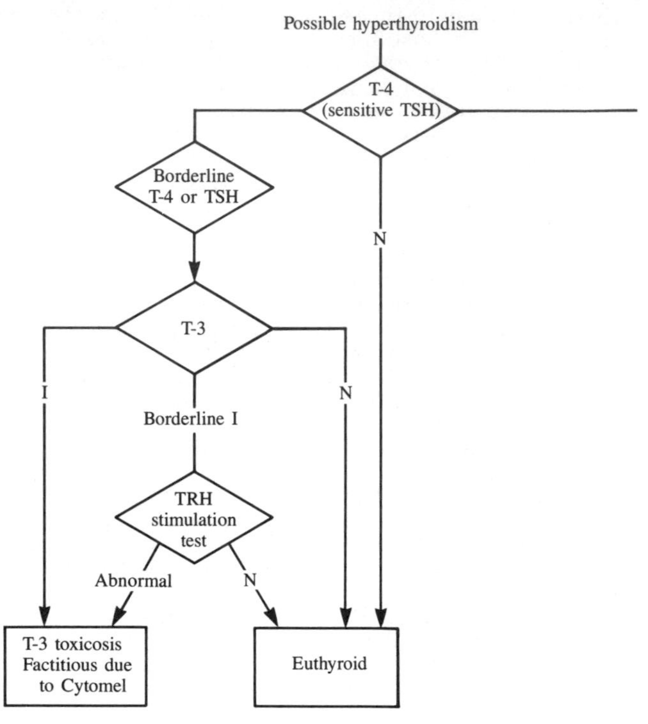

Fig. 14-2. Sequence of laboratory tests for diagnosis of hyperthyroidism. D = decreased; I = increased; N = normal.

Proteinuria is seen in about 8% of cases.

Serum myoglobin is significantly increased in 90% of untreated, long-term hypothyroid patients; inversely proportional to serum T-3 and T-4. Gradual decrease after T-4 therapy begins with return to normal before TSH becomes normal.

Adequate levothyroxine treatment results in normal serum T-4 and TSH levels. When hypothyroidism is due to thyroid failure, the dose is gradually in-

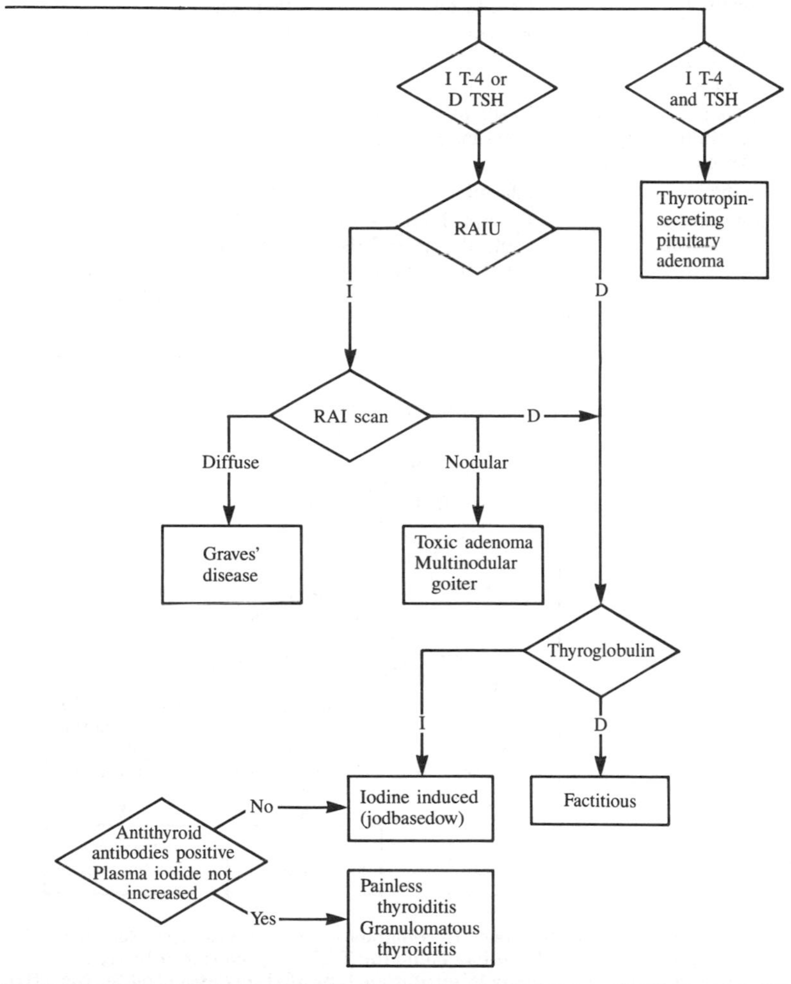

creased, and adequate therapy is indicated when serum T-4 increases to normal and TSH decreases to normal. TSH response to TRH also returns to normal if originally abnormal, but this test is generally not necessary. When hypothyroidism is secondary or tertiary, serum T-4 is used to judge adequacy of therapy, as the TSH is not useful. When levothyroxine is used for TSH suppression in patients with thyroid cancer, nodular disease, or chronic thyroiditis, the decreased TSH cannot be distinguished from normal levels; therefore levothyroxine dose is increased until serum T-4 is normal and TSH is undetectable, or an abbreviated TRH test is performed with a single TSH measurement 15 minutes after injection of TRH—if TSH is undetectable, then TSH secretion is considered adequately suppressed.

Table 14-3. Laboratory Tests in Differential Diagnosis of Primary and Secondary Hypothyroidism

Test	Panhypopituitarism	Primary Myxedema
Serum TSH	Decreased	Increased
Serum TSH response to TRH administration	Absent	Normal or exaggerated
Response to administration of thyrotropic hormone	Responds with increase in RAIU	No response
Urine 17-ketosteroids	Absent	Low
Response to insulin	Prompt decrease in blood sugar; fails to return to normal	Usually delayed fall in blood sugar and sometimes delayed return to normal

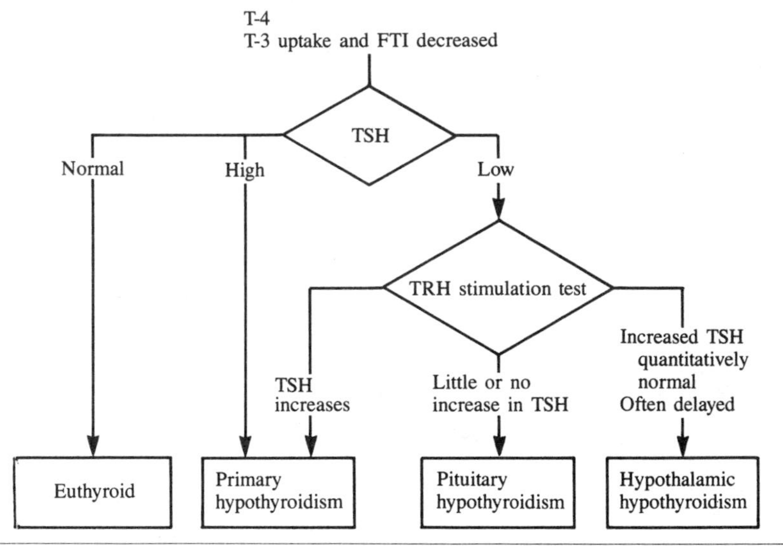

Fig. 14-3. Sequence of laboratory tests for diagnosis of hypothyroidism. Recent availability of a more sensitive TSH test has made the TSH the preferred primary screening test for thyroid disease in many laboratories. Low TSH obviates need for the TRH stimulation test in most patients.

Thyroid hormone status should be reassessed at least yearly in treatment of hypothyroidism.

Myxedema coma—hypoglycemia, hyponatremia, and findings due to adrenocortical insufficiency may be found. Serum creatinine may be increased. Arterial PCO_2 may be increased and PO_2 decreased. Increased WBC and shift to left may occur.

THYROID FUNCTION DURING PREGNANCY

Thyroid function test values are very different in normal pregnancy.

Serum TBG is increased.

Serum T-4 rises from nonpregnant level of 4–8 μg/dl to 10–12 μg/dl from 12th week of gestation until 6 weeks postpartum.
Serum free T-4 is unchanged.
T-3 uptake is decreased; FTI remains normal.
Increased serum T-3, reverse T-3
TSH is increased by 16th week; increased TSH response to TRH stimulation. Sensitive TSH (IRMA) is normal.
RAIU is increased but is contraindicated.

In hyperthyroidism, both serum T-3 uptake and T-4 are increased, but in the pregnant euthyroid patient or euthyroid patient taking birth control pills or estrogens, the T-4 is increased and the T-3 uptake is decreased. Hyperthyroidism may be indicated by the failure of the T-3 uptake to decrease during pregnancy.

T-3 uptake gradually decreases (as early as 3–6 weeks after conception) until the end of the first trimester and then remains relatively constant. It returns to normal 12–13 weeks postpartum. Failure to decrease by the eighth to tenth week of pregnancy may indicate threatened abortion (one should know the patient's normal nonpregnant level).

Maternal hypothyroidism is relatively uncommon because of spontaneous abortion and menstrual irregularities. Most often is iatrogenic or due to Hashimoto's disease. Serum T-4 in the *normal nonpregnant* range of 4–8 μg/dl should suggest hypothyroidism.

Maternal hyperthyroidism: Serum T-4 is increased above the normal range for pregnancy (>12 μg/dl) with T-3 uptake increased to normal nonpregnant range.

EUTHYROID SICK SYNDROME

(wide variety of nonthyroidal acute and chronic conditions such as infection, liver disease, cancer, starvation, renal failure, heart failure, severe burns, trauma, surgery may be associated with abnormal thyroid function tests in euthyroid patients)

Increased T-4 syndrome is most common in acute psychiatric admissions (20%), especially in the presence of certain drugs (e.g., amphetamines, phencyclidine); increased values tend to decrease during first 2 weeks after admission as patient improves. Is rarer in acutely ill patients (e.g., acute hepatitis).
Increased serum T-4, FTI (T-7), and T-3
TSH is usually normal in mild to moderate illness.
TRH test is often not useful due to flat TSH response commonly seen in melancholia patients.
50% of patients with hyperemesis gravidarum show elevated total and sometimes free T-4 that persists until hyperemesis abates.
Symptomatic hyponatremia shows transient increase until low sodium is corrected.

Decreased T-4 in >50% of severe or chronic illness. TSH is transiently (few days or weeks) increased during recovery.

Low T-3 syndrome is the most common.
T-3 is decreased in ~70% of hospitalized patients without intrinsic thyroid disease and is normal in 20–30% of hypothyroid patients; therefore is not indicated.
Increased reversed T-3 (rT-3; performed by reference laboratories)
With progressive illness, tendency is for fall in total T-4 and T-4 binding globulin with increase of free T-4. Thus T-3 uptake increases, and FTI (T-7) tends to remain normal. There is a strong correlation with low T-4 (<3 μg/dl) and high mortality in hospitalized patients.
Serum TSH is typically normal, as is TSH response to TRH.

See Table 14-4, Differential Diagnosis of Euthyroid Sick Syndrome.

Table 14-4. Differential Diagnosis of Euthyroid Sick Syndrome

	Euthyroid Sick Syndrome	Primary Hypothyroidism	Primary Hypothyroidism with Concomitant Illness
Serum T-4	N or D	D	D
Serum T-3 uptake	I	D	
Serum T-3	D	N or D	D
T-7 (FTI)	I, N, or D	D	D
Reverse T-3	I	D	D, N, or I
Serum TSH	N	I	I, occasionally N
TSH response to TRH	N or D	I	I

N = normal; D = decreased; I = increased.

Definitely increased T-3 uptake associated with decreased serum T-4 strongly indicates euthyroid sick syndrome, whereas in hypothyroidism T-3 uptake tends to be decreased.

In hypothyroidism with concomitant illness, T-3 uptake tends to increase into normal range but not above normal.

Serum TSH is increased in primary hypothyroidism as the earliest and most specific test; in contrast, basal and TRH-stimulated TSH are typically normal in euthyroid sick syndrome.

Reverse T-3 may be a useful discriminator in many euthyroid sick patients without renal failure, but it is not as useful as serum TSH.

Pituitary hypothyroidism may be difficult to distinguish, since serum TSH is low and not responsive to TRH, which is a common pattern in euthyroid sick patients.

2% of hospitalized elderly patients have unsuspected hyperthyroidism, and another 2% have unsuspected hypothyroidism; 0.5% of psychiatric hospital admissions have unsuspected hypothyroidism. In addition, thyroid function tests can be affected by the common use of diuretics and low-salt diet (causing iodine deficiency and spurious increase of RAIU) and by many factors that change protein binding of thyroid hormone (see Serum Thyroxine-Binding Globulin, pp. 447–448). These are not included in euthyroid sick syndrome.

No single test is clearly diagnostic, especially in elderly and acutely or severely ill patients.

HASHIMOTO'S THYROIDITIS (CHRONIC LYMPHOCYTIC THYROIDITIS)

Thyroid function may be normal; occasionally a patient passes through a hyperthyroid stage. 15–20% of patients develop hypothyroidism, but Hashimoto's disease is a very unlikely cause of hypothyroidism in the absence of thyroglobulin and microsome antibodies.

Microsomal antibodies are found in 60–70% of these patients. Antithyroglobulin antibodies are frequently present but are less sensitive than microsomal antibodies and are seldom positive if microsomal antibodies are negative. High titers are pathognomonic.

Serum TSH is earliest indicator of hypothyroidism; is increased in one-third of persons who are clinically euthyroid and in those with clinical hypothyroidism, many of whom have normal T-4, T-3, and T-7.

Abnormal iodide-perchlorate discharge test exceeding 10% of gland radioiodine in 60–80% of cases (indicates an underlying organification defect)

RAIU is variable; may be higher than expected in hypothyroidism.

Radioiodine scan may show involvement of only a single lobe (more common in younger patients); "salt and pepper" pattern is classic.

Response to TSH distinguishes primary and secondary hypothyroidism. If thyroid uptake for each lobe is measured separately after TSH, a difference between the lobes may demonstrate lobar thyroiditis when total uptake is apparently normal.

Laboratory findings of hypothyroidism, when present

Biopsy of thyroid may be performed.

LYMPHOCYTIC (PAINLESS) THYROIDITIS; SILENT THYROIDITIS

This is a form of hyperthyroidism described recently that comprises up to 25% of all cases of hyperthyroidism; hyperthyroidism resolves spontaneously in several weeks to months and is often followed by a transient hypothyroidism during recovery period; common in postpartum period; multiple episodes may occur. Pathologic changes are less severe than in Hashimoto's thyroiditis, but the latter cannot be ruled out in biopsy specimens.

Hyperthyroid phase is briefer in postpartum (up to 3 months) than sporadic type (up to 12 months).

- Increased serum T-4, T-3, T-3 resin uptake, FTI (T-7). T-3/T-4 ratio < 20:1. Become normal in 10 days with prednisone therapy.
- RAIU is very low (<3%); not increased after TSH administration.
- Serum TSH is low and fails to respond to TRH.
- Antithyroglobulin antibodies are increased in most patients; antimicrosomal antibodies are increased in about 60% of patients. High titers are rarely in the very high ranges of Hashimoto's thyroiditis.
- Nonspecific markers of inflammation are generally normal in contrast to granulomatous thryoiditis. Erythrocyte sedimentation rate (ESR) is increased in 50% of patients to range of 20–40 mm/hour. WBC and serum proteins are normal.
- Urine iodide level is 2–5 times higher than normal (due to leakage of iodinated material from thyroid).

Recovery phase; is complete in about 50%; rest go on hypothyroid phase.

- Serum T-4 and T-3 fall into normal range, but RAIU and TSH response to TRH remain suppressed.

Hypothyroid phase (occurs in 20–30% of patients; lasts 1–8 months; most recover completely but few develop permanent hypothyroidism; recurs in >10% of sporadic type and more often in postpartum type)

- Antithyroid antibody titers are highest during this phase (especially in postpartum patients). Gradually decrease with time; 50% become negative within 6 months.
- Serum T-4 and T-3 gradually return to normal.
- RAIU, serum TSH, TRH test begin to normalize toward the end of this phase, and urinary iodide falls to normal levels (50–200 μg/day).

SUBACUTE GRANULOMATOUS (DE QUERVAIN'S) THYROIDITIS

(probably of viral origin)

Four sequential phases may be identified: hyperthyroid, euthyroid, hypothyroid, recovery.

Hyperthyroid phase lasts 1–2 months.

- ESR is markedly increased.
- Increased total and free T-4, T-3 may be only mildly increased; T-3/T-4 ratio <20:1.
- Serum TSH is very low and does not respond to TRH.
- Decreased RAIU is the characteristic finding and differentiates it from

acute thyroiditis; may be <5% with bilateral involvement; is not increased by TSH administration. It may be >50% for several weeks after recovery.

Euthyroid phase lasts 1–2 weeks.

RAIU remains low.

Hypothyroid phase lasts 2–6 months.

TSH increases

Recovery

Return of ^{131}I trapping is the first indication.

24-hour RAIU may rise above normal.

Thyroid hormone levels rise to normal.

TSH and RAIU fall to normal.

Relapses occur in up to 47% of patients, usually in first year.

ESR is increased.

WBC is normal or decreased.

Biopsy of thyroid confirms diagnosis.

Antithyroglobulin antibodies may be present for up to several months, but the titer is never as high as in Hashimoto's thyroiditis. The level falls with recovery.

ACUTE SUPPURATIVE THYROIDITIS

WBC and polymorphonuclear leukocytes (PMNs) are increased in 75% of cases; absence may indicate anaerobic infection.

ESR is increased.

The 24-hour RAIU is decreased in <50% of cases.

Thyroid function tests are normal in 80% of cases.

Staphylococcus causes one-third of cases; other organisms include *Streptococcus pyogenes, Streptococcus pneumoniae,* Enterobacteriaceae, *Hemophilus influenzae, Pseudomonas aeruginosa,* anaerobes. Fungi are rare and principally occur in immunocompromised patients.

RIEDEL'S CHRONIC THYROIDITIS

Biopsy of thyroid confirms diagnosis.

Hypothyroidism when complete thyroid involvement occurs; otherwise normal laboratory findings

SIMPLE NONTOXIC DIFFUSE GOITER

No specific laboratory findings

SINGLE OR MULTIPLE NODULAR GOITERS

Isotope scanning of thyroid may show decreased ("cold") or increased ("hot") uptake.

Functioning solitary adenoma may produce hyperthyroidism.

In multinodular goiter, TSH level is rarely increased; usually is normal or low-normal range.

Fine-needle aspiration biopsy will produce a definitive diagnosis in 85% of cases of thyroid nodules.

CARCINOMA OF THYROID

Serum T-3, T-4, TSH are almost always normal in untreated patients. Rarely, evidence of hyperthyroidism may be found with large masses of follicular carcinoma.

Basal serum calcitonin may be increased in patients with medullary carcinoma of the thyroid even when there is no palpable mass in the thyroid. Calcium infusion and/or pentagastrin injection are used as provocative tests in patients with normal basal levels in whom there is a high index of suspicion of medullary carcinoma of thyroid; normally should not rise above 0.2 ng/ml. Serum

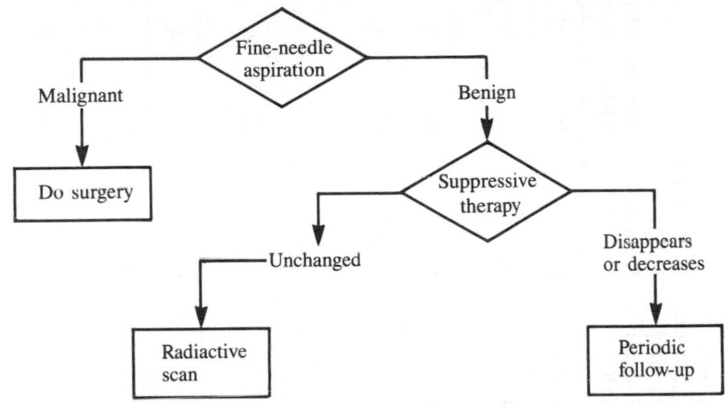

Fig. 14-4. Sequence of tests for solitary nodule of thyroid.

calcitonin levels are also useful to detect incomplete removal, recurrence, or presence of metastases in medullary thyroid carcinoma (see Multiple Endocrine Neoplasia, pp. 553–554).

Serum thyroglobulin levels are increased in most patients with differentiated thyroid carcinoma but not in undifferentiated or medullary carcinoma. May not be increased with small occult differentiated carcinoma. May be useful to detect presence and possibly the extent of residual, recurrent, or metastatic differentiated carcinoma. *Increased levels may be found in patients with nontoxic nodular goiter; presence of autoantibodies interferes with the test.*

Serum carcinoembryonic antigen (CEA) may be increased in medullary carcinoma and may correlate with tumor size or extent of disease.

Laboratory findings due to associated lesions (e.g., pheochromocytoma and parathyroid tumors) (*10–20% of cases of medullary carcinoma of thyroid occur as an inherited familial disease as part of multiple endocrine neoplasia [MEN]* [see pp. 553–554]) and to production of additional substances (e.g., ACTH, serotonin, histaminase) by medullary carcinoma.

RAIU is almost always normal.

Radioactive scan of thyroid

Needle biopsy of thyroid nodule

Tests of Parathyroid Function and Calcium/Phosphate Metabolism

SERUM TOTAL CALCIUM

See pp. 50–52.

SERUM IONIZED CALCIUM

See pp. 52–53.

SERUM PHOSPHORUS

See pp. 53–55.

PHOSPHATE DEPRIVATION

After a diet of 800 mg phosphate/day, determine serum phosphorus and urea nitrogen (BUN) and 12-hour urine phosphorus.

Normal: 6–17 ml/minute

Table 14-5. Thyroid Function Tests in Various Conditions

Disease	Total Serum Thyroxine (T-4)	Serum T-3 (concentration)	Serum T-3 Uptake	Free Thyroxine ("normalized") (FTI, T-7)	Serum Thyroxine-Binding Globulin (TBG)	Radioactive Iodine Uptake (RAIU)	Serum TSH	TRH Test
Hypothyroidism	D	D	D	D	N or I	D	I[a]	A[b]
Euthyroid sick (low T-3) syndrome	N or D	D	I	I, N, or D	N	N	N, I, or D	N or D
Hyperthyroidism	I	I	I	I	N	I	D	A
T-3 thyrotoxicosis	N	I	N or slightly I	N	N	N or I	D	A
Administration of Thyroxine (factitious hyperthyroidism)[c]	I	V	I	I	N	D	D	A
Inorganic iodine	N	N	N	N	N	D	I	A
Radiopaque contrast media[d]	N	N	N	N	N	D	N	
Estrogen and antiovulatory drugs	I	I	D	N	I	I	N	N
Testosterone	D	D	I	N	D	D	N	N

ACTH and corticosteroids	D	N or D	I	N	D	D	N or D	
Dilantin or large doses of salicylates	D	D	I	N	D		N	N
Pregnancy	I	I	D	N	I	X	N or D	N
With hyperthyroidism	I	I	N	I	I	X	N	A
With hypothyroidism	D	D or N	D	D	I	X	I	A
Hereditary increase of TBG in euthyroid state	I	I	D	N	I	I	N	N
Hereditary decrease of TBG in euthyroid state	D	D	I	N	D	D	N	N
Granulomatous thyroiditis	V or I	V or D	V or I	V or I	N	D	V or I	
Adenomatous thyroid goiter	N	N	N	N	N	N	N	
Thyroid neoplasm (nonfunctional)	N	N	N	N	N	N	N	
Nephrosis[e]	D	D	I	N	D	May be I	N	

N = normal; D = decreased; I = increased; A = abnormal; X = contraindicated in pregnancy; V = variable.

[a]Increased serum TSH is diagnostic of primary hypothyroidism; TSH is decreased in secondary and tertiary hypothyroidism.

[b]TRH stimulation test is normal in euthyroid state, increased response in primary hypothyroidism, blunted or no response in pituitary hypothyroidism, delayed response in hypothalamic etiology.

[c]RAIU is decreased when all other thyroid function tests indicate hyperfunction.

[d]Invalidates RAIU results.

[e]Thyroid function tests are altered due to loss of TBG in urine.

Hyperparathyroidism: higher (even with renal dysfunction)
Hypoparathyroidism: lower (e.g., <6 ml/minute), even when hypocalcemia has been corrected

TUBULAR REABSORPTION OF PHOSPHATE (TRP)

After a constant dietary intake of moderate calcium and phosphorus for 3 days, phosphorus and creatinine are determined in fasting blood and 4-hour urine specimens to calculate TRP.

$$\text{TRP} = 100 \times \left(1 - \frac{\text{urine phosphorus} \times \text{serum creatinine}}{\text{urine creatinine} \times \text{serum phosphorus}}\right)$$

Normal: TRP is >78% on normal diet; higher on low-phosphate diet (430 mg/day).
Hyperparathyroidism: TRP is <74% on normal diet; <85% on low-phosphate diet.
False positive result may occur in uremia, renal tubular disease (some patients), osteomalacia, sarcoidosis.

SERUM PARATHYROID HORMONE (PTH)

(see also Fig. 14-5, p. 476)

	PTH Elevated	PTH Not Elevated
Serum calcium low	Secondary hyperparathyroidism (chronic renal disease)	Hypoparathyroidism (surgical or idiopathic)
Serum calcium high	Primary hyperparathyroidism Familial hypocalciuric hypercalcemia Lithium-induced hypercalcemia Some neoplasms (HHM)	Hypercalcemia not due to hyperparathyroidism (e.g., humeral hypercalcemia of malignancy [HHM], milk-alkali syndrome, thiazide diuretics, vitamin intoxication, sarcoidosis, hyperthyroidism, immobilization)
Serum calcium normal	Pregnancy Nephrolithiasis Secondary hyperparathyroidism (chronic renal disease)	Normal

PTH may be normal or elevated in hypercalcemic patients due to acromegaly, vitamin A intoxication, MEN type IIA, renal tubular acidosis, chronic renal failure.
There is considerable overlap of serum PTH levels in normal patients and those with proven hyperparathyroidism. "Normal" level depends on the serum calcium level, which should always be determined simultaneously. Selective catheterization of veins draining the thyroid-parathyroid region for determination of PTH levels may confirm the diagnosis of hyperparathyroidism due to tumor by showing a significant elevation at one site compared to at least one other site.
A low PTH rules out hyperparathyroidism.
PTH >25% above upper limit of normal occurs only in hyperparathyroidism (primary or tertiary), post-acute tubular necrosis, or posttransplant hypercalcemia.
PTH is not increased in humoral hypercalcemia of malignancy (HHM) unless there is coexisting parathyroid adenoma, which occurs in 4% of HHM cases (especially breast or gastric cancer).

Different laboratories assay different parts of PTH molecule:
- C-terminal fragment contains an inactive portion of molecule; is next best (except increases in renal failure) if intact hormone assay is not available; is oldest and most widely available assay.
- N-terminal (mid-region) fragment contains the active portion of molecule, but these assays may not measure intact hormone.
- Intact hormone assay most clearly differentiates hyperparathyroidism from nonparathyroid hypercalcemia.
- Methodologic difficulties are important sources of error and disagreement.

PTH shows diurnal variation with low in morning and peak around midnight.

Diseases of Parathyroid Glands and Calcium, Phosphorus, Alkaline Phosphatase Metabolism

PRIMARY HYPERPARATHYROIDISM (HPT)

Due to parathyroid adenoma in 80%, hyperplasia in 15%, and parathyroid carcinoma in <5% of cases; no laboratory test can differentiate these.

Serum calcium is increased. Repeated determinations may be required to demonstrate increased levels. Rapid decrease after excision of adenoma may cause tetany during next few weeks, especially when serum alkaline phosphatase is increased. Drug-induced hypercalcemia should be reevaluated after discontinuation for 1–2 months; cessation of thiazides may unmask primary HPT. ≤5% of hypercalcemia patients have simultaneous HPT and HHM.

Serum total protein and albumin must always be measured simultaneously, as marked decrease may cause a decrease in calcium.

Normal calcium level may occur with coexistence of conditions that decrease serum calcium level (e.g., high-phosphate intake, malabsorption, acute pancreatitis, nephrosis, infarction of parathyroid adenoma); also beware of laboratory error as a cause of "normal" serum calcium.

High-phosphate intake can abolish increased serum and urine calcium and decreased serum phosphorus; low-phosphate diet unmasks these changes.

Serum PTH level is elevated. Must always be measured concurrently with serum calcium, since PTH level in the upper normal range may be inappropriately high in relation to a distinctly increased calcium level, which is consistent with HPT. PTH level >2 times upper limit of normal is almost always due to primary HPT. Failure to detect PTH in the presence of simultaneous hypercalcemia militates against the diagnosis of primary HPT and surgical exploration of the parathyroid glands. In general, nonparathyroid disease causing hypercalcemia (e.g., sarcoidosis, vitamin D intoxication, hyperthyroidism, milk-alkali syndrome, most malignancies) will have a low or suppressed PTH value. (See Fig. 14-5.)

- PTH C-terminal fragment is not the biologically active one but is more sensitive index of HPT than the active N-terminal fragment; normal ranges vary depending on which fragment is being measured; are more effective to distinguish HPT from normal than from HHM. *Recent immunometric method to measure "intact" PTH is said to be effective, as this is increased only in HPT; this appears to be sufficiently reliable to be used early in the workup of unexplained hypercalcemia.* Lithium-induced hypercalcemia resembles that of familial hypocalciuric hypercalcemia in that both show increased PTH levels and low urine calcium concentrations.

Serum chloride is increased (>102 mEq/L; <99 mEq/L in other types of hypercalcemia). HPT patients tend toward hyperchloremic (nonanion gap) acidosis, whereas other hypercalcemic patients tend toward alkalosis.

Chloride-phosphorus ratio >33 supports the diagnosis of HPT and <30 contradicts this diagnosis.

Serum phosphorus is decreased (<3 mg/dl) in ~50% of patients. It may be normal in the presence of high-phosphorus intake or renal damage with secondary phosphate retention. It may be normal in one-half of patients, even without uremia. Low serum phosphorus supports the diagnosis of primary HPT, an increased level supports the diagnosis of nonparathyroid hypercalcemia, but a normal level is not useful.

Serum alkaline phosphatase is normal in 50% of patients with primary HPT and only slightly increased in the rest; infrequently is markedly increased in the presence of bone disease. There is a slow decrease to normal after excision of adenoma. Increase >2 times upper limit of normal and increased LDH favors HHM rather than HPT.

Urine calcium is increased (>400 mg on a normal diet; 180 mg on a low-calcium diet). Urine calcium increase is found in only 70% of patients with HPT. Urine calcium excretion is often >500 mg/24 hours in malignancy, sarcoidosis, hyperthyroidism. Is <200 mg/24 hours in benign familial hypocalciuric hypercalcemia.

Urine phosphorus is increased unless there is renal insufficiency or phosphate depletion (especially due to commonly used antacids containing aluminum). Phosphate loading unmasks the increased urine phosphorus of HPT.

Polyuria is present, with low specific gravity.

Cortisone suppression test (e.g., administer 40 mg of hydrocortisone 3 times daily for 10 days, then withdraw slowly for 5 days; measure serum calcium at 5, 8, and 10 days). Positive suppression test is fall of corrected serum calcium >1.0 mg/dl.

- Test is positive in 77% of nonparathyroid causes of hypercalcemia (e.g., sarcoidosis, vitamin D intoxication, metastatic carcinoma, multiple myeloma) and in 50% of cases of HPT with osteitis fibrosa.
- Test is negative in HPT without osteitis fibrosa (77% of cases) and therefore is not helpful in this group and in familial benign hypercalcemia.

Serum alpha-2 and beta-1 globulins are slightly increased but return to normal after parathyroidectomy. *Serum protein electrophoresis should be performed in HPT to rule out multiple myeloma and sarcoidosis.*

Serum 1,25-hydroxyvitamin D may be elevated in primary HPT and in sarcoidosis but not in HMM; may be useful to establish vitamin D intoxication, especially in factitious cases.

Urinary cyclic adenosine monophosphate (cAMP) may be high (>4.0 mmol/L) in >90% of cases of primary HPT and of HHM (not increased in hypercalcemia due to osteolytic metastases) but low in vitamin D intoxication and sarcoidosis. Not usually increased in multiple myeloma or other hematologic malignancies. An elevated level that falls to normal range within 6 hours after surgery is said to provide functional confirmation of successful parathyroidectomy. Not widely used because of need for timed samples.

Uric acid is increased in >15% of patients. Uric acid level is not affected by cure of HPT, but a postoperative gout attack may occur. Increased uric acid level favors hypercalcemia due to thiazides, neoplasm, or renal failure rather than HPT.

Increased hydroxyproline in serum and urine may occur with bone disease but is not as useful as serum alkaline phosphatase for detection of bone disease.

Increased ESR is infrequent in HPT (may be due to infection or moderate renal insufficiency). Marked increase occurs in multiple myeloma.

Indirect studies of parathyroid function (e.g., phosphate deprivation, calcium infusion, tubular reabsorption of phosphate) are often borderline, and interpretation is difficult with any significant degree of renal insufficiency (see pp. 465, 468).

HPT must always be ruled out in the presence of

- Renal colic and stones or calcification (2–3% have HPT) (see Table 15-7, p. 581)
- Peptic ulcer (occurs in 15% of patients with HPT)

Calcific keratitis
Bone changes (present in 20% of patients with HPT)
Jaw tumors
Clinical syndrome of hypercalcemia (nocturia, hyposthenuria, polyuria, abdominal pain, adynamic ileus, constipation, nausea, vomiting) (*present in 20% of patients with HPT; only clue to diagnosis in 10% of patients with HPT*)
Multiple endocrine neoplasia (e.g., islet cell tumor of pancreas, pituitary tumor, pheochromocytoma (see pp. 520–523)
Relatives of patients with HPT or "asymptomatic" hypercalcemia
Mental aberrations

A changing clinical spectrum of HPT has resulted from earlier detection of hypercalcemia by multiphasic screening.
50% of patients are asymptomatic (most show only mild elevation of calcium).
20% of patients have renal stones.
6% of patients show osteitis fibrosa cystica.
15% of patients have peptic ulcer.
Two clinical forms:
Mild form detected by multiphasic screening, progresses slowly, total calcium 10.6–11.5 mg/dl, no bone disease, 30% have renal stones.
Severe form progresses rapidly with higher serum calcium that rises faster, serum phosphate is lower than in mild, renal stones are less common.

"Asymptomatic" hypercalcemia is detected by routine multiphasic screening in 1–2% of tests.
21–38% of hospitalized patients had no documented clinical cause found for hypercalcemia.
Malignancy caused one-third to two-thirds of hospitalized causes in different series.
HPT caused 15–50% of cases in different series and is the most common cause in outpatients.

HUMORAL HYPERCALCEMIA OF MALIGNANCY (HHM)

Hypercalcemia occurs in patients with cancer (typically squamous, transitional cell, renal, or ovarian), 5–20% of whom have no bone metastases compared to patients with widespread bone metastases (myeloma, lymphoma, breast cancer). Both groups have large tumor burden and poor prognosis. Occurs in ~20–35% of patients with breast cancer, ~10–15% of cases of lung cancer, ~70% of cases of multiple myeloma, rare in lymphoma and leukemia.

Very high serum calcium (e.g., >14.5 mg/dl) is much more suggestive of HHM than primary HPT; less marked increase with renal tumors.

Serum "intact" PTH is decreased but a parathyroid hormone–like protein can be measured in serum.

Serum 1,25-dihydroxyvitamin D is strikingly decreased in HHM but is increased in HPT.

Urinary cAMP is increased in 90% of cases of HHM and of primary HPT; not increased in hypercalcemia due to bone metastases.

Hypercalciuria much greater than in HPT at any serum calcium level.
Decreased serum chloride
Decreased serum albumin
Alkalosis is present.
Decreased serum phosphorus in >50% of patients.
Alkaline phosphatase is frequently increased.
Serum proteins are not consistently abnormal.
Occult cancer should be ruled out as the cause of hypercalcemia in presence of
Serum alkaline phosphatase > 2 times upper limit of normal.
Increased serum phosphorus

Table 14-6. Laboratory Findings in Various Diseases of Calcium and Phosphorus Metabolism[a]

Disease	Serum Calcium[b]	Serum Phosphorus	Serum Alkaline Phosphatase	Urine Calcium[c]	Urine Phosphorus
Primary hyperparathyroidism[d]	I	D (< 3 mg/dl in 50%)	I slightly in 50% (N if no bone disease)	I in two-thirds	I
Hypoparathyroidism	D	I	N	D	D[e]
Pseudohypoparathyroidism	D	I	N; occasionally D	D	D[e]
Pseudopseudohypoparathyroidism	N	N	N	N	N
Secondary hyperparathyroidism (renal rickets)	V	I	I or N	D or I	D
Vitamin D excess	I	N	D	I	I
Rickets and osteomalacia	D or N	D or N	I	D	D
Osteoporosis	N	N	N	N or I	N
Polyostotic fibrous dysplasia	N	N	N or I	N	N

Paget's disease	N	N or I	I	N or I	I
Metastatic neoplasm to bone	N or I	V	N or I	V	I
Multiple myeloma	N or I	V	N or I	N or I	N or I
Sarcoidosis	N or I	N or I	N or I	I	N
Fanconi's syndrome or renal loss of fixed base	D or N	D	N or I	I	I
Histiocytosis X (Letterer-Siwe, Hand-Schüller-Christian, eosinophilic granuloma)	N	N	N or I	N or I	N
Hypercalcemia and excess intake of alkali (Burnett's syndrome)	I	I or N	N	N	N
Solitary bone cyst	N	N	N	N	N

N = normal; D = decreased; I = increased; V = variable.

[a]See Serum Parathyroid Hormone, p. 469.

[b]Serum calcium. Repeated determinations may be required to demonstrate abnormalities. Serum total protein level should always be known. See also response to corticoids on p. 470.

[c]Urine calcium. Patient should be on a low-calcium diet (e.g., Bauer-Aub).

[d]See Table 14-7, p. 474.

[e]See Ellsworth-Howard Test, p. 477.

Table 14-7. Comparison of Primary Hyperparathyroidism and Humoral Hypercalcemia of Malignancy

	Humoral Hypercalcemia of Malignancy (HHM)	Primary Hyperparathyroidism (HPT)
Etiology	Squamous or large-cell carcinoma of bronchus, hypernephroma of kidney, cancer of ovary, colon	Primary hyperplasia, adenoma, carcinoma of parathyroids
Serum calcium	Very high: >14 mg/dl in 75% of patients	Moderately high: >14 mg/dl in 25% of patients
	Suppressed by cortisone in 25–50% of patients	Suppressed by cortisone in 50% of patients with and 23% of patients without osteitis fibrosa
Serum chloride	Low: <99 mEq/L	High: >102 mEq/L
Serum chloride-phosphorus ratio	<30	>33
Serum bicarbonate	Increased or normal	Normal or low
pH	Alkalosis	Acidosis
Serum alkaline phosphatase	Increased in 50% of patients, even without bone disease	Seldom increased unless bone disease is present
Serum phosphorus	Increased, normal or low	Normal or low
Urine calcium	Often >400 mg/24 hours	Usually <400 mg/24 hours
Serum parathormone	Decreased	Increased
Serum 1,25-dihydroxy-vitamin D	Decreased	Increased
Urine c-AMP	Increased in HHM but not due to bone metastases only	Increased in 90% of patients
ESR	Usually increased	Normal
Anemia	May be present	Absent
Serum albumin	Often decreased	Usually normal
Renal stones	Absent	Common
Pancreatitis	Rare	Occurs
X-ray changes in hand bones	Absent	May be present

Table 14-8. Approximate Sensitivity, Specificity, Positive and Negative Predictive Values (in %) for the Most Commonly Useful Tests*

			Predictive Value	
	Sensitivity	Specificity	Positive	Negative
Cl >99 mEq/L	98	51	18	99
Cl/P ratio >32	95	53	18	99
Cl/P ratio >28	100	53	15	100
Alkaline phosphatase >2 × normal	100	53	19	100
PTH >90 μLeq/ml	100	73	29	100
PTH >180 μLeq/ml (>2 × normal)	56	100	100	95

*Based on a prevalence of 9.7% of primary HPT in hospitalized hypercalcemic patients.

Serum chloride-phosphorus ratio >30
Serum calcium >14.5 mg/dl without florid HPT
Hypercalcemia without increased serum PTH level
Urine calcium >500 mg/24 hours; urine calcium and phosphorus and renal tubular reabsorption of phosphate are not useful in differential diagnosis
Anemia, increased ESR
Positive cortisone suppression test in absence of osteitis fibrosa

Multiple and repeat tests may be necessary in differential diagnosis of some cases of hypercalcemia.
Patients with malignancy, receiving thiazides, or with other causes of hypercalcemia may have concurrent HPT.

SECONDARY HYPERPARATHYROIDISM

This is a diffuse hyperplasia of parathyroid glands usually secondary to chronic advanced renal disease. If HPT becomes autonomous, is termed tertiary type.
Laboratory findings due to underlying causative disease are noted.
Classic findings in renal osteodystrophy
Serum calcium is low or normal.
Serum phosphorus is increased.
Serum alkaline phosphatase is increased.
These levels can also be used to monitor response to treatment with calcitriol or alpha-calcidiol.
Serum PTH level is increased.

FAMILIAL HYPOCALCIURIC HYPERCALCEMIA (FAMILIAL BENIGN HYPERCALCEMIA)

(rare familial autosomal dominant disorder of chronic lifelong, asymptomatic, nonprogressive hypercalcemia with onset before age 10 years without renal stones, kidney damage, peptic ulcer; no response to parathyroidectomy; parathyroid glands are histologically normal)

Has many of same biochemical findings as primary HPT, including
Increased serum total and ionized calcium
Elevated or inappropriately normal PTH level
Serum phosphorus is slightly decreased or normal.
Urinary cAMP is increased in about one-third of patients.

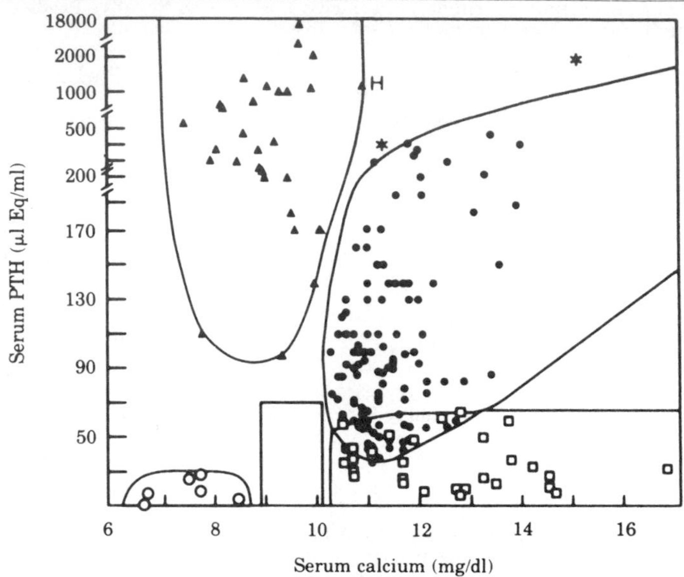

Fig. 14-5. Distribution of patients according to serum calcium and serum PTH. The values of patients with primary hyperparathyroidism are indicated by ●, with malignancies by □, with renal failure by ▲, with parathyroid carcinoma by *, with hypoparathyroidism by ○, and hypernephroma by H. The empty rectangle represents the normal range. (From *Mayo Medical Laboratories Test Catalog, 1984.* Rochester, MN: Mayo Medical Laboratories, 1984.)

Urine calcium excretion is decreased despite hypercalcemia.
- ≤200 mg/24 hours in familial hypocalciuric hypercalcemia; calcium-creatinine clearance ratio is usually <0.01 (but usually >0.02 in primary HPT).
- Up to 300 mg/24 hours in normal adult males
- Increased (often >250 mg/24 hours) in two-thirds of patients with HPT
- Increased (often >500 mg/24 hours) in patients with malignancies

Serum magnesium is mildly increased in 50% of patients; this is the only condition in which serum magnesium and calcium are both increased. Urine magnesium excretion is decreased also.

Renal function is maintained with normal creatinine clearance.

Serum 25-hydroxyvitamin D is normal and 1,25-dihydroxyvitamin D is proportional to parathormone level.

Serum alkaline phosphatase is normal.

MILK-ALKALI (BURNETT'S) SYNDROME

Increased serum calcium (without hypercalciuria)
Increased serum phosphorus
Mild alkalosis

The above findings should suggest the diagnosis in a patient with peptic ulcer

Normal serum alkaline phosphatase
Renal insufficiency with azotemia (increased BUN)
Metastatic calcinosis

HYPERVITAMINOSIS D

Serum calcium may be increased; preceded by hypercalciuria.
Serum phosphorus is normal.
Serum alkaline phosphatase is decreased.
Serum PTH is low or normal.
Urine calcium excretion is increased.
Renal calcinosis may lead to renal insufficiency and uremia.
Serum 1,25-hydroxyvitamin D is increased.
Due to ingestion of >500 μg/day in adults or >50 μg/day in infants

HYPOPARATHYROIDISM

Serum calcium is decreased (as low as 5 mg/dl). Hypocalcemia stimulates PTH secretion in pseudohypoparathyroidism but not in hypoparathyroidism.
Serum phosphorus is increased (usually 5–6 mg/dl; as high as 12 mg/dl).
Serum alkaline phosphatase is normal or slightly decreased.
Urine calcium is decreased (Sulkowitch's test is negative).
Urine phosphorus is decreased. Phosphate clearance is decreased.
Serum parathyroid hormone level is decreased.
Injection of potent parathyroid extract (200 units IV) causes urine phosphorus to increase ≥10 times within 3–5 hours. In a normal person the increase in urine phosphorus is 5–6 times. In pseudohypoparathyroidism, the urine phosphorus is not increased >2 times (Ellsworth-Howard test).
Alkalosis is present.
Congenital form may be associated with thymic aplasia (DiGeorge's syndrome) (see p. 355).
Serum uric acid is increased.
There is a flat oral GTT (due to poor absorption).
CSF is normal, even with mental or emotional symptoms or with calcification of basal ganglia.
Hypoparathyroidism should be ruled out in presence of mental and emotional changes, cataracts, faulty dentition in children, associated changes in skin and nails (e.g., moniliasis is frequent). One-third of these patients may present as "epileptics."

PSEUDOHYPOPARATHYROIDISM

Serum calcium, phosphorus, and alkaline phosphatase are the same as in hypoparathyroidism but cannot be corrected by (or they respond poorly to) administration of parathyroid hormone (see reference to Ellsworth-Howard test in the preceding section).
Serum PTH level is normal or elevated.
Cyclic AMP excretion in urine shows immediate marked increase up to 50 times after IV administration of parathormone in normal persons and in primary hypoparathyroidism but little or no increase in pseudohypoparathyroidism or pseudopseudohypoparathyroidism.

PSEUDOPSEUDOHYPOPARATHYROIDISM

Serum and urine calcium, phosphorus, and alkaline phosphatase are normal.
Response to parathyroid hormone is same as in pseudohypoparathyroidism.
Clinical anomalies are the same as in pseudohypoparathyroidism.

PRIMARY HYPOPHOSPHATEMIA

This is a familial but occasionally sporadic condition of intrinsic renal tubular defect in phosphate resorption.
Serum phosphorus is always decreased in the untreated patient.
Serum calcium is usually normal.
Serum alkaline phosphatase is often increased.
Bone biopsy shows a characteristic pattern of demineralization around osteocyte lacunae.

HYPERPHOSPHATASIA

(autosomal recessive syndrome beginning early in life of fragile bones with multiple fractures and deformities, skeletal x-ray changes, increased serum alkaline phosphatase; also referred to as osteoectasia and osteochalasia desmalis familiaris)

Serum alkaline phosphatase is usually chronically increased, sometimes markedly; electrophoresis indicates bone origin. Serum acid phosphatase is also increased. Indicates increased activity of osteoblasts and osteoclasts.

Serum leukocyte alkaline phosphatase (LAP) may also be increased.

Serum calcium is normal or slightly decreased.

Serum phosphorus is normal or increased.

Serum magnesium, proteins, and electrolytes are usually normal.

Uric acid is increased in blood and urine.

BENIGN FAMILIAL HYPERPHOSPHATASEMIA

Rare familial benign persistent increase of serum total alkaline phosphatase in the absence of any known disease.

Increase is usually of intestinal (but occasionally of bone or liver) origin as shown by monoclonal antibodies. Heat fractionation is generally not useful.

Mild increase of serum acid phosphatase in some family members does not correlate with increase or type of alkaline phosphatase.

BENIGN TRANSIENT HYPERPHOSPHATASEMIA

Sudden transient increase in serum alkaline phosphatase, often to very high levels, that return to normal usually within 4 months. Isoenzymes of bone and liver origin are increased without evidence of liver or bone disease.

Incidental discovery in children usually <5 years old, especially after summer months and following recent weight loss

Plasma 25-hydroxyvitamin D 2 times normal for age and time of year

HYPOPHOSPHATASIA

This rare (1:100,000 live births) autosomal recessive disease of bone mineralization with x-ray changes and at least three different clinical syndromes is found in infants (most severe), children, and adults (least severe).

Serum alkaline phosphatase is decreased to $\sim25\%$ of normal (may vary from 0 to $\leq40\%$ of normal); is not correlated with severity of disease. Due to bone and sometimes liver isoenzymes; normal alkaline phosphatase in intestine and placenta. Is decreased in heterozygotes, but the level cannot distinguish patients from carriers.

Serum calcium may be increased in severe newborn cases.

Serum phosphorus is normal.

Serum and urine levels of phosphoethanolamine are increased (may be increased in asymptomatic heterozygotes and useful for detection).

Treatment with corticosteroids usually causes an increase in serum alkaline phosphatase (but it never attains normal level) with a marked fall in serum calcium; phosphoethanolamine excretion in urine continues high.

Prenatal diagnosis by measurement of alkaline phosphatase in cultured amniocytes, but activity in amniotic fluid is unreliable.

Urine hydroxyproline is low; in contrast is high in vitamin D–resistant rickets or hyperphosphatasia.

PSEUDOHYPOPHOSPHATASIA

(clinical syndrome resembling hypophosphatasia)

Serum alkaline phosphatase is normal.

SYNDROME OF FAMILIAL HYPOCALCEMIA, LATENT TETANY, AND CALCIFICATION OF BASAL GANGLIA

This rare clinical syndrome has features resembling those of pseudohypoparathyroidism, pseudopseudohypoparathyroidism, and basal cell nevus syndrome.

Hypocalcemia is not responsive to parathormone administration.
Parathormone administration produces a phosphate diuresis.

DECREASED TISSUE CALCIUM WITH TETANY

The tetany, associated with normal serum calcium, magnesium, potassium, and CO_2, responds to vitamin D therapy.
Special radioactive calcium studies show decreased tissue calcium pool that returns toward normal with therapy.

MAGNESIUM DEFICIENCY TETANY SYNDROME

Serum magnesium is decreased (usually <1 mEq/L).
Serum calcium is normal (slightly decreased in some patients).
Blood pH is normal.
Tetany responds to administration of magnesium but not of calcium.

Tests for Diagnosis of Diabetes Mellitus and Hypoglycemia

GLYCOHEMOGLOBIN (GLYCATED HEMOGLOBIN)

(may be reported as Hb A_{1c} hemoglobin or as A_{1b}, A_{1a}, A_{1c}; values may not be comparable with different methodologies and even different laboratories using same methodology)

Glucose combines with hemoglobin continuously and nearly irreversibly during life span of RBC; thus glycosylated hemoglobin will be proportional to mean plasma glucose level during previous 6–12 weeks. Therefore, chief use is to *monitor diabetic patients' compliance and long-term blood glucose level control.*

In known diabetics

7% indicates good diabetic control.
10% indicates fair diabetic control.
13–20% indicates poor diabetic control.

When mean annual Hb A_{1c} is <1.1 times upper limit of normal (ULN), renal and retinal complications are rare but occur in >70% of patients when Hb A_{1c} is >1.7 ULN.
Does not require dietary preparation or fasting. Has low sensitivity but high specificity compared to oral GTT, which has high sensitivity but low specificity in diagnosis of diabetes mellitus. Increased level almost certainly means diabetes mellitus if other factors (see list below) are absent (>3 SD above the mean has 99% specificity and ~48% sensitivity), but a normal level does not rule out impaired glucose tolerance. Values less than normal mean are not seen in untreated diabetes. May rise within 1 week after rise in blood glucose due to stopping therapy but may not fall for 2–4 weeks after blood glucose falls when therapy is resumed.

Normal (A_{1a}, A_{1b}, A_{1c}) = 4–8%
For level of 4–20%, this formula may estimate daily average plasma glucose:

Mean daily plasma glucose (mg/dl) = 10 × (glycohemoglobin level + 4)

Increased In

Hb F > normal or 0.5% (e.g., fetomaternal transfusion during pregnancy)
Chronic renal failure with or without hemodialysis
Iron deficiency anemia
Splenectomy
Increased serum triglycerides
Alcohol
Lead toxicity

Decreased In

Hemolytic anemias
- Presence of Hb S, Hb C, Hb D
- Congenital spherocytosis
- Acute or chronic blood loss
- Pregnancy

SERUM FRUCTOSAMINE

Measures concentration of nonlabile glycated serum proteins, giving a reliable estimate of mean blood glucose levels during preceding 1–3 weeks. Most useful to monitor treatment of diabetics.

Correlates with Hb A_{1c} but is not affected by abnormal hemoglobins, Hb F, increased RBC turnover and shows changed glucose levels earlier; is cheaper, faster, less subjective than Hb A_{1c}. Elevated serum bilirubin may interfere with test.

Changes in fructosamine values correlate with significant changes in serum albumin or protein concentrations. Abnormal values also occur during abnormal protein turnover (e.g., thyroid disease) even though patients are normoglycemic. Obviated by using fructose-albumin ratio.

Should primarily be compared with previous values in same patient rather than reference range.

Reference range in nondiabetic persons: fructosamine = 2.4–3.4 mmol/L; fructosamine-albumin ratio = 54–86 μmol/gm).

ORAL GLUCOSE TOLERANCE TEST (OGTT)*

Standards for OGTT: Prior diet of >150 gm of carbohydrate daily, no alcohol, and unrestricted activity for 3 days before test. Test in morning after 10–16 hours of fasting. No medication, smoking, or exercise (remain seated) during test. Not to be done during recovery from acute illness, emotional stress, surgery, trauma, pregnancy, inactivity due to chronic illness; therefore is of limited or no value in hospitalized patients. Certain drugs should be stopped several weeks before the test (e.g., oral diuretics, oral contraceptives, phenytoin). Loading dose of glucose for adults is 75 gm, 1.75 gm/kg for children consumed within 5 minutes. Draw blood at fasting, 30, 60, 90, 120 minutes; 30-minute sample offers little additional information but can confirm adequate gastric absorption when patient is nauseous.

OGTT should be reserved principally for patients with "borderline" fasting plasma glucose levels (i.e., fasting range 110–140 mg/dl).

OGTT is not indicated in
- Persistent fasting hyperglycemia (>140 mg/dl)
- Persistent fasting normoglycemia (<110 mg/dl)
- Patients with typical clinical findings of diabetes mellitus and random plasma glucose >200 mg/dl
- Suspected gestational diabetes
- Secondary diabetes (e.g., genetic hyperglycemic syndromes, following administration of certain hormones)
- Should never be done to evaluate reactive hypoglycemia
- Test is of limited value for diagnosis of diabetes mellitus in children and is rarely indicated for that purpose.

All pregnant women should be tested for gestational diabetes with a 50-gm dose at 24–28 weeks of pregnancy; if that is abnormal, OGTT should be performed after pregnancy.

*Data from National Diabetes Group 1978.

For diagnosis of diabetes mellitus in nonpregnant adults, at least two values of OGTT should be increased (or fasting serum glucose ≥140 mg/dl on more than one occasion) and other causes of transient glucose intolerance must be ruled out. See Classification of Diabetes Mellitus and Other Hyperglycemic Disorders, p. 484.

Decreased Tolerance In

Excessive peak
- Increased absorption (normal IV GTT curve) with normal return to fasting level
  - Mechanical (e.g., gastrectomy, gastroenterostomy)
  - Hyperthyroidism
  - Excess intake of glucose
- Decreased utilization with slow fall to fasting level
  - Diabetes mellitus
  - Hyperlipidemia, types III, IV, V
  - Hemochromatosis
  - Steroid effect (Cushing's disease, administration of ACTH or steroids)
  - CNS lesions
- Decreased formation of glycogen with low fasting levels and subsequent hypoglycemia
  - von Gierke's disease
  - Severe liver damage
  - Hyperthyroidism (normal return to fasting level)
  - Increased epinephrine (stress, pheochromocytoma) (normal return to fasting level)
  - Pregnancy (normal return to fasting level)

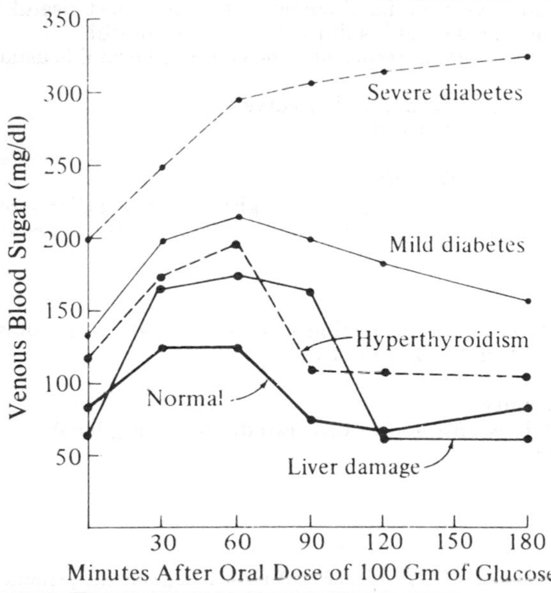

Fig. 14-6. Sample oral glucose tolerance curves in various conditions.

Increased Tolerance In

Flat peak
- Pancreatic islet cell hyperplasia or tumor
- Poor absorption from GI tract (normal IV GTT curve)
  - Intestinal diseases (e.g., steatorrhea, sprue, celiac disease, Whipple's disease)
  - Hypothyroidism
  - Addison's disease
  - Hypoparathyroidism
- Late hypoglycemia
  - Pancreatic islet cell hyperplasia or tumor
  - Hypopituitarism
  - Liver disease

See Serum Glucose, pp. 33–34, and Table 19-1, pp. 750–755, for effect of drugs.

Difficulty in interpretation has caused abandonment of other GTTs, such as IV GTT, cortisone GTT.

TOLBUTAMIDE TOLERANCE TEST

Administer 1 gm of sodium tolbutamide IV within 2 minutes. *Always keep IV glucose available to prevent severe reaction.*

Test is most useful for diagnosis of insulinoma and to rule out functional hyperinsulinism.

In normal persons, glucose is a more potent stimulus for insulin release than tolbutamide, but the opposite is true in insulinoma, which shows an exaggerated early insulin peak (3–5 minutes after injection) with a sustained elevation of insulin and depression of glucose at 150 minutes.

In insulinoma, the fall in blood sugar is usually more marked than in functional hypoglycemia; more important, the blood sugar fails to recover even after 2–3 hours. A mean serum glucose at 120, 150, 180 minutes after tolbutamide ≤55 mg/dl in lean patients and 62 mg/dl in obese patients has a 95% specificity and >95% sensitivity for insulinoma; this is the most useful test.* Other calculations of glucose and insulin levels are less useful.

In functional hypoglycemia, return of blood sugar to normal is usually complete by 90 minutes.

Adrenal insufficiency—normal or low curve

Severe liver disease—low curve

INSULIN TOLERANCE TEST

Administer 0.1 unit of insulin/kg body weight IV. *Use smaller dose if hypopituitarism is suspected. Always keep IV glucose available to prevent severe reaction.*

Normal

Blood glucose falls to 50% of fasting level within 20–30 minutes; returns to fasting level within 90–120 minutes.

Increased Tolerance

Blood glucose falls <25% and returns rapidly to fasting level.

Hypothyroidism

Acromegaly

*Data from MM McMahon, PC O'Brien, and FJ Service, Diagnostic interpretation of the intravenous tolbutamide test for insulinoma. *Mayo Clin Proc* 64:1481, 1989.

Cushing's syndrome
Diabetes mellitus (some patients; especially older, obese ones)

Decreased Tolerance

Increased sensitivity to insulin (excessive fall of blood glucose)
Hypoglycemic irresponsiveness (lack of response by glycogenolysis)
- Pancreatic islet cell tumor
- Adrenocortical insufficiency
- Adrenocortical insufficiency secondary to hypopituitarism
- Hypothyroidism
- von Gierkc's disease (some patients)
- Starvation (depletion of liver glycogen)

INSULIN GLUCOSE TOLERANCE TEST

Administer simultaneously 0.1 unit of insulin/kg body weight IV and 0.8 gm of glucose/kg body weight orally.
Insulin-sensitivity diabetics show little change in blood sugar.
Insulin-resistant diabetics show a diabetic glucose tolerance curve.
Other changes parallel those in the insulin tolerance test.

PLASMA INSULIN

Not clinically useful for diagnosis of diabetes mellitus because of the very wide range in both normal and diabetic patients and because results may be influenced by many other factors.

Increased In

Insulinoma. Fasting blood insulin level >50 μU/ml in presence of low or normal blood glucose level. Intravenous tolbutamide or administration of leucine causes rapid rise of blood insulin to very high levels within a few minutes with rapid return to normal.
Untreated obese mild diabetics. The fasting level is often increased.
Acromegaly (especially with active disease) after ingestion of glucose
Reactive hypoglycemia after glucose ingestion, particularly when diabetic type of glucose tolerance curve is present

Absent In

Severe diabetes mellitus with ketosis and weight loss. In less severe cases, insulin is frequently present but only at lower glucose concentrations.

Normal In

Hypoglycemia associated with nonpancreatic tumors
Idiopathic hypoglycemia of childhood, except after administration of leucine

SERUM C-PEPTIDE

C-peptide is formed during conversion of proinsulin to insulin; C-peptide serum levels correlate with insulin levels in blood, except in islet cell tumors and possibly in obese patients. Therefore test is useful for estimating insulin levels in the presence of antibodies to exogenous insulin. Also useful in factitious hypoglycemia due to surreptitious administration of insulin in which high serum insulin levels will occur with low C-peptide levels.

24-hour urine levels for C-peptide
- Normal: >30 μg
- Type II—obese with insulin resistance: >60 μg
- Type II with some insulin resistance: <30 μg
- Type I: <10 μg (often <2 μg).

Diabetes Mellitus and Other Hyperglycemic and Hypoglycemic Disorders

CLASSIFICATION OF DIABETES MELLITUS AND OTHER HYPERGLYCEMIC DISORDERS*

I and II are idiopathic diabetes mellitus.

- I: Insulin-dependent type (IDDM) (formerly called juvenile diabetes or ketosis-prone or brittle diabetes mellitus)—represents 10–20% of diabetic patients
- II: Non-insulin-dependent type (NIDDM)—represents 80–90% of diabetic patients
  - Not obese NIDDM—represents 15–20% of NIDDM
    - Insulin-treated for hyperglycemia
    - Not insulin treated
  - Obese NIDDM—represents 80–85% of NIDDM
    - Insulin-treated for hyperglycemia (formerly called maturity-onset or ketosis-resistant diabetes mellitus)
    - Not insulin treated
  - Criteria for diagnosis diabetes mellitus: fasting serum glucose $>$140 mg/dl on ≥more occasions or OGTT $>$200 mg/dl at 2 hours and one other sample

III: Gestational diabetes (GDM)—see p. 485.

IV: Impaired glucose tolerance (IGT)—replaces terms "latent" and "chemical" diabetes. Diagnosis in nonpregnant adult is based on fasting glucose $<$140 mg/dl and OGTT at 2-hour glucose = 140–200 mg/dl and OGTT before 2 hours ≥200 mg/dl.

V: Previous abnormality of glucose tolerance (PrevAGT)—this term recognizes the imperfect reproducibility of the OGTT.

VI: Potential abnormality of glucose tolerance (PotAGT)—high-risk subjects without demonstrable abnormality; replaces terms "prediabetes" and "potential diabetes."

VII: Glucose intolerance associated with certain conditions and syndromes (e.g., Cushing's syndrome, acromegaly, chronic pancreatitis, hemochromatosis, pheochromocytoma, miscellaneous drugs and chemicals)

Other causes of transient glucose intolerance must be ruled out before an unequivocal diagnosis of diabetes mellitus is made.

See sections on diabetic nephrosclerosis, papillary necrosis, GU tract infection, serum lipoproteins, etc.

COMPARISON OF INSULIN-DEPENDENT AND NON-INSULIN-DEPENDENT DIABETES MELLITUS

Insulin-Dependent (IDDM) (formerly called juvenile, brittle, or ketosis-prone diabetes)	**Non-Insulin-Dependent (NIDDM) (formerly called adult-onset, stable, maturity-onset, diabetes of youth)**
Deficiency of insulin production due to beta-cell destruction by antibody or cell-mediated mechanisms or some other unknown cause	Possible contributing factors: genetic, environmental, decreased number of beta cells, peripheral insulin resistance
Prone to ketosis	Resistant to ketosis

*Data from National Diabetes Data Group, 1979.

Very low serum C-peptide levels <10 μg; often <2 μg*	Normal or increased C-peptide levels* Some insulin deficiency: <30 μg Obese with insulin resistance: >60 μg

GESTATIONAL DIABETES MELLITUS

Hyperglycemia that develops for the first time during pregnancy; affects 2–3% of pregnant women; most will return to normal glucose tolerance after delivery. 60% become diabetic in next 16 years.

Diagnosis is necessary for short-term identification of increased risk of fetal morbidity (stillbirth, macrosomia, birth trauma, hypoglycemia, hyperbilirubinemia, hypocalcemia, polycythemia). Screening of all pregnant women should include

- Urine test for glucose at each visit
- Random venous blood glucose on first visit
- Serum glucose 1 hour after ingestion of 50 gm of glucose at 24–28 weeks' gestation (earlier if urine or random blood glucose are abnormal). Values <135 mg/dl are considered normal; >182 mg/dl are considered definitely abnormal; 135–182 mg/dl are suspicious and indicate a standard 3-hour GTT should be done. 1-hour, 50-gm test is abnormal in ~15% of pregnant women, ~14% of whom have abnormal 3-hour GTT. Sensitivity ~79%, specificity ~87%.

After overnight fasting, serum glucose >140 mg/dl or postprandial >200 mg/dl is diagnostic of diabetes mellitus and no further tests are required, but intermediate values indicate need for further tests.

Diagnosis is made if at least two of the following glucose levels (venous serum) are found on oral GTT with 100-gm glucose loading dose (see pp. 480–481):

Fasting	>105 mg/dl
1 hour	>190 mg/dl
2 hours	>165 mg/dl
3 hours	>145 mg/dl

If abnormal results during pregnancy, repeat GTT at first postpartum visit; if GTT is normal, diagnose as diabetes only during pregnancy, but blood glucose should be tested at every subsequent visit because of increased risk of developing diabetes mellitus. If postpartum GTT is abnormal, classify as impaired glucose tolerance or diabetes mellitus using standard criteria.

Glycosylated hemoglobin and fructosamine are not reliable tests for detection of gestational diabetes.

For management of diabetes during pregnancy, goal is fasting plasma glucose of 60–110 mg/dl and postprandial levels <150 mg/dl. Measure serum or 24-hour urine estriol for fetal surveillance. Amniotic fluid lecithin-sphingomyelin ratio, phosphatidylglycerol, shake test, or fluorescence polarization to evaluate fetal pulmonary maturity.

During labor, keep maternal glucose at 80–100 mg/dl; beware of markedly increased insulin sensitivity in immediate postpartum period.

DIABETIC KETOACIDOSIS (DKA)

Blood glucose is increased (usually >300 mg/dl); range from slightly increased to very high. Very elevated glucose (>500–800 mg/dl) suggests nonketotic hyperosmolar hyperglycemia (because glucose levels become very high only when extracellular fluid volume is markedly decreased). Glucose <200 mg/

*Normal 24-hour urine C-peptide >30 μg.

dl may occur, especially in alcoholics or pregnant insulin-dependent diabetics. Glucose concentration is not related to severity of DKA.

Plasma acetone is increased (4+ reaction when plasma is diluted 1:1 with water). (Acetone is usually 3–4 times the concentration of acetoacetate but does not contribute to acidosis.) Nitroprusside reagent tests (e.g., Acetest, Ketostix, Chemstrip) react with acetoacetate, not with beta-hydroxybutyrate, weakly with acetone; therefore weak positive reaction with ketone does not rule out ketoacidosis. Beta-hydroxybutyrate–acetoacetate ratio varies from 3:1 in mild up to 15:1 in severe DKA. With correction of DKA, conversion of beta-hydroxybutyrate to acetoacetate gives a stronger nitroprusside test reaction; do not mistake this for worsening of DKA.

Metabolic acidosis (pH <7.3 and/or bicarbonate <15 mEq/L) is mainly due to beta-hydroxybutyrate and acetoacetate. Some lactic acidosis may exist. Whole spectrum of patterns from pure hyperchloremic acidosis to wide anion-gap acidosis. May be obscured by complicating metabolic alkalosis.

Volume and electrolyte depletion (due to glucose-induced osmotic diuresis)

- Absence of volume depletion should arouse suspicion of other possibilities (e.g., hypoglycemic coma, other causes of coma).
- Very low sodium (120 mEq/L) is usually due to hypertriglyceridemia and hyperosmolality although occasionally may be dilutional due to vomiting and water intake. Low in 67%, normal in 26%, increased in 7% of patients. Depleted body stores are not reflected in these initial values, which reflect relative water loss and blood glucose level.
- Serum potassium is normal in 43%, increased in 39% due to potassium exit from cells secondary to acidosis; initial low potassium in 18% of cases indicates severe depletion.
- Serum phosphate decreased in 10%, normal in 18%, and increased in 71% of patients; falls with onset of therapy due to loss by osmotic diuresis. Severe depletion (<0.5 mg/dl may cause muscle weakness, rhabdomyolysis, impaired cardiac function, etc.). Excessive replacement may cause hypocalcemia and hypomagnesemia.

Serum magnesium may be decreased in 7% (in prolonged ketoacidosis), normal in 25%, increased in 68% of patients. Azotemia is present (BUN is usually 25–30 mg/dl); creatinine may be proportionally increased >BUN due to methodologic interference by acetoacetate.

Serum osmolality is slightly increased (up to 340 mOsm/L).

WBC is increased (often >20,000/cu mm) even without infection; associated with decreased lymphocytes and eosinophils.

Hemoglobin, hematocrit, total protein may be increased due to intravascular volume depletion.

Serum amylase may be increased (may originate from salivary glands rather than pancreas) in up to 36% of patients or both sources in 16%.

SGOT, serum glutamic-pyruvic transaminase (SGPT), LDH, and CK are increased in 20–65% of patients partly due to methodologic interference of acetoacetate in colorimetric methods. CK may be increased due to phosphate depletion and rhabdomyolysis.

Thyroid function tests are not reliable (due to sick thyroid syndrome).

Changes due to complications in treatment

- Hypoglycemia
- Hypokalemia
- Alkalosis
- Nonketotic hyperglycemic coma (see p. 487)
- Underlying precipitating medical problem (e.g., myocardial infarction, infection)

See Metabolic Acidosis, p. 393; Lactic Acidosis, p. 397; Hyperosmolar State, p. 487.

Look for precipitating factors, especially infection; also vascular, trauma, pregnancy, emotional, endocrine; not found in 25% of cases.

Follow-up laboratory tests every 2–4 hours initially and less often with clinical improvement. Bedside fingerstick glucose can be determined initially every 30–60 minutes to determine rate of fall of glucose and when to add glucose to IV fluids.

ESR may be increased in diabetic patients even in absence of infection and when serum protein is normal, particularly when glycemic control is poor; does not necessarily indicate underlying infection.

HYPEROSMOLAR HYPERGLYCEMIC NONKETOTIC COMA

Blood glucose is very high, often 600–2000 mg/dl.

Serum osmolality is very high, usually >350 mOsm/L with coma. (See p. 42.)

Acidosis is absent.

Plasma ketones are not usually found.

Serum sodium may be increased, normal, or decreased but is disproportionately decreased for degree of dehydration due to marked hyperglycemia (decreases 1.6 mEq/L per 100 mg/dl increase of serum glucose). Increased sodium with marked hyperglycemia indicates severe dehydration.

Serum potassium may be increased (due to hyperosmolality), low (due to osmotic diuresis with urinary loss), or normal depending on balance of factors.

BUN is increased (70–90 mg/dl) more than diabetic ketoacidosis.

Changes due to preexisting conditions

- Infection
- Renal insufficiency in 90% of cases
- Drugs (e.g., steroids, phenytoin, potassium-wasting diuretics such as thiazides and furosemide, others [propranolol, diazoxide, azathioprine])
- Other medical conditions (e.g., cerebrovascular accident, subdural hematoma, severe burns, acute pancreatitis, thyrotoxicosis, Cushing's syndrome)
- Use of concentrated glucose infusions
- Spontaneous in 5–7% of cases
- Preexisting mild diabetes mellitus Type II

SOME HETEROGENEOUS GENETIC DISEASES ASSOCIATED WITH HYPERGLYCEMIA

Alstrom's syndrome
Ataxia-telangiectasia
Diabetes mellitus
Friedreich's ataxia
Hemochromatosis
Herrmann's syndrome
Hyperlipoproteinemias (three different types)
Isolated growth hormone deficiency
Laurence-Moon-Bardet-Biedl syndrome
Lipoatrophic diabetes
Myotonic dystrophy
Optic atrophy
Prader-Willi syndrome
Refsum's syndrome
Schmidt's syndrome
Werner's syndrome

PRADER-WILLI SYNDROME

This condition is characterized by mental retardation, muscular hypotonia, obesity, short stature, and hypogonadism associated with diabetes mellitus.

Table 14-9. Differential Diagnosis of Diabetic Coma

Condition	Serum Glucose (mg/dl)	Serum Ketones (undiluted)	Arterial pH	Serum Osmolality (mOsm/kg)	Serum Lactate (mmol/L)	Plasma Insulin
Diabetic ketoacidosis	300–1000	+ + + +	D	300–350	2–3	0–L
Lactic acidosis	100–200	0	D	N–300	≧7	L
Alcoholic ketoacidosis	40–200	+ + + +	D	290–310	2–6	L
Hyperosmolar coma	500–2000	0/+	N	320–400	1–2	Some
Hypoglycemia	10–40	0	N	285 ± 6	Low	I

D = decreased; L = low; N = normal; I = increased; 0 = none; + = small amount; up to + + + + = large amount.
Normal serum lactate = 0.6–1.1 mmol/L.

Lactic acidosis occurs in one-third of patients with diabetic ketoacidosis.

Hyperosmolar coma and alcoholic ketoacidosis may occur in diabetic ketoacidosis.

Table 14-10. Comparison of Diabetic Ketoacidosis and Hyperosmolar Hyperglycemic Nonketotic Coma

Findings	Diabetic Ketoacidosis	Hyperosmolar Hyperglycemia Nonketotic Coma
Laboratory		
Serum glucose	Usually <800 mg/dl	>800 mg/dl
Plasma acetone	Positive in diluted plasma	Less positive in undiluted plasma
Serum sodium	Usually low	Normal, increased, or low
Serum potassium	Increased, normal or low	Normal or increased
Serum HCO_3	<10 mEq/L	>16 mEq/L
Anion gap	>12 mEq/L	10–12 mEq/L
Blood pH	<7.35	Normal
Serum osmolality	<330 mOsm/L	>350 mOsm/L
Serum BUN	Not as high	Higher
Blood free fatty acids	>1500 mEq/L	<1000 mEq/L
Clinical		
Dehydration	Less	More
Acidosis	More	Less
Coma	Rare	Frequent
Hyperventilation	Yes	No
Age	Younger	Usually elderly
Diabetes type	I—insulin-dependent	II—Non-insulin-dependent
Previous history of diabetes	Almost always	50% of cases
Prodrome	<1 day	Several days
Neurologic findings	Rare	Very common
Cardiovascular or renal disease	15%	85%
Thrombosis	Very rare	Frequent
Mortality	<10%	20–50%

Diabetes mellitus frequently develops in childhood and adolescence but is insulin-resistant, responds to oral hypoglycemic drugs, and is not accompanied by acidosis.

CLASSIFICATION OF ISLET CELL TUMORS OF PANCREAS

Insulin-secreting beta-cell tumor (may be benign or malignant, primary or metastatic) produces hyperinsulinism with hypoglycemia.

Non-insulin-secreting non-beta-cell tumor (benign or malignant, primary or metastatic) may produce several types of syndromes.

Zollinger-Ellison syndrome

Profuse diarrhea with hypokalemia and dehydration. Profuse diarrhea with hypokalemia (and sometimes periodic paralysis) may occur as a separate syndrome without peptic ulceration. *(Some of the patients have histamine-fast achlorhydria.)* Diabetic glucose tolerance curves may occur in some patients because of chronic potassium depletion. May be associated with MEN.

Nonspecific diarrhea

Steatorrhea (due to inactivation of pancreatic enzymes by acid pH)

PRIMARY ENDOCRINE-SECRETING TUMORS OF PANCREAS

Cell Type	Hormone Secreted	Tumor
B cell	Insulin	Insulinoma (see next section)
D cell	Gastrin	Gastrinoma (see p. 492)
A cell	Glucagon	Glucagonoma (see p. 492)
H cell	Vasoactive intestinal peptide (VIP)	Vipoma (see p. 492)
D cell	Somatostatin	Somatostatinoma (see p. 492)
HPP cell	Human pancreatic polypeptide (HPP)	HPP-secreting tumor (very rare tumor)

Other rare endocrine-secreting tumors have been identified as causing ectopic ACTH syndrome, atypical carcinoid syndrome, syndrome of inappropriate antidiuretic hormone secretion (SIADH), ectopic hypercalcemia syndrome.

INSULINOMA

(tumor of pancreatic islet beta-cell origin; most often benign solitary tumor; occasionally may be part of MEN I [see pp. 553–554]

In patients with fasting hypoglycemia, insulinoma should be considered the cause until another diagnosis can be proved. No single test is certain to be diagnostic; multiple tests may be required.

Fasting 24–36 hours will provoke hypoglycemia in 80–90% of these patients; 72 hours of fasting will provoke hypoglycemia in >95% of these patients, especially if punctuated with exercise. Absence of ketonuria implies surreptitious food intake or excess insulin effect (differentiate by blood glucose level). Low serum glucose and high serum insulin establishes the diagnosis, i.e., insulin level is inappropriately elevated for the degree of hypoglycemia (in normal persons, insulin level becomes <5 μU/ml or undetectable). Serum C-peptide is similarly inappropriately elevated, in contrast to factitious hypoglycemia. In women, serum glucose during fasting can fall to 20–30 mg/dl and return to normal without treatment; in men, a fall in serum glucose to <50 mg/dl is considered abnormal.

Serum insulin-glucose ratio > 0.3 when serum glucose > 50 mg/dl indicates inappropriate hyperinsulinism, and this usually indicates insulinoma if factitious hypoglycemia is ruled out. Ratio may be slightly higher (e.g., ≤0.35) in obese persons.

Serum insulin values are not useful in reactive hypoglycemia but should always be performed in cases of fasting hypoglycemia.

Occasional patients with insulinoma have very low serum insulin levels; their serum shows very high proinsulin level that interferes with the insulin immunoassay, giving falsely low values.

Stimulation tests are usually not necessary and may be dangerous if serum glucose < 50 mg/dl. Too many false positive and negative results make these tests unreliable.

Tolbutamide tolerance test—see p. 482.

Glucagon stimulation test: Administer 1 mg of glucagon IV during 1–2 minutes; measure serum insulin 3 times at 5-minute intervals and then twice at 15-minute intervals. Patients with insulinoma show an exaggerated response of serum immunoreactive insulin. Serum insulin >100 μU/ml after glucagon stimulation in a patient with fasting hypoglycemia and inappropriate insulin secretion strongly suggests insulinoma.

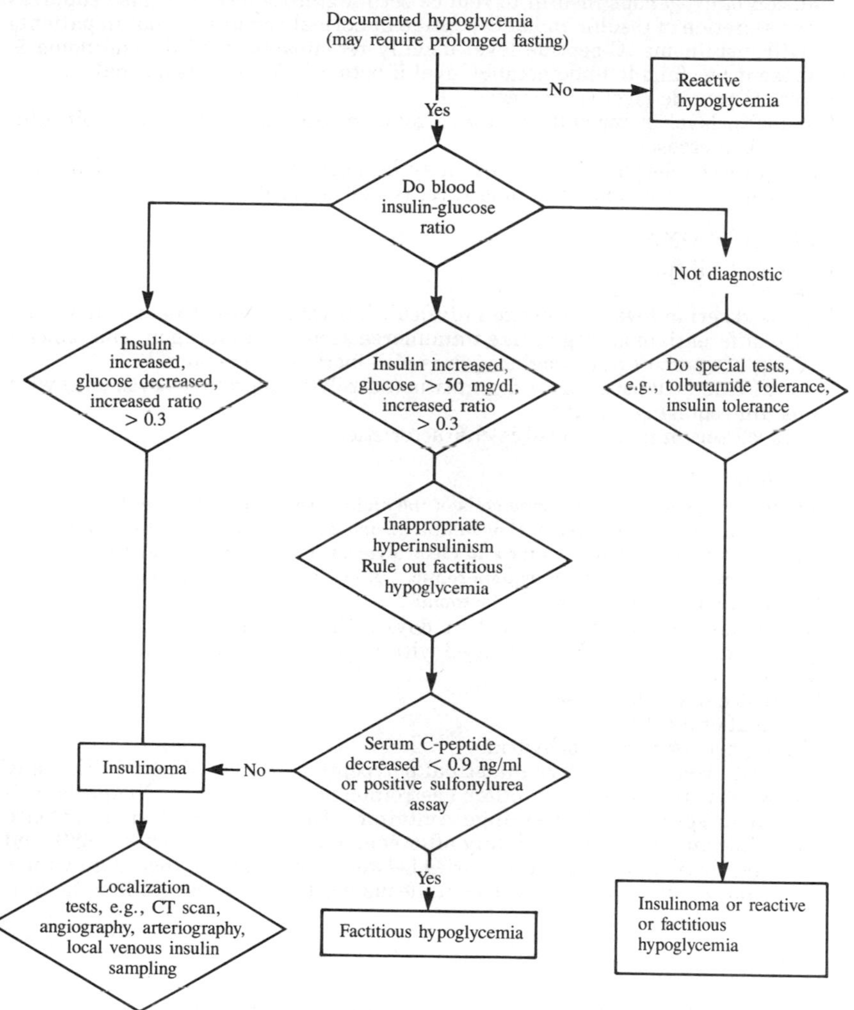

Fig. 14-7. Flow chart for diagnosis of suspected insulinoma.

Infusion of exogenous insulin to reduce serum glucose level will also suppress the secretion of insulin and of C-peptide in normal persons but not in patients with insulinoma. C-peptide level usually remains elevated if insulinoma is present but falls to undetectable level if beta-cell function is normal.

Serum C-peptide level is increased.

Proinsulin level is normally ≤20% of total insulin; in insulinoma, proinsulin level is increased.

Oral glucose tolerance test, which may be normal, flat (in ~20% of normal persons), or show impaired tolerance, is useless for diagnosis.

GLUCAGONOMA

Diabetes mellitus

Anemia

Increased serum level of glucagon (difficult laboratory measurement and must also differentiate glucagon-like immunoreactivity, gut glucagon, and pancreatic glucagon). Serum proglucagon is also increased occasionally.

Clinical clue is association of dermatitis (necrolytic migratory erythema) with insulin-requiring diabetes.

Increased serum insulin level is characteristic.

VIPOMA

(secreted by specialized endocrine cells of the amine precursor uptake and decarboxylation [APUD] system that inhibit gastric acid production and stimulate gastrointestinal secretion of water and electrolytes; most tumors are found in pancreas but about 30% are extrapancreatic, e.g., bronchogenic carcinoma, pheochromocytoma, ganglioneuroblastoma)

Voluminous watery diarrhea (6–10 L/day) with dehydration

Hypokalemia that may be associated with hypokalemic nephropathy

Metabolic acidosis

Hypercalcemia in 50% of cases

Abnormal oral GTT

Achlorhydria or hypochlorhydria

Increased plasma vasoactive intestinal polypeptide (VIP) >75 pg/ml. RIA may show cross reactivity with other gastrointestinal hormones. (Should be collected in special chilled syringe containing EDTA and a plasma protease inhibitor and frozen immediately after centrifugation.) Specificity >88% and positive predictive value 86% (varies between laboratories). Increased values may also occur in patients with cutaneous mastocytoma, severe hepatic failure, or portocaval shunts.

SOMATOSTATINOMA

(rare condition)

Diabetes mellitus that improves after resection of the tumor

Hypochlorhydria

Steatorrhea

Occasionally anemia is present.

ZOLLINGER-ELLISON (Z-E) SYNDROME (GASTRINOMA)

Increased basal serum gastrin. >500 pg/ml is highly suggestive for gastrinoma in absence of achlorhydria or renal failure. <100 pg/ml is unlikely to be gastrinoma. 100–500 pg/ml occurs in ~40% of gastrinoma patients and ~10% of ulcer patients without gastrinoma. For this indeterminate range (half the cases), provocative tests should be performed.

IV injection of secretin (1–2 units/kg body weight) is the most sensitive and accurate provocative test. This will provoke an increase of serum gastrin ≥110 pg/ml within 10 minutes. Some ulcer patients may increase serum gastrin ≤200 pg/ml. Serum gastrin decreases in most nongastrinoma patients. Negative response occurs in ~5% of gastrinoma patients.

Table 14-11. Serum Gastrin Response to Provocative Tests in Hypergastrinemia

Cause	Secretin Injection	Calcium Infusion	Test Meal
Gastrinoma	I >200 pg/ml (95 pM) over basal	I >400 pg/ml (190 pM) over basal	I <50% over basal or NC
Hypochlorhydric states	I <200 pg/ml, D, or NC	Small I or NC	I <50% over basal or NC
Antral–G cell hyperplasia	I <200 pg/ml	Small I or NC	I >100% over basal
Others (e.g., excluded gastric antrum, gastric outlet obstruction, small intestine resection, thyrotoxicosis	I <200 pg/ml, D or NC	Small I or NC	I >50% over basal

I = increase; D = decrease; NC = no change.

Other provocative tests such as IV injection of calcium gluconate (4 mg of Ca^{++}/kg) or a standard test meal are not as sensitive or specific as secretin test. Response after calcium infusion is positive if serum gastrin ≥395 pg/ml.

There is a large volume of highly acid gastric juice in the absence of pyloric obstruction. (12-hour nocturnal secretion shows acid of >100 mEq/L and volume of >1500 ml; baseline secretion is >60% of the secretion caused by histamine or betazole stimulation.) It is refractory to vagotomy and subtotal gastrectomy. Hypochlorhydria or achlorhydria excludes diagnosis of Z-E syndrome (see Gastric Analysis, pp. 149–151).

Basal acid output >15 mEq/hour and ratio of basal acid output-maximal output >0.6 strongly favors gastrinoma, but false positive and false negative results are common. Gastric analysis does not improve the diagnostic ability of the basal serum gastrin and is probably not indicated for diagnosis of gastrinoma in a patient with active ulcer disease. However, if basal acid output determination is not possible, pH <3 excludes Z-E syndrome if patient is not on antisecretory drugs.

Hypokalemia is frequently associated with chronic severe diarrhea, which may be a clue to this diagnosis.

Serum albumin may be decreased.

Steatorrhea occurs rarely due to low pH produced in intestine.

Laboratory findings due to peptic ulcer (present in 70% of patients) of stomach, duodenum, or proximal jejunum (e.g., perforation, fluid loss, hemorrhage) are noted. *25% of these patients have ulcers in unusual locations or have giant or multiple ulcerations. A tendency toward rapid or severe recurrence of ulcer after adequate therapy is a clue to Z-E syndrome.*

Due to gastrinomas (non-beta-cell tumors usually arising in pancreas)

Tumors are multiple in 28% of patients and may be ectopic (e.g., 14% are in duodenal wall; 9% are extrapancreatic and extraintestinal; selective venous sampling for gastrin may be helpful for localizing tumor).

Tumors are malignant in 62% of patients; 44% of patients have metastases.

Diffuse hyperplasia occurs in 10% of patients.

25% of cases of this syndrome are associated with MEN-I (see pp. 553–554). *40–60% of cases of MEN-I have Z-E syndrome.*

CLASSIFICATION OF HYPOGLYCEMIA

Diagnosis requires triad of low blood glucose at the time of hypoglycemic symptoms and alleviation by ingestion of glucose. *(Glucose concentration is 15% lower in whole blood than in serum or plasma.)*

Reactive (i.e., after eating)
- Alimentary (rapid gastric emptying, e.g., after subtotal gastrectomy, vagotomy)
- Impaired glucose tolerance as in diabetes mellitus (mild maturity-onset)
- Functional (idiopathic)
- Rare conditions (e.g., hereditary fructose intolerance, galactosemia, familial fructose and galactose intolerance)

Fasting (spontaneous)—almost always indicates organic disease
- Liver—severe parenchymal disease (including sepsis, congestive heart failure) or enzyme defect (e.g., glycogen storage diseases, galactosemia)
- Chronic renal insufficiency
- Pancreatic
  - Insulinoma (pancreatic islet cell tumor)
  - MEN-I
  - Pancreatic hyperplasia
- Deficiency of hormones that oppose insulin (e.g., decreased function of thyroid, anterior pituitary, or adrenal cortex)
- Nonpancreatic tumors
- Large extrapancreatic tumors (65% are intra- or retroperitoneal fibromas or sarcomas)
- Certain epithelial tumors (e.g., hepatoma, carcinoid, Wilms' tumor)
- Drugs (including factitious hypoglycemia—see next section)
  - Insulin
  - Sulfonylureas
  - Alcohol
  - Salicylates
  - Propranolol (rare)
  - Others may potentiate effect of sulfonylurea (e.g., sulfonamides, butazones, coumarins, clofibrate)
- Artifactual (high WBC or RBC count, e.g., leukemia or polycythemia)
- Insulin antibodies or insulin receptor antibodies

Combined reactive and fasting types
- Insulinoma
- Adrenal insufficiency
- Insulin antibodies or insulin receptor antibodies

Diagnosis of reactive hypoglycemia diagnosis is based on decreased blood glucose at time of signs and symptoms with improvement by eating and a repetitive pattern of occurrence. Diagnosis should not be based on glucose tolerance test since 25% of healthy young men may have postprandial glucose <50 mg/dl and 2–3% of subjects may have <40 mg/dl.

Diagnosis of "nonhypoglycemic syndrome"—normal blood glucose associated with symptoms similar to those in hypoglycemia

Diagnosis of insulinoma by (see pp. 490–492)
- Increased plasma insulin and C-peptide during hypoglycemic episode stimulated by fasting (up to 72 hours may be necessary) or tolbutamide tolerance test. Increased insulin-glucose ratio
- *Serum insulin rarely reaches these high levels in patients with reactive hypoglycemia.*
- Failure to suppress C-peptide by hypoglycemia induced by exogenous insulin administration
- Proinsulin >30% of serum insulin after overnight fast suggests insulinoma. (May also be increased in renal disease.) (*Proinsulin is included in the immunoassay of total insulin and separation requires special technique.*)

Table 14-12. Differentiation of Hypoglycemic Symptoms

Criteria for Diagnosis	Anxiety State	Reactive Hypoglycemia*
5-hour GTT	Blood glucose level not usually < 50 mg/dl	Blood glucose level falls to < 40 mg/dl
Symptoms	Not related to blood glucose level	Coincide with low blood glucose level
Response of plasma cortisol level to low blood glucose level	No plasma cortisol response	Plasma cortisol level doubles within 90 minutes after hypoglycemic symptoms or low blood glucose level occurs

*Reactive hypoglycemia refers to low blood glucose level during 5-hour GTT (not during fasting) and may be due to alimentary conditions (e.g., peptic ulcer) or diabetes mellitus, or it may be idiopathic.

Following overnight fast, normal ranges are
- Serum insulin: 1–25 μU/ml
- Serum proinsulin: <20% of total measurable insulin
- Serum C-peptide: 1–2 ng/ml
- Ratio of insulin to glucose: <0.3 (up to 0.35 in obese persons). During fasting, ratio decreases in healthy persons and increases in insulinoma patients.

FACTITIOUS HYPOGLYCEMIA

Due To Insulin

During hypoglycemic episode, high insulin and low C-peptide levels in serum confirm diagnosis of exogenous insulin administration (diagnostic triad). (Increased endogenous insulin secretion is always associated with increased C-peptide secretion, which is the part of the proinsulin molecule cleaved off when insulin is secreted and therefore is produced in equimolar amounts with insulin.)

Insulin-glucose ratio >0.3 in serum (normal is <0.3). Increased ratio is also seen in autonomous production due to insulinoma. Extreme elevations of serum insulin (e.g., >1000 μU/ml) suggest factitious hypoglycemia (fasting levels in patients with insulinoma rarely >200 μU/ml).

Insulin antibodies appear whenever insulin administration has occurred for more than a few weeks but are almost never present in persons not taking insulin (rarely occurs on an autoimmune basis), although this may be less useful with the future use of more purified and human insulin.

Due To Sulfonylureas

Increased serum C-peptide and insulin levels and therefore mimics insulinoma more closely than insulin abuse.

Specific chemical assay can identify the agent in serum or urine.

Factitious hypoglycemia may also occur as a suicidal manifestation in adolescents who administer their own insulin and as a form of child abuse in younger children.

Laboratory Tests for Evaluation of Adrenal-Pituitary Function

Complete 24-hour urine collections may be difficult to obtain in some patients. Plasma samples are simple to obtain but are altered by diurnal variation, episodic pulsatile secretion, renal and metabolic clearance, stress, protein binding, and effect of drugs. Therefore abnormal screening tests must be confirmed by tests that stimulate or suppress the pituitary adrenal axis.

Increased function is tested by suppression tests, and decreased function is tested by stimulatory tests.

Cortisol measurements have largely replaced other steroid determinations in diagnosis of Cushing's syndrome.

PLASMA ACTH

Decreased In

Cushing's syndrome due to adrenal tumor
Secondary hypoadrenalism
Factitious Cushing's syndrome

Increased In

Pituitary Cushing's syndrome
Primary adrenal insufficiency
Ectopic ACTH syndrome (e.g., carcinoma of lung)—levels very high, with no diurnal variation

SERUM ANDROSTENEDIONE

(one of the major adrenal androgens in serum)

Increased In

Congenital adrenal hyperplasia due to 21-hydroxylase deficiency; marked increase is suppressed to normal levels by adequate glucocorticoid therapy. Suppressed level reflects adequacy of therapeutic control. May be better than 17-hydroxyprogesterone for monitoring therapy because it shows minimal diurnal variation, better correlation with urinary 17-ketosteroid (17-KS) excretion, and plasma levels are not immediately affected by a dose of glucocorticoid.

SERUM DEHYDROEPIANDROSTERONE SULFATE (DHEA-S)

Produced by androgenic zone of adrenal cortex; RIA is specific and relatively easy. Correlates with 17-KS excretion in urine and shows no significant diurnal variation, thereby providing rapid test for abnormal androgen secretion.

Increased In

Congenital adrenal hyperplasia—markedly increased values can be suppressed by dexamethasone. Highest values occur in congenital adrenal hyperplasia due to deficiency of 3-beta-hydroxysteroid dehydrogenase.

Adrenal carcinoma—increased levels cannot be suppressed by dexamethasone.

Cushing's syndrome due to bilateral adrenal hyperplasia shows higher values than Cushing's syndrome due to benign cortical adenoma.

In hypogonadotropic hypogonadism, DHEA-S is usually normal for chronologic age and high for bone age in contrast to idiopathic delayed puberty in which DHEA-S is low relative to chronologic age and normal relative to bone age.

First few days of life, especially in sick or premature infants

SERUM 11-DEOXYCORTISOL

Present in blood as an intermediate in synthesis of cortisol from 17-hydroxyprogesterone; excretion in urine is included in 17-ketogenic steroid (17-KGS) and Porter-Silber 17-hydroxyketosteroid (17-OHKS) measurements.

Used in metyrapone test (see p. 499) in which blood level parallels changes in urine 17-OHKS

- Functioning pituitary-adrenal system shows increase from <200 ng/dl baseline to >7000 ng/dl 8 hours after large dose of metyrapone, whereas in nonfunctioning system there is very little increase in blood level.

TESTS OF PITUITARY-ADRENAL FUNCTION IN PATIENTS WITH ADRENAL INSUFFICIENCY

Plasma ACTH

(see p. 496)

ACTH Stimulation Test

Rapid screening test—administer 0.25 mg of synthetic ACTH (cosyntropin) IM or IV with baseline, 30-, 60-, and 90-minute plasma cortisol levels. If response is not normal, perform long test (see below).

- Normal—baseline plasma cortisol > 5.0 μg/dl with increase to 2 times baseline level ≥ 20 μg/dl is sufficient single criterion of normal adrenal function to preclude need for further workup. Rise in urine 17-OHKS has also been used.
- Addison's disease—is ruled out by a positive response.
- Hypopituitarism—a slight increase is shown the first day and a greater increase the next day.
- Not helpful in diagnosis of Cushing's syndrome.
    - Adrenal carcinoma—little or no response; marked increase in urine 17-KS
    - Adrenal hyperplasia increases 3 to 5 times baseline level.

Long test—daily infusion of ACTH for 5 days, with before and after measurement of serum cortisol, 24-hour urines for cortisol, 17-OHKS. (Protect possible Addison's disease patient against adrenal crisis with 1 mg of dexamethasone.)

- Normal—at least 3-fold increase with maximum >upper reference value
- Complete primary adrenal insufficiency (Addison's disease)—no increase in urine steroids or increase of <2 mg/day
- Incomplete primary adrenal insufficiency—less than normal increases on all 5 days or slight increase on first 3 days that may be followed by decrease on days 4 and 5
- Secondary adrenal insufficiency (due to pituitary hypofunction)—"staircase" response of progressively higher values each day (delayed but normal response)
- Adrenal insufficiency due to chronic steroid therapy—may require prolonged ACTH testing to elicit the "staircase" response; may produce increments only in 17-OHKS but not in 17-KS
- Congenital adrenal hyperplasia (21-hydroxylase and 17-hydroxylase deficiency)—increase 17-KGS and 17-KS, little or no change in 17-OHKS

Do not do metyrapone test until ACTH test proves that adrenals are sensitive to ACTH.

Metyrapone Test

(see p. 499)

May also be used to assess cause of adrenal insufficiency. If secondary to pituitary disease, neither adrenal steroids nor ACTH will rise unless some pituitary reserve exists; in primary adrenal insufficiency, no rise occurs.

TESTS OF ADRENAL-PITUITARY FUNCTION IN PATIENTS WITH HYPERADRENALISM

Dexamethasone (Synthetic Glucocorticoid) Suppression Of Pituitary ACTH Secretion

In low-dose test, 0.5 mg of dexamethasone is given orally every 6 hours for 8 doses; specimen collection as for high-dose test below. A rapid overnight variation for screening uses a single 1-mg dose at 11 P.M. with plasma cortisol collection the following 8 A.M. Normal response is a fall in plasma cortisol to <5 μg/dl, urine 17-OHKS to <4 mg/24 hours, or free cortisol to <25 μg/24 hours. Patients with Cushing's disease of any cause almost always have abnormal suppressibility; few (1–2%) false negative results make this a *good screening test to rule out Cushing's syndrome and to identify cases for further testing;* repeat testing is sometimes needed for accurate diagnosis.

In high-dose test, 2 mg of dexamethasone is given orally every 6 hours for 8 doses, and plasma cortisol is measured 6 hours after last dose and urine free cortisol and 17-OHKS are measured on the second day; baseline specimens for 2 days before test. Suppression occurs in >90% of cases of Cushing's disease but not in 80% of cases of ectopic ACTH syndrome or nodular adrenal hyperplasia; adrenal tumors do not reproducibly suppress. *The high-dose test is the basic test to differentiate Cushing's disease from adrenal tumors or ectopic ACTH production.*

Normal pituitary-adrenal system—urinary 17-OHKS falls to <2.5 mg/24 hours, and plasma cortisol decreases (to <5 μg/dl) after both low- and high-dose dexamethasone tests.

Cushing's disease (pituitary dysfunction causing adrenal hyperplasia)—urinary 17-OHKS and cortisol and plasma cortisol decrease to <50% of baseline level; but up to 25% of cases do not show suppression after high-dose dexamethasone test. Some patients with large ACTH-producing pituitary adenomas have marked resistance to high-dose dexamethasone suppression. In long-standing cases, nodular hyperplasia of adrenal may develop, causing autonomous cortisol production and resistance to dexamethasone test.

Adrenal adenoma or carcinoma or ectopic ACTH syndrome—urinary 17-OHKS and urine and plasma cortisol are not decreased after high or low doses of dexamethasone.

Patients with psychiatric illness may be resistant

Atypical response may also occur due to drugs (e.g., alcohol, estrogens and birth control pills, phenytoin, spironolactone)

Corticotropin-Releasing Factor (CRF) Stimulation Test*

1 μg/kg of body weight or 100 μg of CRF is given IV; blood is then drawn at intervals for 2–3 hours. Sensitivity and specificity are ~90–95%.

Differentiates pituitary and nonpituitary causes of Cushing's syndrome reliably (equal to high-dose dexamethasone suppression test). Is of particular use when the latter test is equivocal or when biochemical data indicate a pituitary source but radiographic examination is normal.

Cushing's syndrome due to pituitary adenoma—positive response is exaggerated increase above baseline of >50% in plasma ACTH and >20% in cortisol concentrations. After surgical removal of adenoma, basal levels of ACTH and cortisol were undetectable, but response to CRF is normal.

Hypercortisolism of adrenal origin—plasma ACTH is low or undetectable before and after CRF without any cortisol response.

*Data from GP Chrousos, et al. NIH Conference: Clinical applications of corticotropin-releasing factor. *Ann Intern Med* 102:344, 1985; TB Kaye and L Crapo, The Cushing syndrome: An update on diagnostic tests. *Ann Intern Med* 122:434, 1990.

Ectopic ACTH syndrome—no ACTH or cortisol response in ~92% of patients; positive response in ~8% of patients.

Psychiatric states associated with hypercortisolism (e.g., depression, anorexia nervosa, bulemia)—in uni- or bipolar depression, both peak and total ACTH responses are decreased; only a small decrease in cortisol occurs (normal); after recovery, response is not distinguishable from normal persons. Similar findings may occur in obsessive-compulsive disorders and alcoholism. Manic patients have response similar to controls.

Overlap in response between control subjects and pituitary Cushing's syndrome patients is too great to permit use for definitive diagnosis.

Metyrapone Test Of Pituitary Reserve

Adrenal suppression of pituitary secretion of ACTH is inhibited by administration of 750 mg of metyrapone (which blocks cortisol production) every 4–6 hours beginning at midnight; draw baseline plasma levels at 8 A.M. and following 8 A.M.

Normal persons and pituitary Cushing's disease—urine 17-OHKS increases by >10 mg/24 hours or to 2.5 times the previous baseline level or plasma 11-deoxycortisol increases >10 μg/dl if cortisol falls to <7 μg/dl and rise in plasma ACTH to >100 ng/L.

Adrenal tumor with excess cortisol production—no increase or fall in urinary 17-OHKS and 17-KS test is positive in 100% of adrenal hyperplasias without tumor, 50% of adrenal adenomas, and 25% of adrenal carcinomas.

Ectopic ACTH syndrome—may not be accurate in this condition

ALDOSTERONE

See Aldosteronism (Primary), p. 503; Aldosteronism (Secondary), p. 510.

PLASMA RENIN ACTIVITY

See Aldosteronism (Primary), p. 503; Aldosteronism (Secondary), p. 510.

Diseases of Adrenal Gland

CUSHING'S SYNDROME*

Definitive diagnosis or exclusion only by laboratory tests

Diagnosis consists of two parts: (1) establish autonomous hypercortisolism and loss of diurnal rhythm, (2) determine etiology (see Fig. 14-8, pp. 504–505).

Diagnosis of excessive cortisol production may include increased plasma cortisol (>30 μg/dl at 8 A.M. and >15 μg/dl at 4 P.M.), 24-hour urine free cortisol, 17-OHKS, 17-KS, low-dose dexamethasone suppression test. More than one test may be needed because these are misleading in up to one-third of patients for various reasons, e.g., impaired renal function; cortisol production is somewhat proportional to obesity or large muscle mass; baseline measurements are increased by stress; some drugs alter ACTH production or interfere with assays; cortisol production is pulsatile rather than uniform; cortisol secretion may not be very increased on every determination; baseline measurements may vary daily and make dexamethasone suppression test difficult to interpret.

Most useful screening test is increased 24-hour urinary free cortisol (best expressed as per gram of creatinine). Found in 95% of Cushing's syndrome. <150 μg/24 hours excludes and >300 μg/24 hours establishes diagnosis of

*Data from NE Dunlap, WE Grizzle, and AL Siegel, Cushing's syndrome: Screening methods in hospitalized patients. *Arch Pathol Lab Med* 109:222, 1985.

Cushing's syndrome. If values are intermediate, low-dose dexamethasone suppression test is indicated. Not affected by body weight; false positives or negatives are very rare; is often more reliable than blood levels, which vary with time of day, require standardized collection, are secreted in pulsatile fashion. Increased values may occur in depression or alcoholism but do not exceed 300 μg/24 hours.

Loss of normal diurnal variation of plasma cortisol is useful screening (normal persons have highest level at 8 A.M. and lowest between 8 P.M. and midnight); this diurnal variation disappears early and may be absent or reversed in 70% of Cushing's syndrome and 18% of patients without Cushing's (due to depression, alcoholism, stress, etc.). False negatives are frequent if blood is drawn before 8 P.M.

Normal urine free cortisol and normal diurnal variation in plasma cortisol virtually exclude Cushing's syndrome.

False positive results with urine free cortisol and low-dose dexamethasone suppression test may occur in acute and chronic illness, alcoholism, depression, and due to certain drugs (e.g., phenytoin, phenobarbital, primidone); estrogens may cause a false positive overnight dexamethasone test.

To determine the etiology of Cushing's syndrome after hypercortisolism has been established, the most useful tests are high-dose dexamethasone suppression, CRF stimulation test, metyrapone test, plasma ACTH level, DHEA-S level. Inferior petrosal sinus sampling identifies ACTH-producing pituitary adenomas in ~88% of cases.

Causes Of Cushing's Syndrome*

Pituitary (Cushing's disease): 50–80% in adults
- Pituitary tumor: 70–90% (may be part of MEN I; see p. 553)
- Pituitary hyperplasia of adrenocorticotropic cells (small %)

Adrenal: 17%
- Adenoma: 9%
- Carcinoma: 8%
- Nodular hyperplasia: ?

Ectopic neoplasms (e.g., oat cell carcinoma of lung; carcinoids): 15%

Iatrogenic
- Therapeutic (glucocorticoids, ACTH)
- Illicit use by athletes
- Factitious

Adrenal cause is predominant in children; adrenal carcinoma is found in 65% of patients less than age 15 years.

Dexamethasone suppression test—see p. 498.
CRF stimulation test—see p. 498.
Metyrapone test—see p. 497.
ACTH stimulation test—see p. 497.

Basal plasma ACTH level (Note that ACTH has diurnal variation, episodic secretion, short plasma half-life, and is a difficult assay to perform.)
- Cushing's syndrome due to autonomous cortisol production (e.g., adrenal tumor or exogenous steroids)—low or undetectable.
- Pituitary Cushing's disease—high or high-normal range but rarely >200 pg/ml.
- Ectopic ACTH production—two-thirds of patients have high levels (>200 pg/ml); the other one-third usually have moderately elevated values (100–200 pg/ml). In these cases, difference in ACTH levels in blood obtained simultaneously from the jugular and peripheral veins suggests pituitary rather than ectopic source of ACTH; this difference can be en-

*Data from PC Carpenter, Cushing's syndrome: Update of diagnosis and management. *Mayo Clin Proc* 61:49, 1986.

hanced by CRH administration. *New immunoradiometric assay (IRMA) for ACTH is more sensitive and specific than RIA method, but some tumors secrete biologically active "big" ACTH fragments not detected by IRMA; therefore RIA is preferred for initial evaluation of cause.*

Urinary steroid findings in different etiologies of Cushing's syndrome
- Increased urinary 17-OHKS >4 times normal in
  - 63% of patients with Cushing's syndrome and 3% of patients without Cushing's syndrome
  - 65% of patients with Cushing's syndrome due to ectopic ACTH syndrome
  - 3% of patients with Cushing's syndrome due to adrenal hyperplasia without tumor
- Urinary 17-OHKS is increased (>10 mg/24 hours) in virtually all patients with Cushing's syndrome but less useful for screening because increased in 20% of persons without Cushing's (e.g., obesity, hyperthyroidism). Night collection sample > day sample (reverse is true in normal persons). ACTH stimulation test produces lowest 17-OHKS in Cushing's syndrome due to adrenal carcinoma and the highest 17-OHKS due to adrenal adenoma.
- Increased urinary 17-KS
  - May be normal in 35% of patients with Cushing's syndrome and increased (>25 mg/24 hours) in 20% of obese persons without Cushing's. Not useful except if virilism or marked hirsutism is present.
  - Normal or low in 70% of adrenal adenomas (<20 mg/24 hours) but increased in 90% of adrenal carcinomas; averages 50–60 mg/24 hours in carcinoma (always >15 mg/24 hours); >4 times normal in 50% of adrenal carcinomas; higher values increase likelihood of diagnosis of adrenal carcinoma, and >100 mg/24 hours is virtually diagnostic.
  - Increased in 15% of cases of ectopic ACTH syndrome
  - In adrenal hyperplasia, increased total 17-KS (in 50% of cases) is due to elevation of all of the 17-KS.
  - In adrenal carcinoma, most of the increase is usually due to DHEA-S, which is markedly increased; DHEA-S is slightly increased in Cushing's disease and often very low in adrenocortical adenoma (<0.4 mg/dl).
  - Increased urinary 17-ketogenic steroids (>20 mg/24 hours).
  - *Isolated measurements of 17-KS or 17-OHKS are not recommended as screening tests for Cushing's syndrome. In general, free cortisol is best for screening, 17-OHKS with free cortisol in dexamethasone suppression tests, 17-KS to screen for possible adrenal carcinoma or to help differentiate adrenal adenoma from pituitary or ectopic ACTH syndrome causes.*

Plasma renin activity is increased; suppressed activity suggests ectopic ACTH syndrome or adrenal adenoma or carcinoma (causing increased secretion of deoxycorticosterone or aldosterone).

Glucose tolerance is diminished in 75% of cases:
- Glycosuria in 50% of patients
- Diabetes mellitus in 20% of cases

Serum sodium is usually moderately increased.

Hypokalemic acidosis is usual, but metabolic alkalosis occurs in ~10% of patients. Hypokalemic alkalosis may indicate extra-adrenal neoplasia (e.g., bronchogenic carcinoma).

Urine potassium is increased; sodium is decreased.

Hematologic changes
- WBC is normal or increased.
- Relative lymphopenia is frequent (differential is usually <15% of cells).

Eosinopenia is frequent (usually <100/cu mm).
Hematocrit is usually normal; if increased, it indicates an androgenic component.

Changes due to osteoporosis. Serum and urine calcium may be increased. Kidney stones occur in 15% of cases.

BUN may be increased.

Urine creatine is increased.

Serum gamma globulins may be decreased, and alpha-2 globulin may be moderately increased.

80% of patients with Cushing's disease have remission after removal of pituitary adenoma; tests of pituitary-adrenal axis may take weeks to months to become normal.

CUSHING'S SYNDROME DUE TO ADRENAL DISEASE

(see Table 14-14 and Fig. 14-8)

Is suggested by

Failure of high-dose dexamethasone test to cause suppression
Very low plasma ACTH
Positive metyrapone test

Adenoma is indicated by low DHEA-S, low or normal 17-KS with increased 17-OHKS.

Adrenal carcinoma is suggested by very high 17-KS. Carcinoma cases show hypercortisolism (50%), virilism (20%), or both (10–15%); are nonfunctioning (10–15%).

Nodular adrenal hyperplasia—ACTH levels are variable, unpredictable response to dexamethasone suppression; therefore is difficult to distinguish from other adrenal causes.

Nonfunctioning adrenal adenoma may be found in 1% of normal persons.

CUSHING'S SYNDROME DUE TO ECTOPIC ACTH PRODUCTION

(by neoplasm, e.g., oat cell carcinoma of lung, thymoma, islet cell tumor of pancreas, medullary carcinoma of thyroid, bronchial carcinoid, pheochromocytoma; occurs in 2% of patients with lung cancer; see Table 14-14 and Fig. 14-8)

Plasma ACTH is markedly increased (500–1000 pg/ml) compared to pituitary Cushing's disease (up to 200 pg/ml) but overlap in 20% of ectopic ACTH cases. Morning basal level in normal persons is 20–100 pg/ml.

Increased plasma and urine free cortisol, which may show marked spontaneous variation; lack of diurnal variation

Marked hypokalemic alkalosis (due to increased desoxycorticosterone and corticosterone occurs in 30–50% of such patients) rather than metabolic acidosis may suggest this diagnosis.

Increased plasma ACTH level (see previous section)

High-dose dexamethasone suppression does not occur in ectopic ACTH production but does occur in >90% of Cushing's disease.

Metyrapone test may not be accurate in distinguishing from Cushing's disease.

Increased urinary 17-OHKS and 17-KS (see previous section).

FACTITIOUS CUSHING'S SYNDROME

Increased plasma and urinary cortisol

Plasma ACTH is low or undetectable.

These findings may also occur in adrenal Cushing's syndrome. Differentiate by history of ingestion or, in some cases, determination of synthetic steroid analogues by specific plasma assays.

ADRENAL FEMINIZATION

This condition occurs in adult males with adrenal tumor (usually unilateral carcinoma, occasionally adenoma) that secretes estrogens.

Urinary estrogens are markedly increased.

17-KS is normal or moderately increased and cannot be suppressed by low doses of dexamethasone when due to adrenal tumor.

17-OHKS is normal.

Biopsy of testicle shows atrophy of tubules.

ALDOSTERONISM (PRIMARY)

Excessive mineralocorticoid hormone secretion by adrenal cortex causes renal tubules to retain sodium and excrete potassium. Classic biochemical abnormalities are increased aldosterone production, suppressed plasma renin activity (PRA), and decreased serum potassium.

Should be *suspected* in any hypertensive patient with spontaneous or easily provoked hypokalemia

Suggestive screening tests are inappropriate kaliuresis, low PRA (<3.0 ng/ml/hour), high plasma aldosterone/PRA ratio (>20).

Confirm diagnosis by nonsuppressible aldosterone excretion with normal cortisol excretion. Discontinue interfering drugs (for at least 2 weeks), and assess plasma volume before beginning testing.

Elevated plasma (reference range = 30–110 ng/L) and/or urinary aldosterone that is relatively nonsuppressible by salt loading or volume expansion. May be normal in 30% of cases (due to episodic secretion or chronic potassium deficiency, which can suppress aldosterone secretion; therefore must replete potassium before measurement if serum <3.0 mEq/L). Reference values decline by 30–50% with increasing age. Plasma aldosterone is normal in recumbent hypertensive and nonhypertensive persons without aldosteronism and increases 2–4 times after 4 hours of upright posture; increases ≥33% in aldosteronism due to adrenal hyperplasia, but no increase occurs if due to adrenal adenoma.

Increased urinary aldosterone (reference range 2–16 μg/24 hours) is best initial screening procedure (normal salt intake, no drugs; not detectable on all days). Cannot be reduced by high sodium intake or deoxycorticosterone (DOC) administration. Therefore high NaCl intake (10–12 gm/day) will cause 24-hour urine aldosterone >14 μg/24 hours and Na >250 mEq/24 hours; 96% sensitivity and 93% specificity for primary hyperaldosteronism.

Saline infusion (2 L normal saline in 4 hours) suppresses plasma aldosterone to <5 ng/dl or by >50% in hypertensive patients without primary aldosteronism but not in patients with primary aldosteronism. (Plasma aldosterone level is first increased by having patient in upright position for 2 hours.) Since plasma aldosterone levels vary from moment to moment, a single specimen may not properly reflect adrenal secretion.

Volume expansion (by high salt intake, NaCl infusion, or DOC) reduces aldosterone level to >50–80% of baseline level in any other condition than primary aldosteronism.

Captopril (angiotensin-converting-enzyme inhibitor that blocks angiotensin II production) administered as 25 mg IV at 8 A.M. decreases aldosterone in plasma 2 hours later in normal persons and essential hypertension but remains elevated in primary aldosteronism.

Hypokalemia (usually <3.0 mEq/L) not related to use of diuretics or laxatives in a hypertensive patient is the first indication. May be normal in cases of shorter duration before classic clinical picture develops (~20% of cases initially). Hypokalemia is usually less in hyperplasia than adenoma, but considerable overlap occurs. Hypokalemia ≤2.7 mEq/L in a hypertensive is usually due to primary aldosteronism, especially adenoma. Normokalemic aldosteron-

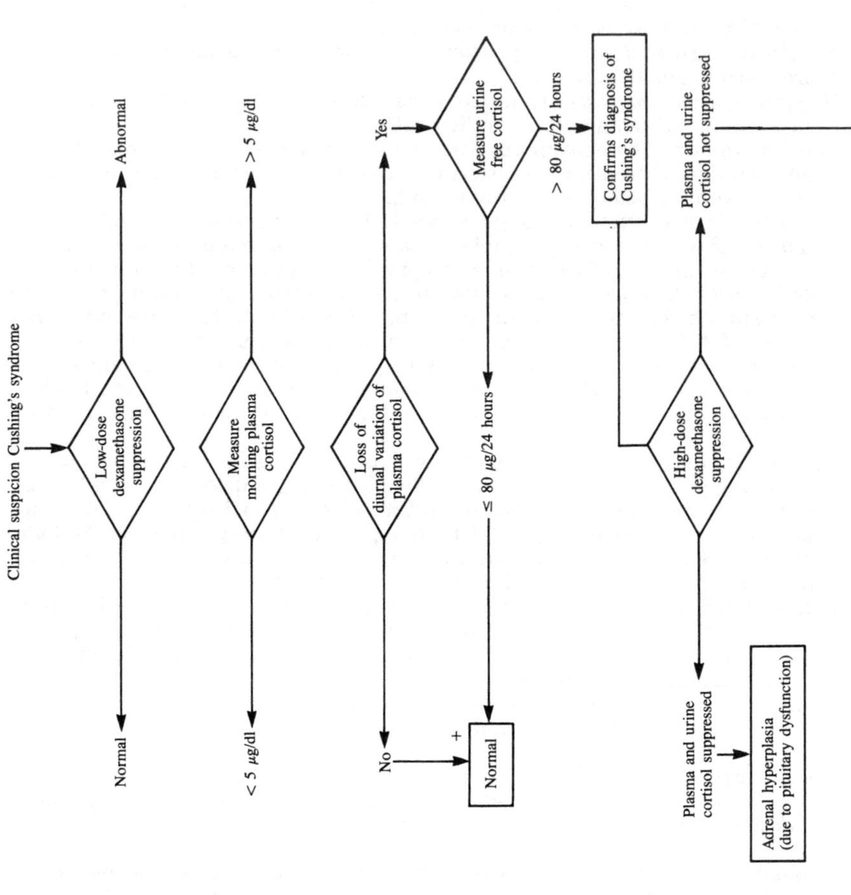
Clinical suspicion Cushing's syndrome
Low-dose dexamethasone suppression
Normal
Abnormal
Measure morning plasma cortisol
< 5 μg/dl
> 5 μg/dl
Loss of diurnal variation of plasma cortisol
No
Yes
+
Normal
Measure urine free cortisol
≤ 80 μg/24 hours
> 80 μg/24 hours
Confirms diagnosis of Cushing's syndrome
High-dose dexamethasone suppression
Plasma and urine cortisol suppressed
Plasma and urine cortisol not suppressed
Adrenal hyperplasia (due to pituitary dysfunction)

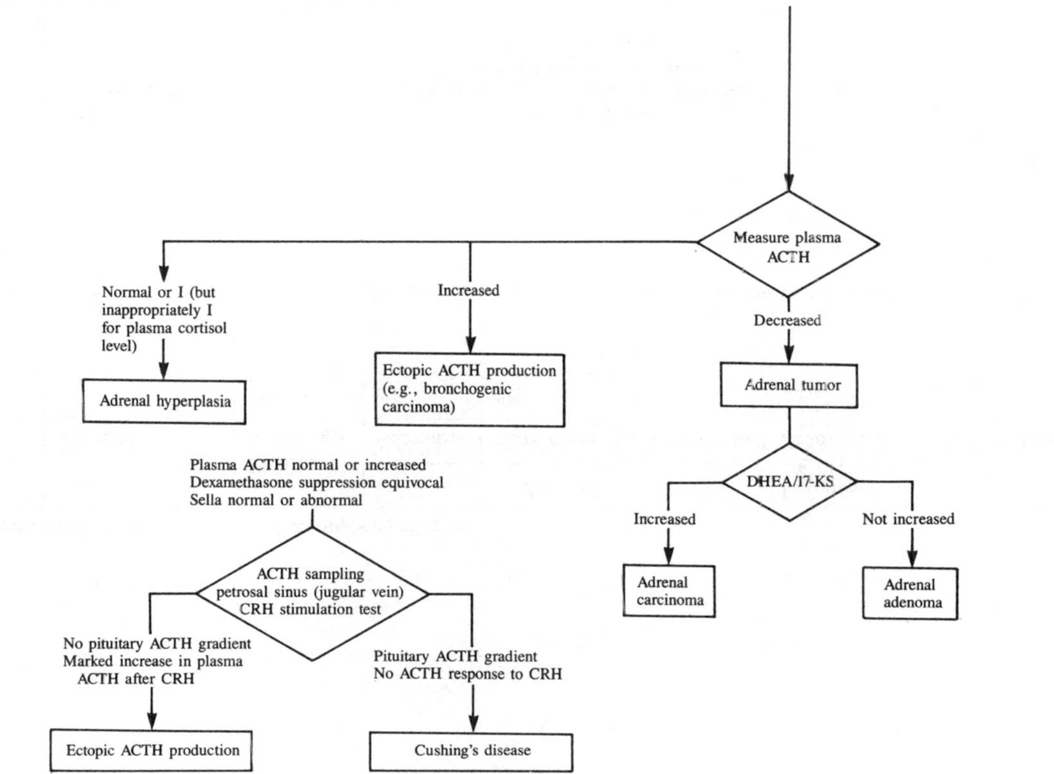

Fig. 14-8. Sequence of laboratory tests in diagnosis of Cushing's syndrome. (More than 90 percent of patients with Cushing's syndrome are found to follow this scheme.)

Table 14-13. Comparison of Different Causes of Cushing's Syndrome

	Normal	Pituitary Cushing's	Adrenal			Ectopic ACTH Production	Other Illness
			Adenoma	Carcinoma	Hyperplasia		
Cause		70%	9%	8%	?	15%	
Free cortisol Urine (μg/24 hrs)	< 120	> 300 establishes diagnosis of Cushing's syndrome if increased					120–300
Plasma (μg/dl)							> 30 at 8 A.M. and > 15 at 4 P.M.
Low-dose dexamethasone suppression Urine free cortisol	Falls to < 25 μg/24 hr	Not suppressed Does not fall to < 25 μg/24 hours in Cushing's syndrome due to any cause					False + may occur in alcoholism, depression drugs, etc.

Plasma cortisol	Falls to <5 µg/dl	Not suppressed				
High-dose dexamethasone suppression	Suppressed in $>90\%$ of cases		Not suppressed but not reproducible	Not suppressed in 80% of cases		
Plasma ACTH (pg/ml)		I or high normal range Not >200	Decreased or not detectable		>200 in 2/3 cases; 100–200 in 1/3 cases	
CRF stimulation		ACTH increases	Flat plasma ACTH response to CRH			
ACTH ratio jugular-peripheral blood		High; enhanced by CRF	Ratio = 1			

ism should be considered when urine potassium is >30 mEq/24 hours when serum potassium is <3.5 mEq/L. Intermittent hypokalemia or normokalemia may occur, especially in adrenal hyperplasia etiologies. In essential hypertensives on diuretic therapy, urine potassium decreases to <30 mEq/L in 2–3 days after cessation of diuretics but continues in primary aldosteronism patients. (This should be checked several times after cessation of diuretics.) Hypokalemia is alleviated by administration of spironolactone and by sodium restriction but not by potassium replacement therapy. (Administration of spironolactone for 3 days increases serum potassium >1.2 mEq/L. It also increases urine sodium and decreases urine potassium. Negative potassium balance reoccurs in 5 days. It increases urinary aldosterone (this is variable in hypertensive and normal people).

Saline infusion causes significant fall in serum potassium and in corrected potassium clearance. This hypokalemia is a reliable screening test.

	Sensitivity (%)	**Specificity (%)**
Potassium <4.0 mEq/L	100	64
Stimulated renin <2.5 ng/ml/3 hours	100	88
Suppressed aldosterone >10 ng/dl	98	92
Sequential 1, 2, and 3	98	99

PRA Is Decreased (<1.5 ng/ml/3 hours) In

98% of cases of primary aldosteronism. Usually absent or low and can be increased less or not at all by sodium depletion and ambulation in contrast to secondary aldosteronism. *PRA may not always be suppressed in primary aldosteronism; repeated testing may be necessary to establish the diagnosis.* Normal PRA does not preclude this diagnosis; not a reliable screening test.

Hypertension due to unilateral renal artery stenosis or unilateral renal parenchymal disease

PRA is particularly useful to diagnose curable hypertension (e.g., primary aldosteronism, unilateral renal artery stenosis).

Increased plasma volume due to high-sodium diet, administration of salt-retaining steroids

18–25% of essential hypertensives (low-renin essential hypertension) and 6% of normal controls

Advancing age in both normal and hypertensive patients (decrease of 35% from the third to the eighth decade)

May also be decreased in congenital adrenal hyperplasia secondary to 11-hydroxylase or 17-hydroxylase deficiency with oversecretion of other mineralocorticoids

Rarely in Liddle's syndrome and excess licorice ingestion

Various drugs (propranolol, clonidine, reserpine; slightly with methyldopa) (see p. 759)

Usually cannot be stimulated by salt restriction, diuretics, and upright posture that deplete plasma volume; therefore measure before and after furosemide and 3–4 hours of ambulation. *Antihypertensive and hypotensive drugs should be discontinued for at least 2 weeks before measurement of PRA; spironolactone may cause an increase for up to 6 weeks; estrogens may cause an increase for up to 6 months.*

Blood should be drawn in an ice-cold tube and the plasma immediately separated in a refrigerated centrifuge. Renin level should be indexed against 24-hour level of sodium in urine.

PRA May Be Increased In

15% of patients with essential hypertension (high-renin hypertension)

Renin-producing tumors of the kidney (see p. 592)

Reduced plasma volume due to low-sodium diet, diuretics, hemorrhage, Addison's disease
Secondary aldosteronism (usually very high levels), especially malignant or severe hypertension (see p. 510)
Some edematous normotensive states (e.g., cirrhosis, nephrosis, congestive heart failure)
Sodium or potassium loss due to GI disease or in 10% of patients with chronic renal failure.
Normal pregnancy
Pheochromocytoma
Last half of menstrual cycle (2-fold increase)
Erect posture for 4 hours (2-fold increase)
Ambulatory patients compared to bed patients
Bartter's syndrome
Various drugs (guanethidine, minoxidil, hydralazine, diazoxide, thiazides, furosemide, spironolactone, nitroprusside, saralasin, estrogens)

In children with salt-losing form of congenital adrenal hyperplasia due to 21-hydroxylase deficiency, severity of disease is related to degree of increase. PRA level may serve as guide to adequate mineralocorticoid replacement therapy.

In diagnosis of renal hypertension, renin is assayed in blood from each renal vein, inferior vena cava, and aorta. The test is considered diagnostic when the level from the ischemic kidney is at least 1.5 times greater than the level from the normal kidney (which is equal to or less than the level in the aorta that serves as the standard). This is due to high PRA in the peripheral blood, increase in PRA in the renal vein compared to the renal artery of the affected kidney, and suppression of PRA in the other kidney. Maximum renin stimulation accentuates the difference between the two kidneys and should *always* be obtained by pretest conditions (avoid antihypertensive, diuretic, and oral contraceptive drugs for at least 1 month if possible; low-salt diet for 7 days; administer thiazide diuretic for 1–3 days; upright posture for at least 2 hours). This is the most useful diagnostic test in renovascular hypertension as judged by surgical results but is not a sufficiently reliable guide to nephrectomy in patients with hypertension due to parenchymal renal disease. *In renovascular hypertension, if renal plasma flow is impaired in the "normal" kidney, surgery often fails to cure the hypertension.*
Renin-aldosterone ratio ≥30 in random blood sample in patient not on medication is said to indicate primary aldosteronism.
Urine is neutral or alkaline (pH >7.0) and not normally responsive to ammonium chloride load. Its large volume and low specific gravity are not responsive to vasopressin or water restriction (decreased tubular function, especially reabsorption of water). There is hyperkaluria even with low potassium intake; <30 mEq/24 hours essentially rules out primary aldosteronism. Sodium output is reduced.
Hypernatremia (>140 mEq/L), hypochloremia, and metabolic alkalosis (CO_2 content >25 mEq/L; blood pH tends to increase >7.42); correlates with severity of potassium depletion. Are clues in all etiologies of primary aldosteronism.
Glucose tolerance is decreased in ≤50% of patients.
Plasma cortisol and ACTH are normal.
Urine 17-KS and 17-OHKS are normal.
Serum magnesium falls.
Total blood volume increases because of increased plasma volume.
Sodium level in sweat is low.
Salivary sodium-potassium ratio <0.65 is consistent with diagnosis, but a higher ratio does not exclude it.

Table 14-14. Differential Diagnosis of Causes of Hypertension and Hypokalemia

Condition	PRA	Aldosterone
Primary hyperaldosteronism	D	I
Cushing's syndrome	D	D
Malignant hypertension	I	I
Renovascular hypertension	I	I
Licorice ingestion	D	D
Exogenous mineralo-corticoids (e.g., in nasal spray or for orthostatic hypotension)	D	D
Liddle's syndrome	D	D
Congenital adrenal hyperplasia (11-beta- or 17-alpha-hydroxylase deficiency)	D	D

D = decreased; I = increased.

Due To

Solitary adrenal cortical adenoma (64% of patients)
Idiopathic bilateral adrenal hyperplasia (32% of patients)
Adrenal carcinoma (rare)
Ectopic production of aldosterone by adrenal embryologic rest within kidney or ovary (rare)
Ectopic production of ACTH or aldosterone by nonadrenal neoplasm (rare)
Glucocorticoid suppressible hyperaldosteronism (rare) (see p. 511)

It is important to distinguish cases due to adenoma (respond to surgical treatment) from idiopathic hyperplasia (treated medically).

ALDOSTERONISM (SECONDARY)

Due To

Decreased effective blood volume
- Congestive heart failure
- Cirrhosis with ascites (aldosteronism 2000–3000 mg/day)
- Nephrosis
- Sodium depletion

Hyperactivity of renin-angiotensin system
- Renin-producing renal tumor (see p. 592)
- Bartter's syndrome (see next section)
- Toxemia of pregnancy
- Malignant hypertension
- Renovascular hypertension
- Oral contraceptive drugs

NORMOTENSIVE SECONDARY HYPERALDOSTERONISM (BARTTER'S SYNDROME)

Hypokalemia with renal potassium wasting associated with juxtaglomerular hyperplasia
Chloride-resistant metabolic alkalosis

Table 14-15. Differentiation of Primary Aldosteronism Due to Adenoma and Hyperplasia

Test	Adenoma	Idiopathic Hyperplasia
During normal sodium intake Plasma renin activity		Tend to higher values than adenoma patients
After salt depletion Plasma renin activity		Significantly higher values than adenoma patients
Urinary aldosterone	Relatively unaffected	Higher than adenoma patients
After saline infusion Plasma aldosterone-cortisol ratio	Increased	Unchanged or decreased (<2.2)
Plasma 18-hydroxy-corticosterone–cortisol ratio	Increased	Unchanged or decreased (<3.0)
Plasma 18-OHB	>100 ng/dl	<50 ng/dl
	(50–100 ng/dl less helpful)	
Plasma aldosterone circadian rhythm correlates with plasma ACTH and cortisol	Yes	No
Effect of posture on plasma aldosterone	Slight/none	Increase ≥33% over baseline
Adrenal vein measurements	See p. 509	

Increased plasma renin is a characteristic feature.

Frequently there is decreased serum magnesium and increased uric acid; often the hypokalemia cannot be corrected without adequate magnesium replacement

Not due to laxatives, diuretics, or GI loss of potassium and chloride

Increased plasma and urine aldosterone in the absence of edema, hypertension, or hypovolemia

Renal concentrating defect resistant to ADH

Also excrete large quantities of Na and Cl in urine

Insensitive to pressor effects of angiotensin II (may occur in patients with prolonged hypokalemia due to any cause)

It is almost impossible to maintain normal plasma potassium levels despite therapy (dietary potassium supplement, limit sodium intake, drugs such as indomethacin or ibuprofen).

GLUCOCORTICOID SUPPRESSIBLE HYPERALDOSTERONISM

(rare autosomal dominant defect of zona glomerulosa where beta-methyloxidase produces aldosterone from precursor arising in zona fasciculata)

Usual findings of primary aldosteronism with hypokalemia, increased aldosterone, and suppressed PRA

Reversal of clinical and laboratory findings by dexamethasone (2 mg/day orally for 3 weeks)

Anomalous decrease in plasma aldosterone response to posture.

Normal CT and MRI of adrenals.

PSEUDOHYPERALDOSTERONISM (LIDDLE'S SYNDROME)

Rare familial nephropathic disorder (? at distal tubule) with clinical manifestations closely resembling those due to aldosterone-producing adrenal adenoma

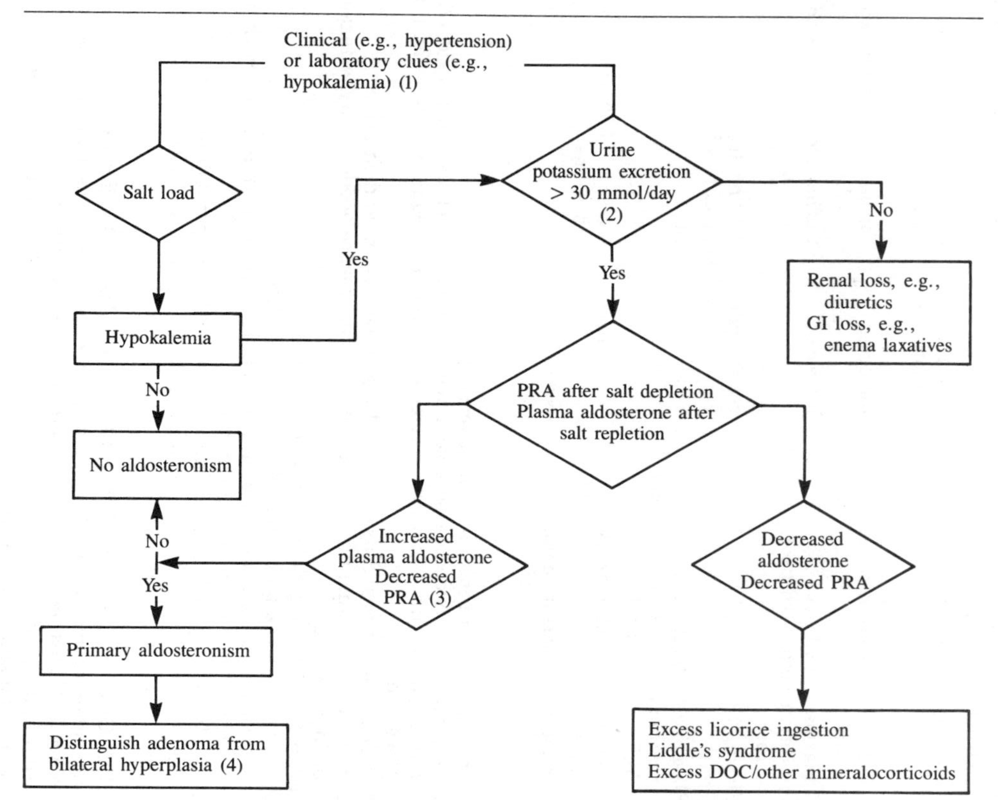

Clinical (e.g., hypertension) or laboratory clues (e.g., hypokalemia) (1)
Salt load
Hypokalemia
Yes
No
No aldosteronism
Urine potassium excretion > 30 mmol/day (2)
No
Renal loss, e.g., diuretics
GI loss, e.g., enema laxatives
Yes
PRA after salt depletion
Plasma aldosterone after salt repletion
Increased plasma aldosterone
Decreased PRA (3)
Decreased aldosterone
Decreased PRA
No
Yes
Primary aldosteronism
Distinguish adenoma from bilateral hyperplasia (4)
Excess licorice ingestion
Liddle's syndrome
Excess DOC/other mineralocorticoids

(1) Hypokalemia may be masked by low-salt diet. Although hypokalemia is found in only 50–80% of patients, it remains the most feasible routine screening test. Metabolic alkalosis.

(2) Loss of potassium in urine.

(3) Salt loading fails to suppress plasma aldosterone level to < 8.0 ng/dl and PRA fails to increase following acute diuretic stimulation (e.g., remains < 2 ng/ml/hour). This is diagnostic in 95% of cases with rare false positive results but is not useful as a screening test.

(4) See Table 14-15.

Measurement of aldosterone in blood from periphery and both adrenal veins confirms the diagnosis by elevated level from side of lesion; opposite side has level close to that in peripheral blood. This also distinguishes unilateral adenoma from bilateral adenomas and hyperplasia and indicates location of lesion for surgeon.

Aldosterone-cortisol ratio measured in blood from each adrenal vein and vena cava (simultaneous measurements verify source of blood and correct for dilution) is > 2 times higher on the side of a unilateral adenoma, and the ratio on the uninvolved side is less (markedly suppressed) than in the inferior vena cava. In hyperplasia, the ratios on both sides are similar and are greater than in the inferior vena cava. Aldosterone is > 5 times higher on the involved side compared to the opposite side in 90% of adenoma patients.

Diagnosis of adenoma rather than hyperplasia is also suggested if plasma aldosterone decreases when patient is in upright posture and by a diurnal rhythm with lower evening plasma aldosterone levels (because adenoma responds to ACTH but not angiotensin II but opposite in hyperplasia). Surgical removal of adenoma cures both hypertension and hypokalemia in ~70% of cases, but in hyperplasia, adrenalectomy seldom cures both conditions.

Visualization of lesions (e.g., radioisotope scans). Adrenal CT scan can localize adenomas >7 mm in size and is now the first test to do after establishing diagnosis of aldosteronism. MRI may become increasingly useful.

Fig. 14-9. Flow chart for diagnosis of aldosteronism.

Hypokalemia due to renal potassium wasting
Metabolic alkalosis
Hypertension
All are corrected by long-term administration of diuretics that act at distal tubule to cause natriuresis and renal potassium retention (e.g., triamterene or amiloride) and by restriction of sodium.
Aldosterone secretion and excretion are greatly reduced and unresponsive to stimulation by ACTH, angiotensin II, or low-sodium diet.
Low plasma renin
Sodium retention

PSEUDOALDOSTERONISM DUE TO INGESTION OF LICORICE (AMMONIUM GLYCYRRHIZATE)

(excessive ingestion causes hypertension due to sodium retention)

Decreased serum potassium
Decreased aldosterone excretion in urine
Decreased plasma renin activity

HYPOALDOSTERONISM (HYPOFUNCTION OF RENIN-ANGIOTENSIN-ALDOSTERONE SYSTEM)

Infrequent condition may be due to
- Addison's disease
- Congenital adrenal hyperplasia (methyl oxidase, type II defect)
- Rare congenital or acquired defect in aldosterone biosynthesis (renin normal or increased)
- Prolonged administration of heparin (very rare)
- Removal of unilateral aldosterone-secreting tumor (usually transient)
- Autonomic nervous system dysfunction; aldosterone deficiency causes impaired renal sodium conservation but without hyperkalemia
- Idiopathic hyporeninism

Hyperkalemia, urinary sodium loss, extracellular volume depletion corrected by administration of mineralocorticoids
Decreased aldosterone and PRA that are not increased by combined diuretic and posture establish the diagnosis.
Normal adrenal glucocorticoid response to ACTH stimulation test
Mild hyperchloremic metabolic acidosis
Most often associated with mild renal insufficiency (especially diabetic nephropathy, some interstitial nephropathies)
Laboratory findings of these associated diseases (e.g., diabetes mellitus, gout, pyelonephritis)

Pseudohypoaldosteronism is a heterogeneous group of disorders with signs and symptoms of aldosterone deficiency, but aldosterone levels are increased, and it is not ameliorated by exogenous mineralocorticoid.

CONGENITAL ADRENAL HYPERPLASIA (CAH)

Inherited inborn errors of metabolism due to specific deficiencies of enzymes needed for normal steroid synthesis of 3 main hormone classes: mineralocorticoids (17-deoxy pathway), glucocorticoids (17-hydroxy pathway), and sex steroids. All forms have decreased cortisol production, which stimulates compensatory secretion of pituitary ACTH that causes the adrenal hyperplasia and hypersecretion of other pathways. The commonest forms are summarized in Table 14-18. The synthetic pathways are shown schematically in Fig. 14-10 to illustrate the altered hormonal levels. Establish diagnoses by increase in specific precursor steroids in blood or urine, which can be suppressed by administration of glucocorticoids. Finding of increased 17-hydroxyprogesterone (17-OHP) or androstenedione in amniotic fluid permits prenatal diagnosis. In U.S., occurs 1:80,000–100,000 live births.

Table 14-16. Comparison of Pathologic Hypofunction of Renin-Angiotensin-Aldosterone System and Low-Renin Hypertension

Pathologic Hypofunction of Renin-Angiotensin-Aldosterone System	Low-Renin Hypertension
Hyperkalemia	Normal or low serum potassium
Urinary sodium loss	Sodium retention
Extracellular volume depletion	Increase in extracellular volume
Hypotension; may be normal	Persistent hypertension
Low renin-angiotensin-aldosterone activity	Low PRA with normal plasma and urine levels of aldosterone

CAH should always be ruled out in infants with
- Ambiguous genitalia and presence of nuclear sex chromatin
- Continued vomiting after pyloroplasty
- Siblings affected with CAH
- Salt loss

21-Hydroxylase Deficiency

(90% of cases of CAH are of this form; 3 types are recognized)

Severe deficiency (salt-losing) form

Severe enzyme deficiency not compensated for by increased ACTH secretion, and cortisol levels are decreased. Excess production of salt-losing steroids plus inability to secrete aldosterone causes characteristic acute adrenal crisis. Salt-wasting crisis usually occurs 1–2 weeks after birth with hyponatremia, hyperkalemia, acidosis, severe dehydration, and shock. Increased ACTH causes hypersecretion of androgens and virilization of female external (ambiguous) genitalia but usually normal internal genitalia. Males do not show abnormal genitals at birth but may show precocious puberty. Both show rapid early growth but premature closure of epiphyses causing shorter stature.

Moderate deficiency (simple virilizing) form (salt wasting mild or absent)

Moderate enzyme deficiency compensated by increased ACTH secretion causing cortisol secretion close to normal and marked increase in androgens (characteristic increase in androstenedione and, to a lesser extent, testosterone) and cortisol precursors some of which (progesterone, 17-OHP) cause some salt wasting, which causes compensatory increase in PRA and increased aldosterone secretion. Androgen ratio in urine of 11-desoxy-17-KS to 11-oxy-17-KS is ~1:1 (normal adult ratio = 1:4). *Urinary excretion of 17-KS and blood steroid secretion can be suppressed by dexamethasone* (1.25 mg/m^2/day for 7 days), which differentiates CAH from virilizing adrenal tumors. Urine 17-OHKS is normal. Normal or low cortisol levels show little or no response to ACTH administration. Karyotype should be done to establish genetic sex whenever ambiguous external genitalia are present.

Mild deficiency (attenuated; late onset) form

At puberty, females show hirsutism and oligomenorrhea; must be differentiated from polycystic ovary syndrome.

Increased 17-OHP (17–hydroxyprogesterone) (20–500 times normal; often >3000 ng/dl) is usually diagnostic; 24-hour urinary metabolite (pregnanetriol) is also increased. Best test is excessive rise (5–10 times) of 17-OHP 30 or 60 minutes after administration of ACTH (cosyntropin) 0.25–1.0 mg IV or 6 hours after 0.40 mg IV (normal <900 ng/dl; late-onset form >2000 ng/dl; severe form >16,000 ng/dl). Exaggerated increase of 17-OHP is used to identify carriers. Monitor glucocorticoid therapy by reduction of 17-OHP to normal.

Table 14-17. Comparison of Different Forms of Congenital Adrenal Hyperplasia

	Sexual Ambiguity in Newborn				
Enzyme Deficiency	Female	Male	Postnatal Virilization	Hypertension	Salt-Wasting
21-Hydroxylase					
Salt-wasting	+	0	+	0	+
Simple virilizing	+	0	+	0	0
Late-onset	0	0	+	0	0
11-Beta-hydroxylase[b]	+	0	+	+	0
3-Beta-hydroxysteroid					
Salt-wasting	+	+	+	0	+
Non-salt-wasting	+	+	+	0	0
Late-onset	0	?	+	0	0
17-Alpha-hydroxylase[b]	0	+	0	+	0
Cholesterol desmolase	0	+	0	0	+

	Urine Hormone Levels				Blood Hormone Levels				
	17-KS	17-OH	Pregnanetriol	Aldosterone	17-OHP	Delta-4	DHEA	Testosterone	Renin
21-Hydroxylase									
Salt-wasting	II	D	II	D	II	II	N/I	I	II
Simple virilizing	II	N/D	II	N/I	II	II	N/I	I	N/I
Late-onset	I	N	I	N/I	I	I	N/I	N/I	N
11-Beta-hydroxylase[b]	II	II	I	D	I	II	I	I	DD
3-Beta-hydroxysteroid									
Salt-wasting	I	DD	N/D	D	N/I	N/I	III	[a]	I
Non-salt-wasting	I	DD	N/D	N	N/I	N/I	III	[a]	N
Late-onset	N/I	N	N	N	N/I	N/I	I	N/I	N
17-Alpha-hydroxylase[b]	DD	DD	DD	D	D	D	D	D	D
Cholesterol desmolase	DD	DD	DD	DD	D	D	D	D	I

I, II, III = degrees of increased; D, DD = degrees of decreased; N = normal.
[a]N/D in males, N/I in females.
[b]Increased 17-deoxycortisol (corticosterone) and 11-deoxycortisol (compound B).
Source: Data from N. Lavin (Ed), *Manual of Endocrinology and Metabolism*. Boston: Little, Brown, 1986.

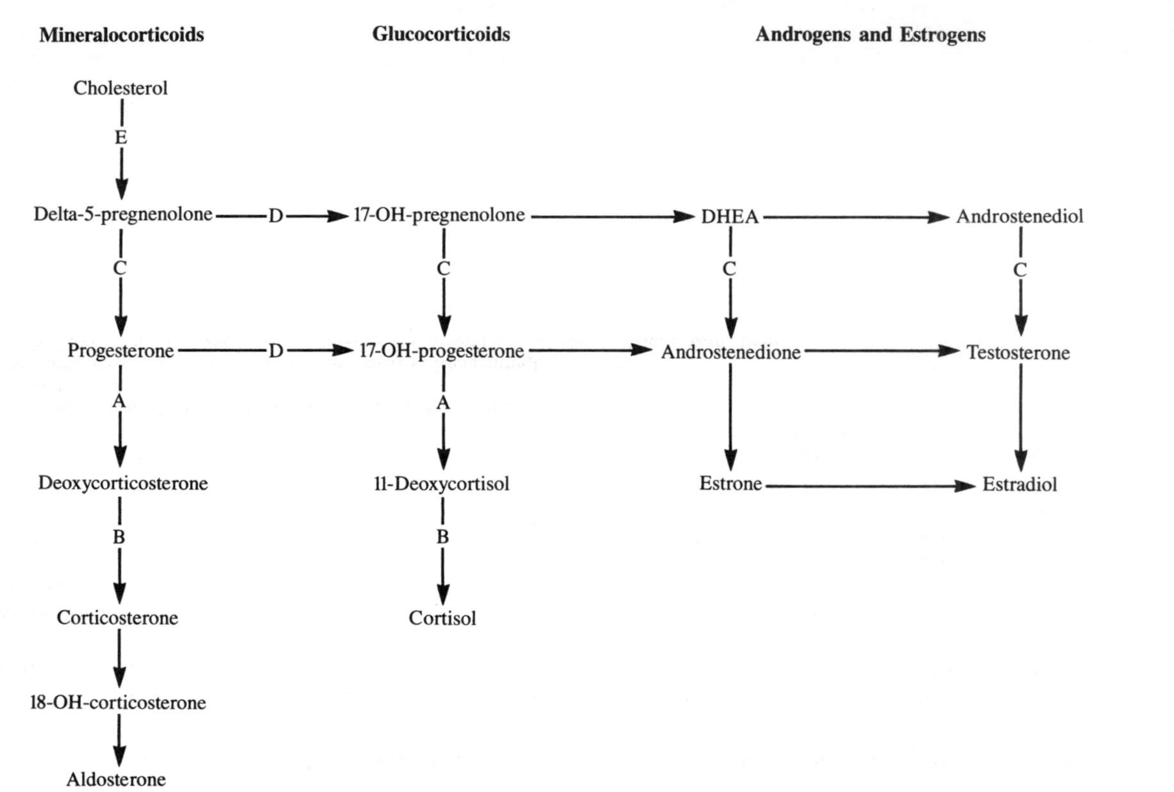
Mineralocorticoids
Glucocorticoids
Androgens and Estrogens
Cholesterol
E
Delta-5-pregnenolone
D
17-OH-pregnenolone
DHEA
Androstenediol
C
C
C
C
Progesterone
D
17-OH-progesterone
Androstenedione
Testosterone
A
A
Deoxycorticosterone
11-Deoxycortisol
Estrone
Estradiol
B
B
Corticosterone
Cortisol
18-OH-corticosterone
Aldosterone

Aldosterone deficiency is also present in salt-wasting form, but not in simple virilizing form. PRA is increased in both forms.
In nonclassical forms, same biochemical pattern occurs (with lower levels) but symptoms of virilization, abnormal growth and puberty, infertility, etc., may be slight or absent.
17-OHP and delta-4 levels are used to monitor therapy.
Cortisol levels are usually fixed and unresponsive.
Excess adrenal androgen production (e.g., androstenedione, DHEA, testosterone, urinary 17-KS), which is suppressed by glucocorticoids.

11-Beta-Hydroxylase Deficiency

(Causes <3% of cases of CAH. Excess mineralocorticoids cause hypertension, which may not appear until adulthood; excess androgen causes female pseudohermaphrodites at birth, postnatal virilism in males and females. Males with mild form may have only hypertension or gynecomastia.)

Increased serum deoxycorticosterone (DOC) causing hypokalemia and suppression of renin and aldosterone
Increased 11-deoxycortisol and 17-OHP
Increase of their metabolites in urine, tetrahydrodeoxycorticosterone, and tetrahydro-11-deoxycortisol
PRA levels can be used to monitor therapy.
Glucocorticoid therapy returns DOC to normal.

3-Beta-Hydroxysteroid Dehydrogenase (3-Beta-HSD) Deficiency

(Rare autosomal recessive; complete deficiency causes death.)

Impaired secretion with decrease of cortisol, aldosterone, androstenedione, and sex steroids
Increased plasma 17-hydroxypregnenolone, pregnenolone, DHEA, increased ratio of delta-5 (pregnenolone, 17-hydroxypregnenolone, DHEA) to delta-4 (progesterone, 17-OHP, delta-4-androstenedione), causing mild virilization.

17-Alpha-Hydroxylase Deficiency

Decreased serum 17-hydroxylated steroids and androgens
Decreased urine 17-KS and 17-OHKS
Increased serum corticosterone and deoxycorticosterone and their urinary metabolites in urine, causing hypertension, hypokalemia
Decreased aldosterone and plasma renin activity. PRA levels can be used to monitor therapy.

Cholesterol Desmolase Deficiency

(complete deficiency incompatible with life)

Mild condition in females may cause short stature, virilization, irregular menses, infertility. Males may show short stature, infertility. (Early diagnosis and therapy may prevent this.)
Virtually no steroids are produced.
Very low urine 17-OHKS is not increased by ACTH stimulation.
Aldosterone is very low in plasma and urine.
Hyponatremia, hyperkalemia, rapid dehydration, shock, and early death if not recognized at birth
Ambiguous or female genitalia in male children

Fig. 14-10. Pathway of adrenal hormone synthesis. Hormones above the level of the deficient enzyme are present in increased amount; those below this level are decreased in amount (see Table 14-18). Shunting to other pathways may occur. Findings depend on completeness of enzyme deficiency, degree of hormone deficiency, or excessive accumulation. A = 21-hydroxylase; B = 11-hydroxylase; C = 3-beta-hydroxysteroid dehydrogenase; D = 17-hydroxylase; E = 20,22-desmolase.

Corticosterone Methyloxidase Deficiency

Type I

- Hyponatremia and hyperkalemia
- Decreased aldosterone and 18-hydroxycorticosterone (18-OHB)
- Increased corticosterone.

Type II

- Ratio of urinary metabolites of 18-OHB to aldosterone is markedly increased (normal is <3.0); is a better marker than 18-OHB levels.

17-Beta-HSD Deficiency

Increased delta-4-testosterone ratios in peripheral and spermatic blood is diagnostic.

During first week of life:

- Urine total 17-KS in normal infants may be as high as in CAH due to maternal steroids. Normally falls to <1 mg/24 hours during second week of life; therefore should do serial determinations in suspected cases. Level <1 mg/24 hours rules out CAH; an increasing level suggests CAH, but a decreasing level does not rule out CAH. Is increased in all virilizing forms except lipoid type.
- 17-OHP is the most valuable test in 21-hydroxylase or 11-hydroxylase deficiency.
- Detectable amounts of pregnanetriol in urine or plasma after first week of life is usually diagnostic of CAH, but in some patients this may not appear until >1 month old.
- 17-OHKS in urine is not particularly useful in diagnosis of CAH.

PHEOCHROMOCYTOMA

Tumor of chromaffin cells of sympathetic nervous system; may secrete epinephrine, norepinephrine, dopamine. Epinephrine is secreted by tumors usually of adrenal medulla and causes characteristic symptoms. Norepinephrine is secreted by almost all extra-adrenal tumors and many adrenal tumors; often associated with sustained hypertension and hypermetabolism. Dopamine secretion is not associated with hypertension. Tumors that secrete both dopamine and epinephrine are more likely to be part of familial syndrome. (Normally, epinephrine is secreted primarily by adrenal medulla and norepinephrine is secreted primarily at sympathetic nerve endings.)

Biochemical diagnosis is based on increased blood or urine levels of catecholamines (norepinephrine and, to a lesser extent, epinephrine) and their metabolites (normetanephrine and metanephrine), which are usual even when patient is asymptomatic and normotensive; rarely are increases found only following a paroxysm. However, the diagnosis is never ruled out by a normal level, and repeated testing may be necessary. Increase of either epinephrine or norepinephrine should be considered positive. Plasma levels are often >2000 pg/dl, which is rarely seen in other conditions and is considered diagnostic. Levels are usually 5–100 times normal, although there is considerable overlap and wide range of normals. Plasma levels <500 pg/dl essentially rules it out; levels >500 pg/dl indicate need for further testing. Plasma levels are particularly useful to compare paroxysm and basal levels and to localize tumors by selective venous sampling. Blood should be drawn in the unstressed supine patient without interfering conditions or drugs. Plasma measurements of norepinephrine and epinephrine are not as sensitive as urine measurements. For diagnosis of pheochromocytoma, 24-hour urine free norepinephrine has 100% sensitivity and 98% specificity, plasma norepinephrine has 82% sensitivity and 95% specificity.* In another study, 24-hour urine meta-

*Data from MW Duncan et al., Measurement of norepinephrine and 3,4-dihydroxyphenylglycol in urine and plasma for the diagnosis of pheochromocytoma. *N Engl J Med* 319:136, 1988.

nephrines had a sensitivity of 79% and specificity of 93%; 24-hour urine vanillylmandelic acid (VMA) had a sensitivity of 42% and specificity of 100%.†

Selective venous catheterization for plasma catecholamine levels on rare occasions when CAT scan or MRI fails to localize a biochemically confirmed tumor.

Plasma Catecholamines May Also Be Increased In

Neural crest tumors (neuroblastoma, ganglioneuroma, ganglioblastoma)
Diabetic ketoacidosis (markedly elevated)
Acute myocardial infarction (markedly elevated)
Acute CNS disturbance (e.g., infarct, hemorrhage, encephalopathy, tumor)
Heavy exercise
After surgery
Hypothyroidism
Thyrotoxicosis
Volume depletion (induced by diuretics)
Renal disease
Heavy alcohol intake
Hypoglycemia
Stress (emotional, physical)
Various drugs (see p. 759)

Plasma catecholamines drop markedly after 5 minutes if RBCs are not separated from plasma. Plasma levels may not be increased when increased secretion is intermittent rather than continuous; for these cases, 24-hour urines are more accurate. Plasma levels are useful if 24-hour urine cannot be collected.

Tumor secretory patterns

- Most common: Norepinephrine predominant with much lesser epinephrine and dopamine
- Less common: equal norepinephrine and epinephrine and some dopamine
- Rare: epinephrine very high with small amounts of norepinephrine and dopamine; usually indicate adrenal rather than extra-adrenal mass
- Malignancy: increased dopamine and almost as much norepinephrine with very low epinephrine

Urine VMA excretion is considerably increased in ~90% of patients. Because this analysis is simpler than for catecholamines, it has been more commonly used but is less sensitive than other tests. Beware of false increase due to foods (e.g., vanilla, fruits, especially bananas, coffee, tea) and drugs (e.g., vasopressor agents) ingested within 72 hours before the test (see p. 743). Beware of nonspecific techniques for VMA assay that fail to detect 30% of cases of pheochromocytoma.

Urinary metanephrines (the single most reliable screening test for pheochromocytoma as false negative = 4% and fewer interferences by drugs and diet than VMA or catecholamines) confirmed by urine catecholamine fraction determinations are an excellent routine to identify pheochromocytoma patients.

Urinary catecholamines are less reliable than VMA or metanephrines in screening for pheochromocytoma due to technical problems; best used to confirm diagnosis (using high-pressure liquid chromatography) when other tests are equivocal. Fractionation that shows predominance of epinephrine suggests tumor in adrenal or organ of Zuckerkandl; rarely bladder or mediastinum. Presence of homovanillic acid is said to suggest malignancy.

Increased catecholamine levels after surgery may indicate recurrence of tumor.

Suppression tests: high plasma catecholamine levels of patients with pheochromocytomas (which secrete autonomously) are not suppressed by pentolinium

†Data from EL Bravo and RW Gifford, Pheochromocytoma: Diagnosis, localization and management. *N Engl J Med* 311:1298, 1984.

(preganglionic blocking agent) or by clonidine, but high basal level in patients without tumor is decreased to normal.

Provocative tests: IV injection of glucagon or histamine causes marked rise in plasma catecholamines in >90% of cases, but false positive and false negative results may occur. Threefold increase or an absolute level >2000 pg/ml within 3 minutes is considered positive.

When other studies are negative, a timed urine specimen or plasma level for catecholamines and metabolites after a typical "spell" may be useful.

Hyperglycemia and glycosuria are found in 50% of patients during an attack.

Glucose tolerance test frequently shows a diabetic type of curve; many develop clinical diabetes mellitus.

Thyroid function tests are normal.

Urine changes are secondary to sustained hypertension.

Plasma renin activity is increased.

Relative erythrocytosis sometimes occurs.

Increased incidence of cholelithiasis.

<15% of pheochromocytomas are malignant; 15% are extra-adrenal; 10% are multiple. 10% occur in children, two-thirds of whom are male. Familial inheritance in 10–20% of patients; 70% of these are bilateral. Associated with certain neurocutaneous syndromes (e.g., von Recklinghausen's disease, tuberous sclerosis, von Hippel-Lindau disease). See MEN II, p. 553, and MEN III, p. 554.

Occurs in 0.1–0.2% of hypertensive population of U.S.

5% of patients with pheochromocytoma have normal blood pressure most or all of the time. Sustained hypertension in 50% of cases.

Indications for laboratory screening for pheochromocytoma:

- Characteristic symptoms
- Familial/hereditary conditions
- Any of the components of MEN type IIa, IIb in patients or relatives
- Neurofibromatosis
- All hypertensive children
- Patients whose hypertension becomes worse on treatment with beta blockers, guanethidine, or ganglionic blockers
- Severe hypertension, especially if resistant to therapy
- Hypertensive episodes during anesthesia, labor, or radiologic procedures

NEUROBLASTOMA, GANGLIONEUROMA, GANGLIOBLASTOMA

Urinary levels of catecholamines (norepinephrine, normetanephrine, dopamine, VMA, and homovanillic acid [HVA]) are increased. Excretion of epinephrine is not increased.

Not all patients have increased urinary levels of catecholamines, VMA, and HVA. If only 1 of these substances is measured, only ~75% of cases are

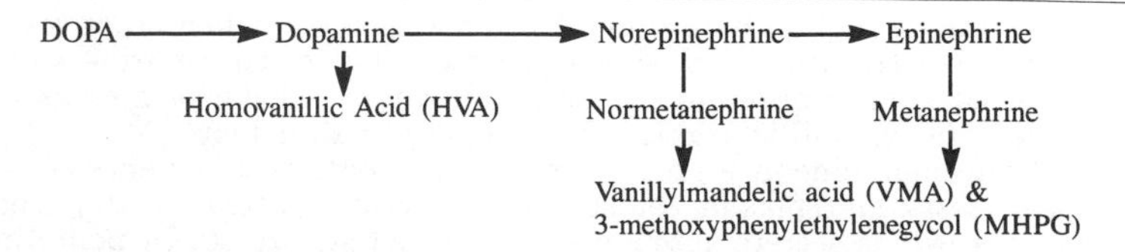

Fig. 14-11. Synthesis and breakdown of catecholamines. Since the hormones are broken down prior to release, metabolites are present in much larger amounts. When excretion of free catecholamines is greater compared to metabolites, it is said that tumor is likely to be very small and difficult to locate.

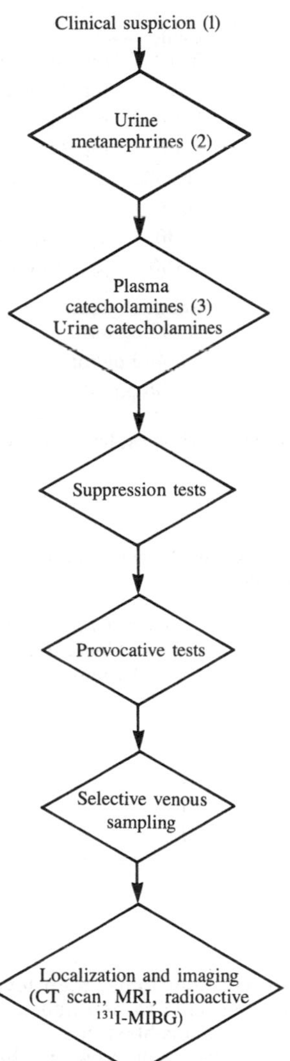

(1) History suggestive of MEA II. <30- year-old hypertensive. Any hypertensive with unusualy symptoms. Only 20% of patients with pheochromocytoma have intermittent hypertension. Pheochromocytoma is more likely in younger patients.

(2) Because of high sensitivity, normal metanephrines in urine virtually rule out pheochromocytoma if MEA II is not suspect. Because of low prevalence of pheochromocytoma, even <10%. Urine metanephrines may be decreased by various drugs (e.g., L-dopa, x-ray contrast media) and may be increased by stress (e.g., MI, CNS trauma) and certain drugs (e.g., MAO inhibitors, hydrazines and prochlorperazine, chlorpromazine, imipramine, methyldopa, oxytetracycline, phenacetin, phenothiazines).

If urine metanephrines are increased, urine VMA should be performed next because of high specificity. Combination of increased metanephrines and VMA in urine is presumptive evidence of pheochromocytoma and should be followed by localizing tests.

(3) Measurement of catecholamines (especially in plasma) should be performed along with localizing tests when MEA II is suspected. Although urinary catecholamine determinations commonly show false negative and false positive results, it may be particularly useful in possible MEA II but must beware of interfering factors (e.g., increased by exercise, stress, emotion, hypoglycemia, certain drugs).

Fig. 14-12. Flow chart of laboratory tests in diagnosis of pheochromocytoma.

diagnosed. If VMA and HVA or VMA and total catecholamines are measured, 95–100% of cases are diagnosed.

These tests are also useful for differentiating Ewing's tumor and metastatic neuroblastoma of bone and to show response to therapy (surgery, irradiation, or chemotherapy), which should bring return to normal in 1–4 months. Continued elevation indicates need for further treatment.

Cystathionine in urine suggests active disease, but absence is not significant since is not normally present.

Table 14-18. Reference Range for Catecholamines and Metabolites

	Urine	
HVA	2–12	mg/24 hours
VMA	2–7	mg/24 hours
MHPG	1.3–4.3	mg/24 hours
Metanephrines	<1.6	mg/24 hours
Dopamine	25–525	μg/24 hours
Norepinephrine	10–64	μg/24 hours
Epinephrine	0–36	μg/24 hours
Norepinephrine + epinephrine	<100	μg/24 hours
	Range Plasma	
Dopamine	<100 pg/ml	
Norepinephrine	65–400 pg/ml	
Epinephrine	15–55 pg/ml	

Source: Data from JM Feldman, Diagnosis and management of pheochromocytoma. *Hospital Practice*, pp. 175–198, Jan 15, 1989.
These data differ depending on source.

Table 14-19. Laboratory Tests in Differential Diagnosis of Benign Pheochromocytoma and Neural Crest Tumors (Neuroblastoma, Ganglioneuroma)

Urinary Levels of	Pheochromocytoma	Neural Crest Tumor (neuroblastoma, ganglioneuroma)
Catecholamines	I	I
VMA	I	I
Metanephrines	I	I
Dopamine	N*	I
HVA	N*	I

I = increased; N = normal.
*I in malignant pheochromocytoma.

Serum neuron-specific enolase may be increased in neuroblastoma; high level is associated with poor prognosis. Ratio of neuron-specific to non-neuronal enolase is reported to improve specificity to >85% for neuroblastoma.

Laboratory findings due to metastases (e.g., tumor in biopsy of marrow or other sites, anemia)

ADRENOCORTICAL INSUFFICIENCY

Acute
- Primary (e.g., due to Waterhouse-Friderichsen syndrome or hemorrhage when on anticoagulant therapy)
- Secondary to pituitary disorders
    - Trauma or surgical removal of pituitary
    - Sheehan's syndrome (postpartum infarction of pituitary)
    - Following cessation of prolonged steroid therapy

Chronic
- Primary
    - Granulomas (e.g., tuberculosis, sarcoidosis)

Metastatic carcinoma
Amyloid
Autoimmune adrenalitis—diagnosed by circulating adrenal antibodies; may be associated with other autoimmune conditions (e.g., Hashimoto's thyroiditis, pernicious anemia)

Secondary
Simmonds' disease (idiopathic atrophy of pituitary)
Destruction of pituitary by granulomas, tumor, etc.

ADDISON'S DISEASE

(chronic adrenocortical insufficiency)

In primary deficiency, both cortisol and aldosterone are deficient with salt loss; in secondary, aldosterone production is maintained but other secondary endocrine deficiencies may appear, e.g., hypothyroidism, hypogonadism)

Serum potassium is increased.
Serum sodium and chloride are decreased.
Sodium-potassium ratio is <30:1.
Blood volume is decreased; hematocrit level is increased (because of water loss).
BUN and creatinine may be moderately increased.
Fasting hypoglycemia is present, with a flat oral glucose tolerance curve and insulin hypersensitivity. IV GTT shows a normal peak followed by severe prolonged hypoglycemia.
Neutropenia and relative lymphocytosis are common.
Eosinophilia is present (300/cu mm). *(A total eosinophil count of <50 is evidence against severe adrenocortical hypofunction.)*
Normocytic anemia is slight or moderate but difficult to estimate because of decreased blood volume.
Increased blood ACTH (200–1600 pg/ml) with wide variation between morning and evening levels in primary adrenal hypofunction but decreased or absent ACTH in pituitary (secondary) hypoadrenalism. Increased ACTH level is quickly suppressed by replacement therapy.
Decreased blood cortisol (<5 μg/dl in 8–10 A.M. specimen) is useful screening test. High or high-normal result excludes both primary and secondary adrenocortical insufficiency. Low or borderline result is indication for ACTH stimulation test.
ACTH stimulation tests (see p. 497)
Metyrapone inhbiition test is performed if ACTH test causes some increase in blood cortisol (see p. 497).
Cortisol treatment will interfere with all of the above tests and must be discontinued for prior 24–48 hours. Dexamethasone will interfere with metyrapone test and plasma ACTH levels.
Laboratory tests for associated conditions
  Primary adrenocortical insufficiency may be caused by congenital adrenal hyperplasia (see pp. 514–530) or associated with hypoaldosteronism.
  Secondary (pituitary) insufficiency may be associated with laboratory findings of hypothyroidism (see pp. 456–459), hypogonadism (see p. 535), etc.
Urine 17-OHKS is absent or markedly decreased.
Urine 17-KS is markedly decreased.
Urine 17-KGS is markedly decreased.
The Robinson-Power-Kepler water tolerance test and the Cutler-Power-Wilder sodium chloride deprivation test have been replaced by the ACTH stimulation tests, which are more direct and avoid the risk of crisis.
Antiadrenal antibodies are found in most cases of idiopathic Addison's disease but in minority of those due to adrenal tuberculosis. Said to have very high sensitivity, specificity, and predictive value for development of adrenocortical failure in women with normal adrenal adrenocortical function.

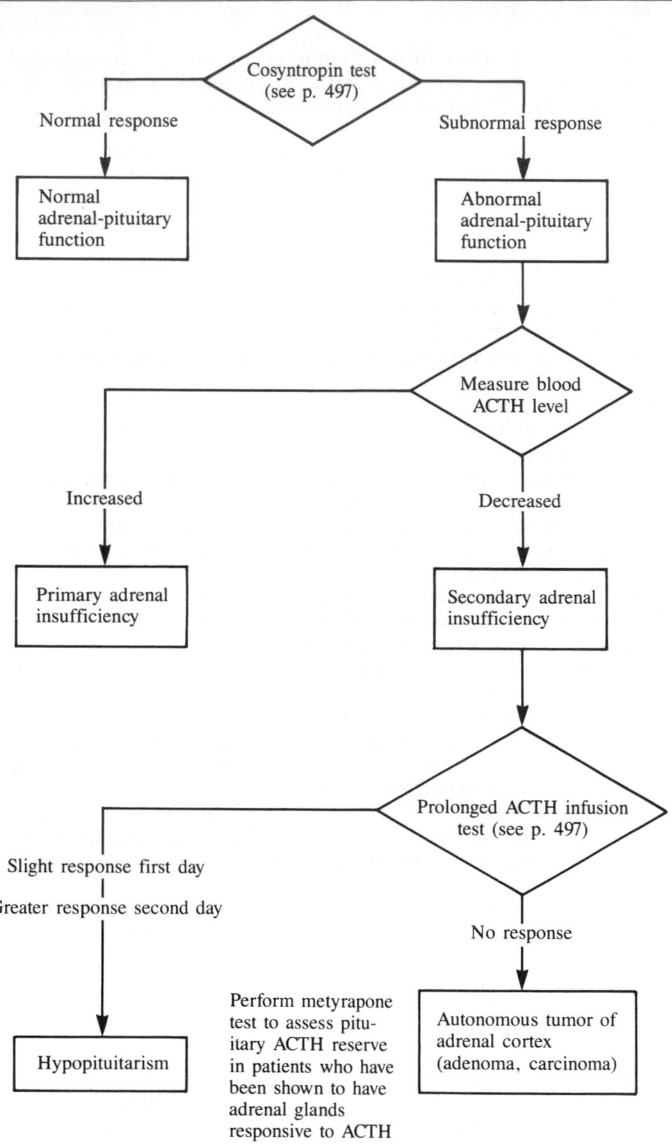

Fig. 14-13. Sequence of laboratory tests in diagnosis of adrenal insufficiency.

WATERHOUSE-FRIDERICHSEN SYNDROME

(acute adrenal insufficiency with degenerative changes in adrenal cortex; patient often dies before progression to cortical hemorrhage)

Dehydration

Azotemia is due to dehydration and shock affecting renal function.

Serum sodium and chloride are decreased and potassium is increased in some patients.

Table 14-20. Laboratory Differentiation of Primary and Secondary Adrenal Insufficiency

Test	Primary Adrenal Insufficiency	Adrenal Insufficiency Secondary to Hypopituitarism
Blood ACTH level	Increased	Decreased
Urine 17-KS and 17-OHKS after ACTH stimulation (see p. 497)	No responsive increase	Marked "staircase" response

Hypoglycemia occurs regularly.
Direct eosinophil count is >50/cu mm (<50/cu mm in other kinds of shock).
Blood cortisol is markedly decreased (<5 μg/dl).

Tests of Gonadal Function

17-KS IN URINE IN MALES (INDICATIVE OF ADRENAL RATHER THAN TESTICULAR STATUS)

Increased In
Interstitial cell tumor

Decreased In
Primary hypogonadism
Secondary hypogonadism

PLASMA TESTOSTERONE

Decreased In (Men)
Primary hypogonadism (e.g., orchiectomy)
Secondary hypogonadism (e.g., hypopituitarism)
Testicular feminization
Klinefelter's syndrome levels lower than in normal male but higher than in normal female and orchiectomized male
Estrogen therapy
Cirrhosis
Chronic renal disease
Massive obesity

Increased In
Premature puberty in boys
Masculinization in women
Drugs that alter thyroxine-binding globulins may also affect testosterone-binding globulins; however, the free testosterone level will not be affected.
Stein-Leventhal syndrome—variable; increased when virilization is present
Adrenogenital syndrome—with virilization (due to tumor or hyperplasia), level is much higher than in normal female; decreases following adrenal suppression
Idiopathic hirsutism—inconclusive
Ovarian stromal hyperthecosis

SEMEN ANALYSIS*

Reference Ranges

Volume	1–5 ml
pH	7.2–8.0
Color	Gray-white
Liquefaction	<30 minutes
Viability	>65%
Motility	>60%
Progressive motility	3+ to 4+
Sperm density	>20 million/ml
Morphology	<30% abnormal
Total motile functional sperm (= volume × % motility × sperm density × % normal morphology)	>40 million
RBCs	0–5/HPF
WBCs	0–5/HPF
Crystals	None
Clumping	None
Mixed antiglobulin reaction	Negative
Bovine cervical mucus penetration	>30 mm
Cultures for bacteria *(Ureaplasma, Chlamydia)*	No pathogens
Antiserum antibodies	Negative

Sterile males usually show

- Volume of <3 ml
- <20 million sperm/ml
- <25% motility
- Abnormal motility or morphology can occur with normal sperm counts but are usually seen with decreased counts. Abnormal forms indicate impaired spermatogenesis. Decreased motility may reflect defects in cilia structure elsewhere (in respiratory and reproductive tracts). Agglutination may indicate antisperm antibodies (which can be measured but relationship to infertility is not established). Normal morphology is >60% normal oval forms, <6% tapered forms, <0.5% immature forms, <8% amorphous forms. Tapered forms and spermatids are often increased in infertility associated with varicocele.
- Inflammatory cells may indicate infection of GU tract.
- Absent fructose (normally produced by seminal vesicles) may indicate absence or obstruction of vas deferens and seminal vesicles. Azospermia, normal semen fructose, and normal serum FSH suggest obstruction proximal to entry of ejaculatory ducts.
- Large numbers of sperm in postejaculation urine in these patients suggest retrograde ejaculation.

Repeated semen analysis is necessary to characterize average spermatogenesis.

Specimens should not be collected within 24 hours of, or >5–7 days later than, previous ejaculation. Should be received in laboratory within 1 hour.

≤40% variability between different semen samples.

*Data from JE Adams, *Infertility in Men: Diagnosis and Treatment.* ASCP Check Sample CC 87-9 (CC-187). 27:1, 1987; SA Rothmann and BW Morgan, Laboratory diagnosis in andrology. *Cleve Clin J Med,* pp. 805–809, Nov–Dec 1989.)

Comparison of split ejaculate specimens is useful in patients with abnormal semen analysis associated with a high volume; specimens may show marked differences.

Antisperm antibodies (may test male serum or seminal fluid or female serum or cervical mucus) may occur in

- Testicular trauma (even minor)
- Almost all vasectomized patients
- Viral orchitis (permanent)
- Bacterial infections of GU tract (usually transient)

Cervical mucus penetration test measures greatest distance traveled by an individual sperm from a small aliquot of semen incubated 90 minutes in a capillary tube of bovine cervical mucus. 68% of infertile men had penetration scores <20 mm, while 79% of fertile men has scores >30 mm.

Hamster egg penetration assay: Hamster oocytes enzymatically treated to remove outer layers of egg (which prevent cross-species fertilization) are incubated with human sperm selected for their motile ability. Penetration rates <15% indicate reduced fertility. Positive test indicates ability of sperm to propel itself to oocyte, bind to oocyte, and penetrate oocyte.

Following vasectomy, spermatozoa are present for some time. To be certain, two centrifuged specimens properly collected 1 month apart should be sperm-free and fructose is absent.

BIOPSY OF TESTICLE

Evidence of atrophy in sterility study
Diagnosis of tumor

Normal spermatogenesis and normal endocrine findings in patient with aspermia and infertility suggest a mechanical obstruction to sperm transport that may be correctable.

FOLLICULAR-STIMULATING HORMONE (FSH) AND LUTEINIZING HORMONE (LH)

(pituitary gonadotropins)

Normal values vary widely according to sex, age, stage of menstrual cycle. Serial determinations may be required.

Increased In

Primary hypogonadism (anorchia, testicular failure, menopause)
Precocious puberty (secondary to a CNS lesion or idiopathic)
Complete testicular feminization syndrome

Decreased In

Failure of pituitary or hypothalamus (secondary hypogonadism)

- Kallmann's syndrome (inherited autosomal isolated deficiency of gonadotropin releasing hormone [GnRH]; occurs in both sexes): Found in ~5% of patients with primary amenorrhea. Causes failure of both gametogenic function and sex steroid production (LH and FSH are "normal" or undetectable but rise in response to prolonged GnRH stimulation).

ESTROGENS

Increased In

Granulosa cell tumor of ovary
Theca-cell tumor of ovary
Luteoma of ovary
Pregnancy
Secondary to stimulation by HCG-producing tumors (e.g., teratoma, teratocarcinoma)

Decreased In

Primary hypofunction of ovary

- Autoimmune oophoritis is the most common cause: usually associated with other autoimmune endocrinopathies, e.g., Hashimoto's thyroiditis, Addison's disease, insulin-dependent diabetes mellitus. May cause premature menopause.
- Resistant ovary syndrome
- Toxic (e.g., irradiation, chemotherapy)
- Infection (e.g., mumps)
- Tumor (primary or secondary)
- Mechanical (e.g., trauma, torsion, surgical excision)
- Genetic (e.g., Turner's syndrome [see p. 533])

Secondary hypofunction of ovary

- Trauma to hypothalamo-pituitary axis

PREGNANEDIOL

Increased In

Luteal cysts of ovary
Arrhenoblastoma of ovary

Decreased In

Amenorrhea
Threatened abortion (some patients)
Fetal death
Toxemia of pregnancy

17-KS IN FEMALES

Increased In

Virilizing ovarian tumors (e.g., adrenal rest tumor, granulosa cell tumor, hilar cell tumor, Brenner tumor, and, most frequently, arrhenoblastoma); increased in 50% of patients and normal in 50% of patients

Decreased In

Primary ovarian agenesis

CYTOLOGIC EXAMINATION OF VAGINAL SMEAR (PAPANICOLAOU SMEAR) FOR EVALUATION OF OVARIAN FUNCTION

Maturation index (MI) is the proportion of parabasal, intermediate, and superficial cells in each 100 cells counted.

- Lack of estrogen effect shows predominance of parabasal cells (e.g., MI = 100/0/0).
- Low estrogen effect shows predominance of intermediate cells (e.g., MI = 10/90/0).
- Increased estrogen effect shows predominance of superficial cells (e.g., MI = 0/0/100) (hormone-producing tumors of ovary, persistent follicular cysts).

Some patterns of maturation index in different conditions

	Index
Childhood	
Normal	80/20/0
Cortisone therapy	0/98/2
Childbearing years	
Preovulatory (late follicular) phase	0/40/60
Premenstrual (late luteal) phase	0/70/30
Pregnancy (second month)	0/90/10
Cortisone therapy	0/85/15

Amenorrhea after ovarian irradiation	0/30/70
Surgical oophorectomy	0/80/20–0/90/10
Bilateral oophorectomy and adrenalectomy	0/98/2
Postmenopausal years, early (age 60)	65/30/5
Postmenopausal years, late (age 75)	
Untreated	100/0/0
Moderate estrogen treatment	0/50/50
High-dose estrogen treatment	0/0/100
Years after bilateral oophorectomy	100/0/0
Postadrenalectomy, bilateral	6/94/0

Karyopyknotic index (KI) is the percent of cells with pyknotic nuclei.
Increased estrogen effect (e.g., KI ≥85%) is seen, as in cystic glandular hyperplasia of the endometrium.
Eosinophilic index is the percent of cells showing eosinophilic cytoplasm; it may also be used as a measure of estrogen effect.
Combined progesterone-estrogen effect: No quantitative cytologic criteria are available. Endometrial biopsy should be used for this purpose.

The pattern may be obscured by cytolysis (e.g., infections, excess bacilli), increased red or white blood cells, excessively thin or thick smears, or drying of smears before fixation (artificial eosinophilic staining).

CHROMOSOME ANALYSIS

(see pp. 108–109)

Turner's syndrome (gonadal dysgenesis)—usually negative for Barr bodies
Klinefelter's syndrome—positive for Barr bodies
Pseudohermaphroditism—chromosomal sex corresponding to gonadal sex

Gonadal Disorders

LABORATORY TESTS IN DIFFERENTIAL DIAGNOSIS OF PATIENTS WITH HIRSUTISM AND DIMINISHED MENSES

Urinary 17-OHKS

Normal
- Constitutional hirsutism
- Stein-Leventhal syndrome
- Mild adrenogenital syndrome
- Masculinizing tumor of ovary

Increased
- Cushing's syndrome

Urinary 17-KS

Normal
- Constitutional hirsutism
- Stein-Leventhal syndrome
- Masculinizing tumor of ovary
- Cushing's syndrome

Slight increase
- Constitutional hirsutism
- Stein-Leventhal syndrome
- Mild adrenogenital syndrome
- Cushing's syndrome

Marked increase
- Masculinizing tumor of adrenal gland
- Adrenogenital syndrome

Urinary 17-KS Decreased By Daily Prednisone

Poor response
- Constitutional hirsutism
- Stein-Leventhal syndrome
- Masculinizing tumor of ovary

Good response
- Adrenogenital syndrome

Urinary 17-KS Further Decreased By Daily Stilbestrol and Prednisone

No response
- Constitutional hirsutism
- Masculinizing tumor of ovary
- Adrenogenital syndrome

Response
- Stein-Leventhal syndrome (testosterone level also decreases)

SOME COMMON CAUSES OF PRIMARY AMENORRHEA/DELAYED MENARCHE

Gonadal disorders (60% of all causes)
- Gonadal dysgenesis (75% of gonadal disorders)
  - Testicular feminization syndrome (most common form of male hermaphroditism; female phenotype with male 46 XY karyotype, testosterone in male range; testes are present)
- Polycystic ovaries
- Resistant ovary syndrome

Structural genital tract disorders (35–40% of all causes)
- Imperforate hymen
- Uterine agenesis
- Vaginal agenesis
- Transverse vaginal septum

Pituitary disorders (rare)
- Hypopituitarism
- Adenomas (prolactin secreting)

Hypothalamic disorders (rare)
- Anatomic lesions (e.g., craniopharyngioma)
- Functional disturbance of hypothalamic-pituitary axis (e.g., anorexia nervosa, emotional stress)

Systemic disorders
- Hypothyroidism
- Congenital adrenal hyperplasia
  - Debilitating chronic diseases (e.g., malnutrition, congenital heart disease, renal failure, collagen diseases)

HORMONE PROFILES IN AMENORRHEA

Normal LH, FSH, prolactin, estradiol, testosterone, T-4 (eugonadal)
- Drugs
- Diet, anorexia
- Exercise
- Stress, illness
- Structural genital tract disorders (see previous section)

Increased LH and normal FSH
- Early pregnancy
- Polycystic ovarian disease (Stein-Leventhal syndrome)
- Ectopic gonadotropin production by neoplasm (e.g., lung, GI tract)
- Increased LH and FSH (>30 mIU/ml), decreased estrogen (<50 pg/ml)
- Primary ovarian hypofunction

Normal or low LH and FSH, decreased estrogen
- Hyperprolactinemia (see pp. 543–544)

Isolated gonadotropin deficiency due to pituitary or hypothalamic impairment
Clomiphene citrate should be administered for 5–10 days; if gonadotropin level rises or menses return, cause is probably hypothalamic.
Administer hypothalamic luteinizing hormone–releasing factor (LRF); normal or exaggerated response in hypothalamic amenorrhea (cause in 80% of patients); smaller or no response in pituitary tumor or dysfunction.
Increased androgen
Polycystic ovarian disease (testosterone level usually <200 ng/dl)
Tumor of adrenal or ovary (testosterone level may be >200 ng/dl)
Testicular feminization
Use of anabolic steroids (e.g., in athletes)

TURNER'S SYNDROME (OVARIAN DYSGENESIS)

Diagnosis is based on karyotype analysis. Chromosomal pattern includes wide spectrum of abnormalities, e.g., 45 chromosomes (monosomy X with XO; or if XX, one X is abnormal; or XO mosaic), various deletions of part of an X chromosome. Female is phenotypic.
Barr bodies are negative (male) in 80% of patients.
Because of the frequency with which 45 X cells are admixed with 46 XX cells, it is impossible to exclude the diagnosis (i.e., 45 X karyotype) by either buccal smear or chromosome analysis alone.
Biopsy of ovary shows connective tissue stroma with rare follicular structure.
Vaginal smear and endometrial biopsy are atrophic.
Increased FSH, LH, and gonadotropins
17-KS and 17-OHKS are normal.
ACTH is normal.
Laboratory findings due to increased prevalence of associated conditions, e.g., Hashimoto's thyroiditis, coarctation of aorta, horseshoe kidneys

About 60% of patients with primary amenorrhea have Turner's syndrome or sometimes testicular feminization. 90% never menstruate. About 10% menstruate for a few years and then present as secondary amenorrhea.

CORPUS LUTEUM DEFICIENCY

(Corpus luteum produces insufficient progesterone for development of endometrium receptive for pregnancy.)

Due to any condition that interferes with follicle growth and development
Severe systemic illness including liver, kidney, or heart dysfunction
Hyperprolactinemia
X-chromosome abnormalities
Polycystic ovarian disease or other causes of inadequate FSH level early in cycle
Deficient LH receptors on corpus luteum cells
LH level inadequate or deficient ovulatory surge

Endometrial biopsy on 26th day of cycle is less developed than on menstrual day.
Serum progesterone measured on three different days during midluteal phase totals <15 ng/ml and random level is <5 ng/ml.

MENOPAUSE (FEMALE CLIMACTERIC)

Serum estradiol <5 ng/dl and FSH >40 mIU/ml confirm primary ovarian failure.
Urinary estrogens are decreased.
Urinary 17-KS is decreased.
Plasma and urinary gonadotropin are increased.

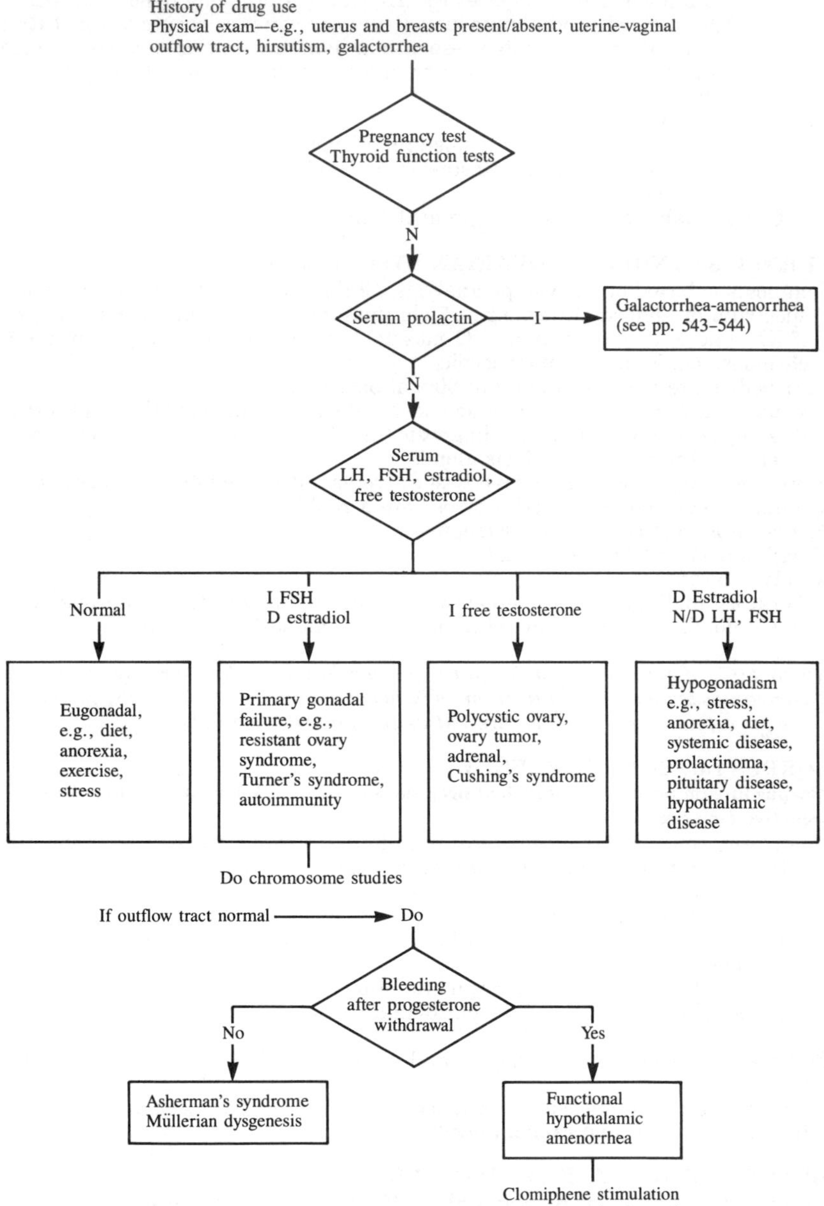
History of drug use
Physical exam—e.g., uterus and breasts present/absent, uterine-vaginal outflow tract, hirsutism, galactorrhea
Pregnancy test
Thyroid function tests
N
Serum prolactin
I
Galactorrhea-amenorrhea (see pp. 543–544)
N
Serum LH, FSH, estradiol, free testosterone
Normal
I FSH D estradiol
I free testosterone
D Estradiol N/D LH, FSH
Eugonadal, e.g., diet, anorexia, exercise, stress
Primary gonadal failure, e.g., resistant ovary syndrome, Turner's syndrome, autoimmunity
Polycystic ovary, ovary tumor, adrenal, Cushing's syndrome
Hypogonadism e.g., stress, anorexia, diet, systemic disease, prolactinoma, pituitary disease, hypothalamic disease
Do chromosome studies
If outflow tract normal
Do
Bleeding after progesterone withdrawal
No
Yes
Asherman's syndrome
Müllerian dysgenesis
Functional hypothalamic amenorrhea
Clomiphene stimulation and reassess in 6 months

Table 14-21. Laboratory Differentiation of Primary and Secondary (to Pituitary Defect) Hypogonadism

Test	Primary Hypogonadism	Hypogonadism Secondary To Pituitary Defect
Level of FSH and gonadotropin in urine	High	Low
After administration of gonadotropins		
17-KS excretion	Does not increase	Increases
Clinical evidence of hypogonadism	Does not subside	Subsides with Increased sperm count or Increased estrogenic effect in Pap smear

SECONDARY OVARIAN INSUFFICIENCY

Due To

Deficient estrogen production, e.g., diseases of the pituitary or hypothalamus (see separate sections)

Normal or increased estrogen production, e.g., ovarian tumors, functional cysts of ovary that suppress LH and FSH secretion

Disorders of adrenal (increased production of cortisol or androgens) or thyroid function.

Urinary gonadotropin is decreased or absent.

Plasma LH <0.5 mIU/ml.

STEIN-LEVENTHAL SYNDROME (POLYCYSTIC OVARIAN DISEASE)

Serum LH is increased ~ 3 times normal (>35 mIU/ml) in approximately 60% of patients in association with normal or slightly low FSH level. Abnormally high LH/FSH ratio (>2) is more consistently abnormal than is either measurement alone. Ratio ≥ 2 is considered highly suggestive; ratio ≥ 3 is considered diagnostic.

Plasma testosterone is increased ≤ 200 μg/dl in 40–60% of cases; (>200 μg/dl usually indicates an androgen-producing tumor).

Plasma androstenedione (DHEA) is increased in up to 50% of cases.

Synthetic estrogens and progestins (as in oral contraceptives) for 21 days with before and after measurement of free testosterone and androstenedione

- Free testosterone and androstenedione decrease by 50% or become normal in LH-dependent hyperandrogenism, e.g., polycytic ovaries.
- No suppression occurs in patients with ovarian tumors or adrenal disorders.
- Change in free testosterone accounts for estrogen-caused increase in sex hormone–binding globulin that could result in unchanged or increased total testosterone level.

Approximately 85% of these patients have one or more abnormalities of serum LH/FSH ratio, testosterone, or androstenedione. Hyperandrogenism does not

Fig. 14-14. Flow chart for workup of amenorrhea. Asherman syndrome is the obliteration of endometrial lining by adhesions due to pelvic inflammatory disease, tuberculosis, postabortal or puerperal endometritis, etc. Normal blood steroid levels that do not respond to progesterone administration by bleeding. Müllerian dysgenesis is a congenital deformity or absence of tubes, uterus, or vagina; normal karyotype and hormone levels. I = increased; D = decreased; N = normal.

differentiate condition from congenital adrenal hyperplasia (CAH), but CAH is more likely if LH/FSH ratio is <2:1 and ovaries are normal in size.

Urinary 17-KS is somewhat increased (higher values occur in congenital virilizing adrenal hyperplasia and hyperadrenalism due to Cushing's syndrome). (DHEA-S is preferable to evaluate adrenal disease.) Dexamethasone administration, 0.5 mg qid for 5–7 days, causes partial suppression in cases of ovarian origin, but complete suppression suggests adrenal origin (e.g., late-onset CAH). Administration of gonadotropin increases urinary 17-KS.

Biopsy of ovary is consistent with increased androgen effect but is not specific; ovarian visualization and biopsy are not routine part of diagnosis.

Plasma cortisol, urinary 17-OHKS, and 17-KGS are normal.

Plasma prolactin is increased in ~30% of patients.

Hyperinsulinemia occurs for unknown reason; correlates with degree of increased androgens.

10–13% of these patients have partial 21-hydroxylase defects.

Increased serum LH (>35 mIU/ml), LH/FSH >2, and mild increase of ovarian androgen level are sufficient for diagnosis in presence of the symptoms and clinical signs. *Because of erratic daily fluctuations of LH and androgens, daily plasma specimens for 3–5 days may be necessary.*

If testosterone is >2 ng/ml or DHEA >7000 ng/ml, ovarian or adrenal tumor should be ruled out.

Laboratory tests may be helpful in defining pathogenesis, following course of treatment, or ruling out adrenal or ovarian tumors.

Increased serum LH with normal or decreased FSH may occur in simple obesity, hyperthyroidism, liver disease.

TURNER'S SYNDROME IN THE MALE

Biopsy of testicle reveals dysgenetic tubules with few or no germ cells.

Chromosomal pattern—46 chromosomes (XY pattern with very defective Y that is equivalent to XO)

SOME CAUSES OF ANDROGEN DEFICIENCY (HYPOGONADISM)

- Primary testicular disease
  - Acquired (e.g., chemotherapy, radiation, castration, orchitis, cryptorchidism, drugs, chronic liver or kidney disease)
  - Chromosomal (Klinefelter's syndrome, true hermaphroditism)
  - Defects in synthesis of androgens due to deficiency of various enzymes (e.g., 20-alpha-hydroxylase, 17,20-desmolase)
  - Agenesis of testicles
  - Miscellaneous (e.g., Noonan's syndrome, streak gonads, myotonia dystrophica, cystic fibrosis)
  - Defects in action of androgens (pseudohermaphroditism)
    - Complete (testicular feminization)
    - Incomplete
      - Type I (defects in testosterone receptors)
      - Type II (5-alpha-reductase deficiency)
  - Secondary to pituitary-hypothalamic disorders
    - Drugs, anorexia nervosa, malnutrition, hyperprolactinemia
    - Panhypopituitarism
    - Isolated FSH or LH deficiency
    - Hypothalamic disorders (Prader-Willi syndrome, Laurence-Moon-Biedl syndrome)

GERMINAL APLASIA

Buccal smears are normal (negative for Barr bodies).

Chromosomal pattern is normal.

Table 14-22. Serum Hormone Levels in Various Types of Androgen Deficiency

Disorder	Follicular Stimulating Hormone	Luteinizing Hormone	Testosterone
Primary testicular disease	I	I	D
Secondary to pituitary-hypothalamic disorders[a]	D	D	D
Testosterone resistance[b]	N to I	I to N	I to N
Isolated germinal cell disease	I to N	N	N

I = increased; D = decreased; N = normal.
[a]Decreased (<2-fold) or absent response of FSH and LH to administration of clomiphene (100 mg/day for 7–10 days) confirms pituitary-hypothalamic cause.
[b]Testosterone receptor defects are the most common cause of testosterone resistance; characteristic pattern is increased serum testosterone and LH.

Urinary gonadotropin is normal.
Urinary pituitary gonadotropin is increased.
17-KS is decreased.
There is azoospermia.
Biopsy of testicle shows that Sertoli's and Leydig's cells are intact and germinal cells are absent.

KLINEFELTER'S SYNDROME

(Patients have 2 or more X chromosomes.)

Buccal smears are helpful if positive for Barr bodies, but a negative does not rule out mosaicism. If negative, chromosome analysis should be performed, but in 70% of patients mosaic pattern may only occur in testes, requiring chromosomal analysis of testicular cells for definite diagnosis.
Abnormal chromosomal pattern. XY males have an extra X; 47 XXY is the classic type; 10% of patients have the mosaic form (46 XY/47 XXY); may have additional X (e.g., XXXY, XXXXY).
Biopsy of testicle shows atrophy, with hyalinized tubules lined only by Sertoli's cells, clumped Leydig's cells, and absent spermatogenesis.
Azoospermia.
Plasma testosterone levels are decreased to normal.
Plasma LH and FSH are increased; high FSH is best demarcator between normal men and Klinefelter's syndrome.
Urinary gonadotropin level is elevated.
Laboratory findings due to associated conditions, e.g., breast cancer, diabetes mellitus, thyroid dysfunction.

MALE CLIMACTERIC

Decreased testosterone level in blood (<300 ng/ml) and urine (<100 μg/day).
Urinary gonadotropin level is elevated. (Gonadotropin is decreased when low testosterone level is due to pituitary tumor, gout, or diabetes.)

OVARIAN TUMORS

Feminizing Ovarian Tumors

(e.g., granulosa cell tumor, thecoma, luteoma)

Pap smear of vagina and endometrial biopsy show high estrogen effect and no progestational activity; no signs of ovulation during reproductive phase.

Urinary FSH is decreased (inhibited by increased estrogen).

Urine 17-KS and 17-OHKS are normal.

Pregnanediol is absent.

Masculinizing Ovarian Tumors

(e.g., arrhenoblastoma, hilar cell tumors, adrenal rest tumors)

Androgen-secreting tumor of ovary or adrenal is highly likely if serum total testosterone >200 ng/dl or DHEA-S > 800 μg/dl. Localization may require androgen measurement in blood from adrenal and ovarian veins.

Pap smear of vagina shows decreased estrogen effect.

Endometrial biopsy shows moderate atrophy of endometrium.

Urine FSH (gonadotropins) is low.

Urine 17-KS is normal or may be slightly increased in arrhenoblastoma. They may be markedly increased in adrenal tumors of ovary ("masculinovoblastoma"). The higher the urine 17-KS level, the greater the likelihood of adrenocortical carcinoma; > 100 mg/24 hours is virtually diagnostic. It may be moderately increased in Leydig cell tumors.

In arrhenoblastoma there may be an increase of androsterone, testosterone, etc., excreted in urine even though the 17-KS is not much increased. Urine 17-KS, normal or slightly increased, associated with plasma testosterone in male range is almost certainly due to ovarian tumor.

In adrenal cell tumors of ovary, laboratory findings may be the same as in hyperfunction of adrenal cortex with Cushing's syndrome, etc.

In some cases there are no endocrine effects from these tumors.

Some cases of arrhenoblastoma with masculinization also show evidence of increased estrogen formation.

Struma Ovarii

About 5–10% of cases are hormone producing. Classic findings of hyperthyroidism may occur. These tumors take up radioactive iodine. *(Simple follicle cysts may also take up radioactive iodine.)*

Primary Chorionepithelioma of Ovary

Urinary chorionic gonadotropins are markedly increased.

Estrogen and progesterone secretion may be much increased.

Nonfunctioning Ovarian Tumors

Only effect may be hypogonadism due to replacement of functioning ovarian parenchyma.

Tumor Markers

(see pp. 706–711)

Serum CA-125 is useful for

- Postoperative monitoring for persistent or recurrent disease; poorer prognosis if elevated 3–6 weeks after surgery. Lower levels in patients with no residual tumor or <2 cm of residual tumor. But a negative test does not exclude residual disease.
- Rising level during chemotherapy is associated with tumor progression, and fall to normal is associated with response. Remains elevated in stable or progressive disease.

Rising level may be indication for second-look operation even in presence of normal clinical examination. Specificity = 99%, sensitivity = 46%, positive predictive value = 97% for second-look cases.

Higher levels are seen in less differentiated tumors (grade 2 and 3) and in serous cystadenocarcinoma. Not increased in mucinous adenocarcinoma.

Sequential determinations are more useful than a single test since levels in benign disease do not show significant change but progressive rise occurs in malignant disease.

Rising level may precede clinical evidence of recurrence by up to 11 months.

Not used for screening since it is negative in 20% of cases at time of diagnosis; normal level does not exclude tumor; greater elevation roughly related to poorer survival.

CA-125 is positive in 80% of cases of common epithelial tumors.

Beta-HCG is positive in almost all cases of choriocarcinoma, 10–30% of seminomas, and 5–35% of cases of dysgerminoma.

Alpha-fetoprotein is present in 80–90% of cases of endodermal sinus tumors or immature teratomas.

Carcinoembryonic antigen (CEA) is present in 50–70% of cases of serous carcinoma. CA-125/CEA ratio is much higher in serous carcinoma (>10 and often >100) than in carcinomas of breast, lung, colon, or pancreas (usually <10), which may also cause increased levels of these markers.

GERM CELL TUMORS OF OVARY AND TESTICLE

Tumor	Alpha-fetoprotein*	Beta-HCG*
Seminoma	−	+
Seminoma with syncytiotrophoblastic giant cells (STGC)	−	+
Embryonal carcinoma	+	−
Embryonal carcinoma with STGC	+	+
Yolk sac tumor	+	−
Yolk sac tumor with STGC	+	+
Choriocarcinoma	−	+
Mature teratoma	−	−

When both markers are positive, both should be assayed after therapy as recurrence or metastases may be reflected by increase of only one marker.

TESTICULAR CANCER

Increased serum HCG (>1–2 ng/ml or >5–10 mIU/ml) is found in 40–60% of patients with nonseminomatous tumors and in some patients with apparently pure seminoma. In the latter case, immunochemical staining of paraffin-embedded tumor should be performed, since isolated syncytiotrophoblastic cells may show the hormone but are not by themselves evidence of choriocarcinoma.

Increased serum alpha-fetoprotein (AFP) (>20 ng/ml) is found in 70% of patients with teratocarcinoma or embryonal carcinoma. Not increased in pure seminoma without teratomatous component.

Both markers should always be measured simultaneously. 40% of patients with nonseminomatous tumors have elevation of only one marker. 90% of patients with testicular tumors are positive for AFP or HCG or both; these are valuable for gauging efficacy of chemotherapy. 30% of patients receiving intensive chemotherapy apparently have a complete clinical remission; AFP levels may remain elevated although lower than pretreatment levels.

*See p. 208.

20–30% of patients have false negative results preoperatively despite tumor (usually microscopic) in the retroperitoneal lymph nodes. Therefore, lymphadenectomy should not be omitted simply because of normal marker levels.
Serum markers for AFP and HCG (beta chain) may be elevated in conditions other than testicular cancer.
False positive elevation of marker levels is rare.
The most important use is for follow-up after surgery or chemotherapy.
Failure of increased preoperative levels to fall after surgery suggests metastatic disease and the need for chemotherapy. Rise of levels that had previously declined to normal suggests recurrent tumor even with no other evidence of disease.
Negative markers are not useful for differential diagnosis of scrotal mass, but elevated levels indicate testicular cancer.

Laboratory Tests for Diagnosis of Disorders of Pituitary and Hypothalamus

SOMATOMEDIN-C

(used in diagnosis of acromegaly and pituitary deficiency; preferable to human growth hormone (HGH) since it is constant after eating and during the day)

Increased In

Acromegaly

Decreased In

Pituitary deficiency
Laron dwarfism
Anorexia or malnutrition. Can be used to monitor effectiveness of nutritional repletion. Is more sensitive indicator than prealbumin, transferrin index, or retinol-binding protein.

GROWTH HORMONE (HGH)

Increased In

Acromegaly and gigantism
Use of estrogens and oral contraceptives
Starvation
2 hours after sleep

Decreased In

Dwarfism
Corticosteroid therapy
Obesity

Low levels must be measured after stimulation (e.g., insulin, arginine).

PROLACTIN

See Prolactinomas, pp. 543–545.

VASOPRESSIN

Increased In

SIADH (inappropriately increased for degree of plasma osmolality)
Nephrogenic diabetes insipidus (or may be normal)

Decreased In

Central diabetes insipidus

Diseases of the Pituitary and Hypothalamus

PITUITARY TUMORS

Findings due to increased production of hormones or effect of growing mass

Most common tumors are

- Prolactin-secreting tumors, which are ~30% of all pituitary tumors (see Prolactinomas, pp. 543–545)
- Growth hormone–secreting tumors (see Acromegaly and Gigantism [next section])
- ACTH-secreting tumors (see Cushing's syndrome, pp. 499–507)
- Nonfunctioning adenomas, which may produce findings of
  - Intracranial mass especially with visual changes
  - Hypopituitarism (sometimes with impaired hypothalamic function) (see p. 545)

Microadenomas (<10 mm in size) may be present in 10–20% of the population by autopsy and x-ray studies ("incidentaloma") but >10 mm in size are quite rare.

ACROMEGALY AND GIGANTISM

Serum somatomedin-C is usually increased in untreated cases.

Serum growth hormone (GH) is increased. (Avoid stress before and during venipuncture because stress stimulates secretion of GH; should perform several random measurements.) Annual random blood GH levels, FTI, and ACTH are used for treatment follow-up.

- Fasting levels >5 ng/ml in men or >10 ng/ml in women are suggestive but not diagnostic of acromegaly.
- Most patients show a fall of <50% or even an increase 60–90 minutes after glucose (50–100 gm orally), whereas normal subjects show almost complete suppression of GH (or to <5 ng/ml) by induced hyperglycemia. This is the most reliable test. Failure to suppress GH to <2 ng/ml after oral glucose load is essential to diagnosis.
- If borderline response to hyperglycemia, perform TRH test. (500 μg TRH IV causes transient increase [>50% over basal levels] of GH in 15–30 minutes in acromegaly patients but little effect in normal persons.)
- Serum insulin-like growth factor I (IGF-I) is uniformly increased; is more precise and cost-effective screening than serum GH, since GH levels fluctuate and have short serum half-life (22 minutes).
- Growth-hormone-releasing hormone (GHRH) excess secretion (e.g., ectopic source such as pancreatic tumor or carcinoid causes <1% of acromegaly cases). Thus GHRH should be measured in all patients with acromegaly.
- All patients with acromegaly should have baseline serum prolactin measured, since up to 40% of these adenomas may secrete both prolactin and GH.
- IV ACTH administration may cause excessive increase in urine 17-KS but normal 17-OHKS excretion.
- Glucose tolerance is impaired in most patients. Mild diabetes mellitus that is insulin-resistant is found in <15% of patients.
- Adrenal virilism and increased urine 17-KS are common in women.
- Urine 17-KS, 17-KGS, and gonadotropins are usually normal or may be slightly changed but not diagnostically useful.
- Rare associated endocrinopathies are hyperthyroidism, hyperparathyroidism, pheochromocytoma, insulinoma.
- Serum phosphorus is increased for age of patient in 40% of cases.
- Serum alkaline phosphatase may be increased.
- Urine calcium is increased.
- Urine hydroxyproline is increased.
- Biopsy of costochondral junction evidences active bone growth.

CBC and ESR are normal.
In inactive cases, all secondary laboratory findings may be normal.
In late stage, panhypopituitarism may develop.

Due To

Excess GH secretion
- Pituitary adenomas, hyperplasia, or carcinoma
- Ectopic pituitary tumor (sphenoid or parapharyngeal sinus)
- Ectopic hormone production (e.g., tumor of pancreas, lung, ovary, breast)

Excess GHRH secretion
- Hypothalamic tumor (e.g., hamartoma, ganglioneuroma)
- Ectopic hormone production (e.g., carcinoid of bronchus, GI tract, pancreas; pancreatic islet cell tumor, small-cell carcinoma of lung, adrenal adenoma, pheochromocytoma)

Other Causes Of Tall Stature In Children

Klinefelter's syndrome (see p. 537)

Marfan's syndrome (inherited disorder with thin limbs, malformation of eyes and ears, medionecrosis of aorta, cardiac valve deformities, hypotonia, kyphoscoliosis)

Beckwith-Wiedemann syndrome (hypoglycemia, omphalocele, macrosomia, macroglossia)

Untreated congenital adrenal hyperplasia (see pp. 514–520)

Precocious secretion of androgens or estrogens

Obesity

PITUITARY GROWTH HORMONE (GH) DEFICIENCY

There may be isolated deficiency with dwarfism or associated with TSH deficiency, with ACTH deficiency, or with TSH and ACTH deficiencies. GH deficiency is usually due to hypothalamic GHRH deficiency.

Serum GH basal levels are decreased (<1.0 ng/ml). Use pooled or average of 3 samples. Stimulation tests have greater sensitivity. Increased basal or random serum level excludes this diagnosis, but low levels do not distinguish normal persons from GH deficiency.

Stimulation (functional) tests
- Draw serum at 0, 30, 60, 90, and 120 minutes.
- Insulin (regular crystalline, IV, 0.05–0.3 unit/kg body weight) should normally produce at least 2 times increase in serum GH level and 3 times increase in serum prolactin level at 60-minute peak. This is the most reliable challenge for GH secretion.
- Levodopa (500 mg orally) should normally produce at least 2 times increase in serum GH level at 60-minute peak.
- Arginine (0.5 gm/kg body weight as 5% solution IV over 30 minutes) should normally produce at least 3 times increase in serum GH and at least 2 times increase in serum prolactin level at 30- to 60-minute peak.
- Failure to produce the minimal responses outlined above indicates a lesion of pituitary or hypothalamus but does not differentiate between them.
- About one-fourth of patients with normal GH secretory capacity are unable to secrete GH in response to provocative tests outlined above, at any given time. Therefore, at least 2 of these tests should be used to confirm diagnosis of GH deficiency. Nonpituitary factors that impair GH response include obesity, primary hypothyroidism, thyrotoxicosis, primary hypogonadism, Kallmann's syndrome, Cushing's syndrome, use of various drugs (e.g., alpha-adrenergic antagonists, beta-adrenergic antagonists, serotonin antagonists, dopamine antagonists). Impaired GH response may even occur in presence of elevated GH basal level. Normal response may also occur in patients with partial deficiency. GH response is normal

or exaggerated in growth failure due to resistance to GH (Laron dwarfism) or resistance to somatomedins (African pygmies).

A normal response is at least 10 ng/ml peak value; 5–10 ng/ml is indeterminate, ≤5 ng/ml is subnormal. (A normal value rules out GH deficiency; in some laboratories the normal level is ≥7 ng/ml.)

Decreased fasting blood sugar (<50 mg/dl) is frequent; responds to GH therapy.

Serum phosphorus and alkaline phosphatase are decreased in prepubertal child but normal in adult-onset cases. TSH deficiency (see serum TSH and TRH stimulation tests, pp. 450–451; Hypothyroidism, pp. 456–459; and Table 14-3, p. 459)

ACTH deficiency (see p. 524)

Gonadotropins are decreased or absent from urine in postpubertal patients (but increased levels occur in primary hypogonadism).

Serum prolactin baseline level is low and does not rise appropriately after TRH or other stimulation. In hypothalamic disease, basal prolactin level is increased and response may be normal or blunted.

PROLACTINOMAS

Reference values for serum prolactin

- Normal <25 ng/ml in females; lower in males and children
- Gradual increase from birth until adolescence
- 13- to 15-year-old boys: 2.5 times adult levels
- 13- to 15-year-old girls: 3 times adult levels

Increased serum prolactin levels are found in 10–25% of women with galactorrhea and normal menses, 10–15% of women with amenorrhea without galactorrhea, 75% of women with both galactorrhea and amenorrhea/oligomenorrhea. Serum samples should be collected under basal conditions with minimal stress and by pooling 3 blood samples collected at 20-minute intervals for one assay; all drugs should be discontinued for at least 2 weeks before testing.

Repeated serum levels in late morning or early afternoon increased 3–5 times normal in men or nonlactating women are usually considered diagnostic of pituitary adenoma or rarely of hypothalamic disease or pituitary stalk section or hypothyroidism. One elevated level is not adequate for diagnosis. Normally increases sharply during sleep.

- 40–85 ng/ml: seen in craniopharyngioma, hypothyroidism, effect of drugs
- 50 ng/ml: 25% chance of a pituitary tumor
- 100 ng/ml: 50% chance of a pituitary tumor
- 200–300 ng/ml: nearly 100% chance of a pituitary tumor; >200 ng/ml may indicate a macroadenoma rather than microadenoma.
- High levels may be seen with simultaneous multiple additive factors that usually cause lesser increases (e.g., chronic renal failure plus methyldopa)
- Immediate postoperative level <7.0 ng/ml indicates long-term cure, but higher levels are associated with recurrence.

Serum Prolactin Also Increased In

Pituitary lesions (e.g., prolactinoma, section of pituitary stalk, empty-sella syndrome, 20–40% of patients with acromegaly, up to 80% of patients with chromophobe adenomas)

Other endocrine diseases (e.g., hypothyroidism [second most common cause of hyperprolactinemia], Addison's disease, polycystic ovaries)

In absence of drug ingestion, most cases of hyperprolactinemia are due to pituitary tumor, hyperplasia, or hypothyroidism. Therefore serum TSH and T-4 should always be performed to rule out compensated hypothyroidism.

Glucocorticoid excess—normal or moderately elevated
Children with sexual precocity—may be increased into pubertal range
Hypothalamic lesions (e.g., sarcoidosis, eosinophilic granuloma, histiocytosis X, tuberculosis, glioma, craniopharyngioma)
Ectopic production of prolactin (e.g., bronchogenic and renal cell carcinoma)
Neurogenic causes (e.g., nursing and breast stimulation, spinal cord lesions, chest wall lesions such as herpes zoster)
Stress (e.g., surgery, hypoglycemia, vigorous exercise)
Pregnancy (increases to 8–20 times normal by delivery, returns to normal in 2–4 weeks postpartum unless nursing occurs)
Lactation
Chronic renal failure (becomes normal after successful renal transplant but not hemodialysis)
Idiopathic causes (some probably represent early cases of microadenoma too small to be detected by CAT scan)
Drugs—most common cause
Neuroleptics (e.g., phenothiazines, thioxanthenes, butyrophenones)
Antipsychotic drugs (e.g., prochlorperazine [Compazine], chlorpromazine [Thorazine], trifluoperazine [Stelazine], thioridazine [Mellaril], haloperidol [Haldol])
Dopamine antagonists (e.g., metoclopramide, sulpiride)
Opiates (morphine, methadone)
Reserpine
Alpha-methyldopa (Aldomet)
Estrogens and oral contraceptives
Thyrotropin-releasing hormone
Amphetamines
Isoniazid

Serum Prolactin May Be Decreased In

Hypopituitarism
- Postpartum pituitary necrosis (Sheehan's syndrome)
- Idiopathic hypogonadotropic hypogonadism

Drugs
- Dopamine agonists
  - Ergot derivatives (bromocriptine mesylate, gergotrile mesylate, lisuride hydrogen maleate)
  - Levodopa, apomorphine, clonidine

Women may also present with hirsutism, infertility. Men may present with decreased libido, impotence, oligospermia, low serum testosterone levels, and sometimes galactorrhea.
Hypothyroidism
Acute fasting and chronic protein-calorie deprivation (when growth hormone often rises)

Interpretation And Usefulness

Normal value in child with growth retardation virtually rules out hypopituitarism, but a low value is not diagnostic. Single blood value may be more reliable than multiple measurements of growth hormone in diagnosis of active acromegaly.

TRH stimulation of patients with increased prolactin not due to pituitary tumors usually doubles serum prolactin level to peak >12 ng/ml in 15–30 minutes, but most patients with prolactinomas do not respond to TRH stimulation (<double baseline level). Enhanced responsiveness in hypothyroidism and blunted prolactin rise in chronic renal failure. Unresponsiveness to TRH (<2 times baseline level) also occurs in panhypopituitarism. Multiple basal prolactin levels have replaced stimulation tests for diagnosis of prolactinoma.

Microscopic examination of breast discharge shows numerous fat globules; if not seen, rule out intraductal breast carcinoma or infection.
Normal or decreased serum FSH, LH, and testosterone may occur in men.

TSH-SECRETING PITUITARY ADENOMAS

(rare type of adenoma that causes hyperthyroidism)

Laboratory findings of hyperthyroidism (see p. 454–456) except serum TSH is detectable or increased and does not respond to TRH stimulation.
Secretion of other hormones (e.g., prolactin, growth hormone) occurs in about one-third of these cases.

HYPOPITUITARISM

Due To

Hypothalamic dysfunction (see p. 546)
Pituitary disease
- Pituitary necrosis secondary to postpartum hemorrhage (Sheehan's syndrome)
- Neoplasms (e.g., craniopharyngioma, chromophobe adenoma, eosinophilic adenoma, meningioma, metastatic tumor [especially breast, lung]); prolactin-secreting tumor is the most common pituitary neoplasm.
- Granulomatous lesions (e.g., sarcoidosis, Hand-Schüller-Christian syndrome, histiocytosis X)
- Head trauma
- Infection (e.g., tuberculosis, fungi)
- Iatrogenic (e.g., hypophysectomy, radiation, section of stalk)
- Hemochromatosis
- Internal carotid artery aneurysm
- Autoimmune inflammation
- Familial pituitary deficiency (deficient hormone production or production of abnormal hormone)
- Partial growth hormone deficiency (some forms of "constitutional short stature" with delayed onset of adolescence)

End-organ resistance to growth hormone (normal or increased serum growth hormone with low somatomedin level)
- Laron dwarfs (somatomedin levels are often undetectable and fail to rise when growth hormone is administered).

Serum somatomedin-C levels are 5–15% of normal in most hypopituitary dwarfs and 4–12 times normal in all active acromegaly patients.

Endocrinologic findings: Diagnosis is based on low serum level of target organ hormone and of the corresponding pituitary stimulating hormone
- Hypogonadism
  - Men: low sperm count, low serum testosterone, inappropriately low serum LH and FSH
  - Women: low serum estradiol, inappropriately low serum LH and FSH
- Low serum T-4 and FTI, inappropriately low serum thyrotropin
- Low serum growth hormone unresponsive to provocative tests
- Low serum cortisol and ACTH
- Low serum prolactin unresponsive to provocative tests
- Usually occurs late in course of hypopituitarism except in Sheehan's syndrome in which it may be the earliest manifestation. Rarely or never due to hypothalamic disease.

  See sections on secondary insufficiency of gonads, thyroid, adrenals. Only one (usually gonadal first) or all of these may be involved.

See Diabetes Insipidus (Central), p. 547.

ANOREXIA NERVOSA

No diagnostic or typical laboratory profile; diagnosis by exclusion. Findings may be compensatory regulatory changes secondary to nutritional deprivation rather than primary hypothalamic dysfunction.

ESR is low.

Vomiting may cause hypokalemic acidosis.

Prerenal azotemia with increased BUN and serum creatinine.

Laboratory findings of hypothyroidism may be found in some patients (decreased or normal T-3 and T-4 but normal TSH; TSH response to TRH may be delayed).

Basal growth hormone levels may be elevated as in other forms of protein-calorie malnutrition; response to stimulation tests is usually normal.

Plasma prolactin level is normal.

Plasma luteinizing and follicle-stimulating hormone may be low with impaired response to LH-releasing hormone.

Adrenal function abnormalities may be found (e.g., normal or increased plasma corticoids, absence of diurnal variation of glucocorticoids, hyperresponsive ACTH test, incomplete suppression by dexamethasone, response to metyrapone may be intact or excessive, low 17-KS and 17-KGS in urine; no adrenal insufficiency).

Atrophic vaginal smear

Elevated serum carotene (>250 mg/dl) and cholesterol

Leukopenia

Anemia is unusual.

With marked loss of body weight, serum protein, potassium, and phosphorus may be decreased.

Vitamin deficiencies are rare.

DISEASES OF HYPOTHALAMUS

Due To

Neoplasms (primary or metastatic cancer, craniopharyngioma)—most frequent cause

Inflammation (e.g., tuberculosis, encephalitis)

Head trauma (e.g., basal skull fractures, gunshot wounds)

Granulomas (e.g., histiocytosis X, sarcoidosis)

Releasing hormone deficiency, genetic or idiopathic

Manifestations

Sexual abnormalities are the most frequent manifestations.

Precocious puberty

Hypogonadism (frequently as part of Fröhlich's syndrome)

Diabetes insipidus is a frequent but not an early manifestation of hypothalamic disease.

Hypopituitarism—differentiate primary hypopituitarism from this secondary form of hypopituitarism by appropriate stimulation tests.

PINEAL TUMORS

Boys—precocious puberty in 30% of patients

Girls—delayed pubescence

Diabetes insipidus occurs occasionally.

CAUSES OF HYPONATREMIAS

(see also Serum Sodium, pp. 37–39)

Isotonic

- Hyperlipidemia (plasma looks milky) "falsely" lowers serum sodium; measured serum osmolality exceeds calculated serum osmolality

$$\text{Calculated serum osmolality} = 2 \times \text{Na} + (\text{serum glucose}/18) + (\text{BUN}/2.8)$$

Hyperproteinemia (e.g., myeloma, macroglobulinemia)

Hypertonic

Hyperglycemia (each increase of blood sugar of 100 mg/dl decreases serum sodium by 1.7 mEq/L)

Excess mannitol treatment

Hypotonic

Hypervolemic usually with clinical edema

With low urine sodium (<10 mEq/L) may be due to congestive heart failure, cirrhosis with ascites, nephrotic syndrome.

With high urine sodium (>20 mEq/L) may be due to acute tubular necrosis or end-stage chronic renal failure where Na and H_2O intake exceeds excretion. Serum uric acid and BUN tend to be increased.

Hypovolemic

Urine sodium <10 mEq/L. Due to extrarenal loss of sodium (e.g., GI tract, fistulas, pancreatitis, exercise, sweating, burns).

Urine sodium >20 mEq/L. Due to renal loss of sodium (e.g., diuretics such as furosemide or osmotic diuresis due to glucose or urea, diabetic ketoacidosis, renal tubular acidosis, salt-losing nephritis, adrenal insufficiency, hyporeninemia, hypoaldosteronism.)

Normovolemic—usually no edema is present.

Large amounts of sodium appear in urine (>20 mEq/L). May be due to SIADH, hypothyroidism, hypopituitarism, low reset osmostat syndrome, physical or emotional stress, potassium depletion, renal failure, water poisoning, certain drugs (e.g., ADH analogues, amitriptyline, carbamazepine, chlorpropamide, cyclophosphamide, diuretics, haloperidol, thioridazine, vincristine).

Hyponatremic patients with BUN <10 mg/dl and uric acid <3.0 mg/dl should be considered to have SIADH or reset osmostat until proved otherwise.

Pseudohyponatremia when sodium is measured with flame photometer rather than ion-selective electrode. May be secondary to hyperlipidemia, hyperproteinemia, increased concentration of osmotically active substances (e.g., glucose in absence of insulin, mannitol). Serum osmolality is normal.

"ESSENTIAL" HYPERNATREMIA

(see also Serum Sodium, pp. 37–39)

This condition is due to a hypothalamic lesion (e.g., infiltration of histiocytes, neoplasm) that causes impaired osmotic regulation but intact volume regulation of antidiuretic hormone secretion.

Serum sodium shows sustained but fluctuating elevations, corrected by administration of antidiuretic hormone but not corrected by fluid administration.

Serum osmolality is increased.

Serum creatinine, BUN, and creatinine clearance are normal.

There is spontaneous excretion of random specimens of urine that may be very concentrated or very dilute and opposite to plasma osmolality.

DIABETES INSIPIDUS (CENTRAL)

Due To

Idiopathic (now causes <50% of cases)

Heredity (causes ~1% of cases)

Supra- and intrasellar tumors

Histiocytosis X (eosinophilic granuloma) is most common.

Neoplasms (e.g., craniopharyngioma, metastatic carcinoma of breast, cyst)

Granulomatous lesions (e.g., sarcoidosis, tuberculosis)

Table 14-23. Comparison of Hyponatremia Due To Various Causes

Cause	Urine Sodium	Urine Osmolarity	BUN
Hypervolemic (e.g., congestive heart failure, cirrhosis, nephrotic syndrome) Early	D (usually < 10–15 mEq/L)	I (usually > 350–400 mOsm/L)	N
Late	D with isotonic urine is ominous finding	(> 200 mmol/kg)	I disproportionate to creatinine
Hypovolemic Extrarenal Gastrointestinal Skin (burns, sweat) Third space	D (< 10 mEq/L)	I (> 400 mOsm/L)	N
Renal Diuretic (most common) Chronic renal disease (especially interstitial) Mineralocorticoid deficiency	I (> 20 mEq/L)	Isotonic to plasma If severe volume contraction, 300–450 mOsm/kg	Usually I
Normovolemic SIADH (almost always) (see p. 551)	I (> 20 mmol/L)	I (> 200 mmol/kg) D in plasma	Often D (< 8–10 mg/dl)
Reset osmostat (see p. 549)	V	V	V (N or D)

I = increased; D = decreased; V = variable.

Trauma, with or without basal skull fracture; neurosurgical procedures
Vascular lesions (e.g., aneurysms, thrombosis)
Infectious (e.g., meningitis, encephalitis)
Others (e.g., hypoxemic encephalopathy)

Urine is inappropriately dilute (low specific gravity [usually <1.005] and osmolality [50–200 mOsm/kg]) in presence of increased serum osmolality (295 mOsm/kg) and increased or normal serum sodium.
Large urine volume (4–15 L/24 hours) is characteristic.
Plasma vasopressin level is decreased.
Dehydration test fails to increase urine specific gravity or osmolality, and serum osmolality remains elevated. After administration of vasopressin, urine osmolality will double.
Partial central diabetes insipidus shows intermediate values between complete central and normal.

See Table 14-24, p. 550.

NEPHROGENIC DIABETES INSIPIDUS

Due To

Chronic renal failure (e.g., glomerulonephritis, pyelonephritis, gout, analgesic nephropathy, polycystic kidneys, nephrosclerosis)
Diuretic phase of acute tubular necrosis
Following renal transplant or relief of urinary tract obstruction
Primary hyperaldosteronism
Sickle cell anemia
Hypergammaglobulinemia (e.g., multiple myeloma, amyloidosis, Sjögren's syndrome)
Drugs (e.g., lithium, demeclocycline)
Prolonged potassium depletion and hypokalemia (condition is reversed by restoring potassium level to normal).
Prolonged hypercalciuria, usually with hypercalcemia (condition is reversed by restoring the calcium level to normal).
Hereditary renal tubular unresponsiveness to vasopressin due to X-linked genetic defect; severe form occurs in males; family history of this condition is frequent.

Laboratory findings are the same as in hypophyseal (central) diabetes insipidus except that nephrogenic type shows
- Normal or increased plasma vasopressin level
- Dehydration test does not cause urine osmolality to rise above plasma osmolality.
- Dehydration test causes the plasma vasopressin level to increase.
- Urine osmolality does not rise with subsequent injection of vasopressin.

See Table 14-23, p. 548.

DIABETES INSIPIDUS DUE TO HIGH-SET OSMORECEPTOR

This is a rare entity in which the set point for stimulating release of ADH is ≥ 300 mOsm/kg instead of the normal 285 mOsm/kg level.
As plasma osmolality rises, patient becomes thirsty and drinks fluids, thereby diluting the plasma before it reaches the higher set level to stimulate release of ADH, initiating cycle of polyuria and polydipsia. If thirst center is also impaired, patient develops essential hypernatremia (see p. 547).

Plasma osmolality after dehydration is significantly higher than in normal state.
Urine osmolality does not change after administration of vasopressin.

Table 14-24. Comparison of Different Types of Diabetes Insipidus

	After Dehydration[a]				
	Urine Specific Gravity	Urine Osmolality (mOsm/kg)	Plasma Osmolality (mOsm/kg)	After Pitressin,[b] Urine Osmolality (% change)	Plasma Vasopressin (pg/ml)
Normal	≧ 1.015	700–1400	288–291	No change (< 5%)	1.3–4.1
Central diabetes insipidus (complete)	< 1.010	50–200	310–320	Doubles (> 100%)[c]	< 1.1
Central diabetes insipidus (partial)	1.010–1.015	250–500	295–305	Increases (9–67%)[c]	
Nephrogenic diabetes insipidus	< 1.010	100–200	310–320	No change[d]	12–13 (> 2.7 in high Ca/low K type)
"High-set" osmoreceptor diabetes insipidus	≧ 1.015	700–1400	300–305	No change	
Primary (psychogenic) polydipsia		700–1200		No change after medullary washout; normal increase after high sodium diet	3.0–7.5

[a]Dehydration test: No fluid intake for 4–18 hours, measure urine osmolality and/or specific gravity hourly, weigh patient (or urine) frequently to avoid loss of >3% of body weight *(if >3% of body weight, measure plasma and urine osmolality, and terminate test to avoid hypotension)*. If 3 successive hourly urine osmolality determinations indicate no further change (i.e., have reached a plateau), administer 5 units of vasopressin (Pitressin) subcutaneously, and 60 minutes later, measure urine osmolality.

[b]1 hour after subcutaneous injection of 5 units of aqueous Pitressin.

[c]Useful to distinguish partial from complete central diabetes insipidus.

[d]Therefore differs from diabetes insipidus.

Plasma vasopressin levels must always be interpreted relative to plasma osmolality.

PSYCHOGENIC POLYDIPSIA

Excessive intake of water causes loss of medullary sodium and urea to renal venous blood and abnormally reduced tonicity of renal medulla.

Should be suspected when large volumes of very dilute urine occur with plasma osmolality that is only slightly decreased or low normal.

Test dose of vasopressin often shows failure to concentrate urine, simulating nephrogenic diabetes insipidus. However, the test will be normal when performed after restoration of normal hypertonicity of renal medulla by a period of high-sodium and low-water intake.

Fluid deprivation test is least reliable in differentiating this from partial central diabetes insipidus; e.g., some increase in urine osmolality after dehydration with an inconclusive (~10%) further increase after vasopressin may be due to either condition.

SYNDROME OF INAPPROPRIATE SECRETION OF ANTIDIURETIC HORMONE (SIADH)

(syndrome of continuing release of vasopressin in presence of low plasma osmolality)

Decreased serum sodium and osmolality (usually <280 mOsm/kg) when urine is not at maximum dilution; this is basis for diagnosis in patient with no evidence of cardiac, liver, kidney, adrenal, pituitary, thyroid disease, or hypovolemia and not on drug therapy (especially diuretics)

Increased urine sodium (>20 mmol/L) with inappropriately high urine osmolality (>500 mOsm/kg) is essential for diagnosis since it excludes hypovolemia as the cause of hyponatremia (in absence of abnormal renal function or causative drugs)

Increased urine osmolality > serum osmolality

Normal serum potassium, CO_2, BUN, and creatinine

Decreased serum chloride

Decreased anion gap

Decreased uric acid (due to dilution)

Increased plasma vasopressin that is inappropriately elevated for the degree of plasma osmolality

Clinical and biochemical response to fluid restriction but not to administration of isotonic or hypertonic saline

Due To

CNS disease of all types (e.g., neoplastic, degenerative, infective, trauma, vascular, psychogenic)

Advanced endocrinopathies (e.g., myxedema, ACTH deficiency, adrenal insufficiency)

Neoplasms (most commonly oat cell carcinoma of lung; adenocarcinoma of lung, carcinoma of pancreas, carcinoma of duodenum, lymphoma), some of which show ectopic production of ADH

Pulmonary infection (e.g., tuberculosis, pneumonia, chronic infections, aspergillosis)

Miscellaneous (e.g., acute intermittent porphyria, postoperative state)

Idiopathic

Various drugs

- Oral hypoglycemic agents (chlorpropamide, tolbutamide, phenformin, metformin)
- Antineoplastic agents (vincristine, cyclophosphamide)
- Diuretics (chlorothiazide)
- Sedatives, analgesics (morphine, barbiturates, acetaminophen)
- Psychotropic drugs (amitriptyline, phenothiazines)
- Miscellaneous (clofibrate, isoproterenol, nicotine)

NONENDOCRINE NEOPLASMS CAUSING ENDOCRINE SYNDROMES

(Tumors secrete proteins, polypeptides, or glycoproteins that have hormonal activity. Diagnosed by arteriovenous gradient of hormone across tumor bed or between tumor and nontumor tissue. Confirm by in vitro demonstration of hormone production by tumor cells and by resolution of endocrine syndrome after successful removal of tumor.)

Cushing's syndrome*
- Bronchogenic oat cell carcinoma (causes ~50% of cases) and carcinoid
- Thymoma
- Hepatoma
- Carcinoma of ovary
- Also medullary carcinoma of thyroid, islet-cell tumor of pancreas, etc.

Hypercalcemia simulating hyperparathyroidism (see Humoral Hypercalcemia of Malignancy, p. 471, and Table 14-7, p. 474)
- Renal carcinoma
- Squamous and large-cell carcinoma of respiratory tract
- Carcinoma of breast (occurs in 15% of patients with bone metastases)
- Malignant lymphoma, myeloma, etc.
- Cancer of ovary, pancreas, etc.

SIADH (see preceding section)
- Especially with oat cell carcinoma of lung

Hypoglycemia—serum insulin is low in presence of fasting hypoglycemia.
- Not associated with decreased serum phosphorus as in insulin-induced hypoglycemia.
- Bronchogenic carcinoma
- Carcinoma of adrenal cortex (6% of patients)
- Hepatoma (23% of patients)
- Retroperitoneal fibrosarcoma (most frequently)

Thyrotoxicosis—signs and symptoms are rare, but laboratory findings are present.
- Tumors of GI tract, hematopoietic, pulmonary, etc.
- Trophoblastic tumors in women
- Choriocarcinoma of testis

Precocious puberty in boys
- Hepatoma

Acromegaly
- Pancreatic tumors producing growth hormone or growth-hormone-releasing factor in presence of normal sella, elevated growth hormone not suppressed by glucose.
- Carcinoid

Erythrocytosis (due to erythropoietin production)
- Carcinoma of kidney, liver
- Fibromyoma of uterus
- Cerebellar hemangioblastoma

See also Carcinoid Syndrome (next section), Secondary Polycythemia (pp. 322–323), Syndrome of Inappropriate Secretion of Antidiuretic Hormone (p. 551).

*Increased blood ACTH level (>200 pg/ml), inability to suppress with high-dose dexamethasone test (except in bronchial carcinoids), loss of diurnal variation of cortisol levels (usually >40 μg/dl). Therefore cannot be distinguished from excessive pituitary secretion of ACTH by use of dexamethasone suppression test. Typically malignant disease causing ectopic ACTH production has acute effects on adrenals manifested predominantly by excess mineralocorticoid production with hypokalemia and hypertension. May sometimes require selective venous catheterization for ACTH levels or in vitro hybridization assay to demonstrate ACTH-encoding messenger RNA to establish the diagnosis. Patients with lung cancer may have elevated ACTH levels without Cushing's syndrome.

CARCINOID SYNDROME

The syndrome in malignant carcinoids (argentaffinomas) includes flushing, diarrhea, bronchospasm, endocardial fibrosis, bronchospasm, arthropathy, glucose intolerance, hypotension. Liver metastases are present in 95% of cases with syndrome except in lung and ovary primary sites.

Urinary level of 5-hydroxyindoleacetic acid (5-HIAA) (a metabolite of serotonin) is increased (>9 mg/24 hours in patient without malabsorption or >30 mg/24 hours with malabsorption; normal <6 mg/24 hours) in 75% of cases, usually when tumor is far advanced (i.e., large liver metastases), but may not be increased despite massive metastases. Useful in diagnosis in only 5–7% of patients with a carcinoid tumor but in ~45% of those with liver metastases. Disease extent and prognosis correlates generally with urine 5-HIAA excretion. May also be increased in Whipple's disease and nontropical sprue; small increases may occur in pregnancy, ovulation, after surgical stress. Increased by various foods (e.g., pineapples, kiwi, bananas, eggplant, plums, tomatoes, avocados, walnuts, pecans, hickory nuts) and drugs (see p. 743). If urine HIAA is normal, check blood level of serotonin or a precursor, 5-hydroxytryptophan.

Blood serotonin may be increased (>0.4 μg/ml).

Platelet serotonin and urine serotonin are increased in 64% of cases.

Some tumors produce histamine, ACTH, gastrin, and bradykinin.

VMA and catecholamine levels in urine are normal.

Laboratory findings due to other aspects of carcinoid syndrome (may include pulmonary valvular stenosis, tricuspid valvular insufficiency, heart failure, liver metastases, electrolyte disturbances).

Nonfunctioning tumors can only be diagnosed by histologic examination.

Some patients may have decreased serum albumin and pellagra (due to diversion of tryptophan to synthesis of serotonin).

MULTIPLE ENDOCRINE NEOPLASIA (MEN SYNDROME)

MEN I (Werner's syndrome)

Hyperparathyroidism (due to hyperplasia or adenoma) in >80% of patients is usual presenting feature; associated renal and bone disease are infrequent. 15% of cases of hyperparathyroidism have MEN; frequently multicentric. 10% of parathyroid tumor patients have relatives with MEN.

Islet cell tumors in >75% of patients; most are functional; usually multiple.
- Gastrinomas with Zollinger-Ellison syndrome occur in ~50% of cases, and ~50% are malignant. 50% of cases of Z-E syndrome have MEN I.
- Insulinomas (beta cells) in ~25% of MEN I patients; usually benign; multiple foci are common.
- Glucagonoma (alpha cells) syndrome of distinctive rash, diabetes mellitus, anemia, weight loss
- Vipomas occur less often (see p. 492).

Pituitary adenomas in >70–80% of cases
- Nonfunctional chromophobe adenomas causing hypopituitarism due to space-occupying effect may be most common.
- ~15% are prolactinomas.
- ~15% are eosinophilic adenomas causing acromegaly.
- ~5% are basophilic adenomas causing Cushing's syndrome.

Adrenal cortical adenomas or hyperplasia in ~40% of cases is incidental and nonfunctional. Adrenal medulla is not involved.

Thyroid disease in ~20% of cases includes benign and malignant tumors, colloid goiter, thyrotoxicosis, Hashimoto's disease.

Uncommon lesions include carcinoids, schwannomas, multiple lipomas, gastric polyps, testicular tumors.

MEN II (or IIa) (SIPPLE'S SYNDROME)

Medullary thyroid carcinoma in >90% of cases is usually multicentric and preceded by C-cell hyperplasia (thereby differing from sporadic type). Produce

calcitonin and sometimes ACTH or serotonin. 25% of these carcinomas occur as part of MEN II. May be asymptomatic but lethal.
Pheochromocytoma in >70% of cases; usually bilateral, often multiple, and may be extra-adrenal. 10% of these tumors occur as part of MEN.
Hyperparathyroidism due to hyperplasia in >50% of cases; occurs late in disease; may occur without medullary thyroid carcinoma.

MEN III (or IIb)
(features in common with MEN II but is a separate genetic syndrome)
Medullary thyroid carcinoma in 75% of cases
Pheochromocytoma in 33% of cases
Hyperparathyroidism is rare (<5% of cases).
Other lesions:
  Multiple mucosal gangliomas in >95% of cases appear early in life.
  Marfan's syndrome habitus, hypertrophy of corneal nerves, ganglioneuromas of GI tract, characteristic retinal changes, and facial appearance are frequent.

All first-order relatives of MEN patients should have appropriate serial testing.

AUTOIMMUNE POLYGLANDULAR SYNDROMES

Type I
(commonly occurs during early childhood; appears as autosomal recessive; often affects siblings; not associated with any major histocompatibility complex)
Requires ≥2 of the following
  Hypoparathyroidism
  Addison's disease
  Chronic mucocutaneous candidiasis
Patient may also have
  Insulin-dependent diabetes
  Premature hypogonadism
  Celiac disease
  Pernicious anemia
  Vertiligo
  Alopecia

Type II
(commonly occurs in early adults through middle age; appears in multiple generations; autosomal dominant; associated with B8 and DR3 major histocompatibility complexes)
Requires ≥2 of the following
  Addison's disease
  Graves' disease
  Primary hypothyroidism
  Insulin-dependent diabetes
  Premature hypogonadism
Patient may also have
  Celiac disease
  Pernicious anemia
  Myasthenia gravis
  Vertiligo
  Alopecia

Genitourinary Diseases

Renal Function Tests

URINE CONCENTRATION TEST

Restrict water intake for 14–16 hours; then collect three urine specimens at 1-, 2-, and 4-hour intervals, and measure specific gravity.

Normal: Urine specific gravity is ≥1.025.

With decreased renal function, specific gravity is <1.020. As renal impairment is more severe, specific gravity approaches 1.010.

The test is sensitive for early loss of renal function, but a normal finding does not necessarily rule out active kidney disease.

The test is unreliable in the presence of any severe water and electrolyte imbalance (e.g., adrenal cortical insufficiency, edema formation), low-protein or low-salt diet, chronic liver disease, pregnancy, lack of patient cooperation.

Fluid deprivation may be contraindicated in heart disease or early renal failure.

VASOPRESSIN (PITRESSIN) CONCENTRATION TEST

The bladder is emptied, and urine is collected 1 and 2 hours after subcutaneous injection of 10 units of vasopressin. Water intake is not restricted, but no diuretics should be administered.

Normal: The specific gravity should reach ≥1.020.

Interpretation is the same as in the urine concentration test.

In diabetes insipidus, urine specific gravity becomes normal after vasopressin administration but not after fluid restriction.

The test may be used in the presence of edema or ascites. It is contraindicated in coronary artery disease and pregnancy.

See Diabetes Insipidus, pp. 547–550.

URINE OSMOLALITY

Measurement of urine osmolality during water restriction is an accurate, sensitive test of decreased renal function.

The patient is on a high-protein diet for 3 days; has a dry supper and no fluids on the evening before the test; empties the bladder at 6 A.M., discards urine, and returns to bed. Test urine specimen is collected at 8 A.M.

Normal: concentration of >800 mOsm/kg

Minimal impairment of renal concentrating ability: 600–800 mOsm/kg

Moderate impairment: 400–600 mOsm/kg

Severe impairment: <400 mOsm/kg

Urine osmolality may be impaired when other tests are normal (Fishberg concentration test, serum urea nitrogen [BUN], phenolsulfonphthalein [PSP] excretion, creatinine clearance, IV pyelogram); may be especially useful in diabetes mellitus, essential hypertension, silent pyelonephritis.

It may be well also to measure serum osmolality and calculate urine-serum ratio (normal > 3).

See Diabetes Insipidus, pp. 547–550.

URINE DILUTION TEST

No breakfast is allowed; 1500 ml of water is taken within 30–45 minutes, and urine is collected every hour for 4 hours.

Normal: Urine volume is >80% of ingested amount (1200 ml).

Specific gravity is 1.003 in at least one specimen.

With decreased renal function there is a smaller volume of urine.

Specific gravity may not fall below 1.010.

Loss of dilution ability occurs later than loss of concentrating ability.

Water loading may be contraindicated in kidney and heart disease.

PHENOLSULFONPHTHALEIN (PSP) EXCRETION TEST

Administer an IV injection of 1 mg/kg body weight or usually 6 mg in 1-ml volume. Collect urine and (sometimes) blood samples at 15-, 30-, and 60-minute intervals.

Normal > 25% in urine in 15 minutes; 55–75% in 2 hours

The test is useful to detect slight to moderate decrease in renal function. It is not useful in chronic azotemia with fixed specific gravity (serum creatinine and creatinine clearance are more useful then).

It is hazardous in severe renal insufficiency or heart failure because adequate prior hydration is required to obtain sufficient urine volume. Using small urine volume magnifies errors.

The test is distorted by residual bladder urine, abnormal drainage sites (e.g., fistulas), and interfering substances (e.g., hematuria).

Hepatic disease may give falsely elevated values (because 20% of the dye is normally removed by the liver). False results may also occur in multiple myeloma (because of excessive protein binding) and in hypoalbuminemia. Certain drugs may interfere with PSP excretion (e.g., salicylates, penicillin, some diuretic and uricosuric drugs, and some x-ray contrast media).

The 15-minute PSP excretion correlates with the glomerular filtration rate (GFR); a normal 15-minute value indicates normal GFR. Progressive decrease of 15-minute value is proportional to decreased GFR (e.g., 15% PSP excretion in 15 minutes approximates a 45% GFR). If the GFR is normal, the PSP test indicates renal blood flow or tubular function; there are better tests available for measuring these two functions, and the PSP test is now rarely used.

Increased dye excretion in later time periods compared to the initial 15-minute period suggests increased residual urine due to obstructive uropathy or incomplete bladder emptying; the latter can be ruled out by indwelling catheterization during the test.

PSP that is normal with increased BUN and serum creatinine and decreased GFR suggests acute glomerulonephritis. PSP parallels these parameters in most chronic renal diseases.

GLOMERULAR FILTRATION RATE (GFR)

(See standard laboratory texts for information on the technical performance of clearance tests.)

Elderly patients with a normal serum creatinine and diminished muscle mass may have a 30% decrease in GFR.

GFR is measured with urea clearance, creatinine clearance, or inulin clearance.

Normal Clearances (corrected to 1.73 sq m body surface area)
Endogenous creatinine*

Age	Mean creatinine clearance (ml/min/1.73 sq m body surface area)		
(years)	Males	Females†	Both males and females
0–1			72
1			45
2			55
3			60
4			71
5			73
6			64
7			67
8			72
9			83
10			89
11			92
12			109
13–14			86
20–29	94–140	72–110	
30–39	59–137	71–121	
40–49	76–120	50–102	
50–59	67–109	50–102	
60–69	54–98	45–75	
70–79	49–79	37–61	
80–89	30–60	27–55	
90–99	26–44	26–42	

Inulin‡

Males	110–150 ml/minute
Females	105–132 ml/minute

Urea§

Maximum	60–100 ml/minute
Standard	40–65 ml/minute

Estimate of creatinine clearance from single serum creatinine clearance may be required for prompt therapy of nephrotoxic drug reaction or because of

*The creatinine clearance test, particularly serial measurements, is the most reliable test of renal function; is independent of rate of urine flow. After baseline urine creatinine has been obtained, serum creatinine levels can be used to calculate clearance. Creatinine clearance overestimates GFR when GFR is <5–10% of normal; in these cases should average with urea clearance, which underestimates GFR. Is excreted by tubules as well as filtered by glomeruli and therefore may overestimate GFR; but is widely used and best measurement of GFR in most clinical instances. Low concentration of creatinine in serum of infants and young children makes laboratory test difficult and inaccurate.

†Data from J Kampmann, et al., Rapid evaluation of creatinine clearance. *Acta Med Scand* 196:517, 1974.

‡Normal inulin clearance = 25–30 ml/minute during first few days of life; ~50–60 ml/minute by end of first month. Adult values by 12–18 months. Considerable individual variation makes interpretation difficult unless clearly abnormal. Is best determinant of GFR but requires continuous infusion to maintain adequate blood concentration during test.

§Urea clearance: marked variability in contributing factors (e.g., BUN, diet, urine flow) makes interpretation difficult and not useful in most clinical situations.

Table 15-1. Laboratory Guide to Evaluation of Renal Impairment

Condition	Renal Clearance of Endogenous Creatinine[a] (glomerular filtration rate)	Urinary Excretion of IV PSP[b] in 15 Minutes (renal tubular transport mechanisms)
Normal	Men: 130–200 L/24 hours (90–139 ml/min)	$\geqq$25%
	Women: 115–180 L/24 hours (80–125 ml/min)	
Slight impairment	75–90 L/24 hours (52.0–62.5 ml/min)	15–25%
Mild impairment	60–75 L/24 hours (42–52 ml/min)	10–15%
Moderate impairment	40–60 L/24 hours (28–42 ml/min)	5–10%
Marked impairment	<40 L/24 hours (<28 ml/min)	<5%

[a] Creatinine clearance is normally less in women than men, and it usually decreases with age, starting at age 20.
[b] Phenolsulfonphthalein.

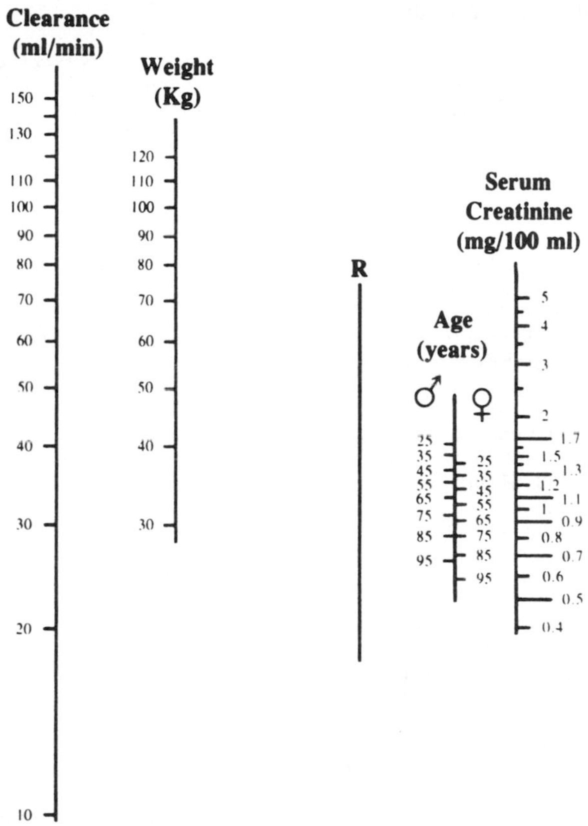

Fig. 15-1. Nomogram for rapid estimation of endogenous creatinine clearance. With a straightedge, join weight to age. Keep straightedge at crossing point of line marked "R." Then move the right-hand side of the straightedge to the appropriate serum creatinine value and read the patient's clearance from the left side of the nomogram. (From GB Appel and HC Neu, Antimicrobial agents in patients with renal disease. *Medical Times* 105(9):116, Sept. 1977.)

difficulty of accurate 24-hour urine collection. This *estimate* may be obtained by the following formulas or by the nomogram in Fig. 15-1.

$$\text{GFR} = \frac{(140 - \text{age in years})(\text{weight in kg})}{72 \times \text{serum creatinine}}$$

(Values for women are 85% of predicted.)

$$\text{Creatinine clearance (ml/min/1.73 sq m)} = \frac{(98 - 0.8) \times (\text{age} - 20)}{\text{serum creatinine}}$$

(Values for women are 90% of predicted.)

Equation may only be accurate in patients with stable renal function who are not massively obese or edematous.

Impairment may be more severe than indicated by laboratory studies if signs and symptoms are more disabling.

Usually there is good correlation between urine concentrating function and GFR. A normal GFR in association with impaired concentrating ability may be found in sickle cell anemia, diabetes insipidus, nephronophthisis, and various acquired disorders (e.g., pyelonephritis, potassium deficiency, hypercalciuria).

OTHER RENAL FUNCTION TESTS

Measure Effective Plasma Flow (RPF) And Tubular Function

Para-aminohippurate (PAH)
- Males 560–800 ml/minute
- Females 500–700 ml/minute

Diodrast 600–800 ml/minute

Filtration fraction (FF) = GFR/RPF
- Males 17–21%
- Females 17–23%

Maximal Diodrast excretory capacity, TmD
- Males 43–59 mg/minute
- Females 33–51 mg/minute

Urea clearance is normal until >50% of renal parenchyma is inactivated. With renal insufficiency, the clearance test parallels the parenchymal destruction.

Urinary acidification is impaired in chronic renal disease with azotemia. It is decreased without parallel impairment of GFR in renal tubular acidosis, some cases of Fanconi's syndrome, and some cases of acquired nephrocalcinosis.

Proximal tubular malfunction is indicated by urinary excretion of substances normally reabsorbed by tubules: in renal glycosuria (blood glucose <180 mg/dl as in Fanconi's syndrome, heavy metal poisoning), aminoaciduria, phosphaturia.

Serum creatinine and BUN are not useful in discovering early renal insufficiency because they do not become abnormal until 50% of renal function has been lost.

Serum creatinine increase occurs in 10–20% of patients taking aminoglycosides and up to 20% of patients taking penicillins (especially methicillin).

SPLIT RENAL FUNCTION TESTS

(for aid in diagnosis of renal artery stenosis)

Affected kidney shows decreased urine volume and sodium excretion and decreased urine concentration of creatinine, inulin, or PAH.

These tests are not useful in presence of GU tract obstruction (e.g., in men over age 50).

Kidney Diseases

RENAL TUBULAR ACIDOSIS

(Glomerular function is either normal or relatively less impaired.)

Primary Proximal Renal Tubular Acidosis

Usually occurs in males

Only clinical manifestation is retarded growth; renal and metabolic complications are absent.

Good prognosis with clinical response to alkali therapy, which is usually not permanently required

Table 15-2. Differentiation of Distal and Proximal Renal Tubular Acidosis

	Distal (type 1)	Proximal (type 2)
Hypokalemia	Severe	Mild–moderate
Response to K^+ therapy	Good	Poor
Bicarbonate Tm	Normal	Decreased
Bicarbonate loss in urine	Small	Large
Serum bicarbonate concentration	May be very low (< 16 mEq/L)	Usually > 16–18 mEq/L
Urine pH when serum HCO_3^-:		
>20 mEq/L	> 5.5	> 5.5
< 15 mEq/L	> 5.5	May be < 5.4
Amount of HCO_3^- needed to correct acidosis	< 2 mEq/kg/day	> 5 mEq/kg/day
Response to alkali therapy	Good	Poor
Glycosuria	Absent	Often present
Aminoaciduria	Absent	Often present
Hypercalciuria	Often present	Usually absent
Urinary citrate	Low	Normal
Fanconi's syndrome	No	Yes
Nephrocalcinosis	Often present	Rare
Nephrolithiasis	Often present	Absent
Renal insufficiency	Often present	Absent
Bone disease	Often present	Absent

Caused by defect in bicarbonate reabsorption

- Low plasma bicarbonate concentration with hyperchloremic acidosis
- Alkaline urine that becomes acid if extracellular bicarbonate level is decreased below the patient's maximum reabsorptive limit
- Normal urine pH in the absence of bicarbonate in the urine

Secondary Proximal Renal Tubular Acidosis May Be Due To

Idiopathic or secondary Fanconi's syndrome (cystinosis, Lowe's syndrome, tyrosinemia, glycogen storage disease, Wilson's disease, hereditary fructose intolerance, heavy-metal intoxication, toxic effect of drugs such as outdated tetracycline)

Vitamin D–deficient rickets

Medullary cystic disease

Following renal transplantation

Nephrotic syndrome, multiple myeloma, renal amyloidosis

Primary Distal Renal Tubular Acidosis
(Butler-Albright syndrome)

Occurs predominantly in females (70%)

Often presents with complications (e.g., nephrocalcinosis, renal calculi, rickets, and osteomalacia) as well as growth retardation

Caused by inability of tubular cell to secrete enough H^+

- Hyperchloremic acidosis, hypokalemia, low plasma bicarbonate concentration

Alkaline urine (pH 6.5–7.0) that persists at any level of plasma bicarbonate
Ammonium loading test shows inability to acidify urine below pH 6.5 and depressed rates of excretion of titratable acid and ammonium.
Absence of other tubular defects
Laboratory findings due to complications (e.g., nephrocalcinosis, nephrolithiasis, interstitial nephritis)

Secondary Distal Tubular Acidosis May Also Be Due To

Increased serum globulins (especially gamma) (e.g., systemic lupus erythematosus [SLE], Sjögren's syndrome, Hodgkin's disease, sarcoidosis, chronic active hepatitis, cryoglobulinemia)
Potassium depletion nephropathy
Pyelonephritis
Medullary sponge kidney
Ureterosigmoidostomy
Hereditary insensitivity to antidiuretic hormone (vasopressin)
Various renal diseases (e.g., obstructive uropathy, hypercalcemia, potassium-losing disorders, medullary cystic disease, polyarteritis nodosa, amyloidosis, Sjögren's syndrome)
A variety of genetically transmitted disorders (e.g., Ehlers-Danlos syndrome, Fabry's disease, hereditary elliptocytosis)
Starvation, malnutrition
Hyperthyroidism
Hyperparathyroidism
Vitamin D intoxication

An incomplete or mixed tubular acidosis may be seen in obstructive uropathy and in hereditary fructose intolerance.

Type 4 Renal Tubular Acidosis (a variety of conditions) Is Characterized By

Mild to moderate renal impairment
Hyperchloremic acidosis
*Hyper*kalemia
Acid urine pH
Reduced ammonium secretion
Frequently, tendency to lose sodium in urine
Some patients have decreased mineralocorticoid secretion due to isolated hypoaldosteronism; others have decreased tubular response to aldosterone.

ACUTE RENAL FAILURE

Early Stage

Urine is scant in volume (often < 50 ml/day) for ≤2 weeks; anuria for >24 hours is unusual. Urine usually bloody (because RBCs and protein are present, specific gravity may be high). Urine sodium concentration is usually >50 mEq/L.
WBC is increased even without infection.
BUN rises ≤20 mg/dl/day in transfusion reaction. It rises ≤50 mg/dl/day in overwhelming infection of severe crushing injuries.
Serum creatinine is increased.
Hypocalcemia may occur.
Disproportionately increased serum phosphorus and creatinine indicate tissue necrosis.
Serum amylase and lipase may be increased without evidence of pancreatitis.
Metabolic acidosis is present.

Second Week

Urine becomes clear several days after onset of acute renal failure, and there is a small daily increase in volume. Daily volume of 400 ml indicates onset of tubular recovery. Daily volume of 1000 ml occurs in several days or ≤2 weeks. RBCs and large hematin casts are present. Protein is slight or absent.

Azotemia increases. BUN continues to rise for several days after onset of diuresis.

Metabolic acidosis increases.

Serum potassium is increased (because of tissue injury, failure of urinary excretion, acidosis, dehydration, etc.). ECG changes are always found when serum potassium is >9 mEq/L but are rarely found when it is <7 mEq/L.

Serum sodium is often decreased, with increased extracellular fluid volume.

Anemia usually appears during second week.

Bleeding tendency is frequent, with decreased platelets, abnormal prothrombin consumption, etc.

Diuretic Stage

Large urinary potassium excretion may cause decreased serum potassium level.

Urine sodium concentration is 50–75 mEq/L.

Serum sodium and chloride may increase because of dehydration from large diuresis if replacement of water is inadequate.

Hypercalcemia may occur in some patients with muscle damage.

Azotemia disappears 1–3 weeks after onset of diuresis.

Later Findings

Anemia may persist for weeks or months.

Pyelonephritis may first occur during this stage.

Renal blood flow and GFR do not usually become completely normal.

Recovery from renal cortical necrosis complicating pregnancy may be followed by renal calcification, contracted kidneys, and death from malignant hypertension in 1–2 years.

If there is complete anuria for >48 hours, suspect urinary tract obstruction, bilateral renal vascular thrombi or emboli, cortical necrosis, or acute glomerulonephritis.

Suspect cortical necrosis if proteinuria is >3–4 gm/L, BUN does not fall, and diuresis does not occur.

Suspect urinary tract obstruction if recurrent oliguria and increasing azotemia occur during period of diuresis.

Urinary Diagnostic Indices In Acute Renal Failure
(see Table 15-3)

These indices may be difficult or impossible to interpret if mannitol or diuretics have been administered.

Urinary sodium levels between 20 and 40 mEq/L may be found in all forms of acute renal failure.

$$\text{Fractional excretion of sodium } (FE_{Na}) = 100 \times \frac{\text{urine sodium/plasma sodium}}{\text{urine creatinine/plasma creatinine}}$$

is an index of renal ability to conserve sodium and represents percent of filtered sodium to reach the urine. Is considered the most reliable test to distinguish prerenal azotemia from acute tubular necrosis with oliguria.

Some causes of $FE_{Na} < 1\%$

- Prerenal azotemia
- Acute glomerulonephritis
- Early (few hours) acute urinary tract obstruction
- Early sepsis

Table 15-3. Urinary Diagnostic Indices in Acute Renal Failure

	Prerenal Azotemia	Acute Oliguric (acute tubular necrosis)	Acute Nonoliguric	Acute Obstructive	Acute Glomerulonephritis
Urine specific gravity	H (>1.015)	L (<1.010)			
Urine osmolality (mOsm/kg H_2O)	H > 500 (518 ± 35)	L < 350 (369 ± 20)	L (343 ± 17)	L (393 ± 39)	L (385 ± 61)
U/P osmolality	>1.5	< 1.2	< 1.2		
Urine Na (mEq/L)	L < 20 (18 ± 3)	H > 40 (68 ± 5)	H > 40 (50 ± 5)	H > 40 (68 ± 10)	(22 ± 6)
U/P urea N	> 8 (18 ± 7)	< 3 (3 ± 0.5)	(7 ± 1)	>8 (8 ± 4)	>8 (11 ± 4)
U/P creatinine	> 40 (45 ± 6)	< 20 (17 ± 2)	< 20 (17 ± 2)	< 20 (16 ± 4)	(43 ± 7)
Renal failure index	< 1 (90% of cases) (0.6 ± 0.1)	> 2 (95% of cases) (10 ± 2)	(4 ± 0.6)	> 2 (8 ± 3)	< 1 (0.4 ± 0.1)
Fractional Na excretion (FE_{Na})	< 1 (85–94% of cases) (0.4 ± 0.1)	> 3 (7 ± 1.4)	> 3 (3 ± 0.5)	> 3 (6 + 2)	< 1 (0.6 ± 0.2)
BUN/creatinine ratio	> 15:1	≅ 10:1	≅ 10:1	> 15:1	≅ 10:1

H = high; L = low.
Source: Data from TR Miller et al, Urinary diagnostic indices in acute renal failure: A prospective study. *Ann Intern Med* 89:47, 1978; DE Oken, On the differential diagnosis of acute renal failure. *Am J Med* 71:916, 1981; and RW Schrier, Acute renal failure: Pathogenesis, diagnosis, and management. *Hosp Pract* (March 1981), p. 93.

Some cases of acute tubular necrosis due to x-ray contrast material or myoglobinuria due to rhabdomyolysis

10% of cases of nonoliguric acute tubular necrosis

Some causes of $FE_{Na} > 1\%$

90% of cases of acute tubular necrosis

Later urinary tract obstruction (days to months)

Diuretic administration

Preexisting chronic renal failure

Diuresis due to mannitol, glycosuria, or bicarbonaturia

Renal failure index (RFI) = urine sodium/(urine creatinine/plasma creatinine)

Measures Na conservation and concentrating ability

Diagnostic indices in patients with reversible acute obstructive uropathy often resemble indices in acute tubular necrosis or prerenal azotemia; indices in obstructive uropathy depend on duration of obstruction and severity of azotemia. Indices are not useful for diagnosis of presence or absence of obstruction in cases of acute renal failure.

These diagnostic indices are often intermediate, and considerable overlapping of values is frequent, especially at time of initial evaluation. Even the total profile may not be useful in the individual case. Indices (especially RFI and FE_{Na}) are chiefly of value in *oliguric* patients for the early differentiation of prerenal azotemia from acute tubular necrosis (values ≤1 for both parameters strongly suggest prerenal azotemia and values ≥ 3 strongly suggest acute tubular necrosis with confidence level of 90%; values of 1–3 are less definitive but usually indicate tubular necrosis); nonoliguric acute renal failure patients frequently have intermediate values between prerenal azotemia and oliguric renal failure. Differences between prerenal azotemia and acute tubular necrosis by these indices are particularly blurred in elderly patients as well as those with hypertensive or diabetic nephrosclerosis or other chronic parenchymal renal diseases. Values usually > 1 in urinary obstruction or acute interstitial nephritis; values usually < 1 in acute glomerulonephritis.

Specimens for urinary indices should be obtained before onset of treatment if possible; several therapies may make results uninterpretable, especially administration of mannitol or furosemide. It is not necessary to obtain a timed 12- or 24-hour urine specimen, since the patient with acute renal failure cannot vary urine sodium or osmolality significantly from hour to hour; a random specimen is sufficient.

Urine sediment in acute renal failure

Renal tubular cells (or cellular casts) and pigmented granular casts indicate acute tubular necrosis; urine Na > 20 mEq/L.

Sediment may be normal in prerenal or postrenal causes with minimal or absent proteinuria.

Eosinophils may be found in acute interstitial nephritis; increased WBC and WBC casts; minimal proteinuria.

RBC casts indicate glomerulonephritis, vasculitis, or microembolic disease; increased RBCs and moderate proteinuria.

RBCs indicate blood from lower GU tract or from glomerulus.

Myoglobin casts indicate myoglobinuria.

WBCs in hyaline casts indicate renal parenchymal infection rather than lower GU tract infection.

In a patient with two functioning kidneys, obstruction of only one ureter should cause serum creatinine to rise ~50% to 2 mg/dl; acute renal failure that is postrenal with creatinine > 2 mg/dl suggests that obstruction is bilateral or patient has only one functioning kidney.

Total anuria for more than 2 days is uncommon in acute tubular necrosis and should suggest other possibilities (e.g., ruptured bladder, GU tract obstruc-

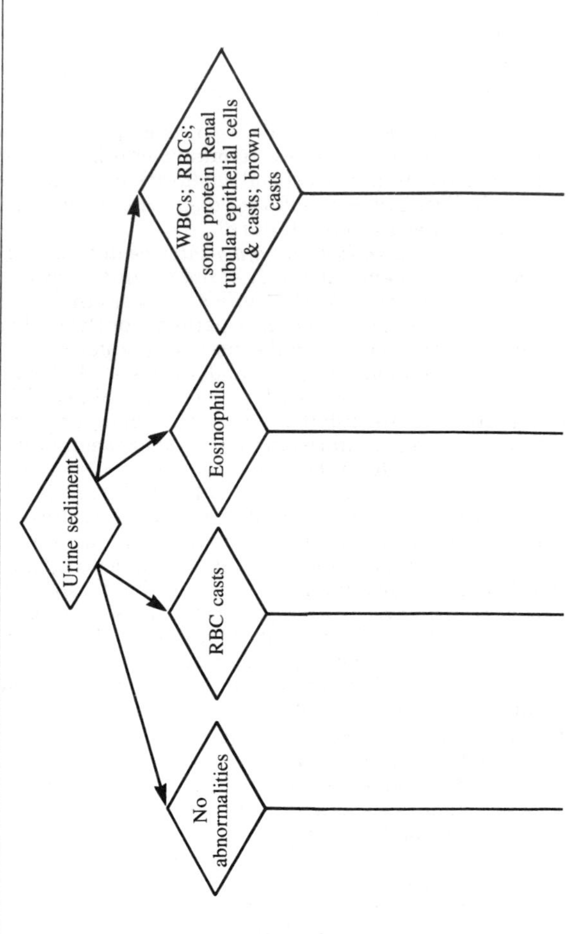
Urine sediment
WBCs; RBCs; some protein Renal tubular epithelial cells & casts; brown casts
Eosinophils
RBC casts
No abnormalities

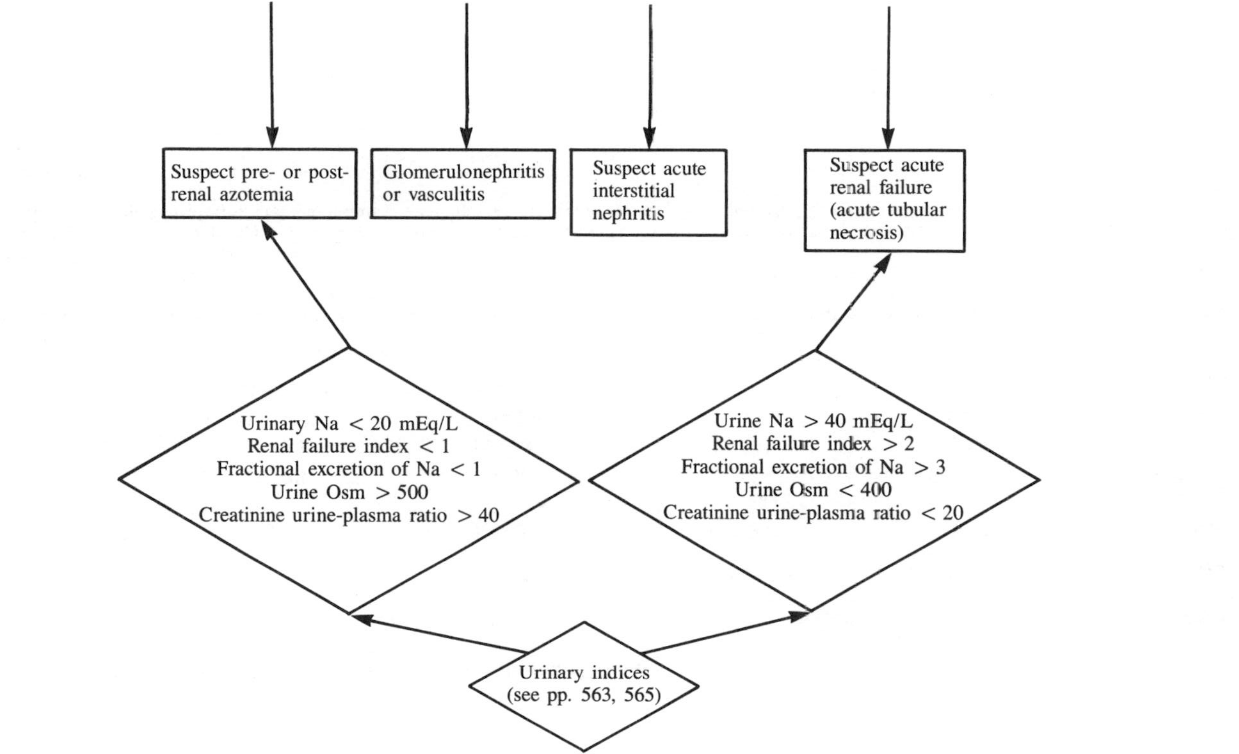

Fig. 15-2. Sequence of laboratory tests in differential diagnosis of acute renal failure. Data from RW Schrier, Acute renal failure: Pathogenesis, diagnosis, and management. *Hosp Pract,* March 1981, p. 93.)

Table 15-4. Some Renal Indices in Three Types of Postischemic Acute Renal Failure

	Type A		Type B		Type C
Postischemic Time	1 hour	3 days	7 days	12 days	21 days
Urine flow rate (ml/min)	2.2–4.4	1.4–2.0	1.3–1.9	1.4–1.6	0.4–0.8
Inulin clear (ml/min/11.731 m^2)	18–28	27–33	10–14	26–32	3–7
U/P inulin	10–18	12–20	9–11	18–26	6–8
U/P osmolality	1.1–1.2	1.3–1.4	1.03–1.09	1.2–1.4	0.96–1.04
FE_{Na}	8.8–17.2	0.6–1.0	4.6–5.6	0.8–2.0	4.6–11.6

U = urine; P = plasma.
Type A: Isolated renal ischemic insult (e.g., suprarenal aortic clamp 15–90 minutes for repair of abdominal aneurysm) with preoperative (volume expansion and mannitol administration) and postoperative (furosemide and dopamine infusion) treatment. When > 50 minutes, acute renal failure is likely to occur.
Type B: More severe and sustained partial renal ischemia (e.g., cardiopulmonary bypass for several days). When >160 minutes, acute renal failure is likely to occur. Recovery after 2–3 weeks. Values during nadir.
Type C: Protracted acute renal failure (e.g., types B or C with additional or prolonged renal ischemia as in rupture of aortic aneurysm) is fatal in >50% of cases.
Source: Data from BD Myers and SM Moran, Hemodynamically mediated acute renal failure. *N Engl J Med* 314:97, 1986)

tion, micro- or large-vessel disease, renal cortical necrosis, glomerulonephritis, allergic interstitial nephritis).

NONOLIGURIC ACUTE TUBULAR NECROSIS

(one-third to two-thirds of all cases of acute tubular necrosis)

CHRONIC RENAL INSUFFICIENCY

BUN and serum creatinine are increased and renal function tests are impaired.

Loss of renal concentrating ability (nocturia, polyuria, polydipsia) is an early manifestation of progressive renal functional impairment. Specific gravity is usually same as that of glomerular filtrate.

Abnormal urinalysis is usually the first finding. Variable abnormalities include proteinuria, hematuria, pyuria, and granular and cellular casts and may be found in asymptomatic patients.

Hypotonic urine unresponsive to vasopressin may occur in

- Obstructive uropathy
- Chronic pyelonephritis
- Nephrocalcinosis
- Amyloidosis
- Familial nephrogenic diabetes insipidus

Serum sodium is decreased (because of tubular damage with loss in urine, vomiting, diarrhea, diet restriction, etc.). The decrease is indicated by increased urine sodium levels (>5–10 mEq sodium/L). It may occur in any renal disease, especially when polyuria is marked, but is more common with obstructive uropathy, chronic pyelonephritis, and interstitial nephritis than with chronic glomerulonephritis.

Serum potassium is increased (on account of dietary sodium restriction and increased potassium ingestion, acidosis, oliguria, tissue breakdown). Decreased serum potassium with increased loss in urine (>15–20 mEq/L) occurs in primary aldosteronism. It may occur in malignant hypertension, tubular acidosis, Fanconi's syndrome, nephrocalcinosis, diuresis during recovery from tubular necrosis.

Acidosis (due to renal failure to secrete acid as NH_4^+ and to reabsorb filtered bicarbonate) is present.

Serum calcium is decreased (because of decreased serum albumin, increased serum phosphorus, decreased calcium absorption in intestine, etc.). Tetany is rare. Secondary parathyroid hyperplasia may occur, but hypercalcemia is not found.

Serum phosphorus increases when creatinine clearance falls to ~25 ml/minute.

Serum alkaline phosphatase may be normal or may be increased with renal osteodystrophy.

Serum magnesium increases when GFR falls to <30 ml/minute.

Increase in serum uric acid is usually <10 mg/dl. Secondary gout is rare. If clinical gout and family history of gout are present or if serum uric acid level is >10 mg/dl, rule out primary gout nephropathy.

Increased serum amylase occurs frequently; baseline level should be obtained in dialysis patients to evaluate episodes of abdominal pain, since these patients have an increased incidence of pancreatitis.

Serum creatine kinase (CK) may be increased; a subset of uremic patients have persistent elevations of CK-MB fraction without evidence of cardiac disease.

Increased serum triglycerides, cholesterol, and very-low-density lipoprotein (VLDL) (prebeta) are common as renal failure progresses.

Blood organic acids, phenols, indoles, certain amino acids, etc., are increased.

Normochromic normocytic anemia is usually proportionate to the degree of azotemia.

Bleeding tendency is evident. There may be decreased platelets, increased capillary fragility, abnormal thromboplastin generation time (TGT) and prothrombin consumption (possible platelet defect), normal bleeding and clotting time.

Gastrointestinal hemorrhage from ulcers anywhere in GI tract may be severe.

Table 15-5. Chief Causes of Chronic Renal Failure Presenting for Dialysis

Glomerulonephritis	44%
Diabetic nephropathy	15%
Nephrosclerosis and renal vascular disease	12%
Congenital or hereditary disease (including polycystic kidney)	10%
Chronic pyelonephritis	6%
Others and unknown	15%

Laboratory findings due to uremic pericarditis, pleuritis, and pancreatitis are noted. (BUN is usually >100 mg/dl.)

Laboratory findings due to uremic meningitis are noted (~50% of these patients have increased CSF protein or leukocytes; protein may be reduced by hemodialysis; pleocytosis is not related to degree of azotemia).

Serum albumin and total protein are decreased. When there is edema without hypoproteinemia or heart failure, rule out acute glomerulonephritis, toxemia of pregnancy, excess fluid intake in oliguria during acute tubular necrosis or terminal renal failure.

Chronic Renal Failure With Normal Urine May Occur In

Nephrosclerosis (e.g., aging, hypertension)
Renal tubular acidosis
Interstitial nephritis
Hypercalcemia
Potassium deficiency
Uric acid nephropathy
Obstruction (including retroperitoneal fibrosis)

RECOMMENDED LABORATORY TESTS FOR MANAGEMENT OF END-STAGE RENAL DISEASE (ESRD) DIALYSIS PATIENTS*

Routine tests to evaluate
- Azotemia†
- Residual renal function†
- Electrolyte and mineral balance†
- Liver function tests‡
- Renal osteodystrophy (osteomalacia)§
- Anemia‖
- Coagulation disorders#

Nonroutine tests (see appropriate separate sections)
- Tests for bleeding or clotting disorders
- Anemia
- Heart disease

*Data from National Center for Health Services Research and Health Care Technology Assessment Reports 1986, Number 5. US Dept HHS, PHS.)

†Weekly creatinine and BUN; monthly serum calcium, potassium, chloride, bicarbonate, phosphorus; semiannual tests for residual renal functions including 24-hour urine volume.

‡Monthly liver function tests (serum total protein, albumin, lactic dehydrogenase [LDH], alkaline phosphatase, serum glutamic-oxaloacetic transaminase [SGOT]), hepatitis B surface antigen [HB_sAg] (if seronegative) or annual if antibodies present after hepatitis B vaccination.

§Monthly serum calcium and phosphorus and quarterly serum parathormone for secondary hyperparathyroidism.

‖Monthly CBC; CBC or hematocrit with each dialysis.

#Clotting time with each dialysis; weekly prothrombin time if on coumadin.

Bone disease
Hepatitis
Symptomatic endocrine problems
Neuropathies
Acute complications associated with dialysis
Tests for aluminum toxicity as cause of encephalopathy, vitamin D–resistant osteodystrophy, and iron-resistant anemia. Histochemical staining of bone biopsy (if serum level > 100 μg/L) or atomic absorption of serum (>200 μg/L = toxic; >100 μg/L "view with concern"; 60–100 μg/L appears to cause no problem). Serum assay every 6–12 months or every 3 months, especially in pediatric patients.
Iron overload (due to frequent transfusions); assay serum ferritin every 3 months.
Special tests for specific conditions (e.g., renal tumors, control of diabetes mellitus)

POSTSTREPTOCOCCAL ACUTE GLOMERULONEPHRITIS IN CHILDREN

Evidence of infection with Group A beta-hemolytic streptococci by
- Culture of throat
- Serologic findings indicative of recent streptococcal infection
  - Antistreptolysin O titers (ASOT) of >250 Todd units (increased in 80% of patients). Rise begins 10–14 days after infection, peaks in 4–6 weeks, declines in next 4–6 months. Titer unreliable after *Streptococcus pyoderma.*

    Increased in ~20% of cases of membranoproliferative glomerulonephritis. Early use of penicillin prevents rise of ASOT in either condition.

  - Usually develops 7–21 days after a beta-hemolytic streptococcal infection
    - Antihyaluronidase
    - Antidesoxyribonuclease-beta
    - Antistreptokinase
    - Antidiphosphopyridine-nucleotidase
    - Antinicotinamide-adeninedenucleotidase, etc.
  - Combined use of serologic tests will establish recent streptococcal infection in virtually all cases.

Urine
- Hematuria—gross or only microscopic. Microscopic hematuria may occur during the initial febrile upper respiratory infection (URI) and then reappear with nephritis in 1–2 weeks. It lasts 2–12 months; usual duration is 2 months.
- RBC casts show glomerular origin of hematuria.
- WBC casts and WBCs show inflammatory nature of lesion.
- Granular and epithelial cell casts are present.
- Fatty casts and lipid droplets occur several weeks later; not related to hyperlipemia.
- Proteinuria is usually <2 gm/day (but may be ≤6–8 gm/day). May disappear while RBC casts and RBCs still occur.
- Oliguria is frequent.

Azotemia is found in ~50% of patients.
GFR usually shows greater decrease than renal blood flow; therefore filtration factor is decreased.
PSP excretion is normal in cases of mild to moderate severity; increases with progression of disease.
Erythrocyte sedimentation rate (ESR) is increased.

Leukocytosis is present, with increased polymorphonuclear leukocytes (PMNs).
There is mild anemia, especially when edema is present (may be due to hemodilution, bone marrow depression, or increased destruction of RBCs).
Serum proteins are normal or there is nonspecific decrease of albumin and increase of $alpha_2$ and sometimes of beta and gamma globulins.
Serum cholesterol may be increased.
Serum complement falls 24 hours before onset of hematuria and rises to normal within about 8 weeks when hematuria subsides.
Antihuman kidney antibodies are present in serum in 50% of patients.
Decreased urinary aldosterone occurs in the presence of edema.
Renal biopsy shows characteristic findings with electron microscopy and immunofluorescence.

Azotemia with high urine specific gravity and normal PSP excretion usually means acute glomerulonephritis.

RAPIDLY PROGRESSIVE NONSTREPTOCOCCAL GLOMERULONEPHRITIS

Preceded by associated systemic diseases in many patients
- Infections
  - Poststreptococcal glomerulonephritis
  - Infective endocarditis
  - Sepsis
  - Hepatitis B
- Multisystem diseases
  - SLE
  - Goodpasture's syndrome
  - Necrotizing vasculitis
  - Polyarteritis nodosa
  - Wegener's granulomatosis
  - Schönlein-Henoch purpura
  - Cryoglobulinemia

No cultural or serologic (e.g., ASOT) evidence of recent streptococcal infection.
Oliguria with urine volume often < 400 ml/day.
Hematuria is often gross.
RBCs, WBCs, and casts are present in urine.
Proteinuria is usually >3 gm/day.
Azotemia is usually marked, with BUN > 80 mg/dl and serum creatinine > 10 mg/dl (in poststreptococcal type, BUN is usually 30–100 mg/dl and serum creatinine 1.5–4.0 mg/dl).
Serum complement levels are normal.
Renal biopsy and immunofluorescent antibody findings
Prognosis is poorer than in poststreptococcal glomerulonephritis.

FOCAL PROLIFERATIVE GLOMERULONEPHRITIS

Attacks of hematuria usually occur at height of upper respiratory infection (bacterial or viral).
Serum IgA is often increased.
Azotemia is usually absent.
Proteinuria is slight or absent.
Prognosis is usually good, especially in children, but progressive nephritis causing renal failure is more common in adults.

MEMBRANOPROLIFERATIVE GLOMERULONEPHRITIS

Marked proteinuria and nephrotic type of syndrome is found in 70% of patients.
Normal serum C4 but prolonged or permanent depression of C3 is found in 60–80% of patients; clinical course is not related to serum complement levels.

Clinical course may be clinically active, or there may be periods of remission; 50% have chronic renal insufficiency in 10 years.
Renal biopsy and immunofluorescent antibody findings.
GFR < 80 ml/min/1.73 sq m in two-thirds of patients.

ACUTE INTERSTITIAL NEPHRITIS

(typical clinical triad of fever, rash, and eosinophilia in patient in acute renal failure and recent exposure to a causative drug is seen in <45% of cases; may occur following infections [especially Group A beta-hemolytic streptococcal, diphtheria, brucellosis, leptospirosis, infectious mononucleosis, disease, toxoplasmosis, Rocky Mountain spotted fever, measles] or as complication of drug therapy [especially antibiotics, diuretics, nonsteroidal anti-inflammatory drugs, miscellaneous drugs such as allopurinol, and street drugs] or idiopathic)

Eosinophilia (in 60–100% of patients) with increased blood IgE
Increased WBC, neutrophils, and bands
Anemia with hemoglobin as low as 6.5 gm/dl; no evidence of hemolysis or iron deficiency; negative indirect Coombs' test; normal bone marrow. Anemia resolves when renal function becomes normal.
ESR is increased.
Serum IgG is usually increased; serum complement is normal.
Varying degrees of renal insufficiency with increased BUN and creatinine, hyponatremia, hyperchloremic metabolic acidosis, decreased serum albumin. May be oliguric or nonoliguric.
Urinalysis
- Urinary indices similar to those seen in acute tubular necrosis
- Eosinophiluria reported in up to 100% of patients
- Microscopic hematuria
- Proteinuria is usually mild to moderate, <1.0 gm/m^2/24 hours, unless nephrotic syndrome is present.
- Sterile pyuria is minimal or absent.
- Casts are uncommon.
- Low osmolality and specific gravity

Glycosuria without hyperglycemia and reduced tubular reabsorption of phosphate (TRP) may occur.
Enlarged, poorly functioning kidneys may be demonstrated by intravenous pyelogram (IVP), ultrasound, or renal scan.
Nephrotic syndrome may occur.
Biopsy of kidney establishes the diagnosis and is usually more severe than indicated by urinalysis and renal studies.

ACUTE TUBULAR NECROSIS

May be oliguric or nonoliguric
Urine sodium is usually >40 mEq/L, but may be <20 mEq/L in nonoliguric patients.
Fe_{Na} is usually >1% in both oliguric and nonoliguric patients.
Usually multiple causes (e.g., hypotension, sepsis, nephrotoxic drugs, x-ray contrast material, volume depletion)
Mortality about 50% in oliguric and 25% in nonoliguric patients

BERGER'S DISEASE (IgA NEPHROPATHY)

(a focal proliferative glomerulonephritis; immunologic mediation; probably the most common form of glomerulonephritis)

Painless recurrent gross hematuria and minimal proteinuria, often associated with (rather than following by 4–10 days) an acute nonstreptococcal URI or GI or GU infection. Recurrent episodes of gross hematuria commonly occur with acute infections. Microhematuria is usually present between acute exacerbations.

Table 15-6. Classification of Glomerulonephritis

Glomerular Disorder	Situations in Which May Be Found	Hematuria		Proteinuria		Renal Function D	Comment
		Micro Present (% of cases)	RBC Casts Present (% of cases)	1–3 gm Present (% of cases)	>3 gm Present (% of cases)		
IgA nephropathy (Berger's disease)	Focal proliferative GN	100	50	75	25	25% or NS; N in 75%	
IgM mesangial nephropathy		50	Rare	50	50	>75% or NS	
Acute GN secondary to infection (focal GN)	SBE, bacterial pneumonia, viral infections, infection of implanted devices	100	50	75	25	100%	
Crescentic (rapidly progressive) GN							
Anti-GBM	Goodpasture's syndrome in 2/3 of patients	100	50	50	50	100%	90% have HLA-DR2 antigen.
Immune complex	SLE, mixed cryoglobulinemia, Schönlein-Henoch purpura	100	50	50	50	100%	

Non-immune complex	Wegener's granulomatosis, polyarteritis						
GN and vasculitis	Wegener's granulomatosis, Schönlein-Henoch purpura, mixed cryoglobulinemia; Goodpasture's syndrome may occur	100	50	50	50	100%	
Systemic lupus erythematosus (SLE)							
Mesangial		15		10		N	Most frequent type in SLE.
Focal proliferative		50		25		N or D	
Membranous		50			85	N or D	
Diffuse proliferative (<25% of SLE patients)		75			75	Usually D; uremia develops in 50–75%	
Minimal change disease	Lipid nephrosis, nil disease	20			100	N	85% respond to steroid therapy. Most common cause of NS in children.
Focal sclerosis		75		25	75	Usually D	Frequent cause of NS.

Table 15-6. (continued)

Glomerular Disorder	Situations in Which May Be Found	Hematuria		Proteinuria		Renal Function D	Comment
		Micro Present (% of cases)	RBC Casts Present (% of cases)	1–3 gm Present (% of cases)	>3 gm Present (% of cases)		
Membranous nephropathy	Usually idiopathic; occasionally due to heavy-metal toxicity (e.g., gold, mercury), persistent hepatitis B infection, other viruses (e.g., measles, varicella, Coxsackie), other infections (e.g., malaria, syphilis, leprosy, schistosomiasis), neoplasias (e.g., colon carcinoma, lymphoma, leukemia), sarcoidosis, SLE, others	50		25	75	N early; D late	Frequent cause of NS. Strong association with HLA-DR3. Spontaneous remission in 25–50%. Persistent proteinuria without progression in 25%. Progressive glomerular sclerosis causing renal failure in 50%. Common in adults; uncommon in children.

Membranoproliferative GN							
Type I (idiopathic)	SBE, essential cryoglobulinemia, Schönlein-Henoch purpura, SLE, sickle cell disease, hepatitis and cirrhosis, C2 deficiency, $alpha_1$ antitrypsin deficiency, infected shunts *(Staphylococcus, Corynebacterium)*	75	25	50	50	Usually D; NS at onset in 75%	Renal failure within 5 years common in adults but may be delayed 10–20 years. Persistent marked proteinuria is poor prognostic sign. Renal vein thrombosis may occur.
Type II (idiopathic)	Infection with streptococci, pneumococci, *Candida,* lipodystrophy						

GN = glomerulonephritis; NS = nephrotic syndrome; SBE = subacute bacterial endocarditis; D = decreased; N = normal.

Goodpasture's syndrome occurs in < 5% of cases of GN.

Source: Data from WA Border and RJ Glassock, Progress in treating glomerulonephritis. *Drug Therapy,* April 1981, p. 97; TR Miller, et al., Urinary diagnostic indices in acute renal failure: A prospective study. *Ann Intern Med* 89:47, 1978; DE Oken, On the differential diagnosis of acute renal failure. *Am J Med* 71:916, Dec. 1981.

Disease may be progressive in up to 10% of adults.
Diagnosis is based on predominant mesangial IgA immunofluorescence on renal biopsy.
May be related to Schönlein-Henoch purpura

NEPHROTIC SYNDROME

Characterized By

Marked proteinuria—usually > 4.5 gm/day; usually exclusively albuminuria in children with lipoid nephrosis, but in glomerulonephritis, high- and low-molecular-weight proteins are present.
Decreased serum albumin (usually < 2.5 gm/dl) and total protein
Hyperlipidemia—increased serum cholesterol (free and esters), usually > 350 mg/dl (low or normal serum cholesterol occurs with poor nutrition and suggests poor prognosis); increased serum phospholipids, neutral fats, triglycerides, low-density beta-lipoproteins, and total lipids
Serum $alpha_2$ and beta globulins are markedly increased, gamma globulin is decreased, $alpha_1$ is normal or decreased. If gamma globulin is increased, rule out systemic disease (e.g., SLE).
Urine containing doubly refractive fat bodies as seen by polarizing microscopy; many granular and epithelial cell casts
Hematuria—may be present in 50% of patients but is usually minimal and not part of syndrome.
Azotemia—may be present but not part of syndrome.
Changes secondary to proteinuria and hypoalbuminemia (e.g., decreased serum calcium, decreased serum ceruloplasmin, increased fibrinogen)
Increased ESR due to increased fibrinogen
Changes due to primary disease
Increased susceptibility to infection (most frequently peritonitis) during periods of edema
Serum C3 complement is normal in idiopathic lipoid nephrosis but decreased when there is underlying glomerulonephritis.
Hypercoagulability with thromboembolism; abnormalities in coagulation factors, clotting inhibitors, fibrinolytic system, platelet function have been described. Associated renal vein thrombosis has been reported in ~35% of patients (≤40% of these will have pulmonary emboli), especially when due to membranous nephropathy, membranoproliferative glomerulonephritis, lipoid nephrosis, rapidly progressive glomerulonephritis.
Associated neoplasm in 10% of adults and 15% > age 60 years
- In adult with minimal-change nephrotic syndrome without evident cause, first rule out Hodgkin's disease. With membranous lesion, carcinoma may be more likely.

Etiology

Renal
- Glomerulonephritis (>50% of patients)
- Lipoid nephrosis (10% in adults; 80% in children)

Systemic
- Diabetic glomerulosclerosis (15% of patients)
- SLE (20% of patients)
- Amyloidosis (primary and secondary)
- Schönlein-Henoch purpura
- Multiple myeloma
- Goodpasture's syndrome
- Berger's disease
- Polyarteritis
- Takayasu's syndrome
- Sarcoidosis

Sjögren's syndrome
Dermatitis herpetiformis
Cryoglobulinemia
Venous obstruction
Obstruction of inferior vena cava (thrombosis, tumor) or renal vein
Constrictive pericarditis
Tricuspid stenosis
Congestive heart failure
Infections
Bacterial (poststreptococcal glomerulonephritis, bacterial endocarditis; syphilis, leprosy, etc.)
Viral (hepatitis B: also cytomegalovirus, infectious mononucleosis, HIV, varicella)
Protozoal (malaria, toxoplasmosis)
Parasitic (schistosomiasis, trypanosomiasis, filiariasis)
Allergic (e.g., serum sickness, bee sting)
Neoplastic (e.g., Hodgkin's disease; carcinoma of colon, lung, stomach, and others; lymphomas and leukemia); paraproteinemia (multiple myeloma, light-chain nephropathy)
Toxic (e.g., heavy metal, heroin, captopril, probenecid, nonsteroidal antiinflammatory drug, penicillamine, mephenytoin, ampicillin, anticonvulsants, chlorpropamide, lithium rifampin)
Hereditary/familial (e.g., Alport's syndrome, Fabry's disease, sickle cell disease). In atypical familial nephrotic syndrome, course is benign; more than 1 sibling is involved.
Miscellaneous
Preeclampsia
Chronic allograft rejection
Others

CHRONIC GLOMERULONEPHRITIS

Various Clinical Courses

Early death after marked proteinuria, hematuria, oliguria, progressive increasing uremia, anemia
Intermittent or continuous or incidental proteinuria, hematuria with slight or absent azotemia, and normal renal function tests (may develop into late renal failure or may subside)
Exacerbation of chronic nephritis (with accentuation of proteinuria, hematuria, and decreased renal function) shortly following streptococcal upper respiratory infection
Nephrotic syndrome

Compared to pyelonephritis, chronic glomerulonephritis shows lipid droplets and epithelial and RBC casts in urine, more marked proteinuria (>2–3 gm/day), poorer prognosis for equivalent amount of azotemia.

NEPHROSCLEROSIS

"Benign" nephrosclerosis ("essential hypertension")
Urine contains little or no protein or microscopic abnormalities.
10% of patients develop marked renal insufficiency.
"Accelerated" nephrosclerosis ("malignant hypertension")
Syndrome may occur in the course of "benign" nephrosclerosis, glomerulonephritis, unilateral renal artery occlusion, or any cause of hypertension.
Increasing uremia is associated with minimal or marked proteinuria and hematuria.

RENAL CALCULI

(autopsy incidence = 1.12%; cause of death = 0.38%)

Calcium oxalate alone or with phosphate is the constituent of kidney stones in 75% of patients in the United States.

- 35% of patients have increased urinary calcium, i.e., >250 mg/24 hours in females and >300 mg/24 hours in males.
- 50–75% of hyperparathyroidism patients have renal calculi; ~5% of patients with nephrolithiasis have primary hyperparathyroidism. (See also Idiopathic Hypercalciuria [next section]).
- 20–30% of patients have
  - Bone diseases—destructive (e.g., metastatic tumor) or osteoporosis (e.g., immobilization, Paget's disease, Cushing's syndrome)
  - Milk-alkali (Burnett's) syndrome
  - Hypervitaminosis D
  - Sarcoidosis
  - Renal tubular acidosis—Type I (hypercalciuria, highly alkaline urine, serum calcium usually normal)
  - Hyperthyroidism
  - Other
- ~50 of patients have idiopathic hypercalciuria (see next section).

Oxalate is a constituent of renal calculi in 65% of all patients, but hyperoxaluria is a relatively rare cause of these calculi and may be due to

- Primary hyperoxaluria (see p. 580)
- Intestinal disease (Crohn's disease, malabsorption)
- Ileal resection
- Jejunoileal bypass
- Vitamin C excess
- Excess dietary oxalate

Magnesium ammonium phosphate is the constituent of renal calculi in 15% of patients. It occurs almost exclusively in patients with recurrent urinary tract infections by urea-splitting organisms, particularly *Proteus* species (but should rule out *Klebsiella, Pseudomonas, Serratia, Enterobacter*), and in patients with persistently alkaline urine.

Cystine stones form when urine contains >300 mg/day of cystine in congenital familial cystinuria. Urine shows cystine crystals. Cyanide-nitroprusside test is positive. Causes 1% of all stones.

Uric acid is present in calculi in 5% of patients.

- Gout—25% of patients with primary gout and 40% of patients with marrow-proliferative disorders have calculi.
- Urine is more acid than normal (e.g., patients with chronic diarrhea, ileostomy).
- >50% of patients with urinary calculi have normal serum and urine uric acid levels.

Xanthine is present in children with inborn error of metabolism.

Hereditary glycinuria is a rare familial disorder associated with renal calculi.

Microscopic hematuria is found in 80% of patients.

In renal colic, hematuria and proteinuria are present, and there is an increased WBC due to associated infection.

Crystalluria is diagnostically useful when there are cystine crystals (occur only in homozygous or heterozygous cysteinuria) or struvite crystals (occur only when urine is infected with urea-splitting bacteria). Calcium oxalate, phosphate, and uric acid should arouse suspicion about possible cause of stones, but they may occur in normal urines.

IDIOPATHIC HYPERCALCIURIA

Increased 24-hour excretion of urinary calcium

- >300 mg in males or >250 mg in females

Table 15-7. Characteristic Features in Differential Diagnosis of Hypercalciuria*

Measurement	Resorptive Hypercalciuria (Primary Hyperpara-thyroidism)	Absorptive Hypercalciuria	Renal Hypercalciuria	Normocalciuric Nephrolithiasis
Serum calcium	I	N	N	N
Urine calcium				
Fasting	I	N	I	N
After calcium load	I	Markedly I	Moderately I	N or I
Urine cyclic AMP				
Fasting	I in 30%	N	Usually I	N
After calcium load	I in 82%	N	N	N
Serum parathormone	I	N	I	N

N = normal; I = increased.
*See reference given as source for normal values and test procedures.
Calcium loading: Overnight fast 9 P.M. to 7 A.M. Collect 2-hour (7 A.M.–9 A.M.) urine for renal hypercalciuria. Then ingest 1 gm of calcium gluconate and collect 4-hour urine (9 A.M.–1 P.M.) to assess intestinal absorption of calcium.
Source: Data from CYC Pak et al., A simple test for the diagnosis of absorptive, resorptive and renal hypercalciurias. *N Engl J Med* 292:497, 1975.

- >4 mg/kg (either sex)
- >140 mg/gm of urinary creatinine is most useful in short or obese patients.

Normal blood calcium levels

Serum 1,25-dihydroxyvitamin D_3 levels are usually high.

Diagnosis requires exclusion of all other causes of hypercalciuria (see p. 101); may be familial. Occurs in ~40% of patients who form calcium renal stones

Occurs in 5–10% of general population

Three types

- Renal: Hypercalciuria persists despite absent dietary calcium in intestine following fasting. One-tenth as common as absorptive type.
- Absorptive: 2-hour urine collection after fasting shows calcium-creatinine ratio < 0.11, but in renal hypercalciuria is >0.15. 24-hour urine falls to <200 mg/24 hours following low-calcium diet (400 mg/day) for 3–4 days.
- Resorptive: due to increased endogenous parathyroid hormone (PTH) production (hyperparathyroidism).

PRIMARY HYPEROXALURIA

Rare, autosomal recessive inherited disorder of glyoxylate metabolism causing

- Calcium oxalate renal lithiasis, interstitial nephritis, uremia
- Urinary oxalate is usually >100 mg/24 hours unless renal function is diminished.

SECONDARY HYPEROXALURIA

Due To

Increased oxalate in diet

Ingestion of oxalate precursors (e.g., ascorbic acid, ethylene glycol)

Methoxyflurane anesthesia

Primary diseases of ileum with normal colon absorption (e.g., bypass surgery, Crohn's disease) causing increased absorption of dietary oxalate. Urinary oxalate is usually 50–100 mg/24 hours.

OBSTRUCTIVE UROPATHY

(unilateral or bilateral; partial or complete)

Partial obstruction of both kidneys may cause increasing azotemia with normal or increased urinary output (due to decreased renal concentrating ability).

Partial obstruction may cause inexplicable wide variations in BUN and urine volume in patients with azotemia. PSP excretion is less in first 15-minute period than in any later period. There is considerable PSP excretion after the 2-hour test period.

In unilateral obstruction, BUN usually remains normal unless underlying renal disease is present.

Laboratory findings due to superimposed infection or underlying disease are noted.

Laboratory findings due to underlying disease

- Obstruction of bladder (e.g., benign prostatic hypertrophy (BPH), carcinoma of prostate or bladder, urethral stricture, neurogenic bladder dysfunction [multiple sclerosis, diabetic neuropathy])
- Obstruction of both ureters (e.g., infiltrating neoplasm [especially of uterine cervix], bilateral calculi, congenital anomalies, retroperitoneal fibrosis)

If ureter is obstructed >4 months, functional recovery is unlikely. When obstruction is relieved, most functional recovery takes place in 2–3 weeks; then there is continued improvement for several months.

TUBULOINTERSTITIAL NEPHROPATHY

Three basic patterns of functional disturbance depending on site of injury: proximal tubular acidosis, distal tubular acidosis, medullary (reduced ability to concentrate urine, causing nephrogenic diabetes insipidus in most severe form)

Due To

Bacterial infection (e.g., acute and chronic pyelonephritis)
Drugs (e.g., acute interstitial nephritis [see p. 573], analgesic nephropathy)
Immune disorders (e.g., acute interstitial nephritis [see p. 573], transplant rejection, associated with glomerulonephritis, Sjögren's syndrome)
Metabolic disorders (e.g., urate, hypercalcemic, hypokalemic, oxalate nephropathies)
Heavy metals (e.g., lead, cadmium)
Physical factors (e.g., obstructive uropathy, radiation nephritis)
Neoplasia (e.g., myeloma kidney, infiltration in leukemia and lymphoma)
Hereditary renal diseases (e.g., medullary cystic disease, familial interstitial nephritis, Alport's syndrome)
Miscellaneous conditions (e.g., granulomatous diseases [sarcoidosis, tuberculosis, leprosy], Balkan nephropathy)

LABORATORY FINDINGS THAT FAVOR CHRONIC TUBULOINTERSTITIAL RATHER THAN GLOMERULOVASCULAR RENAL DISEASE

Minimal or absent proteinuria
Moderate polyuria
Hyperchloremic metabolic acidosis
Severe sodium wasting
Disproportionate hyperkalemia
Mild or absent hypertension

PAPILLARY NECROSIS OF KIDNEY

Findings of associated diseases
- Diabetes mellitus
- Urinary tract infection
- Chronic overuse of phenacetin

Sudden diminution in renal function; occasionally oliguria or anuria with acute renal failure
Hematuria

HORSESHOE KIDNEYS

Laboratory findings due to complications
- Renal calculi
- Pyelonephritis
- Hematuria

POLYCYSTIC KIDNEYS

Polyuria is common.
Hematuria may be gross and episodic or an incidental microscopic finding (50% of patients).
Proteinuria may be an incidental finding of routine analysis (75% of patients).
Renal calculi may be associated (10% of patients).
Superimposed pyelonephritis is frequent (33% of patients).
Death occurs within 5 years after BUN rises to 50 mg/dl (33% of patients). Death usually occurs in early infancy or in middle age when superimposed nephrosclerosis of aging or pyelonephritis has exhausted renal reserve.

Cerebral hemorrhage causes death in 10% of patients; intracranial berry aneurysms are frequently associated.
Autosomal dominant transmission
Diagnosed 1:3000 patients
Accounts for 5% of the hemodialysis population
Increased incidence of gout in patients with polycystic kidneys
Anemia of renal failure is less severe than in other forms of kidney disease.

MEDULLARY CYSTIC DISEASE

Anemia is often severe and out of proportion to degree of renal failure.
Polyuria
Salt-losing syndrome
Death from renal insufficiency (may take many years)

Urinalysis shows minimal or no proteinuria; presence of RBCs, WBCs, casts, or bacteria is rare. Specific gravity may be decreased.
Serum alkaline phosphatase may be increased when bone changes occur.

SPONGE KIDNEY

Findings due to complications (e.g., hematuria, infection, calculi in cysts)
Disease asymptomatic, not progressive

HEREDITARY NEPHRITIS

May be classified into two types
- Angiokeratoma corporis diffusum (familial condition of abnormal glycolipid deposition in glomerular epithelial cells, nervous system, heart, etc.)
  - Proteinuria begins in second decade.
  - Urine may contain lipid globules and foam cells.
  - Uremia occurs by fourth or fifth decade.
- Familial autosomal dominant disease associated with nerve deafness and lens defects (Alport's syndrome) is rare. Renal disease is progressive.
  - Hematuria, gross or microscopic, is common; more marked after occurrence of unrelated infection. Other laboratory findings are the same as in other types of nephritis.

ARTERIAL INFARCTION OF KIDNEY

Microscopic or gross hematuria is usual.
BUN is normal unless other renal disease is present.
In some cases, urine shows no albumin or abnormal sediment at time of analysis.
WBC, SGOT, serum glutamic-pyruvic transaminase (SGPT) are increased if area of infarction is large; peak by second day; return to normal by fifth day.
Serum and urine LDH may be increased markedly.
Increased serum LDH is the most sensitive enzyme abnormality.
C-reactive protein (CRP) and serum LDH peak on third day; return to normal by tenth day.
Changes in serum enzyme levels, WBC, CRP, ESR are similar in time changes to those in myocardial infarction.
Plasma renin activity may rise on second day, peak about 11th day, and remain elevated for more than a month.
Increased serum alkaline phosphatase occurs in about one-third of cases and is the least discriminating enzyme abnormality.
Laboratory findings due to infarction of other organs (e.g., brain, heart)

RENAL VEIN THROMBOSIS

Hematuria
Microscopic pyuria

Proteinuria and decreased creatinine clearance show marked variability from day to day.
Postprandial glycosuria
Nephrotic syndrome (see p. 578)
Hyperchloremic acidosis (renal tubular acidosis)
Hyperosmolarity
Oliguria and uremic death if infarction is extensive
Anemia is common.
Platelet count may be decreased.
Increased fibrin degradation products in blood may be >3 times normal limits (disseminated intravascular coagulation [DIC]).
Laboratory findings due to thromboembolic disease elsewhere (e.g., pulmonary)
Laboratory findings due to underlying causative conditions (e.g., hypernephroma, metastatic cancer, trauma, amyloidosis, diabetic glomerulosclerosis, hypertension, papillary necrosis, DIC, sickle cell disease, polycythemia, heart failure)

RENAL ARTERIOVENOUS FISTULA

Hematuria
Laboratory findings due to congestive heart failure and hypertension

RENAL CHANGES IN BACTERIAL ENDOCARDITIS

There are three types of pathologic changes: diffuse subacute glomerulonephritis, focal embolic glomerulonephritis, microscopic or gross infarcts of kidney.
Laboratory findings due to bacterial endocarditis are noted (see pp. 123–124).
Albuminuria is almost invariably present, even when no renal lesions are found.
Hematuria (usually microscopic, sometimes gross) is usual at some stage of the disease, but repeated examinations may be required.
Renal insufficiency is frequent (15% of cases during active stage; 40% of fatal cases).
  BUN is increased (usually 25–75 mg/dl).
  Renal concentrating ability is decreased.

AZOTEMIA DUE TO CARDIAC FAILURE

(may also occur in other functional forms of acute renal failure [e.g., hepatorenal syndrome, volume contraction])

Parallels the degree of heart failure
Serum creatinine rarely >4 mg/dl even when BUN >100 mg/dl in pure prerenal azotemia.
Urine is hypertonic (increased osmolality) with low sodium concentration (<10 mEq/L).
Protein excretion is frequently increased but rarely >2 gm/24 hours.
Urine sediment may contain granular or hyaline casts, but cellular or pigmented casts are conspicuously absent.
In contrast, *acute tubular necrosis* (may complicate cardiac failure; due to cardiogenic shock, excessive use of diuretics or vasodilators)
  Urine osmolality approaches that of plasma.
  Urine sodium is usually high (40–80 mEq/L).
  Urine sediment contains many renal tubular cells and casts and many narrow (often pigmented) casts.

KIDNEY DISORDERS IN GOUT

Kidney stones occur in 25% of patients with gout; may occur in absence of arthritis.
Early renal damage is indicated by decreased renal concentrating ability, mild proteinuria, and decreased PSP excretion.
Later renal damage is shown by slowly progressive azotemia with slight albuminuria and slight or no abnormalities of urine sediment.

Arteriolar nephrosclerosis and pyelonephritis are usually associated.
Renal disease causes death in ≤50% of patients with gout.
It has been suggested that acute uric acid nephropathy may be differentiated from other forms of acute renal failure if ratio of urine urate–urine creatinine >1.0 in an adult (many children under age 10 years have ratio > 1.0).

KIMMELSTIEL-WILSON SYNDROME (DIABETIC INTERCAPILLARY GLOMERULOSCLEROSIS)

Defined as persistent positive urine protein dipstick test (>0.3 gm/day) in absence of other renal disease. Dipstick assay detects 200–300 mg/L, but normal sedentary male should excrete <20 mg/L or normal ratio urine albumin-creatinine (as mg/dl) < 0.01. In Type I or II diabetes, ratio = 0.02–0.2 or >300 mg/24 hr.
The disease is recognized after diabetes mellitus has been present for years. Occasionally it is associated only with prediabetes.
Proteinuria is usual (may be earliest clinical clue) and may be marked (often >5 gm/day). Periodic dipstick testing of urine should be part of routine treatment of all diabetics; positive test indicates increased risk of end-stage renal disease and cardiovascular disease. Nephrotic syndrome may be associated.
Microalbuminuria is proteinuria below overt level detected by dipstick but definitely above normal. Do not test urine during periods of exercise or prolonged upright posture, in presence of hematuria or blood contamination or GU tract infection, or in glass containers (albumin adheres to glass). Measure by enzyme immunoassay (EIA), radioimmunoassay (RIA), or nephelometry; test only if dipstick is negative. Diagnosed when present in ≥2 or 3 urine collections over 6-month period. Present in ~25% of Type I and 36% of Type II patients with negative dipstick test. In insulin-dependent diabetes mellitus (IDDM), microalbuminuria is 82% sensitive, highly specific (96%) and has 75% positive predictive value for subsequent overt nephropathy; lower values in non-insulin-dependent diabetes mellitus (NIDDM). Compared to normal, microalbuminuria is associated with longer duration of diabetes, poorer glycemic control, higher blood pressure, development of more advanced retinopathy and neuropathy and overt nephropathy and subsequent renal failure, increased vascular damage and risk for cardiovascular disease.

	Normal	Microalbuminuria	Nephropathy
Albumin concentration			
albumin-creatinine ratio	<0.01	0.02–0.2	>0.2
μg/ml			
Volume 1000 ml/day	<15	30	>30
Volume 1500 mg/day	<10	20	>20
Albumin excretion rate			
μg/minute	<10	20–200	>200
mg/day	<15	30–300	>300

Urine shows many hyaline and granular casts and double refractile fat bodies. Hematuria is rare.
Serum protein is decreased.
Azotemia develops gradually after several years of proteinuria.
Biopsy of kidney is diagnostic.
Laboratory findings are those due to frequently associated GU tract infection.
See sections on diabetes mellitus, acidosis, papillary necrosis, urinary tract infection, diabetic neuropathy.

RENAL DISEASE IN POLYARTERITIS NODOSA

Renal involvement occurs in 75% of patients.
Azotemia is often absent or only mild and slowly progressive.
Albuminuria is always present.

Table 15-8. Evolution of Renal Disease in IDDM

Stage	Time of Onset	Laboratory Findings	Morphologic Findings	% of Cases That Progress
Early	At time of diagnosis	I GFR	Kidney size I	100
Renal lesions; no clinical signs	2–3 years after diagnosis	I GFR Albuminuria cannot be detected	I thickness of glomerular and tubular capillary basement membrane Glomerulosclerosis	35–40
Incipient nephropathy	7–15 years after diagnosis	Albuminuria 0.03–0.3 gm/day GFR N/sl I; beginning to decline	Glomerulosclerosis progressing	80–100
Clinical diabetic nephropathy	10–30 years after diagnosis	Albuminuria >0.3 gm/day GFR N/sl D; steady fall	Glomerulosclerosis widespread	>75
End-stage renal disease	20–40 years after diagnosis	GFR $<$ 10 ml/min Serum creatinine $\geq$10mg/dl		

GFR = glomerular filtration rate; I = increased; D = decreased; N = normal; sl = slightly.
Albuminuria $\leq$ 0.3 gm/day is detected only by sensitive assays (e.g., RIA).
When albuminuria is 0.075–0.1 gm/day in IDDM, there is significant renal disease and albuminuria will progress to clinical nephropathy.
GFR declines ~10 ml/min/year after nephropathy is established.
Source: Data from JV Selby, et al., The natural history and epidemiology of diabetic nephropathy. *JAMA* 263:1954, 1990.

Hematuria (gross or microscopic) is very common. Fat bodies are frequently present in urine sediment.
There may be findings of acute glomerulonephritis with remission or early death from renal failure.

Always rule out polyarteritis in any case of glomerulonephritis, renal failure, or hypertension that shows unexplained eosinophilia, increased WBC, or laboratory evidence of involvement of other organ systems.

NEPHRITIS OF SYSTEMIC LUPUS ERYTHEMATOSUS (SLE)

Renal involvement occurs in two-thirds of patients with SLE.
Nephritis of SLE may occur as acute, latent, or chronic glomerulonephritis, nephrosis, or asymptomatic albuminuria or hematuria.
Urine findings are as in chronic active glomerulonephritis.
Azotemia or marked proteinuria usually indicates death in 1–3 years.
Signs of SLE (e.g., positive LE test) may disappear during active nephritis, nephrosis, or uremia.
Examination of needle biopsy should always include immunofluorescent and electron as well as light microscopy. May show normal or minimal disease, mesangial lesions, focal proliferative glomerulonephritis, diffuse proliferative glomerulonephritis, or membranous glomerulonephritis.
Laboratory findings due to drug therapy
- Prednisone
- Cytotoxic drugs (e.g., azathioprine, cyclophosphamide)
  - Leukopenia—nadir WBC kept at 1500–4000/cu mm
  - Infection (e.g., herpes zoster, opportunistic organisms)
  - Gonadal toxicity
  - Hemorrhagic cystitis
  - Neoplasia

RENAL DISEASE IN SCLERODERMA

Renal involvement occurs in two-thirds of patients; one-third die of renal failure.
Proteinuria may be minimal and is usually <2 gm/day; this may be the only finding for a long time.
Azotemia usually signals death within a few months.
Terminal oliguria or anuria may occur.

TOXEMIA OF PREGNANCY

Proteinuria varies from a trace to very marked (≤800 mg/dl, equivalent to 15–20 gm/day). >15 mg/dl may indicate early toxemia.
RBCs and RBC casts are not abundant; hyaline and granular casts are present. BUN, renal concentrating ability, and PSP excretion are normal unless the disease is severe or there is a prior renal lesion. *(BUN usually decreases during normal pregnancy because of increase in GFR.)*
Serum uric acid is increased (decreased renal clearance of urate) in 70% of patients in absence of treatment with thiazides, which can produce hyperuricemia independent of any disease.
Serum total protein and albumin commonly are markedly decreased.
There may be multiple clotting deficiencies in severe cases.
Biopsy of kidney can establish diagnosis; rules out primary renal disease or hypertensive vascular disease.
GFR and renal plasma flow are 10–30% < normal pregnancy but may appear normal, increased, or decreased compared to rates in nonpregnant women. (Normally GFR increases gradually to a maximum of 40% more than nonpregnant level by 32nd week, then decreases slightly until term. Renal plasma flow is not so markedly increased. Therefore the filtration fraction [GFR/RPF ratio] increases slightly.)

Table 15-9. Comparison of Clinical and Morphologic Types of SLE Nephritis

	Mesangial Changes (% of Pts)	Focal Proliferative GN (% of Pts)	Diffuse Proliferative GN (% of Pts)	Membranous GN (% of Pts)
% of total pts	39	27	16	18
Hematuria, pyuria	13	53	78	50
Proteinuria	36	67	89	100
Nephrotic syndrome	0	27	56	90
Azotemia	13	20	22	10
Decreased complement	54	77	100	75
Increased anti-DNA	45	75	80	33
Decreased complement & increased anti-DNA	36	63	80	33
Hypertension	22	40	56	50
Prognosis	Better	Worse	Worse	Better

Source: Appel, GB. The course of management of lupus nephritis. *Intern Med* 2:82, Feb. 1981.

Tubular reabsorption of sodium, water, urea, and uric acid is increased (perhaps on account of decreased GFR). Sodium excretion is decreased ≥ 35%.

Beware of associated or underlying conditions—hydatidiform mole, twin pregnancy, prior renal disease.

KIDNEY IN MULTIPLE MYELOMA

Renal function is impaired in >50% of patients; usually there is loss of renal concentrating ability and azotemia.

Proteinuria is very frequent and is due to albumin and globulins in urine; Bence Jones proteinuria may be intermittent.

There is severe anemia out of proportion to azotemia.

Occasional changes due to altered renal tubular function are present.

- Renal glycosuria, aminoaciduria, decreased serum uric acid, renal potassium wasting
- Renal loss of phosphate with decreased serum phosphorus and increased alkaline phosphatase
- Nephrogenic diabetes insipidus
- Oliguria or anuria with acute renal failure precipitated by dehydration

Changes due to associated amyloidosis are found.

Changes due to associated hypercalcemia are found.

See Multiple Myeloma, pp. 345–347.

PRIMARY OR SECONDARY AMYLOIDOSIS OF KIDNEY

Persistent proteinuria that varies from mild, with or without hematuria, to severe, with nephrotic syndrome

Vasopressin-resistant polyuria is present if the medulla alone is involved (rare).

See Amyloidosis, pp. 702–704.

SICKLE CELL NEPHROPATHY

Gross and microscopic hematuria is common.

Early decrease of renal concentrating ability is evident even with normal BUN, GFR, and renal plasma flow; it occurs in sickle cell trait as well as the disease, but progressive nephropathy occurs only with the disease. The decrease is temporarily reversed in children by transfusion but not in adults.

RENAL DISEASE IN ALLERGIC (SCHÖNLEIN-HENOCH) PURPURA

Urine is abnormal in 50% of patients, but renal biopsy is abnormal in most (usually a focal proliferative glomerulonephritis).

Clinical picture varies from minimal urinary abnormalities to severe, rapidly progressive nephritis that is indistinguishable from glomerulonephritis. Nephrotic syndrome may occur. Chronic course, with remissions and exacerbations and permanent renal damage, may occur. Serum complement is normal.

Platelet count is normal.

HEMOLYTIC-UREMIC SYNDROME

Usually occurs in a child < age 4 years who develops urinary findings of acute glomerulonephritis.

Triad of

- (1) Acute renal failure. BUN may rise 50 mg/dl/day; is often >100 mg/dl. Urine may show blood, protein, casts, or anuria. Progressive renal disease or recovery.
- (2) Severe microangiopathic hemolytic anemia is present at onset or within a few days.
  - Hemoglobin is often <6 gm/dl; may fall 10% in a day. Reticulocytosis
  - Peripheral blood smear always shows fragmented deformed RBCs (e.g., schistocytes, burr cells, spherocytes), anisocytosis
  - Increased serum total and indirect bilirubin, LDH, free hemoglobin
  - Decreased haptoglobin
  - Negative direct Coombs' test
- (3) Platelet count is decreased.

Normal (or only slightly increased) clotting and fibrinogen rule out DIC. Must also be differentiated from thrombotic thrombocytopenic purpura.

WBC is normal.

Serum complement is normal.

Laboratory findings due to associated etiologic events

- Infections (e.g., Coxsackievirus, enteroviruses, salmonella, shigella, *Escherichia coli, Campylobacter*)
- Complications of pregnancy (e.g., eclampsia, abruptio placentae, amniotic fluid embolism)
- Drug therapy (e.g., oral contraceptives, phenylbutazone, cyclosporin, 5-fluorouracil, mitomycin C)
- Underlying systemic diseases (e.g., primary glomerulopathies, rejection of renal transplant, vasculitis, cryoglobulinemia, septicemia, hypertension, adenocarcinoma)

HEPATORENAL SYNDROME

Oliguria is marked.

Azotemia

Urine sodium is decreased to almost absent (<10 mEq/L; often 1–2 mEq/L); serum sodium is usually decreased.

Table 15-10. Comparison of Three Types of Renal Insufficiency

Laboratory Tests	Prerenal Azotemia	Hepatorenal Syndrome	Acute Renal Failure
Urine sodium (mEq/L)	<10	<10	>30 (may be less with sepsis)
Urine-plasma creatinine	>30:1	>30:1	<20:1
Urine osmolality	At least 100 mOsm > plasma osmolality		Same as plasma osmolality
Urine sediment	Normal	Not remarkable	Cell debris, casts

Concentrated urine with high specific gravity, urine-plasma osmolality ratio >1.0.

Urine is acid; small amount of protein, few casts, few RBCs may be found.

Usually appears in patients with decompensated cirrhosis with moderate to marked ascites, especially following fluid loss (e.g., GI hemorrhage, diarrhea, forced diuresis).

Urine indices resemble those of prerenal azotemia and contrast with acute tubular necrosis in which urine has low fixed specific gravity and high sodium content and a characteristic sediment may be found (see Table 15-10).

HYPERCALCEMIC NEPHROPATHY

Diffuse nephrocalcinosis is the result of prolonged increase in serum and urine calcium (e.g., due to hyperparathyroidism, sarcoidosis, vitamin D intoxication, multiple myeloma, carcinomatosis, milk-alkali syndrome).

Urine is normal or contains RBCs, WBCs, WBC casts; proteinuria is usually slight or absent.

Early findings are decreased renal concentrating ability and polyuria.

Later findings are decreased GFR, decreased renal blood flow, azotemia.

Renal insufficiency is insidious and slowly progressive; it may sometimes be reversed by correcting hypercalcemia.

IRRADIATION NEPHRITIS

Exposure (one or both kidneys) to >2300 rads for 6 weeks or less

Latent period is >6 months.

Slight proteinuria is present.

Hematuria and oliguria are absent.

Refractory anemia is present.

Progressive uremia is found; may be reversible later.

Renal biopsy

ANALGESIC NEPHROPATHY

See Phenacetin—Chronic Excessive Ingestion, p. 723.

LABORATORY CRITERIA FOR KIDNEY TRANSPLANTATION

Donor: Three successive urinalyses and cultures must be negative.

Donor and recipient must show

- ABO and Rh blood group compatibility
- Leukoagglutinin compatibility
- Platelet agglutinin compatibility

LABORATORY FINDINGS OF KIDNEY TRANSPLANT REJECTION

Total urine output is decreased.

Proteinuria is increased.

Cellular or granular casts appear.

Urine osmolality is decreased.
BUN and creatinine rise.
Hyperchloremic renal tubular acidosis may be an early sign of rejection or indicate smoldering rejection activity.
Renal clearance values decrease.
Sodium iodohippurate ^{131}I renogram is altered.
Biopsy of kidney shows a characteristic microscopic appearance and is the definitive way to diagnose rejection.
Sequential measuring of subsets of activated T cells by flow cytometry is useful for diagnosis of rejection and monitoring reversibility of rejection.

LEUKOPLAKIA OF RENAL PELVIS

Cell block or Papanicolaou smear of urine shows keratin or keratinized squamous cells.

CARCINOMA OF RENAL PELVIS AND URETER

Hematuria is present.
Renal calculi are associated.
Urinary tract infection is associated.
Cytologic examination of urinary sediment for malignant cells is necessary.

HYPERNEPHROMA OF KIDNEY

Even in the absence of the classic loin pain, flank mass, and hematuria, hypernephroma should be ruled out in the presence of these *unexplained* laboratory findings.

- Abnormal liver function tests (in absence of metastases to liver) found in 40% of these patients, e.g., increased serum alkaline phosphatase, prolonged prothrombin time, altered serum protein values (decreased albumin, increased $alpha_2$ globulin)
- Hypercalcemia
- Polycythemia
- Leukemoid reaction
- Refractory anemia and increased ESR
- Amyloidosis
- Cushing's syndrome
- Salt-losing syndrome

For laboratory assistance in diagnosis

- Exfoliative cytology of urine for tumor cells
- Test for increased urine LDH level
- Radioisotope scan of kidney

Needle biopsy is not recommended.

RENIN-PRODUCING RENAL TUMORS

(hemangiopericytomas of juxtaglomerular apparatus; Wilms' tumor; rarely lung cancer)

Plasma renin activity is increased, with levels significantly higher in renal vein from affected side.
Plasma renin activity responds to changes in posture but not to changes in sodium intake.
Plasma renin activity maintains circadian rhythm despite marked elevation.
Secondary aldosteronism is evident, with hypokalemia, etc. (see p. 510).
Laboratory changes (and hypertension) are reversed by removal of tumor.

PYELONEPHRITIS

Bacteriuria. Colony count of >100,000/ml of urine (properly collected) indicates active infection. If the count is 10,000–100,000/ml, it should be repeated.

<100,000/ml with clinical findings of acute pyelonephritis with no obvious explanation, such as recent use of antibiotics, suggests urinary tract obstruction or perinephric abscess. Bacteria seen on Gram's stain of uncentrifuged urine indicates bacteriuria.

Positive test for antibody-coated bacteria (using fluorescein-conjugated antihuman globulin) is said to indicate bacteria of renal origin and be 81% predictive of upper GU tract infection.

A culture should be performed for identification of the specific organism and determination of antibiotic sensitivity. This antibiogram is useful in subsequently identifying the same organism in relapsing infections.

Microscopic examination of urine sediment: WBC casts are very suggestive of pyelonephritis. Glitter cells may be seen.

Pyuria is present in only 50% of patients with chronic urinary tract infection and asymptomatic bacteriuria. Bacteriuria and pyuria are often intermittent; in the chronic atrophic stage of pyelonephritis, they are often absent. In acute pyelonephritis, marked pyuria and bacteriuria are almost always present; hematuria and proteinuria may also be present during first few days.

Urine concentrating ability is decreased relatively early in chronic infection compared to other renal diseases.

Albuminuria is usually <2 gm/24 hours (≤2+ qualitative) and therefore helps to differentiate pyelonephritis from glomerular disease, in which albuminuria is usually >2 gm/24 hours.

Albuminuria may be undetectable in a very dilute urine associated with fixed specific gravity.

There is a decrease in 24-hour creatinine clearance before a rise in BUN and blood creatinine takes place.

Hyperchloremic acidosis (due to impaired renal acid excretion and bicarbonate reabsorption) occurs more often in chronic pyelonephritis than in glomerulonephritis.

Renal blood flow and glomerular filtration show parallel decrease proportional to progress of renal disease. Comparison of function in right and left kidneys shows more disparity in pyelonephritis than in diffuse renal disease (e.g., nephrosclerosis, glomerulonephritis).

Fluctuation in renal insufficiency (e.g., due to recurrent infection, dehydration) with considerable recovery is more marked and frequent in pyelonephritis than in other renal diseases.

Laboratory findings of associated diseases, e.g., diabetes mellitus, urinary tract obstruction (e.g., stone, tumor), neurogenic bladder dysfunction, are present. Urinary tract infection in infant <1 year old is associated with an underlying GU tract anomaly in 55% of males and 35% of females.

Laboratory findings due to sequelae (e.g., papillary necrosis, bacteremia) are present.

"Cured" patient should be followed with routine periodic urinalysis and colony count for at least 2 years because asymptomatic recurrence of bacteriuria is common.

When urine cultures are persistently negative in the presence of other evidence of pyelonephritis, specific search should be made for tubercle bacilli (e.g., culture).

RENAL ABSCESS

(due to metastatic infection not related to previous renal disease)

Urine
- Trace of albumin
- Few RBCs (may have transient gross hematuria at onset)
- No WBCs
- Very many gram-positive cocci in stained sediment

WBC high (may be >30,000/cu mm)

PERINEPHRIC ABSCESS

Laboratory findings due to underlying or primary diseases

- Hematogenous from distant foci (e.g., furuncles, infected tonsils) usually due to staphylococci and occasionally streptococci
- Direct extension from kidney infection (e.g., pyelonephritis, pyonephrosis) due to gram-negative rods and occasionally tubercle bacilli
- Infected perirenal hematoma (e.g., due to trauma, tumor, polyarteritis nodosa) due to various organisms

Urine changes due to underlying disease

- Urine may be normal and sterile. *(Do acid-fast smear and culture for tubercle bacilli.)*

Increased PMNs

Increased ESR

Positive blood culture (some patients)

RENAL TUBERCULOSIS (TB)

Should be ruled out when there is unexplained albuminuria, pyuria, microhematuria, but cultures for pyogenic bacteria are negative, especially in presence of TB elsewhere

Urine culture for TB

Guinea pig inoculation

See Tuberculosis, pp. 640, 643, for general findings.

BENIGN PROSTATIC HYPERTROPHY

Laboratory findings are those due to urinary tract obstruction and secondary infection.

Prostatic specific antigen may be increased in 55–83% of patients, preventing its use for screening for prostate cancer.

PROSTATITIS

Bacterial form is most frequently due to

- *Escherichia coli*
- *Proteus mirabilis*
- *Pseudomonas*
- *Klebsiella*
- *Streptococcus faecalis*
- *Staphylococcus aureus*

The acute form usually shows laboratory findings of infected urine (WBCs in centrifuged sediment of last portion of voided specimen; positive colony count and culture).

In chronic bacterial prostatitis, prostatic fluid and third-voided bladder urine specimen show a greater (usually 10 times) colony count compared to the first urine specimen.

In chronic nonbacterial prostatitis, prostatic fluid usually shows >10 WBC/hpf with negative cultures of urine and prostatic fluid; do not respond to antibiotic therapy. May be due to organisms that are difficult to culture (e.g., *Ureaplasma,* chlamydiae, trichomonads, cytomegalovirus, or herpes virus) or to treat.

Laboratory findings due to associated or complicating conditions (e.g., epididymitis) may be present.

POSTVASECTOMY STATUS

Sperm count may fall to low levels after 3 or 4 ejaculations and then rise abruptly before falling again.

Ten ejaculations may be required before sperm count reaches 0.

Three consecutive azoospermic specimens are recommended before dispensing with contraception.

Reanastomosis of the vas deferens may occur.

CARCINOMA OF PROSTATE

Increased serum acid phosphatase (PAP) indicates local extension or distant metastases. It is increased in 60–75% of patients with bone metastases, 20% of patients with extension into periprostatic soft tissue but without bone involvement, 5% of patients with carcinoma confined to gland. Occasionally it remains low despite active metastases. Increased PAP shows pronounced fall in activity within 3–4 days after castration or within 2 weeks after estrogen therapy is begun; may return to normal or remain slightly elevated; failure to fall corresponds to the failure of clinical response that occurs in 10% of the patients. Most patients with invasive carcinoma show a significant increase in PAP after massage or palpation; this rarely occurs in patients with normal prostate, benign prostatic hypertrophy, or in situ carcinoma or in patients with prostate carcinoma who are receiving hormone treatment.

- Serum acid phosphatase is also increased in
  - Infarction of the prostate (sometimes to high levels)
  - Operative trauma or instrumentation of the prostate (may cause transient increase) or after prostatic massage
  - Gaucher's disease (only when certain substrates are used in the laboratory determination)
  - Excessive destruction of platelets, as in idiopathic thrombocytopenic purpura with megakaryocytes in bone marrow
  - Thromboembolism, hemolytic crises (e.g., sickle cell disease) due to hemolysis (only when certain substrates are used in the laboratory determination) are said to occur often.
  - Leukemic reticuloendotheliosis ("hairy") cells using a specific assay
- In the absence of prostatic disease, increased acid phosphatase is seen occasionally in
  - Partial translocation trisomy 21
  - Diseases of bone
    - Advanced Paget's disease
    - Metastatic carcinoma of bone
    - Multiple myeloma (some patients)
    - Hyperparathyroidism
    - Other
  - Various liver diseases (≤9 King-Armstrong units)
    - Hepatitis
    - Obstructive jaundice
    - Laennec's cirrhosis
    - Other
  - Acute renal impairment (not related to degree of azotemia)
  - Other diseases of the reticuloendothelial system with liver or bone involvement (e.g., Niemann-Pick disease)
- Decreased values are not clinically significant.

PAP is nearly always increased with a palpable prostatic nodule. Specificity >94% but may be normal in poorly differentiated or androgen-insensitive prostate carcinomas. More frequently increased with advancing stage and grade of cancer and in presence of lymph node or bone metastases. *Is not useful for screening of general or asymptomatic population for prostate cancer.* If PAP assay is elevated in presence of a negative biopsy, the biopsy should be repeated. Elevated PAP assay should return to normal 1 week following surgery or radiotherapy for carcinoma palpable on rectal examination; failure to do so suggests the presence of metastatic lesions; not useful to assess therapy. Not increased in nonprostate diseases listed above.

Prostatic specific antigen not useful for early screening because it is elevated in 55–83% of patients with benign prostatic hypertrophy. Is not useful for staging. Serum level is increased 2 times by prostatic massage, 4 times by cystoscopy and >50 times by needle biopsy or transurethral resection. Chief use is to monitor postoperative recurrence after total prostatectomy for cancer. After complete local excision of prostate, should decline at least to normal range. May also be useful marker when it is elevated and acid phosphatase is normal.

Neither PAP nor prostatic specific antigen is recommended for general screening for occult cancer but should be used together to monitor treatment of prostate cancer. Not used to determine whether to do biopsy.

Alkaline phosphatase is increased in 90% of patients with bone metastases. Increases with favorable response to estrogen therapy or castration and reaches peak in 3 months, then declines. Recurrence of bone metastases causes new rise in alkaline phosphatase.

Anemia is present.

Carcinoma cells may appear in bone marrow aspirates.

Fibrinolysins are found in 12% of patients with metastatic prostatic cancer; occur only with extensive metastases and are usually associated with hemorrhagic manifestations; they show fibrinogen deficiency and prolonged prothrombin time.

Urinary tract infection and hematuria occur late.

Needle biopsy of suspicious nodules in prostate is called for.

Cytologic examination of prostatic fluid is not generally useful.

BACTERIURIC SYNDROMES

(usually associated with pyuria of >8 WBC/cu mm uncentrifuged urine)

Lower GU tract infection	Symptoms + colony count $>10^2$ bacteria/ml
Acute cystitis	Symptoms + colony count $>10^5$ bacteria/ml
Acute urethral syndrome	Symptoms + colony count 10^2–10^5 bacteria/ml or sexually transmitted agent (e.g., *Neisseria gonorrhoeae, Chlamydia trachomatis,* herpes simplex virus) or no agent identified
Acute pyelonephritis	Symptoms + colony count $>10^5$ bacteria/ml (see pp. 592–593)
Asymptomatic bacteriuria	No symptoms + colony count $>10^5$ bacteria/ml
Recurrent bacteriuria	No symptoms or recurrent symptoms + colony count $>10^5$ bacteria/ml
Relapse	Recurrent infection with same agent
Reinfection	Recurrent infection with different agent
Complicated bacteriuria	Structural abnormality of GU tract (e.g., stones, catheter) + colony count $>10^5$ bacteria/ml

SOME CAUSES OF SEXUALLY TRANSMITTED DISEASES

(see also separate sections)

Bacteria

Neisseria gonorrhoeae
Treponema pallidum
Mycoplasma hominis
Calymmatobacterium granulomatis
Campylobacter fetus
Streptococcus Group B (?)
Chlamydia trachomatis
Ureaplasma urealyticum
Haemophilus ducreyi
Shigella sp.
Gardnerella vaginalis (?)

Viruses

HIV
Hepatitis A and B
Papillomavirus (genital wart)
Herpes simplex
Cytomegalovirus
Molluscum contagiosum

Protozoa
Trichomonas vaginalis
Giardia lamblia
Entamoeba histolytica
Ectoparasites
Crab louse
Scabies mite

SEXUALLY TRANSMITTED BACTERIAL DISEASES (INCLUDING URETHRITIS, PELVIC INFLAMMATORY DISEASE, ETC.)

Urethritis is diagnosed if smear of urethral discharge shows >4 PMNs/1000X field.

In absence of urethral discharge, an early-morning urine specimen is collected. An initial 10-ml specimen is centrifuged and compared to the rest of the sample. If the first specimen shows more PMNs (>15 PMNs/400X field) than the later sample, urethritis is diagnosed. If equal numbers of PMNs are present in both specimens, the inflammation is higher up in the GU tract. If no PMNs are present, urethritis is unlikely. Sediment of the first specimen should also be examined for *Trichomonas vaginalis*.

Gram's stains will show gram-negative intracellular diplococci in >95% of cases of gonorrhea. When only some extracellular diplococci are seen, subsequent cultures are positive for *Neisseria gonorrhoeae* in <15% of patients.

In males, a positive gram-stained smear establishes the diagnosis of gonorrhea and a culture is not necessary, but in females, a positive smear should be confirmed by culture on appropriate media (i.e., Gram's stains are highly sensitive and specific in males but not in females).

Chlamydia and *Ureaplasma* cannot be identified on Gram's stains, and cultures must be done at specialized laboratories.

When Gram's stains and cultures for gonorrhea are negative, the presumptive diagnosis is nongonococcal urethritis, and *Chlamydia trachomatis* causes about 50% of such cases. This is the most frequent venereal disease and is estimated to be >2 times more frequent than gonorrhea.

In VD clinics, up to 50% of males with gonococcal urethritis have concomitant *C. trachomatis* present. Chlamydiae are responsible for 70% of postgonococcal urethritis. In VD clinics, *C. trachomatis* can be cultured from 25–50% of females.

In sexually active men with no symptoms or laboratory findings of urethritis, chlamydial infection is found in <3%.

In sexually active young men, acute epididymitis is almost always due to sexually transmitted disease (STD); 10% are due to gonorrhea; 50–80% are due to *C. trachomatis* in heterosexuals but *Escherichia coli* is more common in homosexual men and men > 35 years old. Laboratory findings of urethritis will usually be found even if patient is asymptomatic.

Women infected with *C. trachomatis* show infection of urethra (50% of cases), rectum (25% of cases), and cervix (75% of cases). Present in <50% of women with cervical gonococcal infection.

Sexually active women with symptoms of lower urinary tract infection, pyuria (>15 WBCs/hpf), but sterile urine cultures probably have chlamydial infection. If coliforms or staphylococci are found, bacterial cystitis is likely even if <100,000/cu mm.

Ureaplasma urealyticum probably causes 20–30% of cases of urethritis in males.

Mycoplasma hominis may cause pyelonephritis (5% of cases), pelvic inflammatory disease (10% of cases), and postpartum febrile complications (10% of cases). *U. urealyticum* and *M. hominis* are usually diagnosed by culture; DNA probes are less sensitive. Serologic methods are not widely used for various reasons (e.g., lack of specificity, complexity); diagnosis requires 4-fold rise in IgG titer; increased IgM titer may be reliable in urethritis or salpingitis.

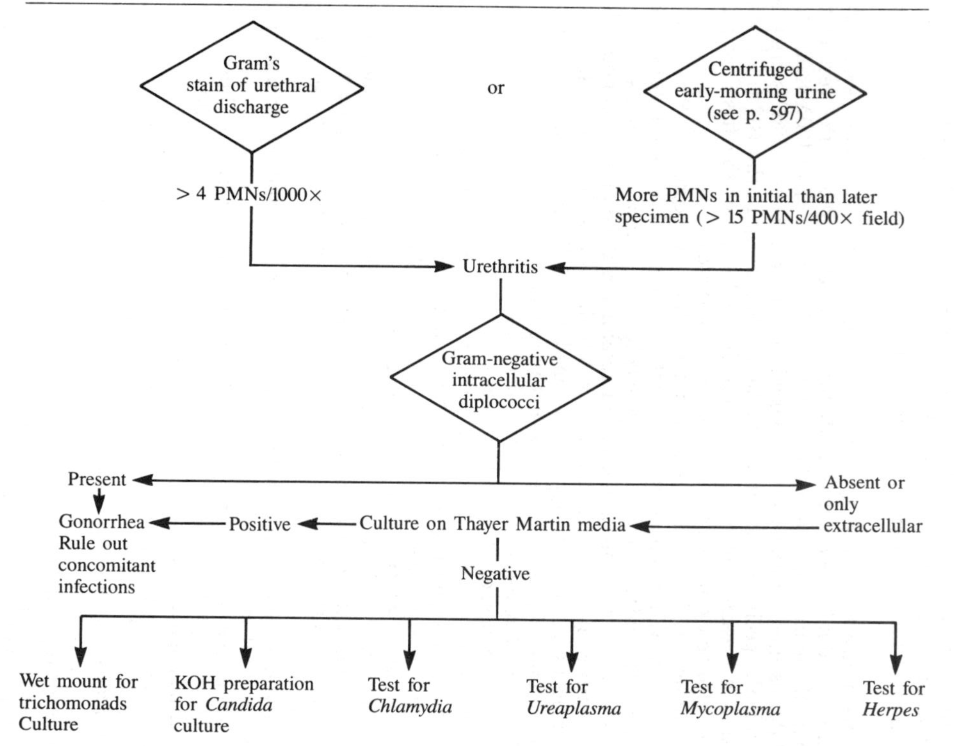

Fig. 15-3. Flow chart for diagnosis of urethritis in males.

Candida albicans, T. vaginalis, herpes simplex, and cytomegalovirus probably cause 10–15% of cases of nongonococcal urethritis.

Laboratory findings of complications
- Prostatitis (20% of patients)
- Epididymitis (<3% of patients)
- Urethral stricture (<5% of patients)
- Reiter's syndrome (2% of patients)
- Cervicitis, cervical erosion, cytologic atypia on Papanicolaou smear, salpingitis
- Sterility
- Acute proctitis

PELVIC INFLAMMATORY DISEASE (PID)

Due To

Chlamydia trachomatis (specific antibodies are found in 80% of acute cases; 20% have specific IgM antibody indicating acute infection and 37% have a 4-fold rise in IgG)
Neisseria gonorrhoeae infection is found in 8% of acute cases.
Anaerobic bacteria
Coliform bacilli
Actinomyces israelii
Mycoplasma hominis
Many cases are polymicrobial.

PID due to C. trachomatis *causes less leukocytosis, fever, less severe symptoms than that due to* N. gonorrhoeae.

Cervicitis
- Cervical Gram's stain > 10 PMNs/hpf (1000 ×) in nonmenstruating women
- Tests for appropriate organism
  - Culture
  - Direct antigen test (e.g., *Chlamydia*)

Human papillomavirus infection (HPV)—suspect in presence of koilocytic changes on Pap smear or cervical biopsy, often with cytologic atypia that varies from mild up to carcinoma of cervix; also present in genital condylomata. Found in 1–4% of routine screening Pap smears and ≤16% of women in STD clinics. May be confirmed by antigen detection staining of tissue or DNA hybridization. Southern blot hybridization detects HPV DNA in ~90% of cases of genital warts and 70–95% of cases of in situ and invasive carcinoma of cervix. HPV also found in 6% of unselected men by DNA studies of cell scrapings from penis. Culture is not available. At present, serologic tests (ELISA) are not clinically useful.
Urethritis—see preceding section.
Vulvovaginitis—see next section.
Perihepatitis (Fitz-Hugh–Curtis syndrome)
- IgM and IgG antibodies for *C. trachomatis*

Laboratory findings due to complications, e.g., infertility, ectopic pregnancy, premature birth, neonatal conjunctivitis, infant pneumonia

VULVOVAGINITIS

Due To

Gonococcus (see p. 620)
Bacterial vaginosis—polymicrobial infection due to increase in anaerobic organisms including *Gardnerella vaginalis* and concomitant decrease in lactobacilli

Vaginal pH > 4.5 (using pH indicator paper) in >80% of cases (found in one-third of normal women)

Wet mount of vaginal discharge shows "clue cells" (vaginal epithelial cells coated with bacilli) found in 90% of cases and curved rods.

Fishy amine odor on addition 10% KOH to vaginal fluid

Positive culture on special media (e.g., chocolate agar) for *G. vaginalis* in 95% of clinical cases (but not recommended for diagnosis or test of cure since it may also be found in 40–50% of asymptomatic women with no signs of infection)

Gram's stain and Papanicolaou smear may also suggest this diagnosis; gram-negative curved rods and decreased to absent gram-positive rods resembling lactobacilli.

Homogeneous adherent discharge; mixed with 10% KOH on slide produces a fishy odor; positive predictive value of 76%

In nongonorrheal cases, smear shows more epithelial cells and fewer WBCs compared to gonorrhea. Gram's stain may show many or few bacteria, which are often mixed (i.e., gram-positive and gram-negative; cocci and bacilli).

Chlamydial urethritis, >10 WBC/1000× without microscopic bacteriuria; hematuria and proteinuria are very unusual. Pap smear may show cytoplasmic inclusion bodies in metaplastic squamous cells of cervix, which have low sensitivity and specificity and positive predictive values 10–40%.

Fungi, especially *Candida albicans,* diagnosed by wet mount in KOH or Gram's stain of vaginal fluid, may not detect 15% of cases. May be seen on Pap smears, but culture on Nickerson's or Sabouraud's medium is needed for definitive identification and is more sensitive. Sexual transmission plays a very minor role.

Trichomonas vaginalis

Recognition of organism in material from vagina

Wet-mount preparation of freshly examined vaginal fluid (sensitivity 50–70% compared to culture) (requires 10^4 organisms/ml)

Frequently an incidental finding in routine urinalysis

Frequently found in routine Papanicolaou smears (sensitivity about same as wet mount, specificity ~95%, positive predictive value > 90%; based on a prevalence of 5%, positive predictive value = 75%, and negative predictive value = 38%). The organism is often not identified but may be associated with characteristic concomitant cytologic changes. Not recommended for screening for *Trichomonas.*

Culture is the most definitive and sensitive test and is the gold standard.

Douching within 24 hours decreases sensitivity of tests. Do not test during first few days of menstrual cycle as number of organisms is low then.

Occasionally detected in material from male urethra in cases of nonspecific urethritis.

Serologic tests are not useful.

On wet mount preparations:

Atrophic inflammatory: >5 PMNs/hpf, parabasal epithelial cells predominate

Nonatrophic inflammatory: >10 PMNs/hpf, mature epithelial cells predominate

Nonatrophic noninflammatory: <10 PMNs/hpf, mature epithelial cells predominate

Atrophic noninflammatory: <5 PMNs/hpf, basal epithelial cells predominate. May be identified in 78% of cases by Pap smear, 85% of cases by wet mount, 94% of cases by culture in one study. Another study of Pap smear alone found sensitivity of 58% and specificity of 40%.

Herpes simplex virus—may be identified in Pap smear of cervix by multinucleated cells showing typical intranuclear inclusions and halo.
Local cause is most common (e.g., endocrine, poor hygiene, pinworms, scabies, foreign body).

Multiple causes may be present and should be sought in each case.

CARCINOMA OF BLADDER

Hematuria may be gross or only microscopic.
Biopsy of tumor should be taken.
Cytologic examination of urine for tumor cells is useful for Grades II, III, and IV carcinoma but not for Grade I, which has a high false positive rate. It may be of value in screening dye workers in chemical industry.

	Sensitivity*	
	First Urine Specimen	**Third Urine Specimen**
Grade I	None	20% (many false positives)
Grade II	30%	80%
Grade III	65%	85%
Grade IV	92%	98%

Flow cytometry of urine quantitatively measures DNA content or ploidy; cells with normal DNA content are diploid and cells with abnormal DNA content are aneuploid, which is found only in neoplastic cells, although diploidy is found in both normal and neoplastic cells. Aneuploidy is early indicator of neoplasia and may be present before microscopic evidence of tumor. 78% sensitivity for bladder cancer; specificity for nonneoplastic disease = 2%.
Urinary LDH level may be useful in screening studies to discover asymptomatic patients with neoplasm of GU tract.
Laboratory findings due to complications will stem from infection or from obstruction of ureter.
Laboratory findings due to preexisting conditions (e.g., schistosomiasis, stone, or infection)

RETROPERITONEAL FIBROSIS

ESR is increased.
Leukocytosis is present.
Occasionally eosinophilia occurs.
Serum protein and albumin-globulin (A/G) ratio are normal; if the person is chronically ill, total protein may be decreased. Gamma globulins may be increased.
Anemia is present.
Laboratory findings due to ureteral obstruction are made.
The condition may be primary, due to angiomatous lymphoid hamartoma, or secondary to administration of methysergide.

CANCER OF UTERUS

Carcinoma Of The Corpus

Cytologic examination (Papanicolaou smear) is positive in ~70% of patients; a false negative result occurs in 30% of patients. Therefore a negative Pap smear does not rule out carcinoma.

*False positives may occur due to atypia in chronic cystitis, calculi, irradiation, chemotherapy (e.g., myleran).

Pap smear from aspiration of endometrial cavity is positive in 95% of patients. Endometrial biopsy may be helpful, but a negative result does not rule out carcinoma.

Diagnostic curettage is the only way to rule out carcinoma of the endometrium.

Carcinoma Of The Cervix

Pap smear for routine screening in the general population may be positive for carcinoma of the cervix in ~6 of every 1000 women (prevalence); only 7% of these lesions are invasive. The prevalence rate is greatest in certain groups:

- Women ages 21–35 years, with peak in 31st to 35th year
- Black and Puerto Rican women
- Women who use birth control pills rather than diaphragm for contraception
- Women with early onset or long duration of sexual activity

Chief use of Pap smear is for routine screening of asymptomatic women to detect carcinoma of cervix or various atypias.

Also used to monitor response to therapy for carcinoma, infections, etc.

Occasionally detects carcinoma from other sites (e.g., endometrium, ovary, tube).

Often detects presence of various previously undiagnosed infectious agents (e.g., *Trichomonas vaginalis,* herpes simplex virus, human papillomavirus, *Candida*)

Useful to estimate hormonal status

Occasionally useful in chromosome studies

Vaginal pool Pap smear has an accuracy rate of ~80% in detecting carcinoma of the cervix. Smears from a combination of vaginal pool, exocervical, and endocervical scrapings have an accuracy rate of 95%.

After an initial abnormal smear, the follow-up smear taken in the next few weeks or months may not always be abnormal; there is no clear explanation for this finding. Biopsy shows important lesions of the cervix in some of these patients. Therefore an abnormal initial smear requires further investigation of the cervix regardless of subsequent cytologic reports.

Late Cases

Laboratory findings due to obstruction of ureters with pyelonephritis, azotemia, etc., may be present.

General effects of cancer are found.

Trophoblastic Neoplasms

Hydatidiform mole—5% progress to choriocarcinoma.

Choriocarcinoma—50% are preceded by molar pregnancy, 25% by term pregnancy, 25% by abortion or ectopic pregnancy.

Amount of human chorionic gonadotropin (HCG) produced correlates with amount of trophoblastic tissue.

HCG is important to identify 15–20% of hydatidiform moles that persist after curettage.

After evacuation of the uterus, HCG is negative by 40 days in 75% of cases. If test is positive at 56 days, 50% have trophoblastic disease. Repeat test every 2 weeks with clinical examination. Disease remits in 80% without further treatment. Plateau or rise of titer indicates persistent disease. Chemotherapy is indicated if disease persists or metastasizes. Repeat negative titer should be rechecked every 3 months for a year. High-risk patients are indicated by initial serum titer > 40,000 mIU/ml. Frequent follow-up titers are indicated after radiation therapy, with lifelong titers every 6 months.

Laboratory findings due to treatment (e.g., hemorrhage, infection, perforation of uterus, radiation, chemotherapy)

Histologic examination of tissue removed by curettage

RUPTURED TUBAL PREGNANCY

WBC may be increased; usually returns to normal in 24 hours. Persistent increase may indicate recurrent bleeding. 50% of patients have normal WBC; 75% of the patients have WBC < 15,000/cu mm. Persistent WBC > 20,000/cu mm may indicate pelvic inflammatory disease.

Anemia depends on degree of blood loss; often precedes the tubal pregnancy in impoverished populations. Progressive anemia may indicate continuing bleeding into hematoma. Absorption of blood from hematoma may cause increased serum bilirubin.

Pregnancy tests are positive in ~50% of patients; however, the beta-subunit HCG assay is positive in ~95% of patients. Qualitative test (ELISA) confirms pregnancy in 30 minutes. Quantitative HCG > 6500 mIU/ml without an intrauterine sac on sonography favors ectopic pregnancy, since at this titer an intrauterine pregnancy should be visualized. HCG < 6000 mIU/ml without a sac = unknown diagnosis. HCG < 6000 mIU with a sac suggests either ectopic or an early normal/abnormal pregnancy. In early pregnancy, serum beta-HCG should double every 1.4–2.1 days.

Urine pregnancy test is variable.

Serum progesterone (by RIA) >15 ng/ml is said to indicate normal intrauterine pregnancy and <15 ng/ml to occur in ectopic or abnormal intrauterine pregnancy.

LABORATORY CRITERIA FOR SEVERE PREECLAMPSIA

Significant proteinuria ≥ 500 mg/24 hours (2+ on dipstick). Proteinuria ≥ 5 gm/24 hours correlates with 3–4+ on dipstick.

Oliguria—urine output < 400 ml/24 hours.

Evidence of microangiopathic hemolysis, abnormal liver function tests, falling platelet count (HELLP syndrome). Lupus anticoagulant, antiphospholipid antibodies may be present.

Laboratory findings due to complications, e.g., cerebral hemorrhage, pulmonary edema, renal cortical necrosis

Weakly creatinine clearance to follow renal function

Laboratory findings due to predisposing conditions, e.g., diabetes mellitus, hydatidiform mole, nonimmune hydrops fetalis

Usefulness of monitoring maternal estriols, human placental lactogen, and other components is questionable.

$MgSO_4$ treatment requires urine output ≥ 100 ml every 4 hours. Therapeutic Mg range = 4–7 mEq/L. Toxicity begins at 7–10 mEq/L; respiratory depression begins at 10–15 mEq/L; cardiac arrest begins at 30 mEq/L.

Eclampsia is indicated by occurrence of generalized seizures. ~20% of women develop eclampsia with only mild hypertension and often without proteinuria or edema.

Amniocentesis to determine fetal maturity if induction of labor is required.

LABORATORY CRITERIA FOR MILD PREECLAMPSIA

Proteinuria of > 300 mg in at least two random clean-catch urine specimens collected 6 hours apart but < 2 gm/24 hours.

Table 15-11. Urinary Findings in Various Diseases

Disease	Volume	Specific Gravity	Protein[a]	RBCs[b]	WBCs and Epithelial Cells[b]	Casts[c,d]	Comment
Normal	600–2500	1.003–1.030	0(0.05 gm)	0–occ. (0–0.130)	0–0.65	0–occ. (2000/24 hrs)	
Acute febrile states	D	I	Trace to +			Few	
Orthostatic proteinuria	N	N	I (up 1 gm)	N (0–0.130)	0–3	V; H & G	Normal when recumbent; abnormalities after upright posture
Glomerulonephritis							
Acute	D	I	2–4+ (0.5–5.0)	1–4+ (1–1000)	1–400	2–4+; H & G; *RBC, epithelial, mixed RBC &* epithelial	Gross hematuria or "smoky" urine
Latent			(0.1–2.0)	(1–100)	1–20	*RBC,* H & G	

Nephrosis ("nephrotic stage")	D	I	4+ (4–40)	0–few (0.5–50)	20–1000	*Epithelial, fatty,* waxy; H & G	Fat-laden epithelial cells, anisotropic fat in epithelial cells and casts
Terminal	I or D	D; fixed	1–2+ (2–7)	Trace–1+ (0.5–10)	1–50	1–3+ *Broad, waxy,* H & G, epithelial	
Pyelonephritis							
Acute	N	N	0–2+ (0.5–2)	Few (0–1)	20–2000	*WBC,* H & G, *bacteria*	Bacteria, many WBCs in clumps
Chronic	N or D	N or D	2–4+ (0–5)	Few (0–1)	0.5–50.0	Same as acute; often few or none	Same as acute; findings may be intermittent
Renal tuberculosis			(0.1–3)	(1–20)	1–50	WBC, H & G	Tubercle bacilli
Disseminated lupus erythematosus	V	N or D	1–4+ (0.5–20.0)	1–4+ (1–100)	1–100	1–4+ RBC, *fatty, waxy;* H & G	

Table 15-11. (continued)

Disease	Volume	Specific Gravity	Protein[a]	RBCs[b]	WBCs and Epithelial Cells[b]	Casts[c,d]	Comment
Toxemia of pregnancy	D	I	3–4+ (0.5–10.0)	0–1+ (0–1)	1–5	3–4+ H & G	
Malignant hypertension	V	D; fixed	1–2+ (1–10)	Trace–1+ (1–100)	1–200	1–2+ H & G, RBC, fatty	Increasing uremia with minimal or marked proteinuria and hematuria
Benign hypertension	N or I	N or D	0–1+	0–trace (1–5)		0–1+ H & G	
Congestive heart failure	D	I	1–2+	0–1+		1+ H & G	

Intercapillary glomerulosclerosis (Kimmelstiel-Wilson syndrome)			1–4 + (2–20)	(0–1)	1–30	Epithelial, fatty, H & G	Frequently associated: pyelonephritis and nephrosclerosis
Lower nephron nephrosis							
Acute	D	I		1–4+	1–4+	RBC; H & G, epithelial	
Diuretic	I		0.5–10.0	(0–1)	1–100	Broad, waxy, epithelial, H & G	

D = decreased; I = increased; occ. = occasionally; N = normal; V = variable; H & G = hyaline and granular casts.
[a]Protein = quantitative values in ( ) given as gm/24 hours.
[b]Quantitative values given as cells × 10^6/24 hours.
[c]Cast requires examination of fresh or preserved urine and acid pH.
[d]Italics denote most important or diagnostic finding.

16

Infectious Diseases

Table 16-1. Organisms Commonly Present in Various Sites

Site	Normal Flora	Pathogens	% of Cases
External ear	*Staphylococcus epidermidis*	*Pseudomonas* sp.	60
	Alpha-hemolytic streptococci	*Staphylococcus aureus*	15
	Enterobacter sp.	Coliform bacilli	2
	Aerobic corynebacteria	Alpha-hemolytic streptococci	1
	Corynebacterium acnes	*Proteus* sp.	5
	Candida sp.	Pneumococci	
	Bacillus sp.	*Corynebacterium diphtheriae*	
		Aspergillus sp.	7
		Candida sp.	3
		Varicella-zoster virus	
		Herpes simplex virus	
		Papovavirus	
		Molluscum contagiosum	
Middle ear	Sterile	**Acute Otitis Media**	
		Hemophilus influenzae	30
		Pneumococci	30
		Beta-hemolytic streptococci	
		Chronic Otitis Media	
		Staphylococcus aureus	15
		Proteus sp.	
		Pseudomonas sp.	
		Other gram-negative bacilli	
		Alpha-hemolytic streptococci	
		Respiratory syncytial virus	
		Influenza virus	
Nasal passages	*Staphylococcus epidermidis*	**Acute Sinusitis**	
	Staphylococcus aureus	*Staphylococcus aureus*	
	Diphtheroids	Pneumococci	
	Pneumococci	*Klebsiella-Enterobacter* sp.	
	Alpha-hemolytic streptococci	Alpha-hemolytic streptococci	
	Nonpathogenic *Neisseria* sp.	Beta-hemolytic streptococci	
	Aerobic corynebacteria		
		Chronic Sinusitis	
		Staphylococcus aureus	
		Alpha-hemolytic streptococci	
		Pneumococci	
		Beta-hemolytic streptococci	
		Mucor, Aspergillus sp. (especially in diabetics)	
Respiratory tract		*Pseudomonas aeruginosa*	24
		Escherichia coli	9
		Klebsiella pneumoniae	9
		Serratia marcescens	9
		Enterobacter sp.	13
		Staphylococcus aureus	7
		Proteus mirabilis	6

Table 16-1 (continued)

Site	Normal Flora	Pathogens	% of Cases
Pharynx and tonsils	Alpha-hemolytic streptococci *Neisseria* sp. *Staphylococcus epidermidis* *Staphylococcus aureus* (small numbers) Pneumococci Nonhemolytic (gamma) streptococci Diphtheroids Coliforms Beta-hemolytic streptococci (not Group A) *Actinomyces israelii* *Hemophilus* spp. *Marked predominance of one organism may be clinically significant even if it is a normal inhabitant.*	Beta-hemolytic streptococci *Corynebacterium diphtheriae* *Bordetella pertussis* *Neisseria meningitidis* *Hemophilus influenzae* Group B *Staphylococcus aureus* *Candida albicans*	
Gastrointestinal tract (see pp. 159–161)			
Mouth	Alpha-hemolytic streptococci Enterococci Lactobacilli Staphylococci Fusobacteria *Bacteroides* sp. Diphtheroids *Neisseria* sp. except *N. gonorrhoeae*	*Candida albicans* *Borrelia vincentii* with *Fusobacterium fusiformis*	
Esophagus		*Candida albicans* Cytomegalovirus Herpes simplex virus	
Stomach	Sterile	*Helicobacter pylori*	
Small intestine	Sterile in one-third Scant bacteria in others *Escherichia coli* *Klebsiella-Enterobacter* Enterococci Alpha-hemolytic streptococci *Staphylococcus epidermidis* Diphtheroids	*Campylobacter jejuni*	
Colon	Abundant bacteria *Bacteroides* sp. *Escherichia coli* *Klebsiella-Enterobacter* Paracolons *Proteus* sp. Enterococci (Group D streptococci) Yeasts	Enteropathogenic *Escherichia coli* *Candida albicans* *Aeromonas* sp. *Salmonella* sp. *Shigella* sp. *Campylobacter jejuni* *Yersinia enterocolitica* *Staphylococcus aureus* *Clostridium difficile* *Vibrio cholerae* *Vibrio parahaemolyticus*	

Table 16-1 (continued)

Site	Normal Flora	Pathogens	% of Cases
		Rotavirus	
		Cytomegalovirus	
		Herpes simplex virus	
		Norwalk virus	
Rectum		*Chlamydia* sp.	
		Neisseria gonorrhoeae	
		Treponema pallidum	
		Lymphogranuloma venereum	
		Herpes simplex virus	
Gallbladder	Sterile	*Escherichia coli*	
		Enterococci	
		Klebsiella-Enterobacter-Serratia	
		Occasionally	
		Coliforms	
		Proteus sp.	
		Pseudomonas sp.	
		Salmonella sp.	
Blood	Sterile	*Staphylococcus epidermidis*	15
		Staphylococcus aureus	10
		Escherichia coli	16
		Enterococci	13
		Pseudomonas sp.	10
		Alpha- and beta-hemolytic streptococci	
		Pneumococci	
		Hemophilus influenzae	
		Clostridium perfringens	
		Proteus sp.	
		Bacteroides and related anaerobes	
		Neisseria meningitidis	
		Brucella sp.	
		Pasteurella tularensis	
		Listeria monocytogenes	
		Achromobacter (Herellea) sp.	
		Streptobacillus moniliformis	
		Leptospira sp.	
		Vibrio fetus	
		Opportunistic fungi	
		Candida sp.	
		Nocardia sp.	
		Blastomyces dermatitidis	
		Histoplasma capsulatum	
		Salmonella sp.	
Eye	Usually sterile	*Staphylococcus aureus*	
	Occasionally small numbers of diphtheroids and coagulase-negative staphylococci	*Hemophilus* sp.	
		Pneumococci	
		Neisseria gonorrhoeae	
		Alpha- and beta-hemolytic streptococci	
		Achromobacter (Herellea) sp.	
		Coliform bacilli	

Table 16-1 (continued)

Site	Normal Flora	Pathogens	% of Cases
		Pseudomonas aeruginosa Other enteric bacilli Morax-Axenfeld bacillus *Bacillus subtilis* (occasionally) *Chlamydia* sp.	
Spinal fluid	Sterile	*Hemophilus influenzae* *Neisseria meningitidis* Pneumococci *Mycobacterium tuberculosis* Staphylococci, streptococci *Cryptococcus neoformans* Coliform bacilli *Pseudomonas* and *Proteus* sp. *Bacteroides* sp. *Listeria monocytogenes*	
Urethra, male	*Staphylococcus aureus* *Staphylococcus epidermidis* Enterococci Diphtheroids *Achromobacter wolffi (Mima)* *Bacillus subtilis*	*Neisseria gonorrhoeae* *Chlamydia* sp. Enterococci *Gardnerella vaginalis* Beta-hemolytic streptococci (usually Group B) Anaerobic and microaerophilic streptococci *Bacteroides* sp. *Escherichia* and *Klebsiella-Enterobacter* *Staphylococcus aureus*	
Urethra, female, and vagina	Lactobacilli (large numbers) Coli-aerogenes Staphylococci Streptococci (aerobic and anaerobic) *Candida albicans* *Bacteroides* sp. *Achromobacter wolffi (Mima)*	Yeasts and *Candida albicans* *Clostridium perfringens* *Listeria monocytogenes* *Gardnerella vaginalis* *Trichomonas vaginalis* *Neisseria gonorrhoeae* *Chlamydia* sp. (See also entries under Urethra, male)	
Prostate	Sterile	*Streptococcus faecalis* *Staphylococcus epidermidis* *Escherichia coli* *Proteus mirabilis* *Pseudomonas* sp. *Klebsiella* sp. Anaerobic and microanaerophilic streptococci (alpha, beta, gamma types) *Bacteroides* sp. Enterococci Beta-hemolytic streptococci (usually Group B)	

Table 16-1 (continued)

Site	Normal Flora	Pathogens	% of Cases
		Staphylococci	
		Proteus sp.	
		Clostridium perfringens	
		Escherichia coli and *Klebsiella-Enterobacter-Serratia*	
		Listeria monocytogenes	
Urine	Staphylococci, coagulase negative	*Escherichia coli*	46
	Diphtheroids	*Klebsiella-Enterobacter-Serratia*	7
	Coliform bacilli	*Proteus* sp.	9
	Enterococci	*Pseudomonas* sp.	15
	Proteus sp.	Enterococci	7
	Lactobacilli	Staphylococci, coagulase positive and negative	10
	Alpha- and beta-hemolytic streptococci	*Alcaligenes* sp.	
		Achromobacter (Herellea) sp.	
		Candida albicans	
		Beta-hemolytic streptococci	
		Neisseria gonorrhoeae	
		Mycobacterium tuberculosis	
		Salmonella and *Shigella* sp.	
Wound		*Staphylococcus aureus*	22
		Staphylococcus epidermidis	15
		Coliform bacilli	10
		Pseudomonas sp.	9
		Enterococci	12
		Streptococcus pyogenes	
		Clostridium sp.	
		Bacteroides sp.; other gram-negative rods	
		Proteus sp.	
		Achromobacter (Herellea) sp.	
		Serratia sp.	
Pleura	Sterile	*Staphylococcus aureus*	
		Staphylococcus epidermidis	
		Pneumococci	
		Hemophilus influenzae	
		Mycobacterium tuberculosis	
		Anaerobic streptococci	
		Streptococcus pyogenes	
		Escherichia coli	
		Klebsiella pneumoniae	
		Actinomyces sp.	
		Nocardia sp.	
		Fungi	
Pericardium	Sterile	*Staphylococcus aureus*	
		Pneumococci	
		Enterobacter sp.	
		Pseudomonas sp.	

Table 16-1 (continued)

Site	Normal Flora	Pathogens	% of Cases
		Hemophilus influenzae *Neisseria meningitidis* *Streptococcus* sp. Anaerobic bacteria *Coccidioides immitis* *Actinomyces* sp. *Candida* sp.	
Peritoneum	Sterile	*Escherichia coli* Enterococci Pneumococci *Bacteroides* sp.; other gram-negative rods Anaerobic streptococci *Clostridium* sp. *Staphylococcus epidermidis* *Staphylococcus aureus* *Pseudomonas* sp. Alpha-hemolytic streptococci *Klebsiella pneumoniae*	
Bones	Sterile	*Staphylococcus aureus* *Hemophilus influenzae* Beta-hemolytic streptococci *Neisseria gonorrhoeae* *Mycobacterium tuberculosis* *Salmonella* sp. in sickle cell disease	
Joints	Sterile	*Staphylococcus aureus* *Staphylococcus epidermidis* Beta-hemolytic streptococci Pneumococci *Klebsiella pneumoniae* Gram-negative pathogens in newborns *Salmonella* sp. in sickle cell disease	

For amebae and parasites, see Table 16-10, pp. 688–689.

Laboratory Tests for Infectious Diseases

RECOMMENDATIONS FOR TAKING OPTIMAL BLOOD CULTURES

As soon as possible after onset of chills or fever
Before antimicrobial therapy is started
Use resin-assisted blood cultures if patient is already on antimicrobial therapy.
Take 2–3 cultures at least 30–60 minutes apart if possible; shorter time interval if urgent need to begin therapy.
Take 2–3 cultures per septic episode or per 24-hour period.
Draw 20–30 ml of blood per culture.
Do not draw blood from IV catheter unless no vein sites are available or umbilical artery catheter in infants.
Special methods should be used if suspected organisms are fungi or mycobacteria; routine methods are negative in 66% of cases of disseminated mycotic disease.
Use strict aseptic technique; contamination rate should be <3%/month.
Suspect contamination if
- Only 1 of several cultures is positive (90% of cases)
- Type of organism
  - True infection is almost always present if organism is streptococci (non-viridans group), aerobic and facultative gram-negative rods, anaerobic cocci and gram negative rods, yeasts (possible exception is *Candida tropicalis*).
  - Common contaminants are *Staphylococcus epidermidis, Bacillus* sp., *Propionibacterium acnes, Corynebacterium* sp., *Clostridium perfringens,* viridans streptococci, *C. tropicalis.*

NONSPECIFIC INDICATORS OF INFECTIOUS DISEASES

Acute-phase reactants (see Serum C-Reactive Protein, pp. 73–76)
Limulus lysate assay detects trace amounts of endotoxin from all gram-negative bacteria (including *Escherichia coli, Neisseria meningitidis, Hemophilus influenzae*). Presence in CSF is sensitive indicator of gram-negative bacterial meningitis, but rapid clearance from blood makes serum test unreliable. (See also p. 221.)

COUNTERCURRENT IMMUNOELECTROPHORESIS (CIE) FOR BACTERIAL ANTIGENS

Provides rapid, specific, reliable detection of certain bacterial antigens in virtually any body fluid obtained from the patient (CSF, serum, urine, joint). In bacterial meningitis, CSF is best specimen; urine is occasionally useful in establishing diagnosis; serum is usually not helpful. Sensitivity may be improved by testing serum, urine, and CSF. Is especially valuable when patient has received antibiotics before cultures and Gram's stains are taken and whenever smear and culture are negative. In contrast to cultures, results can be obtained within several hours. Is most useful for identification of *Hemophilus influenzae* type B, *Streptococcus pneumoniae, Neisseria meningitidis* (Groups A and C), Group B streptococcus. A negative CIE does not, however, unequivocally exclude infection due to that organism. Larger amounts of antigen correlate with more complications and poorer prognosis. *Cross reaction and nonspecific precipitation may occur with some antisera.*

Other Organisms Detected By CIE Include

Staphylococcus aureus in pleural fluid
Listeria monocytogenes in CSF
Klebsiella pneumoniae
Pseudomonas aeruginosa
Pneumocystis carinii pneumonitis
Entamoeba histolytica, especially in liver abscess material

Table 16-2. Etiology of Bacteremia

Organism	% of Cases	Predisposing Factors
Staphylococcus epidermidis	34	Contaminated IV catheters, heart valve prostheses, shunts
Escherichia coli	22	GU indwelling catheters and instruments, perforated bowel, septic abortion
Staphylococcus aureus	15	Abscess, decubitus ulcer, osteomyelitis, staphylococcal pneumonia
Pseudomonas species	6	Burns, immunosuppressive chemotherapy
Alpha streptococcus	6	Dental procedures, gum disease
Streptococcus pneumoniae	6	Alcoholism, chronic obstructive pulmonary disease (COPD), pneumococcal pneumonia
Bacteroides species	3.5	Trauma, GI or GU tract disease
Hemophilis influenzae	3	*H. influenzae* nasopharyngitis
Candida species	1.5	Burns, immunosuppressive chemotherapy, parenteral alimentation
Streptococcus pyogenes	1.4	Streptococcal pharyngitis/tonsillitis
Clostridium species	1.4	Septic abortion, biliary tract disease/surgery
Salmonella species	0.8	Contaminated food/water

One-third of staphylococcal bacteremias are primary; predisposing factors are decreased immune defenses (e.g., diabetes mellitus, neoplasms, steroid therapy, hemodialysis).

Cryptococcus neoformans meningitis in CSF, urine, or serum
Candida precipitin titer = 1:8 or 4 times increase in titer indicates invasive candidiasis rather than *Candida* colonization.

Other sensitive immunologic tests for rapid identification of specific antigens include latex agglutination, coagglutination of *Staphylococcus aureus,* immunofluorescence, ELISA.
For all of these tests, false positives may occur due to a number of different organisms. False negatives can occur early in disease; repeat specimens are often useful. Do not use grossly lipemic or hemolyzed specimens, which may give inaccurate results.

SERUM BACTERICIDAL TITER

That dilution of serum able to kill the responsible organism when patient is on antibiotic therapy (usually for bacterial endocarditis; has also been recommended for osteomyelitis, septic arthritis, empyema, patient receiving multiple antimicrobials, immunosuppressed patients with sepsis). Using CSF or urine instead of serum has been adapted for bacterial meningitis and GU tract infections. Generally correlates with in vitro broth concentration that kills microorganism.

Infectious Diseases

PNEUMOCOCCAL INFECTIONS

Pneumonia

Increased WBC (usually 12,000–25,000/cu mm) with shift to the left; normal or low WBC in overwhelming infection, in aged patients, or with other causative organisms (e.g., Friedländer's bacillus)
Blood culture positive for pneumococci in 25% of untreated patients during first 3–4 days
Gram's stain of sputum—many polymorphonuclear neutrophils (PMNs), many gram-positive cocci in pairs and singly; direct pneumococcus typing using Neufeld capsular swelling method rarely done now
Pleural effusion in ~15% of patients
Laboratory findings due to complications (e.g., endocarditis, meningitis, peritonitis, arthritis, empyema)

Endocarditis

See pp. 123–124.

Meningitis

Is the most common cause of meningitis in adults and children over 4 years old (see pp. 225, 231).
Laboratory findings due to associated or underlying conditions—pneumococcal pneumonia, endocarditis, otitis, sinusitis, multiple myeloma

Peritonitis

Positive blood culture
Increased WBC
Ascitic fluid—identification of organisms by Gram's stain and culture
Children with nephrotic syndrome have increased susceptibility.
See section on laboratory findings in body fluids, p. 139.

Increased susceptibility to pneumococcal infection in hyposplenism (e.g., postsplenectomy, sickle cell disease, congenital abnormalities of spleen).

STREPTOCOCCAL INFECTIONS
(uncommon under age 2)

Classification Of Streptococci

Group	Name	
None	*S. pneumoniae*	See preceding section.
None	Viridans streptococci	Show alpha hemolysis. Cause subacute bacterial endocarditis (see pp. 123–124)
A	*S. pyogenes*	Show beta hemolysis Cause scarlet fever, upper respiratory infection (URI). Are the most frequent type of streptococci causing otitis media, mastoiditis, sinusitis, meningitis, cerebral sinus thrombosis, pneumonia, empyema, pericarditis, bacteremia, suppurative arthritis, puerperal sepsis, lymphangitis, lymphadenitis, erysipelas, cellulitis, impetigo (in older children, is often mixed infection with staphylococci that overgrow the culture plate)

WBC is usually increased (14,000/cu mm) early in scarlet fever and URI. It becomes normal by end of first week. (If still increased, look for complication, e.g., otitis.) Is often more markedly increased ($\leq$20,000–30,000/cu mm) with other sites.

Increased eosinophils appear during convalescence, especially with scarlet fever.

Urine may show transient slight albumin, RBCs, casts, without sequelae.

Antistreptococcal antibody titer (ASOT) (see p. 122)

Streptococci appear in smears and cultures from appropriate sites.

Direct antigen kit for throat swabs for Group A streptococci have specificity $>$97% and sensitivity = 64–100% depending on criteria; allows identification within minutes. (Take 2 swabs: if first is positive, treat as streptococcal pharyngitis; if first is negative, use second swab for routine culture method.)

Blood culture may be positive.

Acute glomerulonephritis follows streptococcal infection after latent period of 1–2 weeks; preceding infection may be pharyngeal or of the skin. Latent period prior to onset of acute rheumatic fever is 2–4 weeks; preceding infection is pharyngeal but rarely of the skin.

See sections on rheumatic fever (p. 122) and acute glomerulonephritis (pp. 571–573).

B	*S. agalactiae*	Especially affects neonates (sepsis, meningitis, puerperal sepsis) and elderly. Most are nosocomial. Involves devitalized soft tissues, decubiti, pneumonia, GU tract
C	*S. equisimilis* and *S. zooepidemicus*	Colonize $<$3% of normal persons. Cause pharyngitis (which may be followed by glomerulonephritis); occasional cases of bacteremia, endocarditis, meningitis, puerperal sepsis, pneumonia
D	*E. faecalis* and *S. bovis*	Both are common cause of endocarditis. (*Half of adults with S. bovis endocarditis have anatomic lesion of colon, e.g., carcinoma, polyp, adenoma.*) *S. bovis* rarely causes other infection. *E. faecalis* causes infections of GU tract, peritoneal cavity, pneumonia in elderly persons, infection of damaged tissues (e.g., decubiti, burns, diabetic tissues), polymicrobial bacteremia
F	*S. milleri,* others	
G	No name	Comprise 5–10% of streptococci in blood cultures. Cause polymicrobial bacteremia, bacteremia with no known primary focus, major underlying diseases, serious infection of compromised skin and soft tissue (e.g., radiation, edema)
Anaerobic streptococci		Associated with coliform bacilli, clostridia, bacteroides in compound fractures and soft-tissue wounds, puerperal and postabortion sepsis, visceral abscesses (e.g., lung, liver, brain). Associated with *Staphylococcus aureus* in gangrenous postoperative abdominal incision. Without associated bacteria in burrowing skin and subcutaneous infection

STAPHYLOCOCCAL INFECTIONS

Pneumonia

(often secondary to measles, influenza, mucoviscidosis, debilitating diseases such as leukemia and collagen diseases, or prolonged treatment with broad-spectrum antibiotics)

WBC is increased (usually >15,000/cu mm).
Sputum contains very many PMNs with intracellular gram-positive cocci.
Bacteremia occurs in <20% of patients.

Acute Osteomyelitis

(due to hematogenous dissemination)

Bacteremia occurs in >50% of early cases.
WBC is increased.
Anemia develops.
Secondary amyloidosis occurs in long-standing chronic osteomyelitis.

Endocarditis

Occurs in valves without preceding rheumatic disease and showing little or no previous damage; causes rapid severe damage to valve, producing acute clinical course of mechanical heart failure (rupture of chordae tendineae, perforation of valve, valvular insufficiency) plus results of acute severe infection
Metastatic abscesses occur in various organs.
Anemia develops rapidly.
WBC is increased (12,000–20,000/cu mm); occasionally is normal or decreased.

From 1–13% of cases of bacterial endocarditis are due to coagulase-negative Staphylococcus albus; *bacterial endocarditis due to* Staphylococcus albus *is found following cardiac surgery in one-third and without preceding surgery in two-thirds of patients.*

Bacteremia is common.
Teichoic acid antibodies are found in titer ≥1:4 in ~two-thirds of patients with *Staphylococcus aureus* endocarditis or bacteremia with metastatic infection, ~one-half of patients with nonbacteremic staphylococcal infections. May be found in ~10% of other infections or in normal persons. Titer ≥1:4 is said to suggest current or recent serious staphylococcal infection; positive result without suppuration at primary site of infection suggests endocarditis or metastatic infection. May also be useful when cultures are negative because of prior antibiotic therapy or when deep-tissue infection is inaccessible to culturing (e.g., osteomyelitis, abscesses of brain, liver). Major value is to determine length of treatment of bacteremia, since lack of rise of titer during 14 days of therapy makes it unlikely that undetected metastatic seeding has occurred.

Food Poisoning

(due to enterotoxin)

Culture of staphylococci from suspected food (especially custard and milk products and meats)

Necrotizing Enterocolitis Of Infancy

As seen in Hirschsprung's disease

Impetigo

Especially in infants between ages 3 weeks and 6 months

Meningitis

See p. 225.

TOXIC SHOCK SYNDROME

(due to toxin-producing strains of *Staphylococcus aureus;* usually associated with use of tampons in healthy menstruating women; may also occur postpartum, in post-operative states, or in patients with burns, boils, or abscesses. Fever, rash, shock, and involvement of at least four organ systems are characteristic.)

Anemia is normocytic, normochromic, nonhemolytic, moderate, progressive and may persist for up to 1 month after onset of illness; resolves without treatment; occurs in ~50% of cases.

Erythrocyte sedimentation rate (ESR) may be normal or very high.

Moderate leukocytosis with predominance of immature granulocytes in 70% of cases and toxic granulation. Usually increases for several days and then rapidly returns to normal.

Thrombocytopenia* (<100,000/cu mm) in about 25% of cases and disseminated intravascular coagulation (DIC) causing hemorrhage are not significant clinical problems.

Decreased serum protein,* total and ionized calcium,* phosphorus.

Hypokalemia, hyponatremia, and metabolic acidosis frequently accompany vomiting and diarrhea.*

Sterile pyuria* in 80% of cases, proteinuria, and RBCs resolve within 2 weeks.

Increased prothrombin time (PT) and partial thromboplastin time (PTT) in two-thirds of patients.

Increased serum bilirubin, serum glutamic-oxaloacetic transaminase (SGOT), lactic dehydrogenase (LDH), creatine kinase (CK), serum urea nitrogen (BUN), and creatinine to 2 times upper limit of normal are found in about 60% of cases about the seventh day of illness, at which time clinical improvement begins to occur and these changes rapidly become normal.

No evidence of other infection (bacterial, viral, rickettsial), drug reaction, or autoimmune disorder.

S. aureus need not be isolated to fulfill criteria for diagnosis.

MENINGOCOCCAL INFECTIONS

Clinical syndromes
- Meningococcemia
- Meningitis (see p. 226)
- Waterhouse-Friderichsen syndrome (see p. 525)

Gram-stained smears of body fluids
- Tissue fluid from skin lesions
- Buffy coat of blood
- CSF. (Pyogenic meningitis in which bacteria cannot be found in smear is more likely to be due to meningococcus than to other bacteria.) Gram's stain is diagnostic in 50–70% of patients with positive cultures.
- Nasopharynx

Culture (use chocolate agar incubated in 10% CO_2)—blood, CSF, skin lesions, nasopharynx, other sites of infection

Latex agglutination and CIE (see p. 221)

Only microbiologic methods are specific; other findings are nonspecific.

CSF (see Table 10-2, pp. 226–229)
- Markedly increased WBC (2500–10,000/cu mm), almost all PMNs
- Increased protein (50–1500 mg/dl)
- Decreased glucose (0–45 mg/dl)
- Positive smear and culture

Increased WBC (12,000–40,000/cu mm)

Urine—may show albumin, RBCs; occasional glycosuria

Laboratory findings due to complications (e.g., DIC, pp. 384–387) and sequelae (e.g., subdural effusion)

*Abnormalities usually become normal by fifth day of illness.

GONOCOCCAL INFECTIONS

Genital Infection

(see also Sexually Transmitted Diseases, pp. 597–600)

Gram's stain of smear from involved site, especially urethra, prostatic secretions, cervix, pelvic inflammatory disease. Consider smear positive only if intracellular, gram-negative diplococci are found; extracellular, gram-negative diplococci are considered equivocal, correlate poorly with culture results, and should always be confirmed with culture. Smear is positive in only 50% of asymptomatic patients; asymptomatic patients should always be cultured. *Smear may become negative within hours of antibiotic therapy*. In women, Gram's stain has sensitivity of 45–65% from endocervical canal and 16% from urethra with >90% specificity; smears from vagina, anal canal, and pharynx are not recommended. Gram's stain from urethra has sensitivity and specificity >95% in symptomatic men, 69% and 86% respectively in asymptomatic men; from anal canal sensitivity = 57% and specificity >87%.

Bacterial culture (*use special media such as Thayer-Martin*) should always be taken at the same time (before beginning antibiotic therapy). In ~2% of male patients, Gram's stain of urethral exudate is negative when a simultaneous culture of the same material is positive.

Fluorescent antibody test on smear of suspected material.

Detection of antigen (EIA) in centrifuged sediment of urine has sensitivity >80% and specificity >97%. Antigen detection is sensitive and specific for urethral infection in men but less sensitive than culture in women. Present methods are useful for screening high-risk patients when distant from the laboratory and should be considered presumptive. Confirm with culture if there are medicolegal implications.

DNA probe tests appear to be highly sensitive and specific but have not yet been sufficiently evaluated; present recommendation for use is to confirm cultures, especially in low-risk patients.

Coexistent *Chlamydia trachomatis* infection is present in 20–60% of cases.

Beware of concomitant inapparent venereal infection that may be suppressed but not adequately treated by antibiotic therapy of gonorrhea.

Proctitis

Is symptomatic in ~5% of cases (see also p. 167)

Gram-stained smears are not sufficiently reliable because of presence of nonpathogenic *Neisseria* species; not recommended unless there is mucopurulent exudate.

Bacterial culture on special media (e.g., Thayer-Martin) is required for confirmation; avoid fecal contamination.

Rectal biopsy shows mild and nonspecific inflammation. In a few cases, Gram's stain of tissue section may reveal small numbers of gram-negative intracellular diplococci after prolonged examination.

Rectal gonorrhea accompanies genital gonorrhea in 20–50% of women and is found without genital gonorrhea in 6–10% of infected women. Therefore rectal cultures for gonococcus should be taken in all suspected cases of gonorrhea.

Oropharyngeal Infection

Is present in 10% of women and 20% of homosexual men. Bacterial cultures are required for diagnosis, as gram-stained smears are not sufficiently reliable because of presence of nonpathogenic *Neisseria* species.

Arthritis

Synovial fluid (see Table 11-4, pp. 252–253)
- Variable; may contain few WBCs or be purulent
- Gonococci identified in about one-third of patients

Gonococcal complement fixation (CF) test for differential diagnosis of other types of arthritis. Not a reliable test in urethritis but may rarely be helpful in arthritis, prostatitis, and epididymitis. Becomes positive at least 2–6 weeks after onset of infection, remains positive for 3 months after cure. If test is negative, it should be repeated; 2 negative tests help to rule out gonococcus infection. False positive test may occur after gonococcus vaccine has been used. Test is of limited value and is seldom used.

Associated nonbacterial ophthalmitis in ≤20% of patients

Rarely, other sites

Ophthalmitis Of Newborn

Acute Bacterial Endocarditis

Toxic hepatitis common.

Gonococcus is the most common bacteria infecting tricuspid or pulmonic valves.

Bacteremia

Resembles meningococcemia; occurs in 1–3% of patients. CNS and cardiac infection occur in 1% of these cases. Only 40% of blood cultures are positive. Gram's stain of skin lesions may be useful.

Peritonitis And Perihepatitis Following Spread From Pelvic Inflammatory Disease (PID)

Cultures should always be done on contacts of known cases of gonorrhea, for suspected extragenital gonorrhea and to evaluate test of cure. Culture for test of cure should be from all sites cultured before therapy and from both endocervix and anal canal in women 3–4 days after treatment; if pharynx culture was positive, at least 2 post-therapy cultures should be taken from this site due to difficulty in eradicating from here.

INFECTIONS WITH COLIFORM BACTERIA

(*Escherichia coli, Enterobacter-Klebsiella* group, paracolon group)

Bacteremia

Secondary to infection elsewhere; occasionally due to transfusion of contaminated blood

Secondary to debilitated condition in 20% of patients (e.g., malignant lymphoma, irradiation or anticancer drugs, steroid therapy, cirrhosis, diabetes mellitus)

Early diagnosis and treatment reduces mortality.

Polymicrobial in 6–21% of cases. Higher mortality than when due to one organism. Most common sources are GI tract and intravascular. Most often mixed gram-negative; occasionally gram-negative and -positive; mixed gram-positive are infrequent.

Gram-negative shock occurs in 20–40% of patients.
- Increased serum potassium
- Decreased serum sodium
- Metabolic acidosis
- Increased serum amylase (decreased renal perfusion)
- Renal findings due to shock (e.g., oliguria, proteinuria, azotemia, acute tubular necrosis). Renal insufficiency in sepsis without shock may be due

to glomerulonephritis, interstitial nephritis, bacterial endocarditis, etc. (see appropriate separate sections).

Hematologic findings: leukocytosis with shift to left, Döhle bodies, toxic granules, eosinopenia. DIC in 10% of cases, usually associated with shock.

Adult respiratory distress syndrome with hypoxemia; tachypnea (an early sign) is usually associated with respiratory alkalosis; metabolic acidosis is much less common and occurrence is usually late.

GI manifestations—stress ulcers of stomach with or without bleeding; mild cholestatic jaundice with increased bilirubin (up to 10 mg/dl), mildly increased alkaline phosphatase and increased SGOT may occur several days before positive blood cultures or clinical recognition of infection.

Hypoglycemia is relatively uncommon; hyperglycemia in diabetics may be early clue to infection.

Infection in most frequently from GU tract, GI tract, uterus, lung (in that order).

E. coli is the most frequent organism; it causes the lowest mortality (45%) and the lowest incidence of shock. *Pseudomonas aeruginosa* has the highest mortality (85%). *Klebsiella-Enterobacter,* paracolon bacilli, and *Proteus mirabilis* are intermediate, with 70% mortality.

GU Tract Infection

(75% of cases due to *E. coli*)

Infections of Intestinal Tract and Biliary Tree

(e.g., appendicitis, cholecystitis)

Wound Infections, Abscesses, etc.

Sepsis Neonatorum

(bacterial infection during the first 30 days of life with primary involvement of blood and, frequently, meninges)

Positive blood culture—*E. coli* and *Klebsiella-Enterobacter* cause ~75% of cases. Group B and Group D streptococci and *Listeria monocytogenes* cause most of the other cases. May also be caused by a large variety of other bacteria. *Incidence of contaminated blood cultures is high in newborns. Negative blood culture does not rule out this condition; should take cultures from umbilical stump, skin lesions, mucous membranes, urine.*

Positive culture of CSF occurs frequently. *There may be no WBC increase early in the course of the disease.*

WBC is variable; leukopenia is often associated with a high mortality.

Anemia and decreased platelets may occur.

Laboratory findings due to involvement of other organs (e.g., kidney, with albumin, cells, or casts increased in urine; liver, with increased direct or indirect bilirubin).

Gastroenteritis

Specific enteropathogenic strains identified by genetic probes

Enterotoxigenic *E. coli* (ETEC)—toxins cause cholera-like secretory diarrhea in third world countries.

Enteroinvasive *E.coli* (EIEC)—cause inflammation of colon; resembles bacillary dysentery.

Enteropathogenic *E. coli* (EPEC)—diarrhea in infants and children

Verotoxin-producing *E. coli* (VTEC)—associated with two separate diseases: hemolytic uremic syndrome and hemorrhagic colitis.

Pneumonia

(1% of primary bacterial pneumonias due to *Klebsiella* [Friedländer's bacilli], especially in alcoholics)

WBC is often normal or decreased.

Sputum is very tenacious; is brown or red. Smear shows encapsulated gram-negative bacilli. (*Gram's stain of sputum in lobar pneumonia allows prompt diagnosis of this organism and appropriate therapy.*) Bacterial culture confirms diagnosis.

Laboratory findings due to complications (lung abscess, empyema) are present.

Rarely chronic lung infection due to Friedländer's bacilli simulates tuberculosis.

PROTEUS INFECTIONS

Proteus infections usually follow other bacterial infections.

- Indolent skin ulcers (decubital, varicose ulcers)
- Burns
- Otitis media, mastoiditis
- Urinary tract infection
- Bacteremia

Characteristic spreading growth on culture plate may obscure associated bacteria since Proteus *infection frequently is part of mixed infection; antibiotic sensitivity testing may not be possible.*

PSEUDOMONAS INFECTIONS

Pseudomonas infections occur in various sites.

Associated With

Replacement of normal bacterial flora or initial pathogen because of antibiotic therapy (e.g., urinary tract, ear, lung)

Burns

Debilitated condition of patient (e.g., premature infants, the aged, patients with leukemia)

Bacteremia is most common in patients with acute leukemia; usually acquired in hospital. Overall mortality ~40%.

- Laboratory findings due to associated factors (e.g., shock and pneumonia each occur in one-third of patients).
- Shock, pneumonia, persistent neutropenia are each associated with poorer prognosis.
- Positive blood culture is usually (80% of cases) only one time.

Decreased WBC during bacteremia in patients with leukemia or burns is more frequently due to Pseudomonas *than to other gram-negative rods.*

BACTEROIDES INFECTION

This is usually a component of mixed infection with coliform bacteria, aerobic and anaerobic streptococci, or staphylococci.

Local suppuration or systemic infection is secondary to disease of the female genital tract, intestinal tract, or tonsillar region.

Laboratory findings due to complications (e.g., thrombophlebitis, endocarditis, metastatic abscesses of lung, liver, brain, joint) are present.

Laboratory findings due to underlying conditions (e.g., recent surgery, cancer, arteriosclerosis, diabetes mellitus, alcoholism, prior antibiotic treatment, and steroid, immunosuppressive, or cytotoxic therapy) are present.

TYPHOID FEVER

(due to *Salmonella typhosa*)

Diagnosis is based on culture.

- Blood cultures are positive during first 10 days of fever in 90% of patients and during relapse; <30% are positive after third week.
- Stool cultures are positive after tenth day, with increasing frequency up to fourth or fifth week. Positive stool culture after 4 months indicates a carrier.
- Urine culture is positive during second to third week in 25% of patients, even if blood culture is negative.

Serologic criteria for diagnosis of ≥4-fold increase in O titer in unvaccinated patients is rarely useful. Serologic diagnosis is unreliable, and Widal's reaction has been largely abandoned for the following reasons:

- Positive Widal's test may occur because of typhoid vaccination or previous typhoid infection; nonspecific febrile disease may cause this titer to increase (anamnestic reaction). False positive may occur in autoimmune disease.
- Early treatment with chloramphenicol or ampicillin may cause titer to remain negative or low.
- Increase in O titer may reflect infection with any organism in the Group D salmonellae (e.g., *Salmonella enteritidis, Salmonella panama*) and not just *Salmonella typhosa.*
- Because of differences in commercially manufactured antigens, there may be a 2–4 times difference in O titers on the same sample of serum tested with antigens of different manufacturers.
- H titer is very variable and may show nonspecific response to other infections; it is therefore of little value in diagnosis of typhoid fever.
- >10% of cases in endemic areas are seronegative.

WBC is decreased—4000–6000/cu mm during first 2 weeks, 3000–5000/cu mm during next 2 weeks; ≥10,000/cu mm suggests perforation or suppuration.

Decreased ESR is found.

Normocytic anemia is frequent; with bleeding, anemia becomes hypochromic and microcytic.

Laboratory findings due to complications

- Increased serum LDH, alkaline phosphatase, and SGOT are frequent; increased CK occurs in some patients.
- Intestinal hemorrhage is occult in 20% of patients, gross in 10%; it occurs usually during second or third week. It is less frequent in treated patients.
- Intestinal perforation occurs in 3% of untreated patients.
- Relapse occurs in ≤20% of patients.
  - Blood culture becomes positive again.
  - Widal's titers are unchanged.
- Secondary suppurative lesions (e.g., pneumonia, parotitis, furunculosis) are found.
- Abnormal liver function tests (e.g., serum bilirubin, SGOT) occur in ~25% of patients as an incidental finding. Hepatitis is the chief clinical feature in ~5% of patients.

INFECTIONS DUE TO OTHER *SALMONELLA* ORGANISMS

Enteritis

Stool culture remains positive for 1–4 weeks, occasionally longer.

WBC is normal.

Paratyphoid Fever

(usually due to *Salmonella paratyphi* A or B or to *Salmonella choleraesuis*)

Cultures of blood and stool and decreased WBC show same values as indicated in preceding section.

Bacteremia

(especially due to *Salmonella choleraesuis*)

Blood cultures are intermittently positive.

Stool cultures are negative.

WBC is normal. It increases (≤25,000/cu mm) with development of focal lesions (e.g., pneumonia, meningitis, pyelonephritis, osteomyelitis).

Local Infections

Meningitis, especially in infants

Local abscesses with or without preceding bacteremia or enteritis

One-third of patients are predisposed by underlying disease (e.g., malignant lymphoma, systemic lupus erythematosus [SLE]). Nontyphoid strains are recognized with increasing frequency as an opportunistic infection in AIDS. Patients with GI salmonellosis at risk for AIDS should be treated with antibiotics even in absence of bacteremia.

Bacteremia and osteomyelitis are more common in patients with sickle hemoglobinopathy. Bacteremia is more common in patients with acute hemolytic Bartonella *infection.*

Agglutination tests on sera from acute and convalescent cases are often not useful unless present in high titer (≥1:560) or rising titer is shown.

BACILLARY DYSENTERY

(due to *Shigella* species)

Stool culture is positive in >75% of patients. Rectal swab can also be used.

Microscopy of stool shows mucus, RBCs, and WBCs.

Serologic tests are not useful.

WBC is normal.

Blood cultures are negative.

Laboratory findings due to complications

- Marked loss of fluid and electrolytes
- Intestinal bleeding
- Relapse (in 10% of untreated patients)
- Carrier state
- Acute arthritis—especially untreated disease due to *Shigella shigae* (culture of joint fluid negative)

CHOLERA

(due to *Vibrio comma*)

Stool culture is positive. One may also identify organism in stool using immunofluorescent techniques.

Serologic tests

- EIA for antitoxin antibodies shows ≥4-fold increase in titer in paired sera. Does not occur due to vaccination. May cross react with some *Escherichia coli* enterotoxins. Not positive with nontoxigenic strains of *Vibrio cholerae.*
- Direct agglutination and vibriocidal antibody tests show ≥4-fold rise in titer in >90% of patients but may not be as available as EIA. Agglutination detects nontoxigenic strains.

Laboratory findings due to marked loss of fluid and electrolytes

- Loss of sodium, chloride, and potassium
- Hypovolemic shock
- Metabolic acidosis
- Uremia

OTHER *VIBRIO* SPECIES INFECTIONS

(Short, curved, gram-negative bacilli; at least 10 species are pathogenic for humans. Often difficult to classify. Most are found in marine or estuarine water.)

Causes three types of infection.

Gastroenteritis Infection

From eating uncooked seafood, especially oysters or clams. Some (e.g., *V. vulnificus*) may rapidly progress to bacteremia with 50% fatality rate.

Due To

V. comma (see preceding section)

Others (e.g., *V. vulnificus, alginolyticus, fluvialis, parahaemolyticus*)

Wound Infection

Usually associated with seawater (e.g., while fishing or swimming). 20% mortality rate. Often rapidly progresses to bacteremia. Superficial localized type of wound infection of eyes, ears, skin due to *V. alginolyticus*.

Systemic Infections

Occur in presence of preexisting disease (e.g., *V. vulnificus, V. hollisae*)

V. vulnificus *septicemia occurs most often (75% of cases) in patients with iron overload (e.g., hemochromatosis, thalassemia major, cirrhosis).*

CAMPYLOBACTERIOSIS

(usually due to *Campylobacter jejuni;* few cases due to *C. coli* and *C. fetus*)

Disseminated Form Without Diarrhea

Meningitis—occurs in infants less than 2 months old, usually premature or with congenital CNS defects; 50% mortality.

Pediatric bacteremia—rare disorder, usually secondary to malnutrition or diarrhea; patients usually recover.

Disseminated adult infection—commonly have predisposing conditions (e.g., immunosuppression, malignancy, cardiovascular, endocrine disease). 90% of cases have positive blood culture. Indirect hemagglutination shows antibody titers of 1:1600–1:6400 in acute phase and 1:40–1:320 six months after cure.

Gastroenteritis

Stool culture using microaerophilic incubation and selective media

Microscopic examination of stool shows "seagull" organisms. Few to moderate number of WBCs

Stools become negative in 3–6 weeks even without therapy, but 5–10% of patients have organisms in stool for a year or longer.

Blood culture positive in $<1\%$ of cases

Newly recognized *C. pylori* is associated with type B gastritis but not with type A gastritis of pernicious anemia.

Peptic Ulcer

C. pylori (now classified in different genus as *Helicobacter pylori*) is found in most persons with duodenal ulcer, 70% of gastric ulcer patients, ~50% of patients with nonulcer dyspepsia. Before therapy, diagnosis should be confirmed by endoscopic antral biopsy. Eradication should be confirmed by another biopsy 1 month after therapy is finished. Noninvasive diagnosis and follow-up in patients without an endoscopic lesion by C-14 breath test or EIA serology.

YERSINIA ENTEROCOLITICA

(facultative anaerobic gram-negative coccoid bacillus; transmitted primarily by ingestion of contaminated food, milk, and water)

Stool may contain WBCs and RBCs; gross blood in $\leq 25\%$ of cases.

Stool culture requires special techniques; should be interpreted cautiously because of low-virulence environmental strains not related to human disease; serotyping may be useful to distinguish these.

Serologic tests

- Tube agglutination, ELISA, RIA rise 1 week after onset of symptoms and peak in second week. Titer $\geq$1:200 present in most cases, but 4-fold increases are rare. Titer ≥1:128 at time of complications is presumptive evidence of *Yersinia* infection.

Limitations

Antibodies may be detected for years after infection.

Cross reactions may occur with *Brucella abortus, Rickettsia* species, *Salmonella* species, *Morganella morganii.*

Titers ≥1:32 present in ≥1.5% of healthy persons with no previous history of infection.

Laboratory findings due to focal infection in many extraintestinal sites without detectable bacteremia (e.g., pharyngitis, lymphadenitis, liver and spleen abscesses, endocarditis).

Laboratory findings due to reactive disease (e.g., arthropathy, erythema nodosum, Reiter's syndrome, myocarditis, glomerulonephritis).

HEMOPHILUS INFLUENZAE INFECTIONS

Clinical types

- Upper respiratory tract infections
- Lower respiratory tract infections
- Otitis media
- Empyema
- Meningitis
- Pyarthrosis, single or multiple

Increased WBC (15,000–30,000/cu mm) and PMNs

Positive blood culture in ~50% of patients with meningitis

Infants less than age 1 commonly have empyema, bacteremia, and meningitis concomitantly; therefore CSF should always be examined in infants with empyema.

PERTUSSIS (WHOOPING COUGH)

(due to *Bordetella pertussis/parapertussis*)

Marked increase in WBC (≤100,000/cu mm; usually 12,000–25,000/cu mm) and ≤90% mature lymphocytes

Negative blood cultures

Positive cultures from nasopharynx or cough plate differentiates organisms; <50% have positive cultures.

Serologic tests

Direct agglutination (correlates with IgG) usually requires paired acute- and convalescent-phase sera 2–4 weeks apart; persists after illness; insensitive in infants <6 months old.

Serum IgM and IgG (EIA) establish diagnosis from first sample in 75% of cases; paired sera are needed before 6 months of age.

Detection of antigen on nasopharyngeal smears by direct fluorescent antibody or CIE is very helpful.

CHANCROID

(due to *Hemophilus ducreyi*)

Biopsy of genital ulcer or regional lymph node is helpful.

Gram's stain of smear from genital ulcer shows bacteria.

Gram's stain and cultures of lymph node aspirate are usually negative; only after rupture is culture likely to be positive. Culture requires special techniques and is of limited practical value.

Serologic tests are not presently available.

Smear of lesion for Donovan bodies is negative.

Syphilis, herpes simplex, and granuloma inguinale should be ruled out in ulcerative genital lesions (see separate sections).

BRUCELLOSIS

(due to *Brucella melitensis, suis,* and *abortus*)

Serologic tests

Agglutination reaction becomes positive during second to third week of illness; 90% of patients have titers of ≥1:160. Rising titer is of diagnostic significance. False negative results are rare. False positive test results may occur with tularemia or cholera or with cholera vaccination or after brucellin skin test. In chronic localized brucellosis, titers may be negative or ≤1:200. They may remain positive long after infection has been cured. Antibodies due to *B. canis* are not detected with the usual antigens; *B. canis* antigen must be used.

EIA is method of choice to detect specific IgM and IgG antibodies.

CF can also be used for screening.

Multiple blood cultures should be performed. (*B. abortus* requires 10% CO_2 for culture.) They are more likely to be positive with high agglutination titer.

Bone marrow culture is occasionally positive when blood culture is negative. It may show microscopic granulomas.

Opsonophagocytic test and CF test are not generally useful.

WBC is usually <10,000/cu mm, with a relative lymphocytosis. Decreased WBC occurs in one-third of patients.

ESR is increased in <25% of patients and usually in nonlocalized type of brucellosis.

Anemia appears in <10% of patients and usually with localized type of disease.

Biopsy of tissue may show nonspecific granulomas, suggesting a diagnosis of brucellosis. Tissue may be used for culture.

Liver function tests may be abnormal.

TULAREMIA

(due to *Francisella tularensis*)

Clinical types

- Typhoidal
- Ulceroglandular
- Glandular
- Pneumonic
- Rarely oculoglandular, gastrointestinal, endocardial, meningeal, osteomyelitic, etc.

Serologic tests

Agglutination reaction becomes positive in 50–70% of patients in second week of infection. Significant titer is 1:160; usually it becomes ≥1:320 by third week. Peaks at 4–7 weeks (≤1:1000), then gradually decreases during next year; appreciable titer persists for many years. ≥4-fold increase strongly supports diagnosis. May cross react with *Brucella* agglutinins.

EIA for specific IgM and IgG is more sensitive than agglutination; may persist for years. Rising titer is diagnostic.

Culture and animal inoculation (positive with ≥5 organisms) of suspected material from appropriate site are performed. (Positive blood culture is rare; regional lymph node and mucocutaneous lesions are usually positive.)

WBC is usually normal.

ESR may be increased in severe typhoidal forms; it is normal in other types.

Biopsy of involved lymph node shows a characteristic histologic picture.

PLAGUE

(due to *Yersinia pestis*)

Clinical types

- Bubonic
- Primary septicemic
- Pneumonic

Identify bacteria by smear, culture, fluorescent antibody technique, or animal inoculation of suspected material from appropriate site (e.g., lymph node aspirate, blood, sputum).
Serum hemagglutination antibodies are present.
WBC is increased (20,000–40,000/cu mm), with increased PMNs.

INFECTIONS WITH *PASTEURELLA MULTOCIDA*

Clinical types
- Localized suppurative infections (e.g., osteomyelitis, cellulitis)
- Bacteremia with endocarditis, meningitis, etc.
- Respiratory tract infection

Gram's stain and culture of bacteria from appropriate sites are performed (e.g., blood, skin, CSF).
WBC is increased.

GLANDERS

(due to *Malleomyces mallei*)

Clinical types
- Acute fulminant
- Chronic disseminated granulomas and abscesses in skin, respiratory tract, etc.

Culture or animal inoculation of infected material from appropriate sites is performed.
Agglutination and CF tests are positive in chronic disease.
WBC is variable.

MELIOIDOSIS

(due to *Pseudomonas pseudomallei*)

Clinical types
- Acute febrile
- Chronic febrile with abscesses in bone, skin, viscera

Infection is occasionally transmitted among narcotic addicts using needles in common.

Culture or animal inoculation of infected material from appropriate sites is performed (e.g., pus, urine, blood, sputum).
Agglutination test is positive in chronic disease; an occasional false positive test occurs.
WBC is normal or increased.

INFECTIONS WITH *MIMAE-HERELLEA*

Clinical types
- Bacteremia, bacterial endocarditis, meningitis, pneumonia, etc.

Often associated with IV catheters or cutdowns.

Bacteria are isolated from appropriate sites (e.g., blood, CSF, sputum).

GRANULOMA INGUINALE

(presumptive etiologic agent is *Campylobacter granulomatis*)

Wright- or Giemsa-stained smears of lesions show intracytoplasmic Donovan bodies in large mononuclear cells in acute stage; they may be present in chronic stages.
Biopsy of lesion shows suggestive histologic pattern and is usually positive for Donovan bodies in acute stage.
Cultures are not useful for routine diagnosis.
No serologic tests are available.

Serologic tests for syphilis are negative unless concomitant infection is present.
Dark-field examination for syphilis is negative.

LISTERIOSIS

(due to *Listeria monocytogenes*)

May occur during pregnancy especially in third trimester, and may cause amnionitis, septic abortion, bacteremic flulike syndrome, etc.

Neonatal infection from maternal infection

- Meningitis
    - Purulent CSF with 100–10,000 WBC/cu mm; 70% show preponderance of PMNs; protein is usually increased; glucose is normal in 60% of cases. Gram's stain is positive in <40%, but cultures are usually positive. Positive blood cultures in 60–75% of cases. CNS involvement without meningitis is based on blood cultures, as <50% of CSF cultures are positive.
- Abscesses of viscera may occur (e.g., endophthalmitis, septic arthritis, osteomyelitis, liver abscess, pleuropulmonary infection). Increased WBC and other evidence of infection are found.
- Gram's stain of meconium may show gram-positive bacilli. *This should be done whenever mother is febrile before or at onset of labor.*

Infection of adult nonpregnant patients is associated with being debilitated or immunocompromised (e.g., alcoholism, diabetes mellitus, adrenocorticoid therapy).

Laboratory findings due to bacteremia, endocarditis (in presence of underlying cardiac lesion), skin infection, etc., are present.

Epidemic cases are usually food-borne. Food role in sporadic cases is unknown.

Monocytosis is rarely found.

Serologic tests are not useful.

Diagnosis requires isolation of organism from a normally sterile site.

Isolation of pure culture from food may require days to weeks. Monoclonal antibodies or nucleic acid hybridizations do not require pure culture; they identify the genus but are not specific for *L. monocytogenes*.

ANTHRAX

(due to *Bacillus anthracis*)

Identification of gram-positive bacillus in material by Gram's stain, culture, and animal inoculation from site of involvement (fluid from cutaneous lesions; sputum and pleural fluid from patients with pulmonary disease; stool or vomitus from patients with intestinal disease; blood from patients with bacteremia)

WBC and ESR normal in mild cases; increased in severe cases

With meningeal involvement

- CSF bloody
- CSF smear and culture positive for bacilli

Precipitin antibodies with high or increasing titer sometimes useful in pulmonary or intestinal disease

DIPHTHERIA

(due to *Corynebacterium diphtheriae*)

Smear from involved area stained with methylene blue is positive in >75% of patients.

Culture from involved area is positive within 12 hours on Loeffler's medium (more slowly on blood agar). *If there has been prior antibiotic therapy, culture may be negative or take several days to grow.* Penicillin G eliminates *C. diphtheriae* within 12 hours; without therapy, organisms usually disappear after 2–4 weeks.

Fluorescent antibody staining of material from involved area provides more rapid diagnosis, with a higher percentage of positive results.

WBC is increased (≤15,000/cu mm). If >25,000/cu mm are found, there is probably a concomitant infection (e.g., hemolytic streptococcal).
Albumin and casts are frequently present in urine; blood is rarely found.
A moderate anemia is common.
Decreased serum glucose occurs frequently.
Laboratory findings of peripheral neuritis are present in 10% of patients, usually during second to sixth week. Increased CSF protein may be of prolonged duration.
Laboratory findings of myocarditis (which occurs in ≤two-thirds of patients) are present.
Serologic tests (EIA) are used for epidemiologic studies or to assess immune function by comparing pre- and postimmunization sera.

TETANUS

(due to *Clostridium tetani*)

WBC is normal.
Urine is normal.
CSF is normal.
Identification of organism in local wound is difficult and not usually helpful.
Serologic tests (EIA) are used to assess immunity and to assay immune function by assay of pre- and postimmunization sera.

BOTULISM

(due to *Clostridium botulinum*)

CSF is normal.
Usual laboratory tests are not abnormal or useful.
Diagnosis is made by injecting suspected food intraperitoneally into mice, which will die in 24 hours unless protected with specific antiserum.

CLOSTRIDIAL GAS GANGRENE, CELLULITIS, AND PUERPERAL SEPSIS

(due to *Clostridium perfringens, C. septicum, C. novyi,* etc.)

WBC is increased (15,000 to >40,000/cu mm).
Platelets are decreased in 50% of patients.
In postabortion sepsis, sudden severe hemolytic anemia is common.
Hemoglobulinemia, hemoglobinuria, increased serum bilirubin, spherocytosis, increased osmotic and mechanical fragility, etc., may be associated.
Protein and casts are often present in urine.
Renal insufficiency may progress to uremia.
Smears of material from appropriate sites show gram-positive rods, but spores are not usually seen and other bacteria are often also present.
Anaerobic culture of material from appropriate site is positive. *Clostridia are frequent contaminants of wounds caused by other agents. Other bacteria may cause gas formation within tissues.*

LEGIONNAIRES' DISEASE

(due to *Legionella pneumophila,* a gram-negative bacillus that is an aerobic, intracellular, opportunistic pathogen widely disseminated in environment; at least 12 serogroups are known)

Organism may be cultured on special media from pleural fluid, lung biopsy, transtracheal or bronchial aspirate, blood; isolate can then only be identified by special tests (e.g., direct immunofluorescent antibody staining [DFA]).
DFA may demonstrate the organism in sputum, pleural fluid, or lung tissue within 2–3 days of onset of clinical disease; sensitivity <50%. May be negative in early or mild cases or after erythromycin treatment. Hence negative test is of little value and does not substitute for culture. Specificity >88% compared to culture or serologic tests.

Serologic tests

Standardized antisera are just becoming commercially available for various serologic tests, e.g., indirect fluorescent antibody (allows detection of IgM versus IgG antibody), ELISA, agglutination. Titers <1:64 are considered negative. Single titers of 1:64–1:256 suggest prior infection at undetermined time. A titer >1:256 or a 4-fold rise in titer 3 weeks after onset is considered evidence of recent infection. (*This rise has been reported in other diseases, e.g., tularemia, plague, leptospirosis.*)

DNA probes have become available as commercial kits. Reported sensitivity = 74% and specificity = 100%. Rapid methodology. Detects all species. Used on clinical specimens or culture material

All methods should be confirmed by culture.

Indicators of acute infection (e.g., WBC)

Elevation of liver enzymes

Hematuria, proteinuria

ANAEROBIC INFECTIONS

Frequently several anaerobic organisms are present simultaneously and are often associated with aerobic bacteria as well. If cultures from suspicious sites are reported as negative, the culturing for anaerobic organisms has not been performed properly.

Mixed aerobic-anaerobic infections are often successfully treated by suppressing only the anaerobes.

The most common anaerobic organisms cultured are *Bacteroides* and *Clostridium* species and streptococci.

The most commonly associated aerobic bacteria are the gram-negative enteric bacteria (*Escherichia coli, Klebsiella, Proteus, Pseudomonas,* enterococci).

Anaerobic organisms should be sought, particularly in cultures from intra-abdominal infections (e.g., bowel perforations, acute appendicitis, biliary tract disease), obstetric and gynecologic infections (e.g., pelvic abscess, Bartholin gland abscess, postpartum, postabortion, post-hysterectomy infections), chest infections (e.g., bronchiectasis, lung abscess, necrotizing pneumonia), urinary tract, soft tissue infections, <5% of endocarditis cases (especially streptococci), 10% of cases of bacteremia.

Bacteremia due to anaerobic organisms is characterized by high incidence of jaundice, septic thrombophlebitis, and metastatic abscesses; the GI tract and the female pelvis are the usual portals of entry (in aerobic bacteremia, the GU tract is the most common portal of entry).

LEPTOSPIROSIS

(most frequently due to *Leptospira icterohaemorrhagiae, L. canicola,* and *L. pomona*)

Normochromic anemia is present.

WBC may be normal or ≤40,000/cu mm in Weil's disease.

ESR is increased.

Urine is abnormal in 75% of patients: proteinuria, WBCs, RBCs, casts.

Liver function tests are abnormal in 50% of patients.

- Increased serum bilirubin
- Increased alkaline phosphatase
- Increased SGOT and serum glutamic-pyruvic transaminase (SGPT), but average levels are not as high as in hepatitis
- Reversed albumin-globulin (A/G) ratio

Increased CK in about one-third of patients during first week may help to differentiate condition from hepatitis.

CSF is abnormal in cases with meningeal involvement (<two-thirds of patients)
- Increased cells (≤500/cu mm), chiefly mononuclear type
- Increased protein (≤80 mg/dl)
- Glucose and chloride normal
- Organisms are not found in CSF.

Blood culture is positive during first 3 days of disease in ≤90% of patients.

Urine cultures may be positive only intermittently and are difficult because of contamination and low pH. They are rarely positive after the fourth week.

Serologic tests
- An increasing titer (≥4 times in 2 weeks) is diagnostic. Titer may last for many years.
- Direct agglutination is often positive within 1 week and lasts several months. An individual titer of 1:100 is suggestive.
- CF is useful for screening, and positives should be confirmed by agglutination because of cross reaction with hepatitis type A, cytomegalovirus, scrub typhus, and mycoplasma antibodies. Appears in 10–21 days. Paired testing is needed.
- EIA for specific IgM should be available; can last several months.

Dark-field examination of body fluids is not helpful.

LYME DISEASE*

(due to *Borrelia burgdorferi;* primary tick vector is *Ixodes dammini* in northeast U.S. and *I. pacificus* in western U.S.)

Stage 1: about 1 week (varies 3–33 days) after tick bite; nonspecific febrile "viral syndrome"; 85% have characteristic erythema chronicum migrans rash. Serologic test is not helpful or necessary at this stage, since only 40–60% sensitive at this stage and diagnosis is not ruled out by a negative test. Early antibiotic treatment often prevents antibody response.

Stage 2: four weeks after tick bite, 10% develop cardiac involvement (causes most deaths); 15% have neurologic findings (triad of aseptic meningitis, Bell's palsy, and peripheral neuropathy is very suggestive).

Stage 3: six weeks to several years after tick bite; occurs in 60% of untreated cases, principally as arthritis frequently mistaken as juvenile rheumatoid.

Reinfection causing recurrence of clinical disease is recognized.

Diagnosis depends on serologic tests.
- ELISA for specific IgM and IgG. IgM antibodies usually take 3–6 weeks to develop; only positive in 40–60% of stage 1 cases; rheumatoid factor may cause false positive for IgM. IgG titers rise more slowly and fall after many months. Almost all patients with complications of stage 2 and 3 have positive IgG on first specimen. False positive IgG: may react at high titers with antibodies from spirochetal diseases (syphilis, yaws, pinta); low titers may be found in infectious mononucleosis, hepatitis B, autoimmune diseases, and 5–15% of normal persons in endemic areas. A single specimen is usually sufficient and is confirmatory. Paired acute- and convalescent-phase sera are principally useful for ill patients without known tick bite or rash who have been in endemic area.
- Western blot method is more sensitive and specific than ELISA and may be of particular value during first month of infection when ELISA is inconclusive and antibiotic therapy is critical to prevent long-term involvement of various organs or for an undiagnosed antibiotic-treated patient. Test is expensive, of limited availability, technically difficult, not standardized, with many cross-reacting antibodies.

*Data from LA Magnarelli, Serologic diagnosis of Lyme disease. *Ann NY Acad Sci* 539:154, 1988; RJ Dattwyler, Lyme borreliosis: An overview of the clinical manifestations. *Lab Med* 21:290, 1990.

Serologic tests cannot judge therapy efficacy or test of cure (unlike VDRL in syphilis).

Antigen testing, polymerase chain reaction (PCR), and other techniques are still under development.

Recovery of spirochete is not generally practical for diagnosis. Culture may take several weeks; organism is infrequently found even using special stains in known positive tissues.

Laboratory findings due to organ involvement

Neurologic: 80% with meningitis may show increased lymphocytes (up to 450/cu mm), increased protein and IgG, oligoclonal bands. Intrathecal antibody may be demonstrateod by comparing simultaneous equivalent dilutions of CSF and serum by ELISA. May have encephalitis (tends to involve white matter), myelitis, radiculitis, cranial or peripheral neuritis in various combinations. IgG and IgM may be present in CSF but not in serum.

Arthritis: joint fluid may show increased WBC (up to 34,000/cu mm), PMNs (up to 96%), and protein (up to 6.6 gm/dl).

Nonspecific findings of mild increase of ESR, lymphopenia, cryoglobulinemia, mild increase of SGOT, increased serum IgM, etc.

Fluorescent treponemal antibody absorption test (FTA-ABS) may be positive, but nontreponemal tests (VDRL, RPR) should be nonreactive.

Morphologic changes in tissues are not specific.

RELAPSING FEVER

(due to *Borrelia recurrentis, B. novyi, B. duttonii; Ornithodoros* is tick vector in western U.S.)

Identification of organism by

Wright's or Giemsa or acridine orange stain or dark-field microscopy of peripheral blood smear or buffy coat

Intraperitoneal injection of rats

Agglutination of *Proteus* OX-K

Biologic false positive serologic test for syphilis in $\leq$25% of patients

Increased WBC (10,000–15,000/cu mm); moderately increased ESR

Protein and mononuclear cells sometimes increased in CSF

Laboratory findings due to complications (e.g., hemorrhage, rupture of spleen, secondary infection)

BABESIOSIS

(due to *Babesia microti* transmitted by bite of nymphal tick)

Hemolytic anemia may last days to months.

Diagnosis is established by

Identification of parasite in RBCs on peripheral blood smear

Serologic studies (immunofluorescent assay $\geq$1:64) may cross react with plasmodia

Isolation in inoculated animals

INFECTIONS WITH *STREPTOBACILLUS MONILIFORMIS* (RAT-BITE FEVER, HAVERHILL FEVER)

Clinical types

Rat-bite fever

Febrile rash with multiple joint type of arthritis

Isolation of bacteria from appropriate sites (e.g., blood, pus, joint fluid) during acute febrile stage

Agglutination antibodies in serum during second to third week; rising titer significant

INFECTIONS WITH *BARTONELLA BACILLIFORMIS*

Oroya Fever

Sudden very marked anemia is found.

Blood smears mayshow gram-negative bacilli in ≤90% of RBCs (Giemsa stain); they are also present in monocytes. Bacteria are also present in phagocytes of reticuloendothelial system.

Blood culture is positive. (Use special enriched media.)

Beware of secondary Salmonella *infection.*

Verruga Peruana

Moderate anemia is found.

Blood smears and blood cultures are positive for bacilli.

SYPHILIS

(due to *Treponema pallidum*)

Primary Syphilis

Direct immunofluorescent staining of smears from lesion has essentially replaced the dark-field examination and allows properly prepared specimens to be mailed to the laboratory.

Dark-field examination of genital lesion is done; if it is negative, regional lymph node aspirate may be used. *Examination will be negative if there has been recent therapy with penicillin or other treponemicidal drugs.*

Serologic test shows rising titer with or without positive dark-field examination. VDRL does not become positive until 7–10 days after appearance of chancre.

Biopsy of suspected lesion for histologic examination is rarely done.

Secondary Syphilis

Dark-field examination of mucocutaneous lesions is positive.

Serologic tests are almost always positive in high titer.

Latent Syphilis

A positive serologic test is the only diagnostic method.

Congenital Syphilis

Dark-field examination of mucocutaneous lesions or scraping from moist umbilical cord is positive.

Serologic tests are positive and show rising or very high titer. *The serologic test may be positive because of maternal antibodies but without congenital syphilitic infection.* Rising infant's titer or titer higher than mother's establishes diagnosis of congenital syphilis. If mother has been adequately treated, infant's titer falls steadily to nonreactive level in 3 months. If mother acquires syphilis late in pregnancy, infant may be seronegative and clinically normal at birth and then manifest syphilis 1–2 months later.

Only the quantitative VDRL is recommended for the diagnosis of congenital syphilis (performed serially to detect rise or fall in titers).

Late Syphilis

CNS (VDRL on CSF is highly specific but lacks sensitivity)
- Meningitis
  - ≤2000 lymphocytes/cu mm
  - Positive serologic test in blood and CSF
- Meningovascular disease
  - Increased cell count (≤100 mononuclear cells/cu mm) in 60% of cases
  - Increased protein (up to 260 mg/dl) in 66% of cases; increased gamma globulin in 75% of cases

Table 16-3. Stages of Syphilis

Stage	Symptom	Time After Exposure	Laboratory Changes	Response to Treatment	
				VDRL	FTA-ABS/MHA-TP
Primary	Chancre	Average 3 weeks (11–90 days)	Dark-field positive Serologic tests often negative Rising titers VDRL and FTA-ABS	Remains negative	Remains negative
	Lymph nodes	Average 4 weeks	Dark-field positive Rising antibody titers	Usually becomes negative within 6 months	After seroconversion, usually remains positive indefinitely without regard for stage of disease or adequacy of treatment
Secondary		6–20 weeks	Dark-field positive Peak antibody titers CSF abnormal in 25–50% of patients without CNS findings	Usually becomes negative within 12–24 months	

			Increased alkaline phosphatase (due to pericholangitis) in 20% Proteinuria	
Latent		Early: 3–12 months Late: >12 months	CSF VDRL negative Serum treponemal test positive Falling VDRL titers	
Late (tertiary)	Neurosyphilis (asymptomatic)	Usually > 4 years	CSF: VDRL positive or increased cells and protein Serum treponemal test positive; nontreponemal test positive or negative Without treatment, CNS disease occurs within 10 years in 20% of patients	
Late (tertiary)	Symptomatic	>4 years	Same as asymptomatic Treatment does not reverse nontreponemal test in 25–75% of patients	Usually remains positive indefinitely with gradually declining titer

Positive serologic test in blood and CSF
Laboratory findings due to cerebrovascular thrombosis

Tabes dorsalis

Early—increased cell count and protein and positive serologic test in blood and CSF (titer may be low). Increased gamma globulin is less marked than in general paresis.

Late—~25% of patients may have normal CSF and negative serologic tests in blood and CSF.

General paresis (CSF always abnormal in untreated patients)

Increased cell count up to 175 mononuclear cells/cu mm

Increased protein up to 10 mg/dl with marked increase in gamma globulin

Positive serologic test (titer usually high)

CSF cell count should return to normal within 3 months after therapy; otherwise retreatment is indicated.

Asymptomatic CNS lues

May have negative blood and positive CSF serologic test

Increased cell count and protein are index of activity.

Cardiovascular syphilis—VDRL is usually reactive, but titer is often low.

Gummatous lesions—VDRL is almost always reactive, usually in high titer.

Cardiovascular, liver, etc., involvement

Biopsy of skin, lymph node, larynx, testes, etc.

Adequately treated primary and secondary syphilis usually show falling titer and become serologically nonreactive in about 9 and 12 months, respectively; 2% of patients remain positive for several years. Therapy causes a negative reagin test in 75% of patients with early latent syphilis in 5 years, but less than 25% of patients with late syphilis become nonreactive, although titers may fall steadily over a long period. In contrast to the VDRL, the FTA-ABS remains reactive once it has become reactive, except for early primary syphilis, and cannot be used to confirm a cure.

If late syphilis of any type is suspected, always do FTA-ABS, even if VDRL is nonreactive.

One-third of patients with only weakly reactive VDRL are reactive with more sensitive test (e.g., TPI); weakly reactive VDRL should always be confirmed with FTA-ABS.

VDRL may be nonreactive in undiluted serum in presence of an actual high titer ("prozone" phenomenon) in 1% of patients with secondary syphilis.

SEROLOGIC TESTS FOR SYPHILIS

Nontreponemal Tests (e.g., VDRL, RPR, ART)

Simple, convenient for routine screening at local level; frequent local requirement for premarital and prenatal serology. False positive rate of 1–2% in pregnant women.

Does not become positive until 7–10 days after appearance of chancre.

High titer (>1:16) usually indicates active disease.

Low titer (≤1:8) indicates biologic false positive (BFP) test in 90% of cases or occasionally due to late or late latent syphilis.

Quantitation of VDRL should always be performed before onset of treatment. Fourfold drop in titer indicates response to therapy. Treatment of primary syphilis usually causes progressive decline to negative VDRL within 2 years. In secondary, late, or latent syphilis, low titers persist in ~50% of cases after 2 years despite fall in titer; this does not indicate treatment failure or reinfection, and these patients are likely to remain positive even if retreated. Titer response is unpredictable in late and latent syphilis.

Falling titer indicates response to treatment. Adequate treatment of primary and secondary syphilis should cause a 4-fold decline in titer by fourth month and 8-fold decline by eighth month. Treatment of early syphilis usually results in little or no reaction after 1 year.

Rising titer (4 times) indicates relapse, reinfection, or treatment failure and need for retreatment.

Serial titers should be done to differentiate congenital syphilis from passive transfer of maternal antibodies; rising titer during 6-month period of infancy is diagnostic of congenital syphilis, since passively transferred antibodies should not be detected after 3 months. Since infection may occur as early as ninth week of gestation, high-risk women should be tested during first and again during each trimester. In early congenital syphilis, treatment causes VDRL to become nonreactive, but after age 2 years, titer decreases slowly but may never become nonreactive.

May be nonreactive in early primary, late latent, and late syphilis (~25% of cases)

Prozone phenomenon in 1% of patients with secondary syphilis (VDRL negative in undiluted serum in presence of high titer)

Reactive and weakly reactive tests should be confirmed with FTA-ABS.

Treponemal Tests

Are used to confirm nontreponemal tests that conflict with clinical findings. Are qualitative tests that cannot be used to monitor efficacy of treatment. Not to be used for screening. Nonreactive test generally indicates no past or present infection unless treated in early primary stage, when 10% will be nonreactive 2 years later. 1% are false positive (same as nontreponemal). Passively transferred antibodies disappear from noninfected infant in 6–8 months but persist in congenital syphilis.

TPI (treponemal pallidum immobilization) has been replaced by the following tests.

MHA-TP (microhemagglutination) and HATTS (hemagglutination treponemal test)

- Sensitized or unsensitized cells may occasionally be reactive with sera from patients with SLE, autoimmune diseases, viral infections, leprosy, drug addicts.
- Compare well with FTA-ABS in sensitivity and specificity as a confirmatory test with fewer false positive reactions but are less sensitive in early primary syphilis

FTA-ABS-IgG (fluorescent treponemal antibody absorption)

- Most sensitive and specific test
- More sensitive than MHA-TP in primary syphilis; parallels findings in other stages
- Test of choice for confirmation of diagnosis (e.g., BFP)
- Titers not correlated with clinical activity
- Remains positive indefinitely in ~95% of patients, reflecting previous infection
- May be positive in late syphilis when VDRL is negative
- Not used to document adequacy of treatment, as remains positive for 2 years after adequate therapy in 80% of cases of seropositive early syphilis; thus a positive test does not separate active from inactive disease.
- Beaded pattern is common in collagen diseases (e.g., SLE) but is considered negative for syphilis.
- No longer recommended for early detection of congenital syphilis in infants

Enzyme immunoassays (EIA) are now available in kit form for detection of IgG and IgM *T. pallidum*–specific antibodies. IgG test can be used for primary screening; positive test indicates current or past infection. IgM test can be used for confirmation of active syphilis or congenital infection and monitoring course of disease and efficacy of therapy.

Table 16-4. Sensitivity and Specificity of Serologic Tests for Untreated Syphilis at Different Stages

	Sensitivity (%)		Specificity (%)		
Test	Primary	Secondary	Late	Latent	
VDRL	78	97	71	92	98
MHA-TP	76	100	94	97	99
FTA-ABS	85	99	95	95	97

Results of these tests are positive in presence of antibodies of related treponematoses (e.g., yaws, pinta, bejel). Once antibodies develop, the tests may thereafter remain positive despite therapy. (This is the mechanism for one type of BFP.) If therapy is given before antibodies develop, these tests may never be positive.

BFP should be confirmed with FTA-ABS. ≤20% of reactive screening tests may be BFP. Two-thirds of these are low titer (<1:8) and revert to normal within 6 months; patients have usually had recent infections (e.g., viral [infectious mononucleosis, hepatitis, measles], *Mycoplasma pneumoniae, Chlamydia,* malaria) or immunizations. The remaining third that do not become nonreactive in 6 months have serious underlying disease (e.g., SLE, leprosy) in 25% or are shown to have syphilis or other treponemal infections in 50%. BFP occurs in 20–25% of IV drug users. ≤10% of patients over age 70 may show BFP. >20% of patients with BFP also show positive tests for rheumatoid arthritis, antinuclear antibodies, antithyroid antibodies, cryoglobulins, elevated serum gamma globulins.

YAWS (due to *Treponema pertenue*), PINTA (due to *T. carateum*), BEJEL (due to a treponema indistinguishable from *T. pallidum*)

Positive serologic tests for syphilis

Positive dark-field demonstration of a treponema in smears from lesions

TUBERCULOSIS

Acid-fast stained smears and cultures (and occasionally guinea pig inoculation) of concentrates of suspected material from involved sites (e.g., sputum, gastric fluid, effusions, urine, CSF, pus) should be performed on multiple specimens. 10^4 acid-fast bacilli/ml of sputum are required for detection on smear. Maximum correlation of smear with culture is 82%, causing unacceptably high false-negative rate. Animal inoculation of material is rarely used now.

Recently DNA nucleic acid probes have become available with reported sensitivity and specificity >92%. Detects mycobacterium species in clinical specimens. Uses radioactive materials.

Characteristic histologic pattern appears in random biopsy of lymph node, liver, bone marrow (especially in miliary dissemination), or other involved sites (e.g., bronchus, pleura).

WBC is usually normal. Granulocytic leukemoid reaction may occur in miliary disease. Active disseminated disease is suggested by more monocytes (10–20%) than lymphocytes (5–10%) in peripheral smear.

ESR is normal in localized disease; increased in disseminated or advanced disease. It is not used as index of activity.

Moderate anemia may be present in advanced disease.

Urine—rule out renal tuberculosis in presence of hematuria (gross or microscopic) or pyuria with negative cultures for pyogenic bacteria.

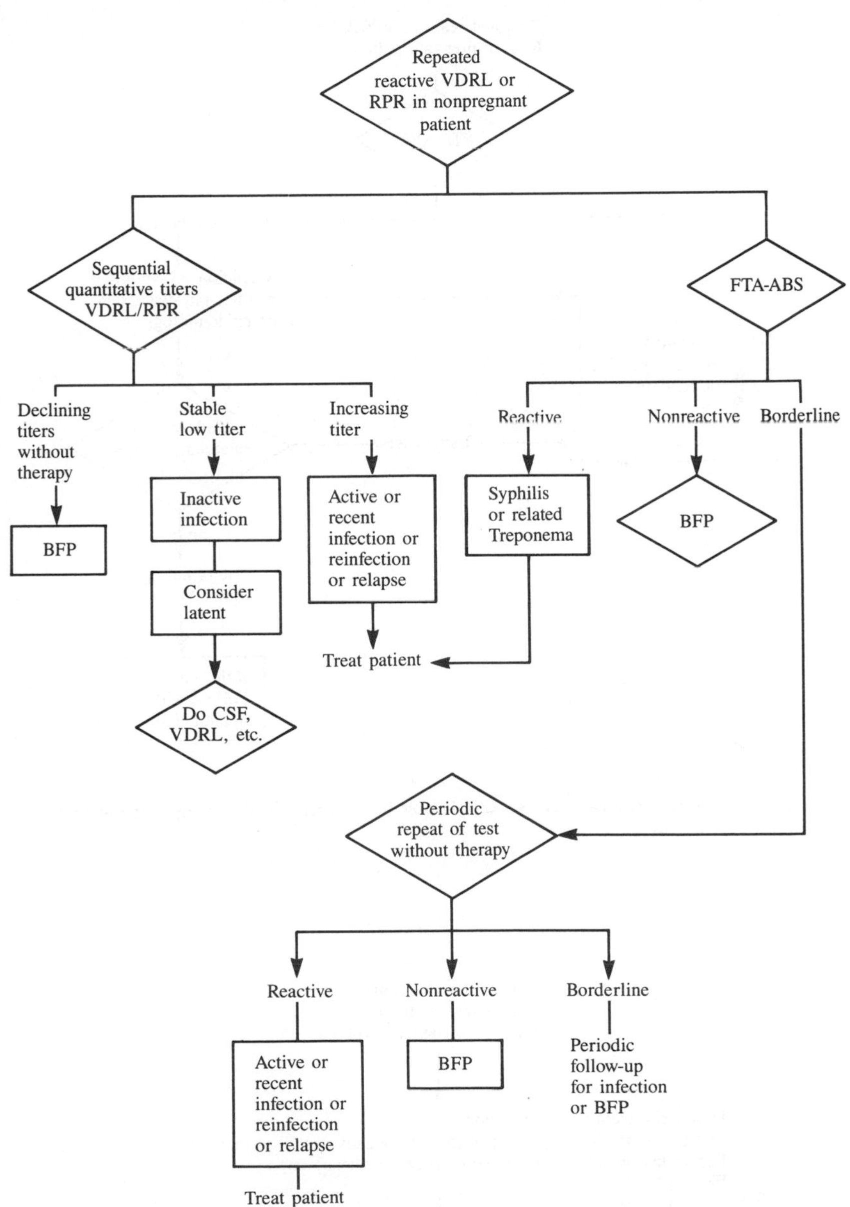

Fig. 16-1. Flow chart for positive serologic test for syphilis. Rule out underlying causes of BFP (see pp. 639–640). BFP = biologic false positive.

Repeated reactive VDRL or RPR in pregnant patient

FTA-ABS

Reactive

Nonreactive

Suspicion of syphilis by history, physical exam, or epidemiology

Yes

Treat for syphilis; follow with quantitative VDRL or RPR titers

Rising titers

Follow with quantitative titers

Titers falling or low and stable

Rule out BFP
Follow with quantitative titers

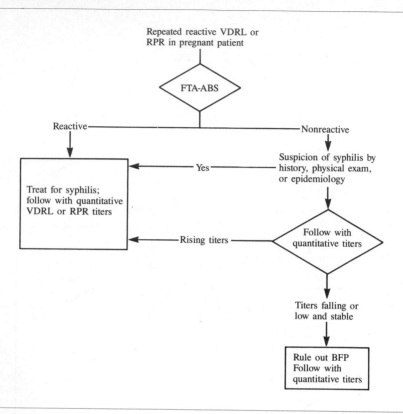

Fig. 16-2. Flow chart for reactive serologic test for syphilis in the pregnant patient.

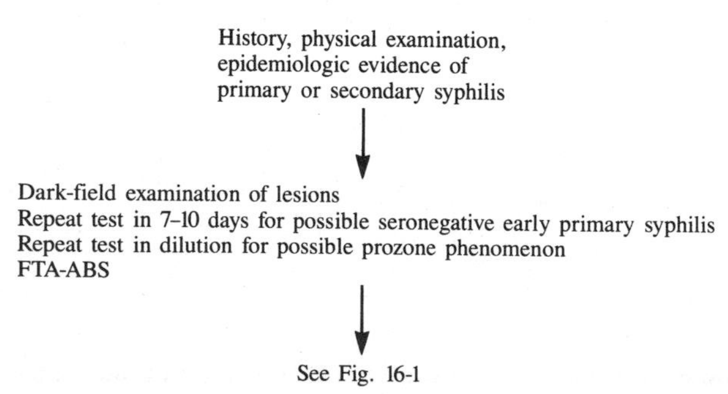

Fig. 16-3. Flow chart for nonreactive serologic test for syphilis in the nonpregnant patient.

Laboratory findings due to extrapulmonary tuberculosis
- Tuberculous meningitis—CSF shows
  - Acid-fast smear and culture from pellicle
  - 100–1000 WBC/cu mm (mostly lymphocytes)
  - Increased protein (slight in early stages but continues to increase; >300 mg/dl associated with advanced disease; much higher levels when block of CSF occurs)
  - Decreased glucose (<50% of blood glucose)
  - Decreased chloride is not useful in diagnosis.
  - Increased tryptophan
  - Serum sodium may be decreased (110–125 mEq/L) especially in aged; may also occur in overwhelming tuberculous infection.
  - Detection of anti-BCG-IgG by ELISA or of antibody-secreting cells by solid immunospot assay has been reported recently.
- Tuberculoma
- Tuberculous pleural effusion (see pp. 131, 138)
  - Sputum is positive on culture in 25% of patients; pleural fluid is positive on culture in 25% of patients.
  - Fluid is an exudate with increased protein (>3 gm/dl) and increased lymphocytes.
- Lymph nodes
  - Culture is important to rule out infection due to other mycobacteria (atypical or anonymous; e.g., *Mycobacterium intracellulare-avium* in AIDS).

Laboratory findings due to complications (see appropriate separate sections)
- Amyloidosis
- Addison's disease
- Other

Laboratory findings due to underlying diseases (e.g., diabetes mellitus, sickle cell anemia, AIDS)

In AIDS, *M. avium* and *M.intracellulare* (MAI) are the major problem (present in 20–60% of AIDS autopsies), but *M. tuberculosis* is also increased. Persistent prolonged bacteremia is characteristic; blood culture is sensitive means of diagnosis; direct examination of Kinyoun stain of buffy coat smear may be helpful; marrow cultures are frequently positive. May involve lymph nodes, spleen, liver, GI tract, lung, and brain.

Environmental Mycobacteria

(soil and water are reservoir for these organisms in contrast to *M. tuberculosis,* which is an obligate human pathogen)

	Diagnosis	Comment
Pulmonary disease		
Common		
M. kansasii	Positive culture, absence of other etiologic agents, compatible clinical picture	Rarely a contaminant
M. avium-intracellulare		
M. chelonae		
Rare		
M. xenopi	Lung biopsy may be needed	
M. szulagai		
M. fortuitum		
M. simiae		
AIDS-associated		
M. avium-intracellulare	May be found in many sites (e.g., lymph nodes, blood, marrow, liver, spleen, GI tract)	Disseminated infection in ~50% of AIDS cases

	Diagnosis	Comment
Lymphadenitis	Histologic examination of tissue	
Common		
M. avium-intracellulare		95% involve unilateral cervical nodes; most common in 2- to 5-year-old children
M. scrofulaceum		
Rare		
M. kansasii		
M. fortuitum		
M. chelonae		
Cutaneous	Culture of skin biopsy	
Common		
M. marinum	Incubate culture at low temperature (28–30°C)	Swimming pool granuloma
M. fortuitum	Culture skin biopsy	Postsurgical or environmental wound contamination
M. chelonae		
Rare		
M. avium complex		
M. kansasii		
M. smegmatis		
M. haemophilum		

LEPROSY (HANSEN'S DISEASE)

(due to *Mycobacterium leprae*)

Mild anemia is found. Sulfone therapy frequently causes anemia, which indicates dosage change is needed.

Serum albumin is decreased, and serum globulin is increased.

ESR is increased.

Serum cholesterol is slightly decreased.

Serum calcium is slightly decreased.

False positive serologic test for syphilis occurs in $\leq$40% of patients.

Acid-fast bacilli are found in smear or tissue biopsy from nasal scrapings or lepromatous lesions. Acid-fast diphtheroids are not infrequently found in nasal septum smears or scrapings in normal persons, and *M. leprae* is not found here in two-thirds of early lepromatous cases. Therefore nasal smear may have very limited diagnostic value. Bacilli may show a typical granulation and fragmentation that precede the clinical improvement due to sulfone therapy. Larger, more nodular lesions are more likely to be positive. During lepra reactions, enormous numbers of bacilli may be present in skin lesions and may be found in peripheral blood smears. Bacilli are usually very difficult to find in skin lesions of tuberculoid leprosy.

Histologic pattern of the lesions is used for classification of type of leprosy.

Laboratory findings due to complications are noted.

- Amyloidosis occurs in 40% of patients in the U.S.
- Other diseases (e.g., tuberculosis, malaria, parasitic infestation) may be present.
- Sterility due to orchitis is very frequent.

RICKETTSIAL DISEASES

Indirect immunofluorescence (IFA) or ELISA detection of rickettsial-specific IgG and IgM. ELISA is more sensitive and specific for IgM and is now the test of choice; specimens taken at 3- to 4-day intervals will show seroconversion.

Complement fixation (CF) or agglutination tests are positive in most cases when group-specific and type-specific rickettsial antigens are used. These tests permit differentiation of various rickettsial diseases. No test is available for trench fever. Rising titer during convalescence is the most important criterion. Early antibiotic therapy may delay appearance of antibodies for an additional 1–4 weeks, and titers may not be as high as when treatment is begun later. Low titers of CF antibodies may persist for years. CF is less sensitive than IFA.

Weil-Felix reaction has poor sensitivity and specificity and has been replaced by ELISA.

Guinea-pig inoculation—scrotal reaction following intraperitoneal injection of blood into male guinea pig.

Test is not often used at present.
Marked in Rocky Mountain spotted fever and endemic typhus
Moderate in boutonneuse fever
Slight in epidemic typhus and Brill-Zinsser disease
Negative in scrub typhus, Q fever, trench fever, and rickettsialpox

Epidemic Typhus (due to *Rickettsia prowazekii*), Brill-Zinsser Disease (recrudescent typhus due to *R. prowazekii*), Murine Typhus (due to *R. typhi*)

Paired sera for specific IgM and ≥4-fold rise in IgG (IFA, ELISA) are best methods and indicate recent infection. Single IFA titer ≥1:128 is strongly suggestive. Specificity of these is close to 100%.

Has replaced Weil-Felix test, which has poor sensitivity and specificity. CF has insufficient sensitivity and specificity.

Presence of IgG generally indicates previous exposure and present immunity.

Rocky Mountain Spotted Fever
(due to *R. rickettsii*)

Paired sera show ≥4-fold increase in IgG or total antibody by IFA or specific IgM is evidence of recent infection. IgM appears by day 3–8, peaks at 1 month, may last 3–4 months. IgG appears within 3 weeks, peaks at 1–3 months, and may last for 12 months or more. Demonstrable IgG usually indicates previous exposure and immunity. Paired sera for both IgG and IgM should always be done early and 10–14 days later.

CF is too insensitive to be used alone and appears too late (8–12 days) for early diagnosis and treatment. CF and IgG titers may be decreased by early treatment.

Direct immunofluorescence of skin biopsy for antigen has sensitivity of ~70% and specificity of ~100%.

Rickettsialpox
(due to *R. akari*)

Paired early and later (2–3 weeks) sera for CF and for IgM and total Ig (IFA) should be used. Should be absorbed with *R. rickettsii* and *R. akari* antigens to prove specificity of reaction.

Q Fever
(due to *Coxiella burnetii*)

Single IgG titer >1:128 or any IgM titer (IFA) is diagnostically significant.

High specific IgM titer suggests hepatitis; high specific IgA titer suggests endocarditis.

≥4-fold increase in CF titer in early and later sera indicates recent infection.

Scrub Typhus
(due to *R. tsutsugamushi*)

Presence of specific IgG and IgM (ELISA, IFA) strongly favors diagnosis.

Diagnostic Weil-Felix agglutination shows ≥4-fold rise in titer to *Proteus* OX-K and no reaction to *Proteus* OX-2 or OX-19 (in 50–70% of patients); a single titer ≥1:160 is also diagnostic; normal is ≤1:40. Better sensitivity and specificity than CF.

Ehrlichiosis

(due to *Ehrlichia canis* or closely related *Ehrlichia* species)

Recently discovered rickettsial disease with clinical picture similar to Rocky Mountain spotted fever or Lyme disease.

IFA showing ≥4-fold change in specific IgG titer suggests recent infection. Peak titer 1:160 during acute or convalescent phases.

CSF may show increased lymphocytes and protein.

Mild brief abnormalities in liver function tests

Microscopic examination of organisms following animal inoculation; test is not often used.

In less severe cases, blood findings are not distinctive.

In severe cases, the following changes are found:

- Early in disease, WBC is decreased and lymphocytes are increased (usually 4000–6000/cu mm; as low as 1200/cu mm in early scrub typhus). Later WBC increases to 10,000–15,000/cu mm with shift to the left and toxic granulation. If count is higher, rule out secondary bacterial infection or hemorrhage.
- Mild normochromic normocytic anemia (hemoglobin as low as 9 gm/dl) appears around tenth day.
- ESR is increased.
- Total protein and serum albumin are decreased.
- BUN may be increased (prerenal).
- Serum chloride may be decreased.
- Urine shows slight increase in albumin; granular casts.
- CSF is normal despite symptoms of meningitis.
- Blood cultures for bacteria are negative (to rule out other tickborne diseases, e.g., tularemia).

Laboratory findings due to specific organ involvement (e.g., pneumonitis, hepatitis) or due to complications (e.g., secondary bacterial infection, hemorrhage) are present.

Acute glomerulonephritis occurs in 78% of patients with epidemic typhus, 50% of patients with Rocky Mountain spotted fever, and 30% of patients with scrub typhus.

DIAGNOSIS OF VIRAL INFECTIONS

Serologic evidence of recent infection may be based on the following:

- Seroconversion from seronegative to seropositive test is conclusive evidence of recent infection if appropriate test method is used.
- ≥4-fold rise in antibody titer in paired serum samples collected 2–4 weeks apart is usually diagnostic. Some exceptions are anamnestic reactions, cross reactions to related antigens, some specific exceptions (e.g., high cytomegalovirus (CMV) antibody titers in influenza A or *Mycoplasma pneumoniae* infections).
- Single serum specimens that show specific IgM antibody within the first few weeks of infection (e.g., Epstein-Barr virus [EBV], CMV, varicella-zoster [VZV], rubella, Coxsackievirus) are useful.
- Various exceptions must be remembered:
    - Some may recur with reactivation or reinfection (e.g., herpes, CMV, EBV, VZV).
    - Some may persist for 6 or more months (e.g., CMV, rubella).
    - Heterotypic response of one virus antibody to another infection (e.g., CMV, EBV).
    - False positives are frequent in sera that contain rheumatoid factor.
    - *Spurious results may also occur in conditions other than rheumatoid arthritis (e.g., bacterial endocarditis, chronic liver disease, tuberculosis and other chronic infections, sarcoidosis, some healthy persons).*

For diagnosis of congenital infection, serial sera from mother and infant should be submitted.

Infants' passive antibody transplacentally acquired decreases markedly in 2–3 months; unchanged or increasing titer indicates active infection.

Specific IgM in neonatal blood or cord blood can diagnose congenital infection, since mother's IgM does not cross placenta.

Single maternal serum negative for IgG may be useful to exclude that particular congenital infection in neonate (e.g., rubella, CMV).

Positive IgG titer that does not rise indicates previous exposure and often immunity. Tests to determine immune status may be used for viruses of rubella (in women of childbearing age), CMV (in women of childbearing age working in high-risk environments, e.g., hemodialysis, transplant, pediatric and nursery units), measles and mumps (IFA indicates prior infection), chickenpox (VZV)

Preferred to culture where virus does not grow well in cell culture (e.g., rubella, EBV) or is too hazardous to handle

Paired sera should always be submitted for diagnosis of viral disease; acute-phase serum should be obtained as early as possible in clinical course; convalescent-phase serum is usually obtained 2–4 weeks later. When the first specimen is submitted, the clinician would be wise to notify the laboratory that a convalescent-phase sera will be sent subsequently.

False negatives may occur in immunocompromised patients, neonates, infants.

Some specific serologic disease or organ system panels are

CNS—herpes simplex virus (HSV), mumps, western equine encephalitis, eastern equine encephalitis, St. Louis encephalitis, California encephalitis, EBV.

Respiratory—influenza A and B; respiratory syncytial virus (RSV); parainfluenza 1, 2, and 3; adenovirus; *Mycoplasma pneumoniae; Chlamydia* (RSV and parainfluenza only in children, not adults).

Exanthems. Measles, rubella. Also HSV and VZV if vesicular

Myocarditis and pericarditis—Group B Coxsackievirus types 1 through 5, influenza A and B

Direct identification of virus or viral antigens in patient tissues by

Cytopathology of inclusion bodies or tissue culture (e.g., CMV, VZV, or herpes) but should further confirm virus identification by immunofluorescent and immunoenzyme specific antibody staining. Isolation of virus is >4 times more sensitive than finding CMV inclusion bodies in urine.

Immunofluorescent and immunoenzyme specific antibody staining

Electron microscopic (EM) identification of viral antigen in patient tissues (e.g., HSV particles in brain biopsy in encephalitis) or specimens (e.g., urine for CMV in congenital infection of infants; feces for rotaviruses, Norwalk agents, adenoviruses, coronaviruses, caliciviruses; vesicle fluid for HSV and poxviruses). Is often enhanced by other techniques (e.g., antibody binding).

DNA hybridization techniques may have a future role.

Viral culture is the "gold standard" for proving etiology but may require 10 or more days. Prompt inoculation and appropriate media are needed. Other constraints are

Some viruses cannot be cultured and require other techniques as in most cases of viral gastroenteritis (e.g., rotavirus in stool requires EM or antigen detection).

Finding enterovirus in stool supports diagnosis but does not prove it is the cause of present illness (e.g., aseptic meningitis, myopericarditis).

Some viruses can be shed for months in asymptomatic persons (e.g., adenoviruses, HSV, CMV), but this is unusual for other viruses (e.g., measles, mumps, influenza, parainfluenza, RSV).

Appropriate source of specimen, e.g.,

- Throat swabs (HSV, enterovirus and adenovirus), nasopharyngeal swabs (RSV, parainfluenza), and nasal swabs (rhinovirus)
- Urine (CMV, mumps, adenovirus)—increased sensitivity by using several specimens. Useful in mumps encephalitis when other sites are negative.
- Rectal swabs and stool—stools are generally more useful (see above).
- Blood—serum for enteroviruses; leukocytes for CMV and arbovirus.
- Tissue—lung (CMV, influenza, adenovirus) and brain (HSV) are the most productive.
- Also CSF, skin vesicles, eye in appropriate cases

VIRAL PNEUMONIA DUE TO EATON AGENT (*MYCOPLASMA PNEUMONIAE*)

(epidemics every 4–6 years; also endemic and sporadic)

WBC is slightly increased (in 25% of patients) or is normal.

ESR is increased in 65% of patients.

Increased cold hemagglutination occurs late in course in 50% of patients (≤90% in severe illness); becomes positive at about seventh day, rises to peak at 4 weeks, then declines rapidly and usually is negative by 4 months. May sometimes be present in other conditions (see p. 81).

Serologic tests

- IgM and IgG (IFA, EIA) are sensitive and specific and are preferred serologic tests; both should be performed in acute and convalescent (2–4 weeks) sera. Presence of IgM (>1:10) or 4-fold rise in IgG indicates recent infection. IgG indicates previous exposure.
- 4-fold increase in CF titer occurs in ~50% of patients; increase begins in 7–9 days; peak at 3–4 weeks may last for 4–6 months, then gradual fall for 2–3 years; if only a convalescent serum is available, a titer >1:64 is suggestive of diagnosis of *Mycoplasma pneumoniae* infection. False positives may occur in acute inflammatory diseases (e.g., bacterial meningitis, pancreatitis).

Culture of organism by special techniques may require several weeks.

Mycoplasma hominis may cause pyelonephritis, pelvic inflammatory disease, and postpartum febrile complications. Mycoplasmas should also be considered in the differential diagnosis of acute arthritis, hemolytic anemia, various dermatologic disorders, myocardial or cerebral disease, as well as severe bilateral pneumonia.

UPPER RESPIRATORY VIRAL INFECTION

Due To Respiratory Syncytial Virus (RSV)

(major cause of bronchiolitis and pneumonia in infants and young children)

ESR and WBC may be increased in children.

Pharyngeal smears may reveal many epithelial cells that contain cytoplasmic inclusion bodies.

Serologic tests

- Presence of serum IgM or ≥4-fold increase in IgG (EIA, IFA) indicates recent infection.
- Rise in titer of CF and neutralizing antibodies occurs during convalescence; have poorer sensitivity and are rarely used.
- These methods are now being replaced by EIA or IFA direct detection of antigen in clinical specimens.

Due To Adenovirus

(may cause at least six clinical syndromes involving pharynx, conjunctiva, and pneumonitis; types 11 and 21 have been associated with acute hemorrhage cystitis)

WBC is slightly decreased after about 7 days.
ESR is increased.
Serologic tests (are often not needed)
CF and neutralizing antibodies appear after 1 week and peak in 2–3 weeks. CF antibody decreases considerably in 2–3 months, but neutralizing antibody may decrease only 2–3 times after 1–2 years. A 4-fold increase in CF antibody titer between acute and convalescent sera is presumptive evidence of infection but does not indicate the type of adenovirus. Only virus isolation or rise in type-specific neutralizing antibody titer during convalescence allows specific diagnosis.
Direct electron microscopy has been useful for diagnosis of gastroenteritis in children.

Due To Rhinoviruses

WBC may be slightly increased.
ESR is increased in ~5% of patients.
Serologic tests are not clinically useful.

Due To Parainfluenza Virus

WBC is variable at first; later becomes normal or decreased.
Specific diagnosis requires recovery of virus in tissue-culture preparation.
Serologic tests include hemagglutination inhibition (HAI) and tissue-culture neutralization; ≥4-fold CF titer in paired sera 2–3 weeks apart is suggestive of diagnosis of appropriate type. Not useful for routine clinical studies.

INFLUENZA A, B

WBC is usually normal (5000–10,000/cu mm) with relative lymphocytosis. Leukopenia occurs in 50% of the patients. WBC >15,000/cu mm suggests secondary bacterial infection.
Presence of IgM or ≥4-fold increase in IgG (EIA, IFA) indicates recent infection. IgM peaks at 2 weeks and IgG at 4–7 weeks. IgG indicates past exposure and immunity. More sensitive and preferred to CF, HAI.
CF and HAI may show 4-fold increase in sera taken during acute phase and 2–3 weeks later. HAI is relatively insensitive.
Direct immunofluorescence detection of antigen in ciliated epithelial cells from nasopharyngeal swab is now available for rapid diagnosis.

CHLAMYDIAE INFECTIONS

(due to *Chlamydia trachomatis;* at least 10 major immunotypes)

Genital tract infection—see Nonspecific Urethritis, pp. 596–600. (Incidence of chlamydial cervicitis and urethritis is 10 times greater than *Neisseria gonorrhoeae* infection. 50% of the latter have concomitant chlamydial infection.)
Isolation in cell culture (obligate intracellular pathogen) is the most sensitive (80–90%) and specific (100%) test but is technically difficult and may not be easily available. Remains the "gold standard" test. Culture requires sample of infected epithelial cells rather than discharges, urine, or semen. Longest turnaround time (2–3 days). Urethral culture increases the diagnostic sensitivity of a single endocervical culture by up to 20%.
Antigen detection provides high sensitivity and specificity by EIA of secretions (>79%, >95%) or staining of smears by direct immunofluorescence (>90%, >95%) in symptomatic or high-prevalence groups; positive and negative predictive values are >80%, >90% and >87%, >98% respectively.*

*Data from WE Stamm, Diagnosis of *Chlamydia trachomatis* genitourinary infections. *Ann Intern Med* 108:710, 1988.

Table 16-5. Methods for Diagnosis of Chlamydial Infections

Method	Application	Sensitivity/Specificity
Culture	All chlamydial infections	"Gold standard"
Cytology	Inclusion conjunctivitis, trachoma	~95% sensitivity
Serology	Invasive infection (pneumonia, psittacosis, lymphogranuloma venereum). Not for superficial infections of eye, urethra	
Complement-fixation	*C. psittaci* infection. Not for infantile pneumonia	
Microimmunofluorescence	Infantile pneumonia (IgM)	
Antigen detection		High sensitivity and specificity
Immunofluorescence	Specimens from GU tract, conjunctiva, rectum, nasopharynx	
EIA	Specimens from GU tract, conjunctiva	81% sensitivity, 99% specificity from endocervix
Nucleic acid hybridization probes	Specimens from GU tract	Very high sensitivity and specificity

Newer DNA hybridization methods are being developed and should be evaluated when available.

Intracytoplasmic inclusions by Giemsa or immunofluorescent staining of scrapings from genital lesions has low sensitivity. Has been replaced by immunologic procedures.

Serodiagnosis is not useful for superficial infections; 4-fold rise in antibody titer between acute and convalescent sera may be useful in diagnosis of invasive and systemic infections, e.g., infantile pneumonia, pelvic inflammatory disease, lymphogranuloma venereum. Microimmunofluorescence (micro-IF) and CF are not routinely available, but ELISA kits are not useful for definitive diagnosis in most oculogenital infections. In neonates, antibody may be derived from mother rather than due to neonatal infection. The only syndrome in which serologic tests are method of choice is neonatal pneumonia, in which high IgM levels should be diagnostic.

Diagnosis should be sought and tests performed on all women in high-risk groups and with mucopurulent cervicitis, endometritis, pelvic inflammatory disease, acute urethritis, acute proctitis or whose male partners have gonorrhea or nongonococcal urethritis. Tests should be performed on men in appropriate groups if resources permit; otherwise treat empirically.

Mucopurulent cervicitis—cervical material shows >10 PMNs/hpf (1000×) in nonmenstruating women, positive culture or direct antigen test.

Acute urethral syndrome in women shows pyuria with bacteriuria, positive culture or direct antigen test from cervix or urethra.

Pelvic inflammatory disease shows findings of mucopurulent cervicitis, acute urethral syndrome; endometrium may show positive culture or direct antigen test and endometritis on biopsy.

Perihepatitis may show findings of pelvic inflammatory disease and high titer of IgM (44% of cases) or IgG antibody to *C. trachomatis.*

Trachoma—see next section.

Ophthalmia neonatorum—occurs in 18–50% of infants of mothers with genital infection (usually cervicitis); fathers often have urethritis.

Adult form of inclusion conjunctivitis is associated with genital tract infections.

Typical intracytoplasmic inclusions in epithelial cells on Giemsa-stained smears from conjunctival scrapings are found in 50% of cases. Immunofluorescent staining of inclusions has sensitivity of 70–95% and specificity of 98% in conjunctival lesions (sensitivity < 50% in genital lesions). Inflammatory response shows both neutrophils and mononuclear cells compared to viral conjunctivitis, which shows predominantly lymphocytes, and allergic conjunctivitis, which shows predominantly eosinophils. Immunofluorescent stains are commercially available and significantly increase sensitivity.

Tissue culture of *Chlamydia* is the most sensitive and specific test, and positive cultures are usually detectable within 48 hours. Requires special techniques and may not be locally available.

Detection of antigen in secretions by EIA or direct immunofluorescent staining of smears

Distinctive pneumonia syndrome of infants (afebrile, chronic diffuse lung involvement, increased serum IgM (>1:32) and IgG, slight eosinophilia, distinctive cough) is the major cause of pneumonia before age 6 months with incidence of 8/1000 live births; occurs in 3–18% of infants of infected mothers.

Psittacosis—see p. 652.

Lymphogranuloma venereum—see p. 652.

Reiter's syndrome—*Chlamydia trachomatis* has been isolated from the urethra in up to 60% of men with Reiter's syndrome, but tetracycline does not change the clinical course, and etiologic role is speculative.

Acute proctitis—see p. 167.

TRACHOMA

(due to *Chlamydia trachomatis*)

Typical cytoplasmic inclusion bodies are in epithelial cells scraped from conjunctiva of upper eyelid (Giemsa stain).

Secondary bacterial infection is common.

Preferred method of diagnosis is presence of serum IgM or rise in IgG (EIA); is more sensitive than CF, which should no longer be used. Presence of IgM in infants with pneumonia is diagnostic of *Chlamydia* pneumonia.

Detection of *Chlamydia* antigen (using EIA, DFA) is becoming increasingly useful.

PSITTACOSIS

(due to *Chlamydia psittaci*)

Positive CF test in early stage is presumptive; is usually also positive with lymphogranuloma venereum and sometimes other infections (e.g., brucellosis, Q fever). Rising titer (≥4 times) between acute and convalescent sera is diagnostic.

Detection of IgM or rising IgG titer (EIA, IFA) indicates recent infection; IgM can last for 4 weeks after infection. May cross react with *C. trachomatis* and lymphogranuloma venereum.

Cold agglutination is negative.

Albuminuria is common.

Sputum smear and culture show normal flora.

WBC may be normal or decreased in acute phase and increases during convalescence.

ESR is increased or frequently is normal.

LYMPHOGRANULOMA VENEREUM

(due to serotypes L1, L2, L3 of *Chlamydia trachomatis*)

High CF titer (>1:64) or increasing (4 times) titers or conversion of negative to positive may indicate recent infection; also present in psittacosis. Fall in titer suggests therapeutic success in acute stage. Persistent negative in the presence of disease is rare.

Detection of antibody to B-complex *C. trachomatis* by microimmunofluorescence.

Biopsy of regional lymph node shows stellate abscesses.

Serum globulin is increased with reversed A/G ratio during period of activity.

Biologically false positive reaction for syphilis that becomes negative in a few weeks appears in 20% of patients. If titer increases, beware of concomitant syphilitic infection.

WBC is normal or increased < 20,000/cu mm. There may be relative lymphocytosis or monocytosis.

ESR is increased.

Slight anemia may be present.

COXSACKIEVIRUS AND ECHOVIRUS INFECTIONS

(These include infections such as epidemic pleurodynia, "grippe," meningitis, myocarditis, herpangina.)

Laboratory findings are not specific.

CSF

- Cell count is ≤500/cu mm, occasionally ≤2000/cu mm; predominantly PMNs at first, then predominantly lymphocytes.
- Protein may increase ≤100 mg/dl.
- Glucose is normal.

WBC varies but is usually normal.

Viral serologic tests may show increasing titer of neutralizing or CF antibodies between acute- and convalescent-phase sera. Are generally not clinically helpful because of many serotypes. With Coxsackie A or B infection, CF antibodies are often increased in acute-phase, making 4-fold rise in titer difficult to demonstrate.

Culture is required for certain syndromes (e.g., chronic meningoencephalitis with agammaglobulinemia may show echovirus 11 in CSF).

VIRAL GASTROENTEROCOLITIS

Suspected by exclusion by negative tests for other causes of the symptoms (e.g., failure to find *Entamoeba histolytica, Shigella, Salmonella*)

See separate sections for specific agents (e.g., rotavirus, echovirus).

Direct electron microscopy of stool can detect and identify all the morphologic types of enteric viruses.

Norwalk virus (especially in raw oysters) can be diagnosed by presence of serum IgM or increasing titer of IgG antibodies (EIA). Chief use is to identify cause of an outbreak.

Detection of viral antigen in stool is usually not useful due to brief period of excretion.

POLIOMYELITIS

CSF

- Cell count is usually 25–500/cu mm; rarely is normal or ≤2000/cu mm. At first, most are PMNs; after several days, most are lymphocytes.
- Protein may be normal at first; increased by second week (usually 50–200 mg/dl); normal by sixth week.
- Glucose is usually normal.
- GOT is always increased but does not correlate with serum GOT; reaches peak in 1 week and returns to normal by 4 weeks; level of GOT does not correlate with severity of paralysis.

CSF findings are not diagnostic but may occur in many CNS diseases due to viruses (e.g., Coxsackie, mumps, herpes), bacteria (e.g., pertussis, scarlet fever), other infections (e.g., leptospirosis, trichinosis, syphilis), CNS tumors, multiple sclerosis, etc.

Blood shows early moderate increase in WBC (≤15,000/cu mm) and PMNs; normal within 1 week.

Laboratory findings of associated lesions (e.g., myocarditis) or complications (e.g., secondary bacterial infection, stone formation in GU tract, alterations in water and electrolyte balance due to continuous artificial respiration) are present.

Increased SGOT in 50% of patients is due to the associated hepatitis.

Serologic tests may show ≥4-fold increase in CF antibody types 1, 2, 3 titer between acute and convalescent sera (after 3 weeks), but titer may have already reached peak at time of hospitalization. Not useful to determine immune status for which neutralization test is useful.

Virus may be cultured from stool up to early convalescence (done by the U.S. Public Health Service's Communicable Disease Center, Atlanta, GA).

ACQUIRED IMMUNE DEFICIENCY SYNDROME (AIDS)

(see appropriate separate section for each disease or test referred to below)

Due to a retrovirus, human immunodeficiency virus (HIV-1)

Laboratory findings that should heighten suspicion in patients at risk

- Lymphopenia
- Anemia
- Idiopathic thrombocytopenic purpura
- Positive serologic test for syphilis
- Increased ESR
- Increased serum globulin
- Increased LDH

Low serum cholesterol
Various infections
Acute (e.g., aseptic meningitis)
Chronic (e.g., oral thrush, chronic vaginitis, "indicator" diseases [see lists below])

Criteria for national reporting are based on combination of laboratory findings (I, II, III) and one or more "indicator" diseases (A, B) (see lists below).

I. Laboratory evidence of HIV infection (any of the following items a–e)
   a. Repeated reactive screening test for HIV antibody (e.g., EIA) confirmed by Western blot or immunofluorescence (IFA) assay
   b. Child <15 months old whose mother had HIV infection during perinatal period with repeated reactive screening test, plus increased serum immunoglobulin levels and at least one of the following abnormal immunologic tests: reduced absolute lymphocyte count, depressed CD4 (T-helper) lymphocyte count, or decreased CD4/CD8 (helper/suppressor) ratio if subsequent confirmatory antibody tests are positive
   c. Positive test for HIV serum antigen
   d. Positive HIV culture confirmed by both reverse transcriptase detection and a specific HIV antigen test or in situ hybridization using nucleic acid probe. Not a standard diagnostic test because expensive, time-consuming, and potentially dangerous; may be useful in unusual cases. Positive in 100% of late stages but 20–60% of early asymptomatic patients.
   e. Positive result with any other highly specific test for HIV (e.g., nucleic acid probe of peripheral blood lymphocytes)

II. Laboratory evidence against HIV infection—nonreactive screening test for serum HIV antibody without any other positive laboratory test for HIV infection (e.g., antibody, antigen, culture), if done.

III. Inconclusive laboratory evidence (item a or b)
   a. Repeatedly reactive screening test for serum HIV antibody (e.g., EIA) followed by a negative or inconclusive test (e.g., Western blot, IFA) without a positive serum antigen or culture if done
   b. Child <15 months old whose mother had HIV infection during perinatal period with repeatedly reactive HIV antibody screening test, even if positive by supplemental test but without additional evidence of immunodeficiency (see item I.b) and without a positive serum antigen or culture if done

List A: Definitively diagnosed "indicator" diseases that are considered evidence of AIDS even if laboratory tests are inconclusive or not performed. If laboratory evidence of AIDS is negative, these diseases are considered evidence of AIDS if other causes of immunodeficiency are excluded (see List C) and patient has either *Pneumocystis carinii* pneumonia or the T-helper/inducer (CD4) lymphocyte count is <400/cu mm and any of the following diseases 2–12 is present:

1. *Pneumocystis carinii* pneumonia (present in >50% of cases)
2. Cytomegalovirus involving organs other than liver, spleen, or lymph nodes in a patient >1 month old
3. Candidiasis of the esophagus, trachea, bronchi, or lungs
4. Cryptococcosis, extrapulmonary
5. Toxoplasmosis of the brain in a patient >1 month old
6. Cryptosporidiosis with diarrhea for >1 month
7. Herpes simplex causing mucocutaneous ulcer for >1 month; or causing bronchitis, pneumonitis, or esophagitis in a patient >1 month old
8. *Mycobacterium avium* complex or *M. kansasii* disease, disseminated beyond lungs, skin, cervical or hilar lymph nodes

9. Kaposi's sarcoma in a patient <60 years old (present in ~25% of cases)
10. Primary brain lymphoma in a patient <60 years old
11. Lymphoid interstitial pneumonia and/or pulmonary lymphoid hyperplasia (LIP/PLH complex) in a child <13 years old
12. Progressive multifocal leukoencephalopathy

List B: "Indicator" diseases that are considered evidence of AIDS when laboratory evidence is present:

1. Child <age 13 years with the following multiple or recurrent bacterial infections: septicemia, pneumonia, meningitis, bone or joint infection, abscess of internal organ or body cavity, due to *Hemophilus, Streptococcus* (including pneumococcus), or other pyogenic bacteria
2. Disseminated coccidioidomycosis other than or in addition to lungs, cervical, or hilar lymph nodes
3. Disseminated histoplasmosis other than or in addition to lungs, cervical, or hilar lymph nodes
4. Isosporiasis with diarrhea for >1 month
5. Any disseminated mycobacterial disease (other than *M. tuberculosis*) other than or in addition to lungs, skin, cervical or hilar lymph nodes
6. Extrapulmonary *M. tuberculosis* disease
7. Recurrent nontyphoid salmonella septicemia
8. HIV wasting syndrome
9. Kaposi's sarcoma at any age
10. Primary brain lymphoma at any age
11. Other non-Hodgkin's lymphoma of B-cell or unknown immunologic phenotype and the following histologic types:
    Small noncleaved lymphoma (Burkitt or non-Burkitt type)
    Immunoblastic sarcoma
    Lymphomas not included are T-cell, lymphocytic, lymphoblastic, small cleaved, plasmacytoid lymphocytic
12. Any disease on List A

List C: In the absence of laboratory evidence of HIV infection, any of these known causes of immunodeficiency disqualify the indicator diseases:

1. High-dose or long-term corticosteroid or other immunosuppressive/cytotoxic therapy within 3 months of onset of indicator disease
2. Genetic (congenital) immunodeficiency syndrome or an acquired syndrome atypical of HIV infection (e.g., with hypogammaglobulinemia)
3. Any of the following diseases diagnosed <3 months after diagnosis of indicator disease: Hodgkin's disease, non-Hodgkin's lymphoma (other than primary brain lymphoma), lymphocytic leukemia, multiple myeloma, any other cancer of lymphoreticular or histiocytic tissue, angioimmunoblastic lymphadenopathy

These criteria are for purposes of national surveillance; for an individual patient, a positive screening test associated with an indicator disease should be confirmed by a supplemental test.

ANTIBODY TO HUMAN IMMUNODEFICIENCY VIRUS TYPE 1 (HIV-1)
(formerly called HUMAN T-CELL LYMPHOTROPIC VIRUS, HTLV III)

HIV appears in plasma and circulating mononuclear cells 1 to several weeks after infection; HIV antibodies usually appear in 1–3 months and, rarely, >12 months after infection. Antigens decline and disappear and viral isolation from blood becomes more difficult as antibodies arise. 80% are asymptomatic and 20% may have nondescript illness with low fever, rash, diarrhea. In late stage, HIV is usually easily recovered from blood and CSF.

Antibody (anti-HIV) develops in all patients infected with this virus and is taken as evidence of past or present infection. Presence of antibody does not cause immunity, however, since virus can be cultured from antibody-positive individuals for years. Thus, antibody-positive persons can transmit the virus to others. Antibodies may appear by 60 days after infection but seroconversion can take >12 months; early reports suggest that 6–20% of HIV-infected persons may be seronegative. Anti-HIV-IgG can cross placenta and enter fetal circulation. Reversion to antibody-negative status can occur but is very rare.

Incidence of HIV antibody in donated blood in the U.S. is about 0.22% by enzyme immunoassay (EIA) and 0.1% by Western blot (WB).

Recommended screening test uses EIA technique, which has a sensitivity and specificity of >99%. Expected false positive rate is 68–89% when HIV prevalence is 0.1% and 17–44% when HIV prevalence is 1.0%. By Feb. 1986, >90% of repeatedly reactive EIA tests on 5.5 million units screened by the American Red Cross were false positive. True rate of false negatives is unknown, but there have been a few reports of positive virus cultures in asymptomatic seronegative persons.

False Negative ELISA Results May Be Due To

Advanced AIDS disease (but there is usually other evidence of AIDS)

Early infection before antibodies are detectable (*This donated blood may transmit HIV.*)

False Positive ELISA Results May Be Due To

Receiving hepatitis B immune globulin within about 6 weeks of testing (antibody is present but gamma globulin cannot transmit the AIDS virus) from products manufactured since early 1980s

Multigravida women (may form antibody to leukocyte antigen components that cross react in ELISA test)

Presence of rheumatoid factor

Test may be positive in persons with subclinical infection who are asymptomatic, in active carriers of viral antigen, in persons with immunity, or due to false positive reactions.

When EIA test is positive or uncertain, EIA must be confirmed using WB or immunofluorescence (IFA) assay, which are more specific but less sensitive and less standardized than EIA. If EIA is negative, a WB is usually not done, and this blood may be used for transfusion if donor does not belong to high-risk groups. If EIA is positive and confirmed by WB or IFA, the individual has been infected with HIV. If EIA is positive and WB is negative, the patient's blood should not be used for transfusion although the diagnosis of AIDS is not confirmed. If EIA is positive and WB and/or IFA is equivocal, infection status with HIV is unknown and WB should be repeated on a subsequent specimen in 4–6 months; this person should not be used as a blood donor. Recently infected persons may have indeterminate WB pattern initially, which becomes positive on repeat in 6 months. Indeterminate WB pattern may also occur in AIDS patients with advanced immunodeficiency because of loss of antibodies. WB is considered the "gold standard" for confirmation of HIV tests but is a technically demanding test.

False Positive WB Test May Be Due To

Presence of antibody to another human retrovirus

Cross reaction with other nonvirus-derived proteins

Indeterminate WB Test May Be Due To

Recent HIV infection. Test will usually become unequivocally positive in 6–12 weeks.

A repeat positive test requires the blood donor facility to inform the donor.

Approximately 22–50% of HIV antibody–positive persons developed AIDS at 5 years and 50–70% at 10 years.

It is not possible to predict which seropositive persons will develop AIDS or show clinical symptoms. Antibody-positive persons are potentially infectious.

The recent recommendations of the USPHS for voluntary blood testing are persons who

- Have a history of IV drug abuse
- Engage in male homosexual activity
- Have identifiable risks (e.g., IV drug use, prostitution, homosexual or bisexual men, infected sex partners) or have sexual partners with such risks
- Are prostitutes
- Are inmates of correctional institutions
- May have a sexually transmitted disease
- Are undergoing medical evaluation or treatment, including tuberculosis
- Received transfusions of blood or blood products (e.g., Factor VIII) between 1978 and 1985
- Are planning marriage
- Are women of childbearing age
- Are patients admitted to hospitals
- Consider themselves at risk

See Fig. 16-4, p. 658, for other tests and criteria for diagnosis of AIDS.

Positive EIA tests referred to above mean that each positive test has been repeatedly positive in duplicate on the same serum specimen.

HIV type 2 is a recently described virus that causes a disease not distinguishable from AIDS in Africans and small numbers of Europeans and South Americans. Current screening tests for HIV-1 do not consistently and reliably detect antibody due to HIV-2 infection (see next section).

Other laboratory findings in AIDS

- Lymphopenia largely due to decreased helper-inducer subset (CD4) and increased suppressor subset of T lymphocytes (CD8) (by flow cytometry). (Normal range of CD4 lymphocytes ≥ 400/cu mm; normal range of CD8 lymphocytes = 200–800; each laboratory should establish their own normal range. Normal CD4/CD8 ratio is 2.0; AIDS patients have reversed ratio of 0.5–1.0; sensitivity about 85% but low specificity since this may be seen in other diseases, particularly in infections with Epstein-Barr virus, herpesvirus, and cytomegalovirus). *CD4 cell count is the most commonly performed and most sensitive marker of immune dysfunction and is often used as indication for antiviral therapy or prophylaxis for Pneumocystis pneumonia.* CD8 count is relatively labile and may devalue the value of the CD4 count alone. Lymphopenia is found in 50% of patients with Kaposi's sarcoma and almost all patients with opportunistic infections. Total B-cell and natural killer–cell counts are usually normal.
- Leukopenia, anemia, and idiopathic thrombocytopenia are common; thrombocytosis also occurs.
- Increased serum gamma globulins early in course of HIV infection, especially IgG and also IgA; slight IgM increase may occur; associated with opportunistic infection.
- Most valuable tests for evaluation of immune status are CD4 and CD8 counts and assay of immunoglobulins.
- Hypoalbuminemia
- Increased serum transaminase
- Complement C3 and C4 levels are usually normal.
- Decreased T-cell function evidenced
  - In vivo by
    - Decreased delayed-type hypersensitivity (skin test reactivity)

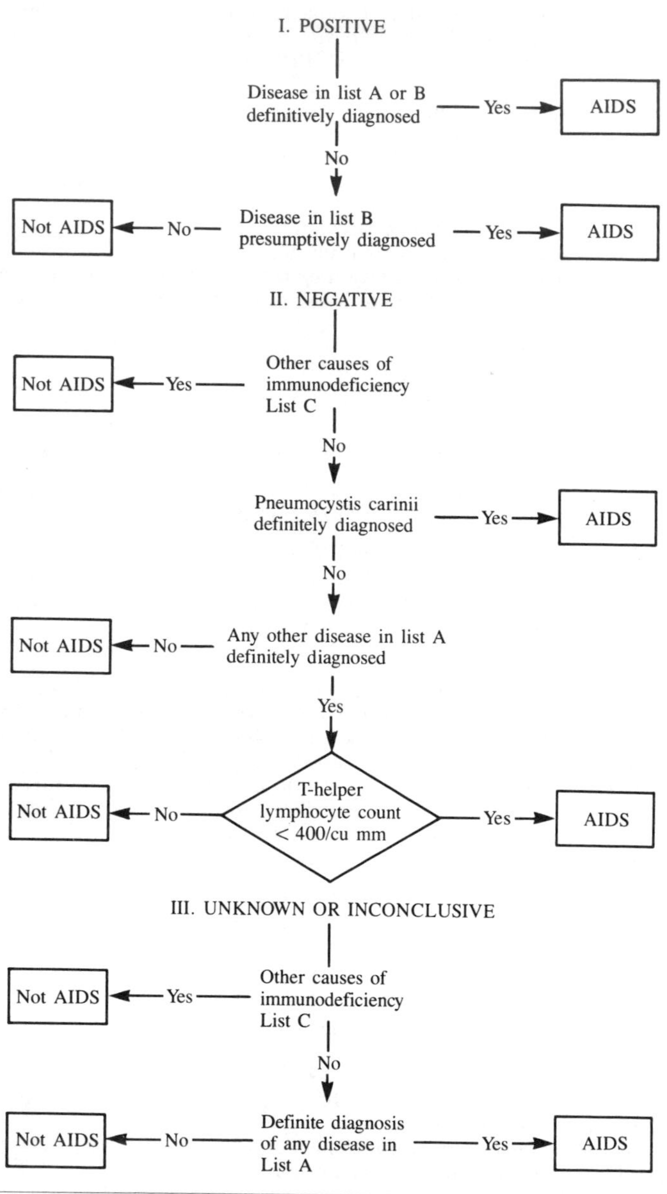

Fig. 16-4. Flow chart of CDC definition of AIDS. I, II, and III refer to criteria on pp. 654–655. (Adapted from revision of the CDC Surveillance Case Definition for Acquired Immunodeficiency Syndrome. Leads from *MMWR. JAMA* 258 (9):1143, 1987.)

        - Opportunistic infections
        - Neoplasms
    - In vitro by various tests not routinely available
- Other serologic findings (not used in clinical diagnosis)—increased levels of
    - Acid-labile alpha interferon (previously known in patients with autoimmune disease; found in 63% of homosexual AIDS patients and 29% without AIDS) (more studies are needed to determine value as screening test)
    - Alpha$_1$ thymosin (found in $<1\%$ of normal persons, 70–80% of AIDS patients, and 60–70% of patients with chronic reactive lymphadenopathy syndrome)
    - Beta$_2$ microglobulins appear to correlate with clinical course of HIV infection (also increased in patients with hepatitis, kidney diseases, B-cell malignancies such as multiple myeloma)
    - Circulating immune complexes
- Laboratory findings due to coexisting diseases
    - Hepatitis B core antigen is positive in $>90\%$ of AIDS patients and 80% of patients with lymphadenopathy syndrome. Rate of hepatitis B is 10–30 times that of general population in U.S.
    - Epstein-Barr virus (EBV) and human T-cell leukemia virus
- No single test establishes or rules out the diagnosis.
- Laboratory findings due to involvement of organ systems
    - Pneumonia
        - Parasites (*Pneumocystis carinii, Toxoplasma gondii*)
        - Viruses (CMV, herpes simplex)
        - Fungi (*Cryptococcus neoformans, Histoplasma capsulatum, Coccidioides immitis, Candida* species)
        - Bacteria (*Mycobacterium tuberculosis, M. avium-intracellulare, Streptococcus pneumoniae, Hemophilus influenzae, Staphylococcus aureus, Legionella* species, *Nocardia asteroides*)
        - Others (lymphoma, Kaposi's sarcoma, lymphocytic interstitial pneumonitis)
    - Nervous system (see Chap. 10)
        - Dementia (subacute encephalitis) occurs in $>50\%$ of cases
        - Aseptic meningitis
        - Meningitis due to various organisms (*Cryptococcus neoformans, Toxoplasma gondii*)
        - Myelopathy
        - Peripheral neuropathy
        - CNS lymphoma
    - Gastrointestinal
        - Oropharyngeal candidiasis
        - *M. avium-intracellulare* causing diarrhea, malabsorption, or hepatitis
        - CMV esophagitis, colitis, or hepatitis
        - Isosporosis causing diarrhea
    - Nephropathy—resembles nephrotic syndrome with rapid progress to end-stage renal disease and very poor prognosis; death usually within 6 months even with dialysis. Acute renal failure may be due to drugs, sepsis, etc.
    - Neoplasms
        - Non-Hodgkin's lymphoma—rapid course, poor prognosis, frequent extranodal and CNS involvement
        - Kaposi's sarcoma
    - Other
        - Infectious mononucleosis–like syndrome (e.g., rash, pharyngitis, enlarged spleen) may occur during initial viremia period with hematologic picture of infectious mononucleosis, but serologic tests for EBV and CMV are negative; meningeal signs with CSF pleocytosis may occur. Most patients are asymptomatic during initial HIV viremia.

When AIDS develops, 20% survive after 2 years and 2% survive after 4 years. Men with only Kaposi's sarcoma have best prognosis; women with opportunistic infection have worst prognosis.

DISTRIBUTION OF CASES OF AIDS BY SEX AND RISK GROUP

	Men (%)	Women (%)
Homosexual/bisexual	71	0
IV drug user	14	50
Homosexual/bisexual + IV drug user	8	0
Haitian	3	8
Hemophiliac	1	0
Transfusion associated	2	10
Heterosexual contact	2	29
None of these	3	17

As of May 1987, 35,318 cases of AIDS were reported to CDC; 58% have died. 498 were <age 13 years; 79% of these had a parent with, or at risk for, AIDS; 12% were transfusion associated.

Among whites, homosexual/bisexual transmission was the major source of infection; IV drug abuse caused 13% of cases. Among blacks and Hispanics, IV drug abuse caused 43% of cases and homosexual/bisexual activity caused 40–48% of cases. Heterosexual transmission was much more common among blacks than among Hispanics or whites. Kaposi's sarcoma is rare in drug users, but tuberculosis is common. Rapid spread of HIV in drug users, especially prostitutes, appears to be a major source for heterosexual transmission throughout the world. Drug use is major source of most pediatric cases. 50–60% of infants born to mothers with HIV infection develop HIV infection. 50–75% of hemophilia patients have HIV antibodies, but only 2% have developed AIDS.

These figures will vary with local population. For example, in New Jersey, 60% of cases occur in IV drug users, 29% occur in homosexual/bisexual men, 35% occur in both groups combined.

In Africa, heterosexual transmission is predominant adult mode of spread, but in U.S. and Europe homosexual/bisexual transmission and IV drug use are predominant modes.

CHRONIC LYMPHADENOPATHY SYNDROME (AIDS-RELATED COMPLEX [ARC])

Found in homosexual men with lymphadenopathy for >3 months involving >2 extrainguinal sites without other illness or drug use known to cause lymphadenopathy. If lymph node is biopsied, shows reactive hyperplasia.

ANTIBODY TO HUMAN T-LYMPHOTROPIC VIRUS TYPE I (HTLV-I)

May Be Positive In

Adult T-cell leukemia/lymphoma (see p. 336). Risk of disease estimated at 2–4% after infected 20 years

Degenerative neurologic disease called tropical spastic paraparesis in Caribbean and HTLV-I–associated myelopathy in Japan. Latent period of clinical disease about 4 years after blood transfusion.

In U.S. in female prostitutes, recipients of multiple blood transfusions, up to 49% of IV drug users. Rare in homosexual men, patients in sexually transmitted disease clinics; nonexistent in hemophiliacs. 0.025% incidence in random blood donors.

In Caribbean islands in 5% of general population and 15% of older persons

In Japan, up to 15% of general population and 30% of older persons

Table 16-6. Commonly Associated Pathogens in Patients with Immunosuppression (e.g., Organ Transplantation, Treatment of Malignancies, AIDS)

Immune Response Depressed	Underlying Condition	Commonly Associated Pathogens
Humoral	Lymphatic leukemia Lymphosarcoma Multiple myeloma Congenital hypogammaglobulinemias Nephrotic syndrome Treatment with cytotoxic or antimetabolite drugs	Pneumococci *Hemophilus influenzae* Streptococci *Pseudomonas aeruginosa* *Pneumocystis carinii*
Cellular	Terminal cancers Hodgkin's disease Sarcoidosis Uremia Treatment with cytotoxic or antimetabolite drugs or corticosteroids	Tubercle bacillus *Listeria* *Candida* species *Toxoplasma* *Pneumocystis carinii*
Leukocyte bactericidal	Myelogenous leukemia Chronic granulomatous disease Acidosis Burns Treatment with corticosteroids Granulocytopenia due to drugs	Staphylococci *Serratia* *Pseudomonas* species *Candida* species *Aspergillus* *Nocardia*

Positive screening test (by EIA) should always be repeated in duplicate and then confirmed by more specific tests (e.g., Western blot), which have not yet been licensed. Sensitivity and specificity of EIA >97%. Neither the screening nor more specific tests distinguish between antibodies to HTLV-I and HTLV-II (a closely related human retrovirus). Disease associations of HLTV-II are unknown.

EIA test recommended for screening for whole blood and cellular components. Source plasma need not be screened for HTLV-I. Repeatedly positive donors should be permanently deferred and counseled against blood donation, sharing needles, breast-feeding, etc.

Seroconversion occurs in 63% of blood transfusion recipients containing cells but not plasma fractions, 25% of breast-fed infants of seropositive mothers, and fewer non-breast-fed infants. Smaller percentage in sexual partners.

HTLV-I is a retrovirus but not closely related to HIV that causes AIDS. HTLV-I does not cause depletion of T-helper lymphocytes and is not generally associated with immunosuppression. HTLV-I does not cause AIDS, and presence of antibody does not imply HIV infection or risk of AIDS.

HTLV-I and HIV antigens do not cross react.

Table 16-7. Commonly Associated Pathogens in Patients with Neoplasms

Neoplasm	Infection	Commonly Associated Pathogens
Acute nonlymphocytic leukemia	Sepsis with no apparent focus, pneumonia, skin, mouth, GU tract, hepatitis	*Enterobacter*, *Pseudomonas*, staphylococci, *Corynebacterium*, *Candida*, *Aspergillus*, *Mucor*, NANB hepatitis
Acute lymphocytic leukemia	Disseminated disease, pneumonia, pharyngitis, skin	Streptococci, *Pneumocystis carinii*, HSV, CMV, VZV
Lymphoma	Disseminated disease, sepsis, GU tract, pneumonia, skin	*Cryptococcus neoformans*, mucocutaneous *Candida*, HSV, HZV, CMV, *Pneumocystis carinii*, *Toxoplasma gondii*, mycobacteria, *Nocardia*, *Strongyloides stercoralis*, *Listeria monocytogenes*, *Brucella*, *Salmonella*, staphylococci, *Enterobacter*, *Pseudomonas*
Multiple myeloma	Sepsis, pneumonia, skin	*Hemophilus influenzae*, *Streptococcus pneumoniae*, *Neisseria meningitidis*, *Pseudomonas*, *Enterobacter*, HZV, *Candida*, *Aspergillus*

HSV = herpes simplex virus; CMV = cytomegalovirus; VZV = varicella-zoster virus; HZV = herpes zoster virus.

CYTOMEGALIC INCLUSION DISEASE (CMV)

(limited to salivary gland involvement in 10% of infant autopsies; disseminated in 1–2% of childhood autopsies)

Intranuclear inclusions in epithelial cells in urine sediment and liver biopsy (more useful in infants than adults)

Hemolytic anemia with icterus and thrombocytopenic purpura in infants

Evidence of damage to liver, kidney, brain

Laboratory findings due to predisposing or underlying conditions (e.g., AIDS, malignant lymphoma, leukemia, refractory anemia, after renal transplant) or after receiving many transfusions of fresh blood; may be associated with *Pneumocystis carinii* pneumonia in adults

May cause a syndrome of heterophil-negative infectious mononucleosis in immunologically competent adults characterized by

- Hematologic and hepatic test findings identical with those in heterophil-positive infectious mononucleosis due to Epstein-Barr virus (see pp. 323–324). CMV causes two-thirds of all heterophil-negative mononucleosis-like illness in patients over age 14 years.

Immunologic findings

- Increased cold agglutinin titer (same as in heterophil-positive patients)
- Cryoglobulinemia is common (mixed IgG-IgM).
- Increased rheumatoid factors (cold-reactive more common than warm-reactive)
- Positive direct Coombs' test is common.
- Polyclonal hypergammaglobulinemia is common.
- False positive serologic test for syphilis in <3% of cases
- Antinuclear antibodies (speckled pattern) commonly present transiently.

Confirmatory tests for CMV

- Presence of CMV-IgM within 1–2 weeks allows rapid diagnosis of primary infection using a single test during acute illness (>1:32); titer <1:16 may persist for 12 months in 24% of patients. Only IgG appears during reactivation. IgM in adults indicates acute infection, reinfection (within past 3–4 months) or reactivation but in newborns indicates in utero infection, as IgM does not cross placenta. False positive and false negative rate in newborns each >20%.
- 4-fold increase in serial CMV-IgG antibody titer in 2–4 weeks in primary but only occasionally in reactivation or reinfection.
- Serologic tests for antibodies include CF, immunofluorescence, HAI, EIA, and neutralization, which vary in sensitivity, specificity, cost, speed. Heterotypic responses to other herpesviruses are known to occur. Nucleic acid hybridization is being evaluated.
- Identification of CMV inclusion bodies or CMV antigen in infected tissue (e.g., bronchoalveolar lavage) by IFA is more rapid but less sensitive than culture.
- Virus may be isolated from fresh urine (100% of cases), throat swabs (50% of cases), saliva, semen, cervical and vaginal secretions during acute phase. Since virus may be shed in urine in absence of disease for up to 2 years after primary infection, must be interpreted carefully. In neonate, presence of virus or inclusions usually means CMV infection. Peripheral blood leukocytes are frequently positive in immunocompromised patients and those with CMV mononucleosis.

LYMPHOCYTIC CHORIOMENINGITIS

WBC is slightly decreased at first; normal with onset of meningitis.

ESR is usually normal.

Thrombocytopenia develops during first week.

CSF

- Cell count is increased (100–3000 lymphocytes/cu mm, occasionally <30,000).
- Protein is normal or slightly increased.
- Glucose is usually normal.

Viral serologic tests

- IgM (IFA) may be detected in serum and CSF within first week of illness.
- Increasing CF antibody titer between acute and convalescent sera (2–3 weeks). Disappears in a few months. IgG (IFA) may appear very early, making 4-fold increase in titer difficult to detect; therefore sera should be drawn early.

Viral isolation by animal inoculation is not routinely performed.

ARBOVIRAL ENCEPHALITIDES

(including LaCrosse, eastern and western equine, and St. Louis encephalitis)

Marked decrease occurs in WBC with relative lymphocytosis.

CSF findings (see Table 10-2, pp. 226–229)

Serologic tests for arboviruses

- IFA detects infection early and is more sensitive than CF.

Antibody capture ELISA detects IgM in serum and CSF; becomes positive in <1 week and lasts a few weeks; persists ≤8 months in 29% of St. Louis encephalitis cases.

Paired sera detect IgG (EIA, IFA) in sera and establish diagnosis.

RABIES (HYDROPHOBIA)

(due to bite of rabid animal; in U.S., skunks [62%], bats [12%], raccoons [7%], cattle [6%], cats [4%], dogs [3%]; in Africa and Asia, dog rabies is endemic. *Immediate notification of state and local health departments is required for prompt, expert evaluation of patient and suspected animal.*)

WBC is increased (20,000–30,000/cu mm), with increased PMNs and large mononuclear cells.

Urine shows hyaline casts; reaction for albumin, sugar, and acetone may be positive.

CSF is usually normal or has a slight increase in protein and an increased number of mononuclear cells (usually <100/cu mm).

Microscopic examination of brain tissue sections or imprint smears of rabid animal shows Negri bodies (intracytoplasmic inclusions) in ~80% of cases. Rabid animal dies within 7–10 days. Demonstration of Negri bodies (50–80% sensitivity) has largely been supplanted by following tests.

Brain tissue of suspected animal is inoculated into brain of white mouse, which is later examined by immunofluorescent antibody (IFA) sections. >96% sensitivity and specificity. IFA staining of corneal smears (only in research laboratories) is positive in ~50%; skin and buccal mucosa biopsies and brain biopsy material can also be used for diagnosis during clinical phase.

Positive CF or ELISA detection of antibody in CSF is conclusive evidence of infection; serum antibodies usually require rising titer for accurate diagnosis. Antibody does not appear until >8 days (50% of cases) after onset of clinical symptoms, which may be months after exposure and is sometimes delayed or absent; almost all patients have antibodies by 15 days. Antibody in CSF appears 1–8 days later than serum; does not occur due to immunization.

Viral culture from brain or saliva may be positive and can sometimes be reported in 48 hours.

Intradermal prophylactic immunization may not be adequate and should be checked with serologic tests. Preferred is rapid fluorescent focus inhibition neutralization test.

ENCEPHALOMYELITIS (VIRAL AND POSTINFECTIOUS)

CSF

- Early (first 2–3 days)
  - Cell count is usually increased (≤100/cu mm), mostly PMNs (higher total count and more PMNs in infants).
  - Protein is usually normal.
  - Glucose and chloride are normal.
- Later (after third day)
  - Increased cell count is >90% lymphocytes.
  - Protein gradually increases after first week (≤100 mg/dl).
  - Glucose and chloride remain normal.

Serologic tests for specific virus identification and additional laboratory tests, see separate sections for each agent (e.g., CMV, mumps, measles, rabies, psittacosis, poliomyelitis, Coxsackie and echovirus, lymphocytic choriomeningitis, equine encephalomyelitis)

MUMPS

Uncomplicated salivary adenitis

- WBC and ESR are normal; WBC may be decreased, with relative lymphocytosis.
- Serum and urine amylase are increased during first week of parotitis; therefore increase does not always indicate pancreatitis.

Serum lipase is normal.
Serologic tests
Serum IgG and IgM should be taken as early as possible and again in 10–14 days (EIA, IFA). ≥4-fold rise in IgG (88% sensitivity) or presence of IgM indicates recent infection. IgM (EIA) is present by day 2 in 70% of patients and by day 5 in 100% of patients. Presence of IgG indicates past infection or vaccination and hence immunity. Simultaneous CSF specimens should be tested for possible mumps meningitis. Have largely replaced serum neutralization, CF, and hemagglutination inhibition tests that become positive later and are much less sensitive.

Complications of mumps
Orchitis (in 20% of postpubertal males but rare in children)
WBC is increased, with shift to the left. ESR is increased.
Sperm are decreased or absent after bilateral atrophy.
Ovaries are involved in 5% of adult females.
Pancreatitis (pp. 211–213) is much less frequent in children. Serum amylase and lipase are increased. Patient may have hyperglycemia and glycosuria.
Meningitis or meningoencephalitis (pp. 233–234)—mumps causes >10% of cases of aseptic meningitis. The disease may be clinically identical with mild paralytic poliomyelitis. WBC is usually normal. Serum amylase may be increased even if no abdominal symptoms are present. CSF contains 0–2000 mononuclear cells/cu mm.
Thyroiditis, myocarditis, arthritis, etc.

MEASLES (RUBEOLA)

WBC shows slight increase at onset, then falls to ~5000/cu mm with increased lymphocyte count. Increased WBC with shift to the left suggests bacterial complication (e.g., otitis media, pneumonia, appendicitis).

Mild thrombocytopenia in early stage

Wright's stain of sputum or nasal scrapings shows measles multinucleated giant cells, especially during prodrome and early rash.

Papanicolaou's stain of urine sediment after appearance of rash shows intracellular inclusion bodies; more specific is fluorescent antibody demonstration of measles antigen in urine sediment cells.

Viral serologic tests: IgG and IgM (EIA), CF, and HAI. Within 3 days after onset of rash, antibodies are found in 35–85% of cases (HAI is most sensitive). Maximum titers are reached in 2–3 weeks. Almost all paired sera show significant increases in titer. IgM is used for diagnosis of recent infection and IgG for screening for immunity.

Serum IgM (IFA, EIA) is detectable with onset of rash and usually persists for 4 weeks; 50% become negative by 4 months (beginning by 2 months). Presence of IgM or ≥4-fold rise in IgG indicates recent infection. Presence of IgG generally indicates previous exposure and present immunity.

Measles encephalitis: There is a marked increase in WBCs. CSF may show slightly increased protein and ≤500 mononuclear cells/cu mm. ≤10% of all measles patients have a significant increase in cells in CSF.

Persistent CNS infection causes subacute sclerosing panencephalitis (progressive fatal illness in children 5–14 years old). Diagnosed by presence of IgM or ≥4-fold rise in IgG titers in CSF.

Measles may cause remission in children with nephrosis.

RUBELLA (GERMAN MEASLES)

Viral serologic tests: IgM and total (IFA, EIA), hemagglutination inhibition (HAI), latex agglutination.

It is important to identify exposure to rubella infection and susceptibility status in pregnant women because infection in the first trimester of pregnancy is associated with congenital abnormalities, abortion, or stillbirth in about 30% of patients; during first month, up to 80% of patients show this association.

To determine antenatal immunity, test for IgG (EIA, HAI); IgM should also be tested if rubella is present in the community. In some laboratories, EIA has replaced HAI, which was the "gold standard" for antibody testing, and is the best documented test to establish immunity. IgG titer >1:10 confirms immunity. Up to one-third of persons show no detectable IgG 10 years after vaccination.

IgM is detected 11–25 days after onset of rash in all patients, 15–25 days after vaccination in 60–80% of cases, 2–12 weeks after birth in 90–97% of infants with congenital rubella; IgM often persists for 20–30 days. During first 6 months of life, IgM is the best test for congenital or recent infection. After age 7 months, persistence of IgG is assessed by HAI and EIA. IgG appears 15–25 days after infection and >25–50 days after vaccination. Absence of IgG in infant excludes congenital infection.

Low levels of IgM may occur in infectious mononucleosis; cross reaction may occur with parvovirus IgM. Some pregnant women with IgM antibodies to rubella may also have IgM to CMV, varicella-zoster, and measles virus.

With rubella rash, diagnosis is established if acute sample titer is >1:10 or if convalescent-phase serum taken 7 days after rash shows increase in titer.

Even if no rash develops in a patient exposed to rubella, a convalescent-phase serum taken 14–28 days after exposure that shows >4-fold increase in titer compared to the earlier sample indicates rubella infection.

Reinfection (occurs occasionally but usually asymptomatic) can be suspected if sera drawn ≥2 weeks apart show ≥4-fold increase in IgG titer and IgM does not develop.

HERPES SIMPLEX

(due to herpes simplex virus [HSV])

Culture of lesions establishes the diagnosis; is most sensitive and specific method; may take up to 7 days but usually within 4 days. Immune assay studies confirm that isolate is HSV and differentiate HSV-1 and HSV-2.

Antigen detection (EIA or direct fluorescence) in clinical specimen (e.g., skin vesicles) is more rapid but less sensitive (~60%) in asymptomatic persons than culture and is significantly more sensitive and specific than Tzanck test or direct electron microscopy. Distinguishes HSV-1 and HSV-2 and permits rapid diagnosis.

DNA hybridization identifies HSV in tissue or cell samples, is specific and rapid, and equals sensitivity of direct antigen detection if sufficient cells are collected.

Direct cytologic examination of scrapings of lesions (Wright-Giemsa stain) shows multinucleated giant cells with intranuclear inclusions (Tzanck smear). Skin vesicles produce a positive smear in 66% and positive viral culture in 100% of cases; pustules produce a positive smear in 50% and a positive viral culture in 70% of cases; crusted ulcers produce a positive smear in 15% and a positive viral culture in 34% of cases. Permits rapid diagnosis. Also positive in herpes zoster and varicella. (Positive smear refers to multinucleated giant cells not necessarily showing inclusions.) May also be seen on Pap stain. Direct electron microscopy can also be used. Other microscopy-based tests include indirect IFA and immunoperoxidase that approach sensitivity of viral isolation.

Serology is not useful clinically except in primary genital herpes. Primary infections show seroconversion or an increased (4 times) titer of CF, EIA (IgG or IgM), and neutralizing antibodies in convalescent-phase compared with acute-phase sera. In recurrent infections, a high titer is present in acute-phase sera and thus is rarely useful (5% of patients). May help in retrospect. May also use EIA, HAI, RIA, latex agglutination methods. False positive IgM may occur in presence of rheumatoid factor. CF does not distinguish HSV-1 and HSV-2. Western blot is accurate for subtyping.

Presence of IgG does not indicate reinfection, recurrent infection, or immunity. Presence or absence in newborn is not related to severity of CNS infection. IgM can be demonstrated for weeks after primary infection. Treatment status (e.g., acyclovir) should be known, as it may affect titers.
Specificity of positive tests should be checked by assay for VZV antibody.
Serologic tests are much less useful than detection of antigen in infected tissue (e.g., brain) by culture, microscopy, or immunoassay.
Type-specific serologies include neutralization tests and Western blot assay.
Findings of encephalitis if this complication occurs. High-titer serologic tests in CSF may be useful to establish the diagnosis. Antigen detection in CSF is not reliable. CSF viral culture may be useful in diagnosis of congenital infection. Causes 5% of cases of aseptic meningitis.
WBC is normal.

VIRAL GASTROENTERITIS
See pp. 160–161.

VIRAL HEPATITIS
See pp. 186–192.

EXANTHEMA SUBITUM (ROSEOLA INFANTUM)
WBC is increased during fever, then decreased during rash, with relative lymphocytosis.
Human herpesvirus-6 (a newly recognized virus) can be isolated from these patients (and also from some patients with HIV-1, HIV-2, and HTLV-1, and some lymphoproliferative disorders in which it may be a cofactor).
Antibody titer to HHV-6 rises in convalescent serum 3 weeks after disease onset. High prevalence during first 4 years of life with decline in prevalence thereafter.

ERYTHEMA INFECTIOSUM (FIFTH DISEASE)
WBC is normal. Some patients have slight increase in eosinophils.

CHICKENPOX (VARICELLA) AND HERPES ZOSTER (SHINGLES)
(Shingles is reactivation of latent varicella virus.)
Demonstration of varicella-zoster virus (VZV) antigen by immunofluorescent staining in material from a lesion is diagnostic of acute infection; is more sensitive than culture (in contrast to HSV and CMV), especially in crusted lesions. Allows prompt diagnosis.
Isolation of VZV by culture of vesicle fluid or scrapings of lesion; is insensitive, may take up to 2 weeks.
Serologic tests (IFA, EIA, CF) to confirm prior infection and immunity; often not helpful in acute infection because antibody increases late. Antibody may not prevent clinical infection, especially in immunocompromised persons. Heterotypic rise in antibodies is very frequent in primary HSV infection. Useful for diagnosis of fetal infection. Presence in CSF is diagnostic of aseptic meningitis due to VZV even without skin lesions.
- CF usually appears 7–10 days and peaks 2–3 weeks after varicella rash; appears 1–2 days after zoster. Not reliable to determine immunity, as only 50% of sensitivity of EIA. Not reliable in childhood leukemia. Acute and convalescent sera with ≥4-fold increase in CF titer are diagnostic of acute infection. CF disappears in >50% of patients.
- EIA titers of IgG and IgM usually appear within 5 days of varicella rash; IgM disappears in weeks to months, but IgG persists for indeterminate time. Significant titer increase is diagnostic.

Nucleic acid probes may be useful in the future.
Microscopic demonstration of very large epithelial giant cells with intranuclear inclusion in fluid or base of vesicle may occur in herpes.

WBC is normal; may increase with secondary bacterial infection.
40% of zoster patients show increased cells (<300 mononuclear/cu mm) in CSF.

SMALLPOX (VARIOLA)

Microscopic findings of cytoplasmic elementary bodies (Guarnieri bodies) in scrapings from base of skin lesions
Fluorescent antibody staining of virus from skin lesion
Viral serologic tests
- Increased titer of neutralizing antibody in acute-phase and convalescent-phase (2–3 weeks later) sera
- Rapid technique using vesicular fluid in hemagglutination, precipitation, or CF tests

WBC decreased during prodrome, increased during pustular rash

VACCINIA

(vaccine virus skin infection during vaccination against smallpox)

Guarnieri bodies (cytoplasmic inclusions) in skin lesions
Complications
- Progressive vaccinia. Rule out malignant lymphoma, chronic lymphatic leukemia, neoplasms, hypogammaglobulinemia, and dysgammaglobulinemia
- Superimposed infection (e.g., tetanus)
- Postvaccinal encephalitis

CAT-SCRATCH DISEASE

Microscopic examination of excised lymph node suggests this diagnosis and rules out other lesions; culture is sterile.
ESR is usually increased.
WBC is usually normal but occasionally is increased ≤13,000/cu mm; eosinophils may be increased.
Skin test with cat-scratch antigen is positive; test is sensitive but not specific; positive in 20% of veterinarians and 4–6% of general population. Frei test is negative.

YELLOW FEVER

Decreased WBC is most marked by sixth day, associated with decreased leukocytes and lymphocytes.
Proteinuria occurs in severe cases.
Laboratory findings are those due to GI hemorrhage, which is frequent; there may be associated oliguria and anuria.
Liver function tests are abnormal, but serum bilirubin is only slightly increased.
Biopsy of liver is taken for histologic examination.
Serum is positive by mouse intracerebral inoculation ≤ the fifth day; serum during convalescence protects mice.

DENGUE

(due to arbovirus or flavivirus)

Serologic tests show increased titer (CF if IFA or EIA is not available) in acute- and convalescent-phase sera or presence of specific IgM. Cross reaction with other viruses may occur (e.g., St. Louis encephalitis, Japanese encephalitis).
WBC decreased (2000–5000/cu mm) with toxic granulation of leukocytes in early stage; often increased during convalescence
Children commonly have decreased platelets.

VIRAL EPIDEMIC HEMORRHAGIC FEVER

WBC is increased, with shift to the left.
Platelet count is decreased (<100,000/cu mm) in 50% of patients.

Laboratory findings due to renal damage
- Proteinuria
- Oliguria with azotemia and hemoconcentration and abnormal electrolyte concentrations

Return of normal tubular function may take 4–6 weeks.

Other viral hemorrhagic fevers (e.g., Philippine, Thailand, Singapore, Argentinian, Bolivian, Crimean, Omsk, Kyasanur Forest) show much less severe renal damage, and WBC is normal (Philippine, Thailand) or decreased.

COLORADO TICK FEVER

(due to an orbivirus)

WBC is decreased (2000–4000/cu mm). The number of PMNs is decreased, but with shift to the left.

Serologic tests show an increase in antibodies (EIA, IFA, CF, and neutralizing) in acute- and convalescent-phase sera. EIA and IFA titers are larger and appear earlier, often within 10 days, and persist for life. IFA for IgG is 90% sensitive and for IgM is 66% sensitive. CF antibodies last only a few months, so presence of CF suggests recent infection.

Direct fluorescent antibody method can demonstrate antigen in peripheral RBCs in 40% of cases 8 weeks after onset and sometimes up to 6 months. During first week, 50% of cases show false negative.

Virus isolation is the most reliable test.

Blood should be inoculated into suckling mice.

PHLEBOTOMUS FEVER (SANDFLY FEVER)

Decreased WBC and lymphocytes with shift to the left of PMNs are most marked when fever ends.

CSF is normal.

Liver function tests are normal.

Urine is normal.

CRYPTOCOCCOSIS

(due to *Cryptococcus neoformans.* Usual manifestation is CNS, although lung is usual portal of entry.)

Serologic tests for antigen detection are very useful. Antibody detection (IFA, direct agglutination) is most useful in early disease when antigen production is small. Beware of false positives due to IgM rheumatoid factor and other fungi and false negatives due to immune complexes, prozones, nonencapsulated variants, very early disease.

- Latex slide agglutination on serum and CSF detects specific cryptococcal *antigen.* Measurement of cryptococcal antigen in serum and CSF is the most valuable test. Use for screening of suspected cryptococcosis, since it is more sensitive (95%) than India ink smears of CSF; may be positive in 30% of cases without meningitis. Serum or CSF is positive in most cases; when negative, agglutination test may be positive. Antigen titers reflect extent of disease; is rarely positive with local involvement other than CNS (e.g., lung, skin); increasing titer suggests progressive disease, and failure to decrease with treatment suggests insufficient therapy. When available, ELISA antigen detection may be more sensitive.
- Use whole yeast cell agglutination test for presence of *antibodies* in serum and CSF. It is positive only in early CNS disease or no CNS involvement; may become positive only after institution of therapy. May be found in normal persons. Rising titer may be a favorable prognostic sign.

Culture of CSF for *C. neoformans* on Sabouraud's medium becomes positive in 1–2 weeks (positive in 97% of cases) followed by mouse inoculation; 20% of cases require multiple cultures. Culture is commonly positive even without chemical changes in CSF. Repeated fungal cultures are often necessary; cisternal fluid is sometimes superior to lumbar CSF. One may also get positive cultures from blood (25%), urine (37%), stool (20%), sputum (19%), and bone marrow (13%). Sputum cultures are most often positive when there is no x-ray evidence of pulmonary disease. Urine cultures are commonly positive with little kidney involvement. Positive blood culture indicates extensive disease and an extremely poor prognosis. Cultures should always be done because false positive antigen tests may occur due to other fungi (e.g., *Trichosporon beigelii*).

India ink slide of CSF is positive in ~50% of meningitis patients (usually more acute onset); thus one-half of cases will be missed if India ink preparations are used as the sole criterion; rarely seen in other fungal types. Requires 10^5 organisms/cu ml. Latex agglutination of CSF is more sensitive (99%).

CSF cell count is almost always increased to ≤800 cells (more lymphocytes than leukocytes). Protein is increased in 90% (<500 mg/dl). Glucose is moderately decreased in ~55% of patients. Relapse is less frequent when increase in protein and cells is marked rather than moderate. Poor prognosis is suggested if initial CSF examination shows positive India ink preparation, low glucose (<20 mg/dl), low WBC count (<20/cu mm). Positive serologic test without other CSF changes should be viewed with suspicion except in AIDS or other causes of serious immunosuppression. Should always confirm low-titer serology with culture. Repeat CSF examination to evaluate therapy.

In biopsy material, mucicarmine stain is positive; also positive on intraperitoneal injection of white mice.

CBC and ESR usually remain normal.

Increased risk of failure of amphotericin B treatment if positive culture from sites other than CSF (e.g., blood, sputum, urine), anticryptococcal antibodies are absent, CSF or serum cryptococcal antigen titer initially is >1:32 or posttreatment is ≥1:8, immunosuppressed states.

There is evidence of coexisting disease affecting T-lymphocytes in ~50% of patients (e.g., AIDS, diabetes mellitus, steroid therapy, Hodgkin's disease, lymphosarcoma, leukemia). Occurs in up to 9% of patients with AIDS. In AIDS, cryptococcal disease most commonly appears as meningitis but typical signs in only ~50% of cases; dissemination to lungs, marrow, skin is common. In AIDS patients, are more likely to find organisms in blood cultures and blood smears; CSF changes may be very slight and organisms may have smaller capsules, making recognition with India ink more difficult; while CSF antigen titer declines with treatment, serum antigen level often remains constant or increases.

COCCIDIOIDOMYCOSIS

(due to *Coccidioides immitis*)

Serologic tests are especially useful in this disease for both diagnosis and prognosis. Tube precipitin, immunodiffusion, and latex agglutination are used to detect IgM antibodies during first few weeks of infection with >90% specificity reported. CF detects later antibodies (primarily IgG) that persist throughout disease course.

Precipitin antibodies (by immunodiffusion) appear early, decrease after the third week, are uncommon after the fifth month. They occur at some stage of the disease in 75% of patients and usually indicate early infection. In primary infection, they are the only demonstrable antibodies in 40% of patients. If tests are negative, repeat 3 times at intervals of 1–2 weeks. *Beware of occasional cross reaction with primary histoplasmosis and cutaneous blastomycosis.*

CF antibodies appear later (positive in 10% of patients in first week), and the titer rises with increasing severity. Less than one-third of cases are positive in the first month; most positive reactions occur between the fourth and fifth weeks. Antibodies decrease after 4–8 months but may remain positive in low titer for years. The titer parallels severity of infection and is useful for following the course. Low titers may be found early in disease and are significant; low titers may be seen in pulmonary, limited extrapulmonary, or inactive disease. 1:16–1:32 are highly suggestive of disease. Titers >1:32 indicate active disease and suggest extensive, disseminated disease. Fall in titer suggests effective therapy, but rising titer is diagnostic and denotes disease progression. May be found in other body fluids, usually 1–2 dilutions less than serum. In CSF, is diagnostic of meningitis (occurs in 75% of these cases).

Latex particle agglutination test shows 6% false positive reactions. Chief value is for screening. A positive result should be confirmed with CF and precipitin antibody tests. A negative test does not rule out coccidioidomycosis.

IgG and IgM by EIA appear to be the most sensitive serologic test.

Smear (wet preparation in 20% KOH) and culture are taken from sputum, gastric contents, cerebrospinal fluid, urine, marrow biopsy, liver biopsy, exudate, skin scrapings, etc., on Sabouraud's medium or intraperitoneal injection of mice.

Biopsy of skin lesions and affected lymph nodes is made.

Skin test conversion strongly indicates recent infection; skin testing does not cause serologic response.

CSF in meningitis shows 100–200 WBCs/cu mm (mostly mononuclear), increased protein, frequently decreased glucose. Positive antibody test is diagnostic in undiluted CSF; any titer is significant. CF antibodies are present in 75% of meningitis patients; latex agglutination parallels CF. IgG-specific by EIA is strong evidence of meningitis.

Eosinophilia is ≤35%; >10% in 25% of patients.

WBC (with shift to the left) and ESR are increased.

HISTOPLASMOSIS

(due to *Histoplasma capsulatum*)

Culture of skin and mucosal lesions, sputum, gastric washings, blood, or bone marrow may be difficult (Sabouraud's medium at room temperature; blood agar at 37°C not specific). Blood and bone marrow cultures are positive in 50–70% of patients. Culture is positive in <10% of asymptomatic self-limiting cases, 65% of cavitary pulmonary cases, and 75% of disseminated cases. Large volumes of CSF (30–40 ml) may be needed. Mouse inoculation, especially from sputum, may give a positive subculture from spleen on Sabouraud's medium in 1 month.

Serologic tests: screen sera using latex agglutination and immunodiffusion; follow disease course with CF titers. False positive serologic tests are reported in ~10% of cases.

CF titers (against yeast antigen or mycelia antigen) show high sensitivity but low specificity; positive in 90% of chronic cases and in 50% of acute pulmonary cases. They appear during the third to sixth week. 4-fold increase in titer is presumptive of infection but may occur in ~one-third of cases. In epidemic histoplasmosis, 70% of patients have titers ≥1:32 and 90% have titers ≥1:8 to both antigens. Higher titers tend to be found in chronic pulmonary cavitary disease and lower titers in disseminated disease. Positive titers persist for months or years if disease remains active. Prognosis is not indicated by level or changes in titers. Titers may be negative in severe disease. Cross reaction may occur in leishmaniasis and some fungal infections (e.g., blastomycosis, coccidioidomycosis).

Latex agglutination titers become positive in 2–3 weeks and revert to negative in 5–8 months, even with persistent disease; is commonly negative in chronic disease. Less sensitive than EIA. False positives may occur in other diseases (e.g., rheumatoid arthritis, tuberculosis, lung cancer). A titer of 1:32 or more indicates active or very recent disease.

Immunodiffusion demonstrates precipitin antibody (H antigen) in ~25% of cases, which provides strong but not definitive evidence of disease; M antigen is found in 75% of cases but does not distinguish active from inactive disease and may result from skin testing. Negative in 10% of patients with positive CF and positive in only 1% of patients with negative CF.

IgG and IgM by EIA and RIA are more sensitive and show fewer cross reactions with other fungi but still significant (e.g., blastomycosis 40%, coccidioidomycosis 16%).

A positive skin test can cause conversion of serologic titers within 1 week. Negative in 50% of disseminated cases. Frequent cross-reactivity with blastomycosis and coccidioidomycosis. Not helpful in clinical diagnosis but useful in epidemiologic studies.

Antigen detection (by RIA)

- In urine in 90% of disseminated cases, ~20% of acute self-limited disease, <10% of chronic pulmonary cavitary disease. Especially useful in disseminated disease, in which patients may not show significant antibody response
- In serum in 50% of disseminated cases
- In CSF in <50% of meningitis cases; may cross react with coccidioidal meningitis (CSF antibodies may also cross react).

Biopsy of skin and mucosal lesions, bone marrow, and reticuloendothelial system provides initial diagnosis in ~45% of cases.

Demonstration of *H. capsulatum* (special stains) in peripheral blood smears, bone marrow, or tissues is often the most rapid method of diagnosis.

Anemia, leukopenia, and thombocytopenia are more common (60–80% of cases) in acute than in subacute or chronic disseminated types.

Laboratory findings due to involvement of various organ systems, e.g., meningitis, endocarditis, adrenal insufficiency, which are occasionally seen in subacute and less often in chronic disseminated histoplasmosis.

ACTINOMYCOSIS

(due to *Actinomyces israelii*)

Recognition of organism in tissue or drainage material (e.g., sinus tracts, abscess cavities, empyema fluid; may be found normally in sputum) from sites of involvement (especially jaw, lung, cecum)

Sulfur granules show radial gram-positive bacilli or filaments with central gram-negative zone.

No growth is seen on Sabouraud's medium.

Anaerobic culture methods (e.g., thioglycolate medium) are positive. Anaerobic growth on blood agar shows small colonies after 4–6 days. Hold 2–4 weeks before consider negative.

Histologic examination is suggestive; the diagnosis may be confirmed if a "ray fungus" is seen.

Serologic tests are not useful.

Animal inoculation is negative.

WBC is normal or slightly increased (≤14,000/cu mm); high WBC indicates secondary infection.

ESR is usually increased.

Normocytic normochromic anemia is mild to moderate.

NOCARDIOSIS

(due to *Nocardia asteroides*)

Clinical types

- Lung abscess; metastatic brain abscesses in one-third of patients
- Maduromycosis

Recognition of organism
- Direct smear—gram-positive and acid-fast (*may be overdecolorized by Ziehl-Neelsen stain for tubercle bacilli*)
- Positive culture on Sabouraud's medium and blood agar (*Beware of inactivation by concentration technique for tubercle bacillus.*)
- Positive guinea pig inoculation

Serologic tests
- CF (titer = 1:16–1:32 3–4 weeks after infection; sensitivity = 80%) and immunodiffusion (positive 2 weeks after infection; sensitivity = 50–70%) are sometimes useful in systemic nocardiosis.

May be saprophytic in sputum or gastric juice.

Rule out underlying pulmonary alveolar proteinosis, Cushing's syndrome.

BLASTOMYCOSIS

(North American blastomycosis due to *Blastomyces dermatitidis;* South American blastomycosis due to *Paracoccidioides brasiliensis*)

Clinical types
- South American—involvement of nasopharynx, lymph nodes, cecum
- North American—involvement of skin and lungs
- Later, visceral involvement may occur in both types.

Recognition of organism in material (e.g., pus, sputum, biopsied tissue)
- Positive culture on Sabouraud's medium at room temperature and blood agar at 37°C; slow growth of *P. brasiliensis* on blood agar ≤1 month. Culture of organism from tissue is the only certain diagnostic method. Seeing typical yeasts in tissue sections is less satisfactory.
- Wet smear preparation in 20% KOH
- Negative animal inoculation

Serologic tests for *B. dermatitidis*
- EIA is most sensitive and specific, especially in early disease; is initial test of choice.
- Immunodiffusion assay for precipitin antibodies against antigen A is ~80% sensitive and 95% specific; may be negative in early disease.
- CF test is positive in high titer with systemic infection and high titer is correlated with poor prognosis, but test is not useful for diagnosis; sensitivity <25%. CF and immunodiffusion show extensive cross reaction with histoplasmosis and are positive in only a small proportion of cases proven by culture.

WBC and ESR are increased.

Serum globulin is slightly increased.

Mild normochromic anemia is present.

Alkaline phosphatase may be increased with bone lesions.

Skin tests are positive in 40% of patients; false positives may occur in other fungal diseases (e.g., histoplasmosis) due to cross reactivity.

MONILIASIS

(due to *Candida albicans*)

Positive culture on Sabouraud's medium and on direct microscopic examination of suspected material

In vaginitis, rule out underlying diabetes mellitus.

In skin and nail involvement in children, rule out congenital hypoparathyroidism and Addison's disease.

In septicemia with endocarditis, rule out narcotic addiction.

In GI tract overgrowth, rule out chemotherapy suppression of normal bacterial flora.

In positive blood culture, which is rare, rule out serious underlying disease (e.g., malignant lymphoma), multiple therapeutic antibiotics, and plastic IV catheters.

Table 16-8. Summary of Laboratory Findings in Fungus Infections

		Source of Material												Diagnostic Methods									
Disease	Causative Organism	Blood	Cerebrospinal fluid	Stool	Urine	Nasopharynx, throat	Sputum, lung	Gastric washings	Vagina, cervix	Exudates, lesions, sinus tracts, etc.	Skin, nails, hair	Bone marrow	Lymph node	Microscopic Examination	Fresh unstained material	Stained material	Culture	Animal inoculation	Serologic tests	Complement-fixation	Agglutination	Precipitin	Histologic examination
Cryptococcosis	*Cryptococcus neoformans*	+	+	+	+		+				+	+				+	+	+			+		+
Coccidioidomycosis	*Coccidioides immitis*		+				+	+			+				+		+	+		+		+	+
Histoplasmosis	*Histoplasma capsulatum*	+					+	+			+	+	+				+	+		+	+	+	+
Actinomycosis	*Actinomyces israelii*						+			+						+	+						+

Nocardiosis	*Nocardia asteroides*						+				+					+	+	+					+
North American blastomycosis	*Blastomyces dermatitidis*						+				+				+		+			+			+
South American blastomycosis	*Paracoccidioides brasiliensis*					+					+		+		+		+			+			+
Moniliasis	*Candida albicans*	+				+			+		+					+	+						
Aspergillosis	*Aspergillus fumigatus*, others						+								+		+						+
Geotrichosis	*Geotrichum candidum*						+										+						+
Chromoblastomycosis	*Phialophora pedrosi*, *compactum*, etc.										+				+		+						+
Sporotrichosis	*Sporotrichum schenckii*										+						+	+		+	+	+	+
Rhinosporidiosis	*Rhinosporidium seeberi*					+																	+

ASPERGILLOSIS

(due to *Aspergillus fumigatus* and other species)

May be invasive septicemic aspergillosis in immunocompromised individuals with invasion of bronchial wall; more commonly, a saprophytic aspergilloma superimposed on an anatomic abnormality called allergic bronchopulmonary aspergillosis; or may be a fungus ball (pulmonary aspergilloma).

Serologic tests

- CF is useful for detecting recent or active disease; has good specificity but less sensitive than immunodiffusion
- Immunodiffusion has high specificity but is often negative in invasive disease in immunocompromised patients for whom EIA for IgG is best choice.

Recognition of organism in material (especially sputum) from sites of involvement (especially lung; also brain, sinuses, orbit, ear)

Positive culture on most media at room temperature or 35°C

Organisms occur as saprophytes in sputum and mouth. Confirm by staining organisms in biopsy specimens.

Laboratory findings due to underlying or primary disease

- Superimposed on lung cavities caused by tuberculosis, bronchiectasis, carcinoma
- Underlying condition (e.g., malignant lymphoma; irradiation, steroid, or antibiotic therapy; cystic fibrosis)

Allergic patients show

- Eosinophilia (>1000/cu mm; often >3000/cu mm)
- Serum IgE antibody is markedly increased; significantly greater than in uncomplicated bronchial asthma
- Serum precipitating IgE and IgG for *A. fumigatus* is present but not diagnostic (also present in 27% of patients with farmer's lung, 12% of patients with allergic asthma, 9% of hospital patients, 3% of normal persons)
- Positive skin test

TOXOPLASMOSIS

(due to *Toxoplasma gondii*)

Recognition of trophozoite in appropriate material (CSF, lymph node, muscle)

Cysts may be incidental finding of chronic asymptomatic infection.

Smears stained with Wright's or Giemsa stain

Mouse inoculation or tissue culture (e.g., from tissue, blood, or CSF)

Histologic examination of tissue (e.g., lymph node, muscle, brain)

Serology (~one-third of U.S. population has evidence of past infection; causes 15% of unexplained lymphadenopathy. In immunosuppressed patients, serologic titers may show no evidence of reactivated infection and are not reliable; 30–80% of domestic cats have evidence of past infection.)

- Sabin-Feldman dye test (detects primarily IgG antibodies) is benchmark for evaluating new tests but is superceded by other tests due to complexity and need for live organisms. Dye test detects antibodies 1–2 weeks after onset of infection, and titer rapidly rises to ≥1:1000 in the next few weeks, then declines during months or years to low level (1:4–1:64) for life of patient; false positive or false negative tests are rare.
- Indirect hemagglutination titer (detects IgG antibodies) follows the same course but lags by a few days. Is useful for screening and population studies but not helpful in diagnosis of acute infection. Is less sensitive than IFA or CF tests.
- IgM (IFA) appears in first week of infection, peaks within 1 month, disappears in 2–3 months (as early as 1 month). A negative test rules out infection of <3 weeks' duration but does not exclude infection of longer duration. A single high titer or serial rise in titer (>2 dilutions) indicates

recent, new, or reactivated infection. (High titer ≥1:16, low titer <1:16, negative titer <1:8; levels; titers vary with laboratory.)

IgM and IgG may also be tested by EIA, which has fewer false positives or negatives.

IgG (IFA) (major test currently in use), Sabin-Feldman dye test, indirect hemagglutination test, or CF test that shows a 2-dilution rise in titer at 3-week interval indicates acute infection. IgG peak occurs within 1–2 months, so initial specimen must be drawn early to demonstrate the rise in titer. Titers will eventually reach 1:1000; IgG or dye test is rarely <1:1000 in acute toxoplasmosis. IgG antibodies may persist for many years. Flat IgG titers in absence of IgM titers suggests chronic or latent infection.

CF detects IgG later than IFA test, returns to normal earlier, is less sensitive than other tests, and is not widely used now.

IgM test should be done if the IgG or dye test is positive at any titer in a pregnant woman; if not available, do serial IgG or dye tests. If IgM is negative and IgG <1:1000, further evaluation is unnecessary.

Antinuclear antibodies and rheumatoid factor may cause false positive IgM-IFA test; CF and dye tests do not show false positive reactions.

In AIDS, serologic tests are often not helpful, since IgM is usually negative and IgG is often moderately elevated and 4-fold rise is uncommon. Titer = 1:1024 strongly supports the diagnosis but is not usually found. Disease activity does not correlate with antibody titer or with changes in titer. Absence of IgG in serum occurs in <3% of AIDS patients with toxoplasmic encephalitis.

Recently described specific antigen in serum, CSF, and urine.

Adult Patients

WBC varies from leukopenia to leukemoid reaction; atypical lymphocytes may be found.

Anemia is present.

Serum gamma globulins are increased.

Heterophil agglutination is negative, but hematologic picture may exactly mimic infectious mononucleosis; eosinophilia in 10–20% of patients.

Laboratory findings are those due to involvement of various organ systems.

Lymph node shows distinctive marked hyperplasia; organism may be identified in histologic section.

CNS shows CSF changes (typically mild increase in number of mononuclear cells, normal glucose, moderate increase in protein, and organism can be identified in smear of sediment). Occasionally biopsy of brain may be needed. Immunoperoxidase stain may be very valuable when histopathology is not definitive.

Disseminated form is an important complication of the immunologically compromised patient (e.g., lymphoma, leukemia, immunosuppressive drugs), but positive or changing titers may not be present.

If ocular findings are the only clinical disease, many patients show only very low titers that are not useful.

PNEUMOCYSTIS PNEUMONIA

(due to *Pneumocystis carinii;* variously classified as protozoa, fungus, or yeast)

There are no specific laboratory tests.

No culture techniques are available.

Diagnosis requires demonstration of organism. Transbronchial lung biopsy is very effective way to make a definite diagnosis. Also allows diagnosis of other infections (e.g., fungi) or diseases (e.g., lymphoma), use of various stains, touch preparations. Open lung biopsy is rarely needed.

Bronchoalveolar lavage is equally successful in diagnosis (sensitivity ~95%).

Induced sputum (nebulization with saline) is also effective for diagnosis, is inexpensive, and can be done as outpatient. Use of immunofluorescent stain allows diagnosis in up to 95% of cases.

The organism is rarely found in routine sputum, bronchial washings or brushings.

Organisms are found in postmortem histologic preparations.

The morphology of the lung lesions suggests the diagnosis.

Organism does not stain with routine H & E stains; requires immunofluorescence or special stains (e.g., Giemsa, Schiff).

Serologic tests are generally not useful at present.
- Immunofluorescent tests have a reported sensitivity of 71% (titer = 1:16) in acute cases and 97% (titer = 1:16) in convalescent cases with overall sensitivity of 30–40%. High specificity with few cross reactions. CF is positive in <20% of patients.

Laboratory findings of associated diseases; found in >55% of sputum specimens from patients with various types of immunosuppression.
- Is the primary presenting opportunistic infection in 55–65% of AIDS cases; is twice as common in IV drug users than in homosexuals.
- Administration of cytotoxic drugs and corticosteroids
- Premature or debilitated infants
- Underlying diseases (e.g., malignant lymphoma, leukemia, immunoglobulin defects)
- Other infections, especially cytomegalic inclusion disease, systemic bacterial infections (especially *Pseudomonas* or *Staphylococcus*), tuberculosis, cryptococcosis
- 25% of patients who die after renal transplant

Laboratory findings due to organ system involvement (e.g., hypoxemia and hypercapnia due to pulmonary disease)

Leukopenia indicates a poor prognosis.

GEOTRICHOSIS
(due to *Geotrichum candidum*)

Recognition of organisms from material from sites of involvement (respiratory tract; possibly colon)
- Positive culture on Sabouraud's medium (room temperature). *Organisms occur as saprophytes in pharynx and colon.*
- Microscopic visualization of organisms in biopsy material

CHROMOBLASTOMYCOSIS
(due to *Phialophora pedrosi, P. compactum,* etc.)

Recognition of organism from sites of involvement (usually skin; rarely brain abscess)

Wet smear preparation in 10% KOH

Positive culture on Sabouraud's medium (slow growth)

Biopsy of tissue

SPOROTRICHOSIS
(due to *Sporotrichum schenckii*)

Recognition of organism in skin, pus, or biopsy
- Positive culture on Sabouraud's medium from unbroken pustule
  - Intraperitoneal mouse inoculation of these colonies or of fresh pus produces organism-containing lesions.
- Direct microscopic examination is usually negative.

Serum agglutinins, precipitins, and CF (titer ≥1:16) antibodies can be demonstrated in extracutaneous disease (e.g., pulmonary, disseminated).
- Serial paired specimens of sera and CSF should be tested for suspected CNS disease.

Latex agglutination shows 94% sensitivity; persistent elevation or rising titer is common in pulmonary disease. Low titer (e.g., <1:16) in nonfungal disease (e.g., leishmaniasis). CSF titer of 1:32 in meningeal infection.

RHINOSPORIDIOSIS

(due to *Rhinosporidium seeberi*)

Recognition of organism in biopsy material from polypoid lesions of nasopharynx or eye (cannot be cultured)

MUCORMYCOSIS

(due to *Zygomycetes* species)

Clinical types
- Cranial (acute diffuse cerebrovascular disease and ophthalmoplegia in uncontrolled diabetes mellitus with acidosis)
- Pulmonary (findings due to pulmonary infarction)
- In abdominal blood vessels (findings due to hemorrhagic infarction of ileum or colon)

Mycologic cultures from brain and spinal fluid are negative; may be positive from infected nasal sinuses or turbinate.

Serologic tests
- EIA for IgM and IgG gives best sensitivity and specificity.
- Immunodiffusion is positive in ~70% of patients.

Laboratory findings of underlying disease (e.g., diabetes mellitus with acidosis, leukemia, irradiation or cytotoxic drugs, uremic acidosis) are present.

Laboratory findings due to complications (e.g., visceral infarcts) are present.

MALARIA

(due to *Plasmodium vivax, P. malariae, P. falciparum, P. ovale*)

Identification of organism is made in thin or thick smears of peripheral blood or bone marrow.

Anemia (average 2.5 million RBCs/cu mm in chronic cases) is usually hypochromic; may be macrocytic in severe chronic disease. Reticulocyte count is increased.

Monocytes are increased in peripheral blood; there may be pigment in large mononuclear cells occasionally.

WBC is decreased.

There is increased serum indirect bilirubin and other evidence of hemolysis.

Bone marrow shows erythroid hyperplasia, RBCs containing organisms, and pigment in RE cells. Marrow hyperplasia may fail in chronic phase. Agranulocytosis and purpura may occur late.

Serum globulin is increased (especially euglobulin fraction); albumin is decreased.

ESR is increased.

Biologic false positive test of syphilis is frequent.

Osmotic fragility of RBCs is normal.

Acute hemorrhagic nephritis due to *P. malariae*
- Albuminuria
- Hematuria

Blackwater fever (massive intravascular hemolysis) due to *P. falciparum*
- Severe acute hemolytic anemia (1–2 million RBCs/cu mm) with increased bilirubin, hemoglobinuria, etc.
- May be associated with acute tubular necrosis with hemoglobin casts, azotemia, oliguria to anuria, etc.

Parasites absent from blood

Laboratory findings due to involvement of organs
- Liver—vary from congestion to fatty changes to malarial hepatitis or central necrosis; moderate increase in SGOT, SGPT, and alkaline phosphatase

Table 16-9. Serologic Tests in Diagnosis of Parasitic Diseases

Disease	Indirect Hemagglutination	Complement Fixation	Direct Agglutination	Indirect Immunofluorescence	Bentonite Flocculation	Counterimmunoelectrophoresis	ELISA (enzyme-linked immunosorbent assay)	Tests are performed by CDC, Atlanta, Ga. (titers are expressed as ≧)
Malaria				1:64				
Chagas' disease	+	1:8	+					
Leishmaniasis	+	1:8	1:64					
Toxoplasmosis	+			1:256				IgM-IFA ≧ 1:16
Pneumocystis carinii				+				

Amebiasis	1:256					+		
Ascariasis	+				+			
Toxocariasis							+	
Strongyloidiasis	+							
Trichinosis					1:5	+		
Filariasis	1:128				+			
Schistosomiasis		+		1:16			+	
Paragonimiasis		+						
Cysticercosis	1:64				+			
Echinococcosis	1:256				+			

Source: Data from DD Despommier, The immune system and parasitism. *Infect Dis* 9:4, 1979; WL Drew, Serologic tests—Diagnosing viral, fungal, and parasitic infections. *Consultant,* March 1983, pp. 123–141.

Pigment stones in gallbladder
Cerebral malaria
Serologic tests—useful when there are few parasites in blood or when smears are obtained after therapy; not useful to determine species.
Indirect fluorescent antibody test (for IgG) shows high sensitivity (99%) and specificity and is useful for diagnostic purposes. Titer >1:256 suggests recent infection (>1:64 in nonendemic areas). Titers disappear 6 months after cure except in endemic areas, where 1:64 may be present with clinical infection.
Indirect hemagglutination can detect antibody many years after infection and is useful for prevalence studies.
Research method presently being studied identifies rRNA of individual species using autoradiography.

TRYPANOSOMIASIS

Sleeping sickness
Acute (Rhodesian) due to *Trypanosoma rhodesiense*
Chronic (Gambian) due to *Trypanosoma gambiense*
Identification of organism in appropriate material (blood, bone marrow, lymph node aspirate, CSF) by thick or thin smears or concentrations, animal inoculation, rarely culture
Anemia
Increased serum globulin producing increased ESR, rouleaux formation, etc.
Increased monocytes in peripheral blood
CSF
Increased number of cells (mononuclear type)—≤30/cu mm during second month; later 100–400/cu mm
Increased protein (use as index to severity of disease and to therapeutic response)—60–100 mg/dl with considerable increase in gamma globulin
Organisms may be identified by microscopic examination of CSF sediment.
CF test specific for *T. gambiense*
Chagas' disease (American trypanosomiasis) due to *Trypanosoma cruzi*
Identification of organism
Blood concentration technique during acute stage
Biopsy of lymph node or liver (shows leishmanial forms)
Culture on blood broth at 28°C from lymph node aspirate
Xenodiagnosis (laboratory-bred bug fed on patient develops trypanosomes in gut in 2 weeks)
Serologic tests
CF test positive in 50% of acute cases; specific and positive in >90% of chronic cases. Less sensitive but more specific than indirect hemagglutination. Titer >1:8 suggests acute Chagas' disease; usually negative in chronic disease.
Indirect hemagglutination titer = 1:128 in 96% of chronic cases. Frequently cross react in leishmaniasis.
Laboratory findings due to organ involvement (e.g., heart, central nervous system, skeletal muscle)

LEISHMANIASIS

Kala-azar (due to *Leishmania donovani*)
Organism identified in stained smears from spleen, bone marrow, peripheral blood, liver biopsy, lymph node aspirate
Culture (incubate at 26°C) from same sources
Serologic tests should be done in immunosuppressed patients from endemic areas with appropriate clinical findings. Are positive only in visceral type when indirect hemagglutination titer >1:64. Cross reaction in trypano-

somiasis. Should confirm positive test with CF and indirect fluorescent tests.
Anemia due to hypersplenism and decreased marrow production
Leukopenia
Thrombocytopenia
Markedly increased serum globulin (IgG) with decreased albumin and reversed A/G ratio
Increased ESR, etc., due to increased serum globulin
Frequent urine changes
Proteinuria
Hematuria
Laboratory findings due to amyloidosis in chronic cases
American mucocutaneous leishmaniasis (due to *Leishmania brasiliensis*)
Organism identification by direct microscopy, culture, or histologic examination in scrapings from lesions often fails.
Anemia sometimes present
Oriental sore (cutaneous leishmaniasis) (due to *Leishmania tropica*)
Organisms identified by direct microscopy and culture in scrapings from lesion

AMEBIASIS

(due to *Entamoeba histolytica*)

Microscopic examination of stool for *E. histolytica*. Six daily consecutive stools concentrated and stained will identify 90% of positive cases. *(Beware of interfering substances in feces, e.g., bismuth, kaolin, barium sulfate, soap or hypertonic-salt enema solutions, antacids and laxatives, sulfonamides; antibiotic, antiprotozoal, and antihelmintic agents.) Abundant RBCs but minimal WBCs on microscopic examination of stool help to differentiate condition from bacillary dysentery (see pp. 623–625).*
Direct detection of *E. histolytica* antigen in stool by commercial kit
Biopsy of rectum may show *E. histolytica*.
Serologic tests
Indirect hemagglutination test (>1:256) is sensitive and specific; positive in ~95% of patients with liver abscess or invasive intestinal disease but cannot distinguish these from noninvasive intestinal infection.Immunofluorescence, CIE, and EIA are also available.
When severe diarrhea is due to *E. histolytica*, serologic tests will be positive in >90%; when diarrhea has never been present, <50% of carriers will have positive serologic tests.
Negative tests are unlikely with invasive disease if patient is not immunosuppressed.

Liver abscess
Normochromic, normocytic anemia
Leukocytosis (5000–33,000/cu mm)
Eosinophilia is not usually present.
ESR is markedly increased.
Increased SGOT and SGPT (2–6 times normal)
Increased alkaline phosphatase (usually 2–3 times normal)
Serum albumin may be decreased and globulin increased.
Total bilirubin may be increased if complications occur.
Liver scanning
Serologic tests—see above.

GIARDIASIS

(due to *Giardia lamblia*)

Recognition of organism in stools or duodenal washings stained with iodine. Chronic infection may cause malabsorption syndrome.

Serologic tests by CF, immunofluorescence, and EIA are available. Presence of antibodies indicates prior infection but not useful for current diagnosis except to rule out giardiasis in malabsorption.
Detection of *Giardia* antigen in stool by ELISA in recently developed test has sensitivity and specificity each >87%.

BALANTIDIASIS

(due to *Balantidium coli*)

Recognition of organisms in stool. (*Intermittent appearance requires repeated examinations.*)
No serologic tests are available.

COCCIDIOSIS

(due to *Isospora hominis* or *I. belli*)

Recognition of organism in $ZnSO_4$-concentrated stool specimens

ASCARIASIS

(due to *Ascaris lumbricoides*)

Stools contain ova. Occasionally adults are spontaneously excreted in stool.
Eosinophils are increased during symptomatic phase, especially pulmonary phase.
Serologic tests are not useful.

TRICHURIASIS

(due to whipworm—*Trichuris trichiura*)

Stools contain ova.
Increased eosinophils (≤25%), leukocytosis, and microcytic hypochromic anemia may be present.
Serologic tests are not useful.

PINWORM INFECTION

(due to *Enterobius vermicularis*)

Ova and occasionally adults are found on Scotch tape swab of perianal region, which *should be taken on first arising early in morning*. Three tests will find 90% and five tests will find 95% of cases.
Stool is usually negative for ova and adults.
Eosinophil count is usually normal; may be slightly increased.
Serologic tests are not useful.

VISCERAL LARVA MIGRANS

(due to roundworms *Toxocara canis* or *T. cati;* past exposure in humans is ~10%)

WBC is increased; increased eosinophils (usually >30%) may be vacuolated and contain fewer than normal granules; persists for several months.
Serum gamma globulin is often increased, especially IgE.
Tissue biopsy showing larvae is only definite way to make diagnosis; usually from liver, which shows granulomas.
ELISA is 78% sensitive and 92% specific; positive test supports diagnosis. May be less sensitive in ocular than in visceral disease. Indirect hemagglutination and bentonite flocculation tests are insensitive and nonspecific.
Elevated anti-A and anti-B antibodies in most cases due to stimulation of isohemagglutinins
Laboratory findings due to organ system involvement (e.g., liver in 85% and lung in 50% of cases—may cause Loeffler's syndrome).

CUTANEOUS LARVA MIGRANS

(due to *Ancylostoma caninum* and *A. braziliense* from dogs, cats, other carnivores)

Serologic tests and biopsy are not useful.

TRICHOSTRONGYLOSIS

(due to *Trichostrongylus* species)

Stools contain ova. Usually a concentration technique is required; *worm may be mistaken for hookworm.*

There is an increase in WBC and eosinophils (≤75%) when patient is symptomatic.

STRONGYLOIDIASIS

(due to *Strongyloides stercoralis;* found in ~4% of rural Kentucky schoolchildren)

Stools contain larvae (sensitivity = 30–60% for direct examination, 70–80% for Baermann examination). Larvae may also be found in duodenal washings (sensitivity = 60–70%). String test (Entertest) sensitivity is 60–80%. Filariform larvae may suggest hyperinfection.

Larvae appear in sputum with pulmonary involvement; indicates hyperinfection.

Serologic tests (ELISA and indirect immunofluorescence) for IgG antibodies against filariform larvae show sensitivity >85% and high specificity. Thus a positive test may indicate need for workup when a patient is to be treated with cytotoxic or immunosuppressive therapy. A negative test without symptoms or other laboratory findings suggests no infection. Titers slowly decrease over several months after treatment.

Leukocytosis is common. Increase in eosinophils is almost always present, but the number usually decreases with chronicity; is most marked in patients with prominent skin manifestations; may be absent with immunosuppression. Leukopenia and absence of eosinophilia are poor prognostic signs.

Condition is especially common in orphanages and mental institutions.

HOOKWORM DISEASE

(due to *Necator americanus* or *Ancylostoma duodenale*)

WBC is normal or slightly increased, with 15–30% eosinophils; in early cases, ≤75% eosinophils are present.

Anemia due to blood loss is hypochromic microcytic. When anemia is more severe, eosinophilia is less prominent.

Hypoproteinemia may occur with heavy infestation.

Stools contain hookworm ova. Stools are usually positive for occult blood. Charcot-Leyden crystals are present in >50% of patients.

Serologic tests are not useful.

Laboratory findings are those due to frequently associated diseases (e.g., malaria, beriberi).

TRICHINOSIS

(due to *Trichinella spiralis*)

Eosinophilia appears with values of ≤85% on differential count and 15,000/cu mm on absolute count. It occurs about 1 week after the eating of infected food and reaches maximum after third week. It usually subsides in 4–6 weeks but may last up to 6 months and occasionally for years. Occasionally it is absent; it is usually absent in fatal infections.

Stool may contain adults and larvae *only* during the first 1–2 weeks after infection (during the stage of enteritis and invasion).

Identification of larvae is made in suspected meat by acid-pepsin digestion followed by microscopic examination.

Muscle biopsy may show the encysted larvae beginning 10 days after ingestion. Direct microscopic examination of compressed specimen is superior to routine histologic preparation.

Serologic tests become positive 1 week after onset of symptoms in only 20–30% of patients and reach a peak in 80–90% of patients by fourth to fifth week. Rise in titer in acute- and convalescent-phase sera is diagnostic. Titers may remain negative in overwhelming infection. False positive results may occur in polyarteritis nodosa, serum sickness, penicillin sensitivity, infectious mononucleosis, malignant lymphomas, and leukemia.

CF test becomes positive ~2 weeks after occurrence of eosinophilia. It may remain positive for 6 months.

Bentonite flocculation test may remain strongly positive for 6 months; less strongly positive for another 6 months; becomes negative in 2–3 years.

Precipitin and latex fixation tests are also used.

More recently developed tests (immunodiffusion, immunofluorescence, CIE, and especially ELISA) are more sensitive.

Decrease in serum total protein and albumin occurs in severe cases between 2 and 4 weeks and may last for years.

Increased (relative and absolute) gamma globulins parallel titer of serologic tests. The increase occurs between 5 and 8 weeks and may last 6 months or more.

ESR is normal or only slightly increased.

Decreased serum cholinesterase often lasts 6 months.

Serum muscle enzymes may be increased (e.g., creatine kinase).

Urine may show albuminuria with hyaline and granular casts in severe cases.

With meningoencephalitis, CSF may be normal or up to 300 lymphocytes/cu mm with increased protein.

FILARIASIS

(due to *Wuchereria bancrofti* or *W. malayi*)

Microfilariae appear in peripheral blood smear (Wright's or Giemsa stain) or wet preparation.

Eosinophils are increased.

Biopsy of lymph node may contain adult worms.

CF test may not be reliable.

Chyluria may occur.

Tropical eosinophilia due to filaria

Eosinophilia is extreme (usually >3000/cu mm) and persists for weeks.

Serum IgE levels are markedly elevated (usually >1000 U/ml).

High titers of antifilarial antibodies are detected by CF, hemagglutination, and especially EIA in up to 80% of patients.

No microfilaria can be found in blood but may be found in enlarged lymph nodes when adenopathy is present.

Other laboratory abnormalities (e.g., elevated ESR) are not diagnostically useful.

LOAIASIS

(due to *Loa loa*)

Marked increase of eosinophils (50–80%) may occur.

Serologic tests—see Filariasis, preceding section.

PULMONARY DIROFILARIASIS

(due to dog heartworm *Dirofilaria immitis*)

Insect transmission (usually mosquito; rarely some species of fleas or ticks)

Filariform larvae transmitted by bite of intermediate host mosquito migrate to heart and die, resulting in pulmonary emboli and infarcts.

Diagnosis is made by open lung biopsy.

Eosinophilia is not significant.

Cross reactions make serologic tests difficult to interpret.

TAPEWORM INFESTATION

Due To *Taenia saginata* (beef tapeworm)

In stool, ova cannot be distinguished from those of *Taenia solium*.

Proglottids establish diagnosis. Stool examination is positive in 50–75% of patients.

Scotch tape swab of perianal region is positive in ≤95% of patients.
Eosinophils may be slightly increased.

Due To *Taenia solium* (pork tapeworm)

Stool and Scotch tape swab of perianal region are examined.
Eosinophils may be slightly increased.
CSF may show increased eosinophils with cysticercal meningoencephalitis.

Due To *Hymenolepis nana* (Dwarf tapeworm)

Stool shows ova, occasionally proglottids, etc.

Due To *Diphyllobothrium latum* (fish tapeworm)

Stool shows ova.
Macrocytic anemia (see p. 275) may occur when worm is in proximal small intestine.
Increased eosinophils and leukocytes are found.

Due To *Echinococcus granulosus* (multilocularis)

Cystic lesion appears, especially in liver (see Space-Occupying Lesions of Liver, pp. 205–206). 65% of cysts occur in lung, and the remaining 10% of cysts are widely scattered.
Identification of scoleces and hooklets is made in cyst fluid and histologic examination.
Eosinophils are occasionally increased; the number rises dramatically in cyst leaks.
Stool examination is not helpful.
Serologic tests

- High titers (>1:256) indirect hemagglutination in 88% of cases with hydatid cysts of liver or peritoneum; <5% false positives (in cysticercosis, schistosomiasis, collagen disease, neoplasia); titers can persist for years after surgical removal. 10% of cases of calcified cysts or lung cysts are positive.
- EIA but not indirect hemagglutination can differentiate granulosus from multilocularis in test for antigen on cyst fluid.
- CIE is recommended to confirm antibodies to *E. granulosus*.
- CF test is also used by some laboratories.

SCHISTOSOMIASIS

(due to *Schistosoma mansoni, S. japonicum, S. haematobium*)

Acute

- Eosinophilia occurs; may be 20–60%.
- ESR is increased.
- Serum globulin is increased.

Chronic

- Ova appear in stools; only viable eggs indicate active infection. Quantification by egg count per gram of feces or per 10 ml of urine gives some indication of severity of infection.
- Unstained rectal mucosa examined microscopically may show living or dead ova when stools are negative.
- Serologic tests are particularly useful for chronic infections when stools contain no ova; they are not useful to assess chemotherapeutic cure.
    - Indirect fluorescent antibody test is useful when indirect hemagglutination titer <1:64.
    - Indirect hemagglutination titer >1:256 in >90% of acute *S. mansoni* cases; cross react with other schistosoma, filariasis, trichinosis.
- Rectal biopsy of mucosal fold may show parasites and granulomatous lesions.
- Multiple granulomatous lesions appear in uterine cervix.

Table 16-10. Summary of Laboratory Findings in Protozoan Diseases

		Source of Material										Diagnostic Procedures									Other Significant Laboratory Abnormalities									
Disease	Causative Organism	Blood	Cerebrospinal fluid	Stool	Urine	Vagina	Urethra	Exudates, ulcers, skin lesions	Bone marrow	Spleen	Lymph node aspirate	Microscopic examination: Fresh unstained material	Microscopic examination: Stained material	Culture	Animal inoculation	Xenodiagnosis	Serologic tests	Complement-fixation	Others	Histologic examination	Anemia	WBC decreased	Monocytosis	Serum globulin increased	Cerebrospinal fluid abnormalities	Renal function abnormalities	Liver function abnormalities	Skeletal muscle abnormalities	Cardiac abnormalities	Other
Malaria	*Plasmodium* species	+							+				+						+		+	+	+	+	+	+	+			
Trypanosomiasis																														
Acute sleeping sickness	*T. rhodesiense*	+	+						+		+		+	rare	+						+		+	+	+					
Chronic sleeping sickness	*T. gambiense*	+	+						+		+		+		+			+			+		+	+	+					
Chagas' disease	*T. cruzi*	+											+	+		+		+		a					+			+	+	

Leishmaniasis																															
Kala-azar	*L. donovani*	+							+	+	+			+	+				+			+	+		+		+				
American muco-cutaneous	*L. brasiliensis*							+						+	+							+									
Oriental sore	*L. tropica*							+						+	+																
Toxoplasmosis	*T. gondii*		+								+			+		+			+	b	c	+			+						
Interstitial plasma cell pneumonia	*Pneumocystis carinii*																		+	+	+										d
Amebiasis	*Entamoeba histolytica*													+					+	+	e										
Giardiasis	*G. lamblia*			+	f									+																	
Balantidiasis	*B. coli*			+										+																	
Coccidiosis	*Isospora hominis* or *belli*			+										+																	
Trichomoniasis	*T. vaginalis*				+	+	+						+																		

[a]Liver, lymph node.
[b]Hemagglutination, Sabin-Feldman dye test.
[c]Lymph node, muscle.
[d]Special stains.
[e]Rectum.
[f]Also duodenal washings.
Serologic tests can be performed at the Centers for Disease Control (Atlanta, Ga.) on specimens submitted through state health department laboratories that do not perform such tests.

Table 16-11. Identification of Parasites

Organism	Stool	Other Body Sites
Nematodes		
Ascaris lumbricoides	O, A	Rarely L in sputum early
Trichuris trichiura	O	
Enterobius vermicularis	Usually neg.; A after enema	Scotch tape, perianal region—O and A
Strongyloides stercoralis	L	Occasionally L in sputum and duodenal contents
Ancylostoma duodenale	O, rarely L	
Necator americanus	O, rarely L	
Trichinella spiralis	Occasionally A and/or L	
Wuchereria bancrofti, W. malayi	None	Microfilariae in blood
Loa loa	None	Microfilariae in blood; adult under conjunctiva
Onchocerca volvulus	None	Adult in subcutaneous nodules
Dracunculus medinensis	None	L in fluid from ulcer
Cestodes		
Taenia solium	G, O, S; A after treatment	
Taenia saginata	G, O, S	Scotch tape, perianal region—O
Hymenolepis nana, H. diminata	O	
Diphyllobothrium latum	O	
Echinococcus multilocularis	Not found	Histologic examination of biopsy specimen
Trematodes		
Schistosoma mansoni, S. japonicum,	O	See p. 687
S. haematobium	None	O in urine
Clonorchis sinensis	O	O in duodenal contents
Opisthorchis felineus	O	O in duodenal contents
Paragonimus westermani	O	O in sputum
Fasciola hepatica	O	
Fasciolopsis buski	O, occasionally A	

O = ova; A = adult; L = larvae; G = gravid segments; S = scolex.

Changes appear that are secondary to clay pipestem fibrosis of liver with portal hypertension, esophageal varices, splenomegaly, etc. Liver function changes are quite minimal; increased serum bilirubin is rare, even with advanced cirrhosis. Increased serum globulin is frequent. Serum alkaline phosphatase is elevated in 50% of adult patients but is not useful in children.

Changes secondary to pulmonary hypertension are seen.

Ova appear in urine sediment and in biopsy of vesical mucosa in infection with *S. haematobium.*

PARAGONIMIASIS

(due to *Paragonimus westermani*)

Eosinophilia is usual.

Ova appear in sputum, which may contain blood.

Serologic tests

CF titer >1:8 supports diagnosis; titer falls several weeks after successful therapy.

EIA is more sensitive but less useful for monitoring effect of treatment.

CLONORCHIASIS

(due to *Clonorchis sinensis*)

Ova appear in stool or duodenal contents.

CF test may be positive.

Clonorchiasis may cause laboratory findings due to biliary obstruction or recurrent cholecystitis.

OPISTHORCHIASIS

(due to *Opisthorchis felineus*)

Ova appear in stool or duodenal contents.

FASCIOLIASIS

(due to *Fasciola hepatica*)

Ova appear in stool or duodenal contents.

Eosinophils are increased.

Liver function tests are abnormal.

Serologic tests

Indirect fluorescent antibody is positive in ~80% of cases; frequent cross reaction with other helminth infections, *Clonorchis sinensis,* and *Opisthorchis* species.

EIA, CF, CIE methods are under study.

FASCIOLOPSIASIS

(due to *Fasciolopsis buski*)

Ova appear in stool.

OPPORTUNISTIC INFECTIONS

Laboratory findings due to underlying diseases (e.g., AIDS [see pp. 653–661], malignant lymphoma and leukemia, diabetes mellitus, immunoglobulin defects, following renal transplant, uremia, hypoparathyroidism, hypoadrenalism)

Laboratory findings due to administration of drugs (antibiotics, corticosteroids, cytotoxic and immunosuppressive drugs)

Associated with other factors (e.g., plastic intravenous catheters, narcotic addiction)

Table 16-12. Some Human Diseases That May Be Transmitted By/From Animals

	Dogs	Cats	Birds	Farm animals	Poultry	Rodents	Reptiles	Monkeys
Bacterial								
Campylobacter jejuni	+	+	+	+	+	+	+	+
Salmonella infections	+	+	+	+	+	+	+	+
Bacillary dysentery								+
Yersinia infections	+	+		+	+	+		
Anthrax	+			+				
Brucellosis	+	+		+	+	+		
Tularemia	+	+				+		
Leptospirosis	+		+	+		+		
Tuberculosis	+	+		+				
Viral								
Rabies	+	+		+				
Cat-scratch disease		+						
Psittacosis			+		+			
Encephalomyelitis			+	+				
Lymphocytic choriomeningitis	+					+		
Fungal								
Ringworm	+	+		+		+		
Parasitic								
Roundworm infestation	+	+						
Tapeworm infestation	+	+		+				
Visceral larva migrans	+	+						
Cutaneous larva migrans	+	+						
Scabies	+	+						
Toxoplasmosis	+	+						
Echinococcus	+	+						

Anisakiasis (nematode) from eating raw fish (e.g., sashimi)

Trichinosis from eating poorly prepared pork or exotic meats (e.g., bear, walrus, wild boar)

Blastomycosis (*Blastomyces dermatitidis*) occurring at same time as pet dog's illness

California encephalitis (caused by arboviruses)—squirrel is principal reservoir; primary insect vector is woodland mosquito

Hemorrhagic fever with renal syndrome (Hantaan virus carried by mice and other rodents)

Capnocytophaga canimorsus (gram-negative bacteria) transmitted by dog bite or saliva causing acute overwhelming cellulitis, septicemia, meningitis, endocarditis; diagnosis by culture of blood, CSF, or tissue

Plague (due to *Yersinia pestis*) transmitted from wild rodents by bite of rat flea or direct contact with infected tissues, inhalation or animal bites

Epidemic typhus (*Rickettsia prowazekii*) now transmitted from eastern flying squirrel

Rickettsialpox (due to *Rickettsia akari*) transmitted from house mice by mites

Canine ehrlichiosis (due to rickettsia *Ehrlichia canis*)—human illness similar to Rocky Mountain spotted fever transmitted from dogs by tick bite

Lyme disease (due to *Borrelia burgdorferi*) transmitted by various ticks from white-tailed deer, white-footed mouse, and various medium-sized mammals (e.g., dog, raccoon, opossum)

Giardiasis (due to *Giardia lamblia*) by fecal contamination of water by wild animals (e.g., beavers, muskrats)

Pulmonary dirofilariasis (dog heartworm) due to bite of intermediate host mosquito

---

Laboratory findings due to particular organism (see appropriate separate sections)

- *Cryptococcus neoformans*
- *Candida albicans*
- *Aspergillus*
- *Mucorales* fungi
- *Staphylococcus aureus*
- *Staphylococcus albus, Bacillus subtilis, Bacillus cereus,* and other saprophytes
- Enteric bacteria (*Pseudomonas aeruginosa, Escherichia coli, Klebsiella-Enterobacter, Proteus*)

17

Miscellaneous Diseases

SYSTEMIC LUPUS ERYTHEMATOSUS (SLE)

Criteria for classification of SLE (American Rheumatism Association, 1982)

Presence of ≥4 criteria at same or different times allows the diagnosis of SLE and excludes other disorders.

	Sensitivity (%)	**Specificity (%)**
Malar rash	57	96
Discoid lupus	18	99
Oral/nasopharyngeal ulcers	27	96
Photosensitivity	43	96
Arthritis	86	37
Proteinuria (>0.5 gm/day) or cellular casts	51	94
Seizures or psychosis	20	98
Pleuritis or pericarditis	56	86
Cytopenia (any of these 4 findings)	59	89
Autoimmune hemolytic anemia		
Neutropenia (<4000/cu mm on 2 or more occasions)		
Lymphopenia (<1500/cu mm on 2 or more occasions)		
Thrombocytopenia (<100,000/cu mm in absence of causative drugs)		
Immunologic findings (any of these 4 findings)	85	93
Anti-nDNA antibodies		
Anti-Sm antibodies		
LE cells		
Chronic false positive serologic test for syphilis (>6 months' duration)		
Positive antinuclear antibodies (ANA) in the absence of known causative drugs	99	49
Overall =	96	96

LE cells occur in

- 60–75% of patients with SLE; occur in 70–90% of SLE patients at some time during the course of disease
- 10% of patients with rheumatoid arthritis (only half of these have multisystem disease)
- 10% of patients with scleroderma
- 100% of patients with lupoid hepatitis
- 100% of drug-induced lupus (e.g., due to procainamide, hydralazine, isoniazid, various anticonvulsants)
- Some infections

Specificity in SLE is as low as 80%. Should be performed only when ANA is positive because it is more specific than ANA, but ANA is more sensitive. Is rarely performed now because newer tests are more specific.

The test becomes negative in about 4–6 weeks in 60% of patients treated successfully but is not useful as a guide to therapy; it is not correlated with the clinical picture.

The test is positive when two typical LE cells are found; it may be repeated for verification. Because of gradual changes in LE cell factor, repetition in <3 weeks is not useful; instead a more sensitive technique or a serologic test for antinuclear or anti-DNA antibodies should be used.

Rosettes (clusters of polymorphonuclear neutrophils [PMNs] surrounding an extracellular hematoxylin body) are usually found in association with LE cells.

Hematoxylin bodies (homogeneous round extracellular material) may be found in SLE, rheumatoid arthritis, multiple myeloma, cirrhosis. In SLE, they may be found without LE cells in the same sample.

ANA is the most sensitive laboratory test for SLE (detects up to 95% of cases) (see Table 17-1, p. 697, and 17-2, p. 699). Specificity is as low as 50% in rheumatic disease in general. May be present in healthy persons, aged, other rheumatic and nonrheumatic diseases, family of SLE patients. Negative ANA in patient with active multisystem disease is strong (but not absolute) evidence against SLE; positive ANA without other manifestations is not diagnostic. High titers are most often associated with SLE. Persistently negative ANA tests occur in about 5% of SLE patients due to congenital deficiency of early complement component (usually C4 or C2); detected by absent total hemolytic complement (CH50). These patients tend to have prominent skin disease and low incidence of serious renal and CNS disease. ANA may also become negative during remission. Pattern of ANA immunofluorescence is of limited value in discriminating SLE from other collagen vascular diseases. Homogeneous (diffuse or solid) pattern is associated with antibodies to deoxyribonucleoprotein; high titers are more strongly associated with SLE than with other diseases and correlate with activity of SLE. Rim (peripheral) pattern is associated with anti-dsDNA and has the highest specificity for SLE. Speckled pattern detects numerous antigens (e.g., extractable nuclear antigen [ENA], Smith [SM], native ribonucleoprotein [nRNP], Sjögren's syndrome A and B [SS-A and SS-B]); antibodies to these antigens should be ordered when a speckled pattern is found.

Anti-ENA (passive hemagglutination assay) detects only 2 ENAs—ribonucleoprotein (RNP) and Sm.

Anti-RNP is found in 25–30% of SLE, 10% of rheumatoid arthritis, 22% of scleroderma, 100% of mixed connective tissue disease (MCTD) patients. Anti-Sm is found in 25–30% of SLE patients and is the most specific diagnostic test for SLE (speckled immunofluorescence pattern).

Anti-DNA (native double-stranded DNA) is found in 40–80% of SLE patients and rarely in other diseases; high specificity is almost the same as anti-Sm (rim or peripheral nodular immunofluorescence pattern). Absence of anti-dsDNA throughout clinical course is associated with improved prognosis, and severe clinical disease frequently correlates with a high initial titer that declines with clinical improvement; however it may be present for prolonged periods without clinical activity. High titers are characteristic of SLE; low titers (e.g., 1–10 to 1–20) are found in other rheumatic diseases.

Anti-SS-DNA (single-stranded DNA) is found in all other rheumatic diseases and many chronic inflammatory conditions, is not specific for SLE, but presence in almost all SLE patients makes it a sensitive indicator.

Lupus band test (LBT) (direct immunofluorescence on biopsy of normal skin in SLE patients) is positive in 50% of all SLE patients and up to 80% with active multisystem (especially renal) disease; in discoid lupus is found only in skin lesions. May be positive in dermatomyositis, undifferentiated collagen-vascular disease, and other nonrheumatic diseases but usually only one immunoglobulin is found. Specificity for SLE increases with the number of immunoglobulins and complement components found. May be diagnostically useful (1) in patients without sufficient clinical manifestations (e.g., only renal or CNS findings), (2) in patients whose symptoms and other laboratory tests show remission due to steroid therapy, or (3) in differentiation of early SLE from rheumatoid arthritis.

DNA-histone (deoxyribonucleoprotein) antibodies are found in drug-induced SLE due to procainamide, hydralazine, phenytoin, and other drugs and many connective tissue diseases.

Most patients with SLE will have multiple (3 or more) antibodies present but drug-induced lupus and other connective tissue diseases are likely to have fewer ANA present (see Table 17-1, p. 697).

Traditional parameters of disease activity (hemoglobin, WBC, erythrocyte sedimentation rate [ESR], urinalysis, serum creatinine) do not distinguish activity from superimposed infection or drug toxicity and may not be sensitive enough to detect early exacerbation.

Current parameters of disease activity

- Decrease in early complement components (C3, C4; C4 is most sensitive). Depressed levels of total hemolytic complement are not specific for diagnosis but are helpful in managing patients who are at risk for renal and CNS involvement; treat to normalize complement level.
- Increasing titers of anti-DNA
- Presence of circulating immune complexes
- Presence of cryoglobulins (see pp. 349–350) correlates well with disease activity.
- Monoclonal rheumatoid factor assay
- C1q binding
- Raji cell assay is not recommended as indicator of SLE disease activity.

These parameters do not predict which manifestations are likely to become active or the time interval (may be weeks to months), and some patients with these laboratory abnormalities never manifest active disease. The strongest correlation is with active nephritis, but these tests may be normal in 10–25% of cases and in any case do not substitute for renal biopsy.

Combination of positive ANA test, positive dsDNA antibodies, and hypocomplementemia has diagnostic specificity of virtually 100%.

SLE may present as "idiopathic" thrombocytopenic purpura, but serious thrombocytopenia occurs in <10% of patients.

Abnormal serum proteins frequently occur.

- Biologically false positive (BFP) test for syphilis is very common; occurs in <20% of patients. *(This may be the first manifestation of SLE and may precede other features by many months; 7% of asymptomatic individuals with BFP tested for syphilis ultimately develop SLE.)*
- Serum gamma globulin is increased in 50% of patients; a continuing rise may indicate poor prognosis. Alpha$_2$ globulin is increased; albumin is decreased. Immunoglobulins may be abnormal on immunoelectrophoresis.
- C-reactive protein (CRP) may be increased.

Circulating lupus anticoagulants are found in 34% of SLE patients, and 80% of these are associated with a BFP. Indicated by prolonged partial thromboplastin time (PTT) and thromboplastin time not corrected by normal plasma (see p. 389).

"Antiphospholipid antibody syndrome" comprising presence of anticardiolipin (present in 44% of SLE patients) and lupus anticoagulants associated with clinical findings of venous and arterial thrombosis, neuropsychiatric disorders, recurrent fetal wastage, thrombocytopenia. Antiphospholipid antibodies may be important risk factors for these complications. Both antibodies may also be found in drug-induced lupus, nonautoimmune diseases (e.g., syphilis, acute infection), and elderly persons, but clinically significant bleeding is rare without thrombocytopenia. Anticardiolipin present in 0–7.5% of normal persons.*

*Data from PE Love and SA Santoro, Antiphospholipid antibodies: Anticardiolipin and the lupus anticoagulant in SLE and in non-SLE disorders. Prevalence and clinical significance. *Ann Intern Med* 112:682, 1990.

Laboratory findings reflecting specific organ involvement

Urine findings indicate acute nephritis, nephrotic syndrome, chronic renal impairment, secondary pyelonephritis. Patients with azotemia and marked proteinuria usually die in 1–3 years. Sediment is the same as in chronic active glomerulonephritis. With uremia, nephrotic syndrome, or active nephritis, the LE test may become negative. High antibody titer to native DNA associated with decreased serum complement indicates lupus nephritis.

CSF findings are of aseptic meningitis (increased protein and pleocytosis are found in 50% of these patients). *(Rule out complicating tuberculosis and cryptococcosis.)*

Cardiovascular, pulmonary, etc., findings may be present. Pleural effusions are exudate in type.

Joint involvement occurs in 90% of patients.

Laboratory findings reflecting diseases due to autoantibodies

Hashimoto's thyroiditis

Sjögren's syndrome

Myasthenia gravis

Tissue biopsy of skin, muscles, kidney, and lymph node may be useful. Drug-induced lupus syndromes (see p. 744) due to prolonged administration of

Procainamide (15–100% develop ANA within 1 year and 5–30% develop SLE; does not induce antibodies to dsNDA)

Hydralazine (24–50% develop ANA and 8–13% develop SLE)

Isoniazid and birth control pills may induce ANA without symptoms

Various anticonvulsants (e.g., phenytoin)

ANA PROFILE IN SLE

(see Table 17-1)

Multiple antibodies are characteristic of SLE.

High titers of native DNA are characteristic of SLE; very specific for SLE; occur in 50–60% of patients.

Table 17-1. ANA Disease Profiles (reported frequency of ANAs in various diseases in %)

ANAs	SLE	Drug-Induced LE	MCTD	Scl	CREST	SS	DM/PM	RA
ANA screen	>95	>95	>95	70–90	70–90	75–90	40–60	R
Native DNA	*60*	R	R	R	R	R	R	40
Histones	70	*>95*	R	R	R	R	R	R
Sm	*30*	R	R	R	R	R	R	R
Nuclear RNP	40–50	R	*>95*	15	10	R	15	10
Scl-70	R	R	R	*20–60*	R	R	R	R
SS-A(Ro)	25	R	R	R	R	*70*	10	R
SS-B(La)	15	R	R	R	R	*60*	R	R
Centromere	R	R	R	*30*	*70–85*	R	R	R
Nucleolar	25	R	R	*60–70*	R	R	R	R
PM-Scl (PM-1) & Jo-1	R	R	R	R	R	R	*30–50*	R

Italics indicate significant correlation.

SLE = systemic lupus erythematosus; MCTD = mixed connective tissue disease; Scl = scleroderma; SS = Sjögren's syndrome; DM = dermatomyositis; PM = polymyositis; RA = rheumatoid arthritis; R = rare.

Source: Data from EM Tan, CA Robinson, and RM Nakamura, ANAs in systemic rheumatic disease: Diagnostic significance. *Postgrad Med* 78:141, 1985.

High titers of anti-Sm are specific but not sensitive. Sm antigen in 30% of patients is very specific for SLE.
DNP in up to 70% of patients
Histones in up to 60% of patients
SS-A in 25% of patients
SS-B in 15% of patients
RNP in 40–50% of patients

DRUG-INDUCED LUPUS
(see Table 17-1 and p. 744)

Histone antibodies in up to 95% of patients without other antibodies.

ANA PROFILE IN SJÖGREN'S SYNDROME
(see Table 17-1)

SS-A in 70% of patients, SS-B in 60% of patients without other antibodies indicates probable Sjögren's syndrome; with other ANA probably indicates SLE.

ANA PROFILE IN MIXED CONNECTIVE TISSUE DISEASE (MCTD)
(see Table 17-1)

High titer of RNP in >95% of patients without other antibodies.

ANA PROFILE IN SCLERODERMA AND CREST
(see Table 17-1)

Centromere is only antibody in 70–85% of CREST (acronym for calcinosis, Raynaud's syndrome, esophageal dysmotility, sclerodatyly, telangiectasia) syndrome patients.
Scl-70 in 10–20% of patients is specific for scleroderma.
High-titer nucleolar antibodies in 40–50% of patients
RNP, SS-A, SS-B at low titers

ANA PROFILE IN POLYMYOSITIS AND DERMATOMYOSITIS
(see Table 17-1)

PM-1 antigen in 50% of polymyositis and 10% of dermatomyositis patients without other antibodies

ANA PROFILE IN RHEUMATOID ARTHRITIS
(see Table 17-1)

Rheumatoid arthritis nuclear antigen (RANA) in 85–95% of patients
Histones in 20% of patients
Rheumatoid factor (RF) present
ANAs absent; low-titer native DNA may be present.

POLYARTERITIS NODOSA

Increased WBC (≤40,000/cu mm) and PMNs. A rise in eosinophils takes place in 25% of patients, sometimes very marked; it usually occurs in patients with pulmonary manifestations.
ESR is increased.
Mild anemia is frequent; may be hemolytic anemia with positive Coombs' test.
Urine is frequently abnormal.
- Albuminuria (60% of patients)
- Hematuria (40% of patients)
- "Telescoping" of sediment (variety of cellular and noncellular casts)

Uremia occurs in 15% of patients.
Tissue biopsy
- Random skin and muscle biopsy is confirmatory in 25% of patients; most useful when taken from area of tenderness; if no symptoms are present, pectoralis major is the most useful site.

Table 17-2. Comparison of Idiopathic and Drug-Induced Lupus

	Idiopathic SLE	Drug-Induced
Renal, CNS involvement	Common	Rare
ANA pattern	Rim	Homogeneous
Immune complexes	Present	Rare
Low complement level	50–70%	<5%

Drug-induced ANA is histone dependent, but in idiopathic SLE, histone dependence is found in only 30% of patients and histone-dependent are never the only ANA.
Source: Data from JJ Condemi, The autoimmune diseases. *JAMA* 258:2920, 1987.

Testicular biopsy is useful when local symptoms are present.
Lymph node and liver biopsies are usually not helpful.
Renal biopsy is not specific; often shows glomerular disease.
Serum globulins are increased.
Abnormal serum proteins occasionally occur. BFP test occurs for syphilis, circulating anticoagulants, cryoglobulins, macroglobulins, etc.
Laboratory findings due to organ involvement by arteritis may be present—e.g., genitourinary system, nervous system, pulmonary.

WEGENER'S GRANULOMATOSIS

(necrotizing granulomatous vasculitis affecting respiratory tract; disseminated form shows renal involvement)

Diagnosis is established by biopsy of affected tissue.
Immunofluorescent autoantibodies to cytoplasm of neutrophils (C-ANCA) are recently described highly specific (99%) tests for Wegener's granulomatosis. Sensitivity > 93% with active generalized disease and 30% in full remission. May also be useful to assess activity, response to therapy, and early detection of relapse. Perinuclear pattern (P-ANCA) is seen in other types of vasculitis and connective tissue diseases (e.g., polyarteritis, idiopathic necrotizing and crescentic glomerulonephritis).
Following laboratory findings are not specific:
Normochromic anemia, thrombocytosis and mild leukocytosis occur in 30–40% of patients; eosinophilia may occur but is not a feature. Leukopenia or thrombocytopenia occurs only during cytotoxic therapy.
ESR is increased in 90% of cases, often to very high levels; CRP correlates with disease activity even better than ESR.
Serum globulins (IgG and IgA) are increased in up to 50% of cases.
Serum C3 and C4 complement levels may be increased.
Rheumatoid factor may be present in low titer in one-third of cases.
ANA and lupus preparations are normal.
Laboratory findings reflecting specific organ involvement
Renal—hematuria, proteinuria, azotemia. Nephrosis or chronic nephritis may occur. Most patients develop renal insufficiency. Biopsy most frequently shows focal necrotizing glomerulonephritis with crescent formation; coarse granular pattern with immunofluorescent staining. Biopsy is important to define extent of disease.
Central nervous system
Respiratory tract
Heart

GIANT CELL ARTERITIS

(systemic panarteritis of medium-sized elastic arteries)

Biopsy of involved segment of temporal artery is diagnostic.
Classic triad of increased ESR, anemia, increased alkaline phosphatase is strongly suggestive of giant cell arteritis.

Mild to moderate normocytic normochromic anemia is present in 20–50% of cases.
ESR is markedly increased in virtually all (97%) patients; average Westergren = 107. A normal ESR excludes the diagnosis when there is little clinical evidence for temporal arteritis.
Serum alkaline phosphatase is slightly increased in ~25% of patients.
WBC is usually normal or slightly increased with shift to the left.
Platelet count may be nonspecifically increased.
Serum protein electrophoresis may show increased gamma globulins. Rouleaux may occur.
Serum creatine kinase (CK) is normal.
Laboratory findings reflecting specific organ involvement
- Kidney (e.g., glomerulonephritis)
- CNS (e.g., intracerebral artery involvement may cause increased CSF protein; stroke; mononeuritis of brachial plexus)
- Heart and great vessels (e.g., myocardial infarction, aortic dissection, Raynaud's disease)
- Liver disease
- Syndrome of inappropriate secretion of antidiuretic hormone (SIADH)
- Microangiopathic hemolytic anemia
- Polymyalgia rheumatica is presenting symptom in one-third of patients and ultimately develops in 50–90% of cases.

PROGRESSIVE SYSTEMIC SCLEROSIS (SCLERODERMA)

Biopsy of skin, esophagus, intestine, synovia may establish diagnosis.
Antinuclear antibodies are found in low titers in 40–90% of patients. High titer of anti-nRNP alone may indicate risk of developing scleroderma.
Antinucleolar pattern is most specific for scleroderma; is highly specific when no other antibody is present. Is rarely found in early scleroderma. May be found in 20% of other rheumatic diseases in association with other antibodies.
Anticentromere antibody is sensitive and specific for CREST syndrome (calcinosis, Raynaud's phenomenon, esophageal dysfunction, sclerodactyly, telangiectasia). May be present in early stage when only Raynaud's phenomenon is present.
Scl-70 antibody (precipitation technique) occurs in 25% of cases and is highly specific but occurs late in disease when diagnosis is obvious.
ESR is normal in one-third of patients, mildly increased in one-third of patients, markedly increased in one-third of patients.
Eosinophilia is described in all scleroderma syndromes.
Mild hypochromic microcytic anemia may be present in 10% of patients.
Serum gamma globulins are increased in 25% of patients (usually slight increase) and have no predictive value.
Abnormal serum proteins occasionally occur, as revealed by BFP test for syphilis (5% of patients), positive LE test, positive rheumatoid arthritis (RA) test (35% of patients), cold agglutinins, cryoglobulins, etc.
Laboratory findings reflect specific organ involvement.
- Malabsorption syndrome due to small intestine involvement
- Abnormal urinary findings, renal function tests, and uremia due to renal involvement
- Myocarditis, pericarditis, secondary bacterial endocarditis
- Pulmonary fibrosis, secondary pneumonitis
- Other

EOSINOPHILIC FASCIITIS

(may be a scleroderma variant)

Diagnosis is confirmed by characteristic findings in a deep biopsy of skin down to and including muscle.
Eosinophilia
Hypergammaglobulinemia

SCLEREDEMA

WBC, ESR, and other laboratory tests are usually normal.

WEBER-CHRISTIAN DISEASE (RELAPSING FEBRILE NODULAR NONSUPPURATIVE PANNICULITIS)

Biopsy is taken of involved area of subcutaneous fat.
WBC may be increased or decreased.
Mild anemia may occur.

DISCOID LUPUS

Some patients may show
- Decreased WBC
- Decreased platelet count
- Increased ESR
- Increased serum gamma globulins
- Positive LE cell test (<10% of patients)

See SLE, lupus band test, p. 695.

SARCOIDOSIS*

Kveim reaction (skin biopsy 4–6 weeks after injection of human sarcoid tissue shows histologic picture of sarcoid at that site is positive in 80% of patients with sarcoidosis; many false negatives are seen in patients who are later proved to have sarcoidosis; a positive reaction is less frequent if there is no lymph node involvement, if the disease is of long standing and inactive, and during steroid therapy; false positive reactions occur in 2–5% of patients. Positive Kveim tests may occur in other diseases with enlarged lymph nodes (e.g., tuberculosis, leukemia). Kveim test material is not available commercially; a few medical centers have limited quantities with variable specificities.

Diagnosis is established by tissue biopsy that shows noncaseous granulomas at several sites for which a specific cause (e.g., fungal, acid-fast bacillus infection, or berylliosis) has been excluded. Kveim test may be used in place of another tissue biopsy.
- Needle biopsy of liver shows granulomas in 75% of patients even if there is no impairment of liver function.
- Lymph node biopsy is likely to be positive if lymph node is enlarged.
- Muscle biopsy is likely to be positive if arthralgia or muscle pain is present. Skin lesions occur in 35% of cases.
- Other sites of biopsy are synovium, eye, lung, minor salivary glands of lower lip.

Serum globulins are increased in 75% of patients, producing reduced albumin-globulin (A/G) ratio and increased total protein (in 30% of patients). Is often the first clue to diagnosis.

Serum protein electrophoresis shows decreased albumin and increased globulin (especially gamma) with characteristic "sarcoid-step" pattern.

Serum angiotensin-converting enzyme (ACE) is increased in 85% of patients with active pulmonary sarcoidosis but only 11% with inactive disease (increase is >35 units/ml by radioassay in adults and >50 units/ml if <19 years old; *values vary between laboratories even with same method*). May also be increased in other conditions—e.g., Gaucher's disease (100%), diabetes mellitus (>24%), hyperthyroidism (81%), leprosy (53%), chronic renal disease, cirrhosis (25%), silicosis (>20%), berylliosis (75%), amyloidosis, tuberculosis. Normal levels are found in lymphoma, lung cancer; false positive rate = 2–4%. Thus is not diagnostic but is primarily useful to monitor activity of disease and response to therapy.

Bronchioalveolar lavage and radioactive gallium (^{67}Ga) scans of lung (show

*Data from J Lieberman, Enzymes in sarcoidosis: Angiotensin-converting enzyme (ACE). *Clin Lab Med* 9:745, 1989.

distribution of inflammatory granulomatous lesions) have also been used to assess disease activity.
WBC is decreased in 30% of patients.
Eosinophilia occurs in 15% of patients.
Mild normocytic, normochromic anemia occurs.
ESR is increased.
Serum calcium may be mild to markedly increased in ~10% of patients; often transiently.
Increased urine calcium occurs twice as often as hypercalcemia and may be found even with normal serum calcium. Increased frequency of renal calculi is found and of nephrocalcinosis in some series of patients.
Serum and urine calcium abnormalities are frequently corrected by cortisone; often within normal range in 1 week.
Increased sensitivity to vitamin D is often present.
Increased serum 1,25-hydroxyvitamin D in hypercalcemic patients.
Steroids rapidly lower serum 1-alpha, 25-hydroxyvitamin D.
Serum phosphorus is normal.
Increased serum uric acid may occur even with normal renal function in ≤50% of patients.
Mumps complement-fixation test, which is positive in presence of negative mumps skin test (due to dissociation between normal circulating antibodies and defective cellular antibody response), supports the diagnosis but is not specific.
Serum lysozyme (muramidase) is increased in ~70% of cases but does not distinguish stable from progressive disease. Also increased with other chest diseases (e.g., tuberculosis, lung cancer).
Laboratory findings reflect specific organ involvement.
- Liver—serum alkaline phosphatase is increased.
- Spleen—hypersplenism may occur (anemia, leukopenia, thrombocytopenia).
- CNS—CSF may be normal or may show moderate to marked increase in protein and pleocytosis (chiefly lymphocytes). Sugar is sometimes decreased.
- Pituitary—diabetes insipidus, hypopituitarism, or hyperprolactinemia may occur.
- Kidney—renal function is decreased (because of hypercalcemia or increased uric acid with resultant nephrocalcinosis or renal calculi).
- Lung—diagnosis requires demonstration of noncaseating granulomas in biopsy; method of choice for intrathoracic tissue is transbronchial biopsy.
- Bronchoalveolar lavage shows 3–5 times increase in cells; T-lymphocytes are increased to 36%; B-lymphocytes = 4%; macrophages decreased to 55%; neutrophils and eosinophils are <5%.
- ^{67}Ga scan is usually positive with a diffuse lung pattern and uptake in lymph nodes and other organs with active disease. Gas exchange is usually normal early in disease; later PO_2 is decreased with marked fall after exercise.

AMYLOIDOSIS

Biopsy of tissue may be done at several sites.
- Electron microscopy is the most specific diagnostic method.
- Gingival biopsy is positive in one-half to two-thirds of patients.
- Rectal biopsy is positive in one-half to two-thirds of patients.
- Needle biopsy of kidney is useful when gingival and rectal biopsies are not helpful and there is a differential diagnosis of nephrosis.
- Bone biopsy is positive in 30% of patients; useful to identify multiple myeloma.
- Needle biopsy of liver is often positive, but beware of intractable bleeding or rupture.

Skin biopsy is taken from sites of plaque formation.

Tissue from carpal-tunnel decompression is positive in 90% of amyloidosis cases.

Other areas of involvement include GI tract, spleen, respiratory tract.

Congo red test is positive in one-third of patients with primary amyloidosis and approximately two-thirds of patients with secondary amyloidosis. *One should use Congo red stain of tissue under polarized light (apple-green birefringence) as well as transmitted light.*

Evans blue dye is retained in serum.

Classification

(AL) Light-Chain Amyloid

(Bence Jones proteinuria occurs; derived from malignant clone of plasma cells in neoplastic type or small nonproliferative population of plasma cells in nontumor type)

One-third of cases show overt myeloma; occurs in ~15% of cases of multiple myeloma. Primary when there is no evidence of associated disease, e.g., myeloma. May also be associated with Waldenström's macroglobulinemia, heavy-chain disease, etc.

One organ usually shows predominant involvement.

Cardiovascular system—involved in almost all cases; presenting symptom in 26% of cases

Proteinuria and azotemia occur in most cases; nephrotic range proteinuria (>3 gm/day) occurs in 45% of cases. Amyloidosis should always be ruled out in patients >age 30 years with unexplained nephrotic syndrome.

Tongue is enlarged in 20% of cases.

Peripheral neuropathy in 16% of cases; CNS is not involved by amyloidosis.

Respiratory system is usually involved, but decreased pulmonary function is rare.

Others

Serum protein electrophoresis shows hypogammaglobulinemia in 40% and an abnormal immunoglobulin in another 56% of cases.

Immunoelectrophoresis detects a monoclonal protein in two-thirds of cases. ~25% of patients have a free monoclonal light chain in serum (Bence Jones proteinemia). Lambda light chains are more common (65%) than kappa light chains (35%) in contrast to multiple myeloma.

Urine contains free light chains in >75% of cases; two-thirds of these are lambda-type BJ proteins; monoclonal peak is often hidden by nephrotic protein loss, requiring immunoelectrophoresis. Sensitivity for detection of free light chains is increased by concentration of urine (100–500 times) and by immunoelectrophoresis and immunofixation. Low levels of urine monoclonal light chains (<200 mg/24 hours) may indicate an immunocytic malignancy (multiple myeloma, chronic lymphocytic leukemia, or non-Hodgkin's lymphoma) even when serum is negative for M proteins, and thus occult malignancy should be ruled out. An M protein is found in urine and/or serum in ~80% of cases. *Monoclonal proteins are not found in secondary, senile, familial, or localized amyloidosis.*

Serum creatinine > 1.3 mg/dl is associated with a shorter survival time.

Mild anemia in 50% of cases.

Platelet count may be elevated.

WBC is frequently increased.

ESR is increased.

Bone marrow shows >5% plasma cells in 50% of cases.

See Multiple Myeloma (pp. 345–347).

(AA) Reactive (Secondary) Systemic (Amyloid A Protein)

(no Bence Jones proteinuria)

Due to

Rheumatoid arthritis (10–15% of cases)

Juvenile rheumatoid arthritis (9–15% of cases)
Ankylosing spondylitis (9–15% of cases)
Chronic infections
- Osteomyelitis, burns, decubital ulcers (25% of cases)
- Leprosy (6–31% of cases)
- Tuberculosis (was most common cause prior to antibiotic era)
- Heroin use with chronic infection of skin injection sites

Chronic inflammation (e.g., bowel disease)
Neoplasms
- Hodgkin's disease
- Nonlymphoid solid tumors (e.g., renal and bladder adenocarcinoma)

Heredofamilial systemic amyloidosis
- Familial Mediterranean fever (25% of cases) (AA type)
- Neuropathic types (I, II, III, IV)—serum protein electrophoresis and immunoelectrophoresis are normal.

Local Amyloidosis Types
(no Bence Jones proteinuria)

(SSA) Senile cardiac amyloid (formed from prealbumin)—found in 24% of patients > 70 years old; may cause heart failure
(AF) Familial amyloid (formed from prealbumin)—autosomal dominant with cardiac, renal, neuropathic involvement
(CAA) Cerebral amyloid (subunit protein is called A4 or beta)—in cerebral vessels, plaques and neurofibrillary tangles in senile dementia and Down's syndrome
(A-beta$_2$-M) Dialysis amyloid (from beta$_2$ microglobulin)
(IAPP) Amyloid of type II diabetes (from islet polypeptide)
(AE) Amyloid of medullary cancer of thyroid (from calcitonin)

Laboratory findings due to associated diseases (see above)
Laboratory findings due to involvement of specific organs (e.g., liver, kidney, GI system, endocrine, skin, synovia and tendons in carpal tunnel syndrome, lung, bladder, skin, larynx; see appropriate separate sections)

HEREDITARY ANGIOEDEMA
(due to autosomal dominant congenital deficiency of inhibitor of first component of complement [C1 INH])

Long history of clinical syndrome of episodes of upper airway obstruction, cramping abdominal pain, absence of urticaria, attacks precipitated by trauma, positive family history in 75–85% of cases

Serum C4 is the single most reliable screening test; is decreased even when patient is asymptomatic. If borderline, repeat at height of attack, since C4 falls during episode.
Low (0–30% of normal) C1 INH is necessary to confirm diagnosis. Do not use for screening. (Radioimmunoassay [RIA] will not detect the 15% of cases of variant form in which C1 INH antigen is present but nonfunctioning; for these cases, more difficult functional assay for C1 INH is needed.)

KAWASAKI SYNDROME

Recently described acute febrile illness of unknown etiology, occurring primarily in infants and young children with high incidence of cardiac complications; diagnosis is based on clinical criteria.

Leukocytosis (20,000–30,000/cu mm) during first week; lymphocytosis thereafter

Anemia reaches nadir about end of second week; improves during recovery.

Thrombocytosis is a hallmark; peaks at end of second week.

Acute-phase reactants are increased (e.g., ESR, CRP, $alpha_1$ antitrypsin).

Elevated serum interleukin-2 receptor molecules; marked increase by second week predicts development of coronary aneurysms.

ALLERGIC DISORDERS

Nasal cytology smears stained with Wright-Giemsa showing >5% eosinophils, >1% basophils, and/or >50% goblet/epithelial cells suggest allergic disease of respiratory tract. Significant number of false positive and false negative results occur.

Blood eosinophil count > 450/cu mm in adults and 750/cu mm in children suggests allergic disorders. Significant number of false positive and false negative results occur.

Increased serum total IgE may also occur in parasitic infections, immune deficiency, bronchopulmonary aspergillosis.

RAST (radioallergosorbent test) measures IgE specific for individual allergens. It is useful when skin testing cannot be done (e.g., children, risk of anaphylaxis).

MULTIPLE ORGAN FAILURE SYNDROME

Sequela of certain severe conditions especially in surgical ICU (e.g., ruptured aneurysm, acute pancreatitis, septic shock, surgical complications, burns, trauma) with four clinical stages with 40% mortality in early stage ranging to 90% in late stage

- Episode of physiologic shock
- Active resuscitation lasting up to 24 hours
- Stable hypermetabolism (hyperglycemia, hyperlacticemia, polyuria, urine urea nitrogen > 15 gm/day) lasting 7–10 days with appearance of acute lung injury and repeated septic episodes
- Onset of liver and kidney failure (serum bilirubin > 3 mg/dl after 7–10 days with progressive rise followed by increase in serum creatinine); encephalopathy, consumption coagulopathy, GI bleeding, recurrent infection

Progressive increase in blood glucose, lactate, urine nitrogen excretion and fall in serum albumin, transferrin and other liver proteins

Increasing consumption coagulopathy and thrombocytopenia

Failure of immune system marked by bacteremia (especially gram-negative organisms) and positive cultures from urine, wounds, tracheal aspirate, invasive lines. *Candida* species, viruses (especially herpes simplex virus [HSV]), and cytomegalovirus (CMV) can be cultured.

In one clinical variant, there is no clinically evident lung injury. In another clinical type (usually associated with a primary lung injury such as aspiration), liver and kidney failure does not manifest until a few days before death.

Poor prognostic findings are

- Initial mean PaO_2/FIO_2 ratio < 250 (normal = 400)
- Serum lactate on day 2 ≥ 3.4 mg/dl (normal <1.5 mg/dl)
- Liver failure by day 6 with mean serum bilirubin = 8.5 mg/dl and rising
- Kidney failure by day 12 with mean serum creatinine = 3.9 mg/dl and rising

SWEAT COLOR

Brown—ochronosis

Red—rifampin overdose

Blue—occupational exposure to copper

Blue-black—idiopathic chromhidrosis (in black persons, axillary chromhidrosis may also be yellow, blue-green)

Malignant Diseases/Tumor Markers

BIOCHEMICAL DETECTION OF CANCER (TUMOR MARKERS)

Decreased

Serum glucose
Serum protein and albumin (e.g., due to malnutrition, blood loss)
Anemia (e.g., due to hemorrhage, malnutrition, hemolysis, anemia of chronic disease, myelophthisis)

Increased

Serum uric acid
Serum calcium—occurs in about 20% of cancer patients, usually due to bone metastases, which sometimes cannot be detected. >14 mg/dl suggests cancer rather than hyperparathyroidism. (See Hypercalcemia of Malignancy, p. 471.)
Serum globulin (e.g., multiple myeloma), especially $alpha_2$ globulin
Serum lactic acid
Development of autoantibodies, hemolytic anemia, etc.
Tumor cells in bone marrow, liver biopsy, etc.
Occult blood in stool
ESR is often normal in patients with cancer and therefore is not a good test for screening, and a normal value does not exclude metastases. In patients with known cancer, ESR > 100 mm/hour is usually associated with metastases.
WBC may be increased due to tumor necrosis, secondary infection, etc.
Laboratory findings due to metastatic tumor masses (e.g., liver, brain)
Laboratory findings due to obstruction (e.g., ureters, bile ducts, intestine)
Laboratory findings due to metastases that interfere with endocrine secretion (e.g., adrenal, pituitary)
Laboratory findings due to fluid in body cavities (pleural, abdominal, CSF)
Laboratory findings due to complications of anticancer therapy
- Blood dyscrasias including secondary leukemia
- Bladder cancer after prolonged Cytoxan therapy
- Cardiotoxicity (e.g., doxorubicin hydrochloride [Adriamycin])
- Pulmonary fibrosis (e.g., methotrexate, bleomycin)
- Sterility
- Teratogenic effects

Diseases that occur with particular frequency in association with neoplasms (e.g., polymyositis)

Tumor Markers

These changes in blood are not generally useful to establish a definite diagnosis or for screening but may be useful to monitor effect of therapy or recurrence of lesion, to follow the clinical course, to pinpoint the tissue of origin. May sometimes be useful to assess the extent of tumor and to estimate prognosis. (See appropriate separate sections for each.)

Enzymes increased
- Serum alkaline phosphatase and gamma-glutamyl transferase (GGT) in liver metastases; increase is predictive of positive liver scan but not of positive bone scan for metastases from breast cancer. Also in bone metastases, osteogenic sarcoma, myeloid leukemia. Placenta-like isoenzyme of alkaline phosphatase increased in 30% of ovarian cancers (especially serous cystadenocarcinoma), some cancers of endometrium, lung, breast, and 40% of seminomas (75% in metastatic seminoma)
- 5′-Nucleotidase in metastatic carcinoma of liver but not bone
- Serum GGT in metastatic carcinoma of liver
- Serum lactic dehydrogenase (LDH) in metastatic carcinoma of liver, acute leukemia, lymphomas

- Serum CK-BB in various cancers (e.g., prostate, breast, ovary, colon, small-cell carcinoma of lung) in ~30% of early cases and ~45% of extensive cancers
- Serum acid phosphatase in 80% of men with metastatic prostate cancer and 25% of those without metastases
- Neuron-specific enolase (NSE) in APUD tumors including small-cell carcinoma of lung, neuroblastoma, medullary carcinoma of thyroid; 32% accompanied by increased CK-BB
- Serum amylase in 8–40% of cases of carcinoma of pancreas
- Terminal deoxynucleotidyl transferase (Tdt)—large amounts in blast cells of acute lymphoblastic leukemia but little or none in nonlymphoid leukemia or nonleukemic cells; useful to differentiate acute lymphoid and acute myeloid leukemia

Oncofetal antigens

- Serum alpha-fetoprotein in hepatoma, teratoblastoma, yolk sac tumor
- Serum carcinoembryonic antigen (CEA) in carcinoma of GI tract, breast, >40% of small-cell carcinoma of lung

Specific products of hormone-producing tumor

- Renin-producing tumor of kidney
- Parathormone
- Vanillylmandelic acid (VMA), catecholamines in pheochromoblastoma, neuroblastoma
- Urinary 17-ketosteroids in adrenal cortical carcinoma, androgenic arrhenoblastoma
- Hydroxyindoleacetic acid (HIAA) in carcinoid
- Erythropoietin in paraneoplastic erythrocytosis
- Serum thyroglobulin in patients with total thyroidectomy; detectable level indicates recurrent thyroid cancer
- Serum calcitonin in medullary carcinoma of thyroid
- Prolactin
- Adrenocorticotropic hormone (ACTH) in Cushing's syndrome (e.g., due to adrenal tumor, due to oat cell carcinoma)
- Beta-HCG subunit (in blood or urine) for early detection of hydatidiform mole or choriocarcinoma as well as early detection of recurrence of these tumors
- Serum gastrin (gastrinoma, gastric carcinoma)
- C-peptide in insulinoma
- Estrogen and progesterone receptors (see Steroid Receptor Assays, pp. 712–713)

Other proteins

- Prostate specific antigen
- CA-125
- CA 19-9
- Immunoglobulins in multiple myeloma, lymphomas, Waldenström's macroglobulinemia

Paraneoplastic syndromes

- One-third of these patients show ectopic hormone production (e.g., bronchogenic carcinoma).
- One-third show evidence of connective tissue (e.g., polymyositis, dermatomyositis) and dermatologic (e.g., acanthosis nigricans) disorders.
- One-sixth show psychiatric and neurologic syndromes.
- Remainder show immunologic, gastrointestinal (e.g., malabsorption), renal (e.g., nephrotic syndrome), hematologic (e.g., anemia of chronic disease, disseminated intravascular coagulation [DIC]), paraproteinemias (e.g., multiple myeloma), amyloidosis.

SERUM HUMAN CHORIONIC GONADOTROPIN (HCG)

Increased In

Trophoblastic tumors, benign or malignant (see Germ Cell Tumors of Ovary and Testicle, pp. 539, 602)

- Hydatidiform mole
- Choriocarcinoma (virtually 100% of cases). Elevated levels are most useful for monitoring remission after treatment; failure to fall to an undetectable level or a rise after an initial fall signals residual tumor or progression of disease and need for another form of therapy. Measure weekly during therapy; every 2 weeks for 6 months after therapy; then less frequently.
- After uterine evacuation, average disappearance times were 99 days for hydatidiform mole, 59 days for partial mole, 51 days for hydropic degeneration; therefore if levels show a steady fall they may become negative by 100 days regardless of chemotherapy.
- 10% of patients with pure seminoma of testicle

Pregnancy

- HCG levels double approximately every 48 hours during early pregnancy.
- Serial HCG levels will usually decrease over 48 hours in ectopic pregnancy and in abortion.

False positive results have been found in

- Postorchiectomy patients (decreased testosterone causes secondary increase in LDH)
- Marijuana smokers

Not Increased In

Endodermal sinus tumors

NEURON-SPECIFIC ENOLASE (NSE)

Increased In

Small-cell carcinoma of lung in 68% of patients with limited disease and 87% with extensive disease.

Other lung cancers in 17% of cases

20% of cancers of breast, GI tract, prostate

Neuroblastoma, Wilms' tumor, malignant lymphoma

SERUM ALPHA-FETOPROTEIN (AFP)

Normal (<40 ng/ml)

Absent after first weeks of life

Increased In

(>50 ng/ml is essentially diagnostic of AFP-producing tumor)

Increases associated with nonmalignant conditions are usually temporary and levels subsequently fall, but in malignant disease, elevations continue to rise. High initial levels indicate a poor prognosis. Failure to return to normal after surgery indicates incomplete resection or presence of metastases. Changes in level can indicate effects of chemotherapy.

Primary cancer of liver (hepatoma) in 50% of whites and 75–90% of nonwhites; levels may be markedly elevated (>1000 ng/ml in ~50/% of cases; this level usually indicates tumor > 3 cm in size). Elevated in almost 100% of cases in children and young adults. Useful tumor marker. 90% of cases of hepatoma have AFP > 200, and 70% have levels > 400 ng/ml, but in benign liver diseases AFP > 400 ng/ml is extremely rare. More likely to be increased in immature type of hepatoma compared to mature type. Has been used for screening in high-prevalence areas (e.g., China, Eskimos).

Germ cell tumors of ovary and testis (see p. 539)

- Embryonal carcinoma (in 27% of cases)
- Malignant teratoma (in 60% of cases)

Should be used in conjunction with HCG for these tumors; more often elevated with advanced disease. These are useful to monitor chemotherapy; predict relapse before clinical or x-ray evidence.

Neonatal hepatitis. Most patients with this disorder have levels > 40 ng/ml, but in neonatal biliary atresia most patients have levels < 40 ng/ml.
Pregnancy: increased above normal level in fetal neural tube defects (e.g., 80% of open spina bifida or 90% of anencephaly cases; <5% of closed spina bifida cases). (*Increased blood levels of AFP in pregnancy are a valuable screening test, but diagnosis should be confirmed by finding of increased levels in amniotic fluid; serum should be drawn after the 15th week of gestation.*) May also be increased in omphalocele, gastroschisis, congenital nephrosis, fetal hemorrhage.
Some patients with liver metastases from carcinoma of stomach or pancreas
Ataxia-telangiectasia
Hereditary tyrosinemia

False Positive In
Twin pregnancy
Dead fetus
Overestimated gestation age
Congenital nephrosis
Congenital anomalies with viscera outside fetal body (e.g., exomphalos)
0.5% of normal fetuses

Absent In
Various types of cirrhosis and hepatitis in adults
Seminoma of testis
Choriocarcinoma, adenocarcinoma, and dermoid cyst of ovary

Decreased In Maternal Serum
Down's syndrome (useful for screening; see pp. 442–443)
Death of fetus
Incorrect dates of gestation
Choriocarcinoma
Maternal diabetes mellitus
Increased maternal weight
Other unknown factors

SERUM CARCINOEMBRYONIC ANTIGEN (CEA)

Is primarily used in patients with colon carcinoma; less often for other sites

Monitoring after surgery: Primary use is monitoring for persistent, metastatic, or recurrent cancer of colon and less frequently of breast, indicated by sustained and progressive increase; not usually useful for diagnosis of local recurrence. Failure to fall to normal levels postoperatively makes diagnosis of incomplete resection likely. Predicts recurrence earlier than other methods, but for most patients this is not useful therapeutically, although increasing level may precede clinical evidence of recurrence by 2–6 months. 20% change in plasma level is concordant with change in the tumor. In ~50% of patients with advanced cancer, there may be a latent phase of 4–6 weeks from onset of therapy to change in CEA level.

Screening: Not recommended because of low sensitivity and specificity, especially in early stages of malignant disease.

Diagnosis: Serum levels cannot be used alone to establish the diagnosis but in conjunction with other findings may help decide on active pursuit of diagnostic workup for colon carcinoma.

Prognosis: Serum levels predict recurrence of colon carcinoma independently of stage but cannot be used to improve prognosis. After complete removal of colon cancer, CEA should fall to normal in 0–12 weeks.

Serum level at time of diagnosis is related to prognosis (stage of disease and likelihood of recurrence). CEA level > 5 ng/ml before therapy suggests localized disease and a favorable prognosis, but a level > 10 ng/ml suggests extensive disease and a poor prognosis. With values > 20 ng/ml, plasma CEA correlates with tumor volume in breast and colon cancer. Titers > 20 ng/ml are usually associated with metastatic disease or with a few types of cancer (e.g., cancer of the colon or pancreas); however, metastases may occur with levels < 20 ng/ml. Values < 2.5 ng/ml do not rule out primary, metastatic, or recurrent cancer.

Increased In

Cancer (see preceding paragraph). (There is a wide overlap in values between benign and malignant disease. Increased levels are suggestive but not diagnostic of cancer.)
- 75% of patients with carcinoma of entodermal origin (colon, stomach, pancreas, lung) have CEA titers > 2.5 ng/ml, and two-thirds of these titers are >5 ng/ml. Increased in ~one-third of patients with small-cell carcinoma of lung and ~two-thirds with non-small-cell carcinoma of lung.
- 50% of patients with carcinoma of nonentodermal origin (especially cancer of the breast, head and neck, ovary) have CEA titers > 2.5 ng/ml, and 50% of the titers are >5 ng/ml. Increased in >50% of breast cancer with metastases, 25% of cases without metastases, but not associated with benign lesions.
- 40% of patients with noncarcinomatous malignant disease have increased CEA levels, usually 2.5–5.0 ng/ml.
- Increase in pleural fluids indicates malignant effusion.

Active cases of nonmalignant inflammatory diseases (especially of the GI tract, e.g., ulcerative colitis, regional enteritis, diverticulitis, peptic ulcer, chronic pancreatitis) frequently have elevated levels that decline when the disease is in remission.

Liver disease (alcoholic, cirrhosis, chronic active hepatitis, obstructive jaundice)

Others
- Renal failure
- Fibrocystic disease of breast

Smoking
- 97% of healthy nonsmokers have plasma CEA levels < 2.5 ng/ml.
- 19% of heavy smokers and 7% of former smokers have CEA levels > 2.5 ng/ml.

Do not test heparinized patients or collect plasma in heparinized tubes, since this may interfere with accuracy of CEA assay.

SERUM CA-125

(glycoprotein derived from coelomic epithelium)

Increased In

(upper limit of normal < 35 units/ml)

Malignant disease
- Nonmucinous epithelial ovarian carcinoma (85%)
- Carcinoma of fallopian tube, endometrium, endocervix (22%)
- Liver carcinoma (70%)
- Pancreatic carcinoma (61%)
- Colon carcinoma (15%)
- Breast carcinoma (12%)
- Lung carcinoma (47%)

Healthy persons (1%)

Pregnancy (27%)

Nonmalignant conditions
- Commonly increased in advanced stages of endometriosis

Cirrhosis, severe liver necrosis (66%)
Other diseases of liver, pancreas, GI tract (5–8%)

Primary usefulness in serous carcinoma of ovary
Monitoring for persistent or recurrent disease in postoperative period or during chemotherapy. Remains elevated in stable or progressive disease. Rising level may be indication for second-look operation and may precede clinical recurrence by many months. Greater elevation is roughly related to poorer survival.
Not used for screening since it is negative in 20% of cases at time of diagnosis; normal level does not exclude tumor.
Not increased in mucinous adenocarcinoma

SERUM CA-19-9

Increased In

Carcinoma of pancreas
In a small series of patients with reported sensitivity = 70%, specificity = 87%, positive predictive value = 59%, negative predictive value = 92%. There was no difference in sensitivity between local and metastatic disease.*
Hepatobiliary and gastric cancer
New test, whose utility is still being evaluated. May be a useful adjunct to CEA for diagnosis and to detect early recurrence of these cancers.

TUMOR CHEMOSENSITIVITY TESTING

Assays to predict sensitivity/resistance of a tumor to specific chemotherapeutic agents
Sterile preparation; transported on ice; avoid freezing; in cold tissue transport media; set up in tissue culture media within 24 hours
Clonogenic assay
Minced solid tumor or fluids containing tumor (e.g., malignant effusions, urine, CSF)
Incubated for 1 hour with test drug, then incubated on cell culture plates. Colonies are counted after 10–14 days and compared with control plates to determine percent decrease in tumor-colony-forming units.
Subrenal capsule assay
Tumor fragments (not individual cells) injected into immunocompetent mouse
Reported as percent change in implantation weight
Rotman in vitro chemosensitivity (fluorescent cytoprint) assay
Measures ability of viable human tumor cells in culture to transport and hydrolyze fluorescein diacetate and retain fluorescein. Tumor is incubated with drug in media for 48 hours. Sensitivity = 100% cell death at lowest drug dose currently used.

Neoplastic Diseases

ACUTE TUMOR LYSIS SYNDROME

Caused by effective induction chemotherapy of rapidly growing neoplasms (e.g., acute leukemia, malignant lymphoma, Burkitt's lymphoma). Associated with higher WBC count in leukemias or very large tumors, inadequate urine output, high pretreatment serum LDH levels that rise further. Occurs in one-

*Data from DK Pleskow et al., Evaluation of a serologic marker CA19-9, in the diagnosis of pancreatic cancer. *Ann Intern Med* 110:701, 1989.

Table 17-3. Comparison of Assays for Tumor Chemosensitivity Testing

Assay	Specimen	% of Specimens That Can Be Evaluated	% Accuracy In Determining		Reporting Time (day)
			Resistance	Sensitivity	
Clonogenic	Single cell	40–60	90	70	10–21
Subrenal capsule	Tumor fragments in vivo	80–90	80	80–90	7–10
Rotman Fluorescent Cytoprint	Tumor fragments	95–98	90	90–95	7–10

Source: Data from EA Woltering, Tumor chemosensitivity testing: An evolving technique. *Lab Med* 21 (2):82, 1990.

third of nonazotemic and virtually all azotemic patients. Changes are greater in those with preexisting azotemia or who develop acute renal failure.

Hyperuricemia (often increases above elevation prior to therapy)

Hyperkalemia

Hypocalcemia

Severe hyperphosphatemia—occurs only after chemotherapy; is criterion for dialysis to avoid renal failure. May cause rapid decrease in serum calcium. Pretreatment with allopurinol and diuresis may prevent syndrome unless there is concomitant renal failure.

Changes due to urate nephropathy or renal calcification, which may cause or worsen azotemia and further accentuate the above changes.

BREAST CANCER

Serum CEA increase becomes more frequent with increasing stage and tumor burden. More frequent with bone and visceral involvement than with soft tissue involvement.

A rising level usually reflects disease progression, and a falling level usually reflects remission.

An elevated or rising level may precede recurrence by 1–31 months.

May be increased in CSF in metastases to CNS, meninges, or spine but not in primary brain tumors.

Not useful for screening or diagnosis of early breast cancer

Steroid Receptor Assays

Useful in prognosis and treatment of breast carcinoma.

Determination of both receptors yields best information on response to hormone therapy.

Estrogen receptor (ER) is positive (>10 femtomoles (fmol)/mg cytoplasmic protein) in ~50% of breast tumor specimens; levels are higher in post- than in premenopausal patients, but this is not so for progesterone receptors (PgR).

When ER is negative, there is <10% chance of obtaining a favorable response to any endocrine therapy; thus chemotherapy would be the primary approach. There is a greater likelihood of visceral metastases (>50%) with ER-negative than with ER-positive patients (<6%).

When ER is positive, there is 55–60% chance of favorable response (i.e., tumor shrinkage and/or clinical improvement).

When ER and PgR are both positive, response rate is 75–80%. No response to endocrine therapy in 10–15% of patients with ER/PgR positive tumors.

Predictive value of assay is increased if ER and PgR levels are both high.

ER titer > 100 fmol/mg protein

PR (progesterone receptor assay) is also positive, especially > 100 fmol/mg.

Prognostic value

Recurrence rate is significantly greater for ER-negative tumors, both Stage I (negative axillary lymph nodes) and Stage II (positive axillary lymph nodes).

Overall response rate to endocrine therapy is about 50%.

Response Rate to Endocrine Therapy

ERA > 100 fmol/mg protein	~75%
ERA < 100 fmol/mg protein	~40%
ERA < 3 fmol/mg protein	~12%
ERA positive/PRA positive (60% of total group)	~80%
ERA negative/PRA negative (31% of total group)	~ 5%
ERA positive/PRA negative	~26%
ERA negative/PRA positive (4% of total group; this small group may be due to inaccuracy in assay procedures)	~50%

Receptor assay should also be performed on recurrent carcinoma even when the original tumor has been previously assayed. Initial ER positives are later found negative in 19%, and initial ER negatives are later positive in 13%. Initial PgR negatives are later positive in 8%, and initial PgR positives are later reported negative in 28–44% of cases. These discordance rates may be up to 75% in patients receiving anti-estrogen tamoxifen within 2 months.

Receptor assay may sometimes be useful in differential diagnosis of metastatic undifferentiated carcinoma in women.

Improved utility may result from newer technology using monoclonal antibody assays and immunocytochemical stains of tumor tissue.

Tissue specimen should be unfixed and frozen immediately after removal.

Epidermal growth factor receptor (EGF-R) is an integral membrane protein. Elevated EGF-R correlates with poor prognosis, and no detectable EGF-R is a good predictor of response to tamoxifen therapy.

DNA aneuploidy predicts shorter mean survival, independent of stage. Four-year relapse-free rate is 72% for patients with DNA diploid tumors, compared to 43% for DNA aneuploid tumors. ERA- and PRA-negative tumors are more likely to be DNA aneuploid.

DNA ploidy strongly correlates with histopathologic grade—poorly differentiated tumors are more likely to be DNA aneuploid.

SYSTEMIC MAST CELL DISEASE (MASTOCYTOSIS)

(a rare condition of disseminated mast cell tumor with functional secretion or abnormal proliferation of tissue mast cells)

Abnormal hematologic findings in ≤70% of patients. May include

- Progressive anemia and thrombocytopenia
- WBC may be increased or decreased.
- Eosinophilia and occasionally basophilia may occur.
- Mast cells are uncommon in peripheral blood, which may contain ≤10% mast cells. May progress to mast cell leukemia or develop other leukemias, lymphoma, or carcinoma.

Histamine is increased in blood, urine, and tissues. Increased levels of metabolites of histamine in random and 24-hour urine specimens. Is more specific and sensitive than determination of histamine itself.

Gastric acid is increased; there is a higher incidence of peptic ulcer; but hypochlorhydria and achlorhydria have been reported.

Urinary 5-HIAA is normal.

Diagnosis by biopsy of metastatic sites, e.g., skin (urticaria pigmentosa), lymph nodes, spleen, bone. Marrow biopsy is positive in ~90% of cases, but marrow smears are less useful. Toluidine blue stains mast cell granules.

BASAL CELL NEVUS SYNDROME

Rare disease that shows

- Multiple basal cell tumors of skin
- Odontogenic cysts of jaw
- Bone anomalies (especially of ribs, vertebrae, and metacarpals) and defective dentition
- Neurologic abnormalities (e.g., calcification of dura)
- Ophthalmologic abnormalities (e.g., abnormal width between the eyes, lateral displacement of inner canthi)
- Sexual abnormalities (e.g., frequent ovarian fibromas, male hypogonadism)
- Normal karyotyping by chromosomal analysis
- Hyporesponsiveness to parathormone (Ellsworth-Howard test)

Rule out presence or development of occult neoplasms (e.g., ovarian fibroma, medulloblastoma).

18

Disorders Due to Physical and Chemical Agents

NARCOTICS ADDICTION (usually heroin) AND CHRONIC USAGE; DRUGS OF ABUSE

Persistent absolute and relative lymphocytosis occurs with lymphocytes, often bizarre and atypical, that may resemble Downey cells.

Eosinophilia is seen in 25% of patients.

Liver function tests commonly show increased serum glutamic-oxaloacetic transaminase (SGOT) and serum glutamic-pyruvic transaminase (SGPT) (increased in 75% of patients). Higher frequency of positive tests is evident on routine periodic repeat of these tests. This probably represents a mild, chronic, serum hepatitis. Serum protein electrophoresis is usually normal.

Hepatitis B surface antigen (HB_sAg) is found in 10% of patients.

Liver biopsy shows abnormal morphology in 25% of patients, and foreign particles are particularly suggestive.

Laboratory findings due to preexisting glucose-6-PD deficiency may be precipitated (by quinine, which is often used to adulterate heroin).

Laboratory findings due to malaria transmitted by common syringes may occur. *(Malaria is not frequent; may be suppressed by quinine used for adulteration of heroin.)*

Laboratory findings due to active duodenal ulcer may occur.

Laboratory findings due to tuberculosis, which develops with increased frequency in narcotics addicts, may be present.

Laboratory findings due to staphylococcal pneumonia or septic pulmonary emboli secondary to skin infections or bacterial endocarditis (conditions that are more frequent in narcotics addicts) may be present.

Laboratory findings due to endocarditis

- Right-sided—usually *Staphylococcus aureus* affecting previously normal tricuspid valve
- Left-sided—may be due to *Candida* superimposed on previously normal valve

Laboratory findings due to syphilis and other venereal diseases, which occur with increased frequency in narcotics addicts, may occur. Biologically false positive (BFP) tests for syphilis also occur with increased frequency.

Laboratory findings due to tetanus (which occurs with increased frequency in narcotics addicts because of "skin-popping") may occur. (*Tetanus causes 5–10% of addicts' deaths in New York City.*)

Laboratory findings due to other infections, e.g., pyelonephritis, phlebitis, abscesses.

Laboratory findings due to concomitant use of sedatives, especially alcohol, barbiturates, and glutethimide (Doriden) may occur.

Laboratory findings due to complications of cocaine abuse, e.g., hepatic necrosis, coronary artery spasm with arrhythmias, acute cardiomyopathy or myocardial infarction, stroke, cerebral vasculitis, subarachnoid hemorrhage, hyperthyroidism, sudden death, rhabdomyolysis.

Oral and IV glucose tolerance curves are often flat (explanation for this finding is not known).

Urinalysis is usually normal unless renal failure due to endocarditis occurs.

Complications of drug addiction during pregnancy may also include premature rupture of membranes, abruptio placentae, stillbirth, meconium aspiration.

In screening for detection or to monitor abstinence in a drug abuse treatment program, the clinician should be aware of which drugs are included in the screen, causes of false reactions, and detection levels for the particular methodology.

In urine testing for cannabinoids (marijuana metabolites), enzyme multiplied immunoassay technique (EMIT) lower level of 100 ng/ml failed to detect 25–40% of cases identified by thin-layer chromatography (lower level ~25 ng/ml).

Traces of marijuana may be present by EMIT up to 1 week after use or in a heavy user up to 3 weeks. Cocaine and amphetamines are difficult to detect >48 hours after use. Opiates can be detected 2–4 days after use.

Eating poppy seeds may cause a false positive EMIT for heroin confirmed by gas chromatography/mass spectrometry. Poppy seed ingestion as the only source of urinary morphine and codeine can be ruled out if urine codeine >300 ng/ml, urine morphine >5000 ng/ml, morphine >1000 ng/ml when no codeine is present, and morphine-codeine ratio <2.*

CIGARETTE SMOKING

Cotinine increased in plasma or urine. Use to assess compliance in smoking cessation programs and to identify passively exposed nonsmokers. Has a longer half-life than nicotine, is more sensitive and specific than other markers to distinguish smokers from nonsmokers.

Reference ranges (high-pressure liquid chromatography [HPLC])

	Plasma	**Urine**
Nonsmoker or passive exposure	0–8 μg/L	0.0–0.2 mg/L
Smoker	>8 μg/L	>0.2 mg/L

Blood carbon monoxide increased—see p. 732.

BARBITURATE OVERDOSAGE

Correlation between serum concentrations of barbiturates and state of intoxication in patients who have taken only a short-acting barbiturate, who are not habitual drug users, and who have no medical complications:

<6 μg/ml	Alert
6–10 μg/ml	Drowsy
11–17 μg/ml	Stuporous
16–20 μg/ml	Coma 1
20–24 μg/ml	Coma 2
24–28 μg/ml	Coma 3
28–40 μg/ml	Coma 4

If the serum drug level is less than expected for the state of intoxication, look for medical complications (e.g., aspiration pneumonia, head trauma) or presence of other drugs.

ALCOHOLISM

Laboratory findings due to alcohol ingestion

Blood alcohol level >300 mg/dl at any time or >100 mg/dl in routine examination. (*Blood alcohol level >150 mg/dl without gross evidence of intoxication suggests alcoholic patient's increased tolerance.*) In high-dose coma, blood alcohol should be >300 mg/dl; otherwise rule out other etiologies, especially diabetic acidosis and hypoglycemia.

Rules of thumb to estimate blood alcohol level

Peak is reached 1/2–3 hours after last drink.

Each ounce of whisky, glass of wine, or 12 ounces of beer raises blood alcohol 15–25 mg/dl.

*Data from HN ElSohly, MA ElSohly, and DF Stanford, Poppy seed ingestion and opiates urinalysis: A closer look. *J Anal Toxicol* 14:308, 1990.

- Women absorb alcohol much more rapidly than do men and show a 35–45% higher blood alcohol level. During premenstrual period, peak occurs more rapidly and reaches a higher peak. Birth control pills cause a higher, more sustained level.
- Elderly become intoxicated more quickly than young persons.
- Urine concentration is not well correlated with blood levels; cannot be used to determine level of intoxication or impairment.
- Breath test (Breathalyzer) has certain constraints and limitations.

Saliva alcohol using cotton swab inserted into kit device for use in drug abuse centers, hospital ER, and trauma units colors enzyme strip in 2 minutes, which is compared with a color scale.

Serum osmolality (reflects blood alcohol levels)—every 22.4 increment >200 mOsm/L reflects 50 mg/dl alcohol. Increased osmolar gap (difference between measured and calculated osmolality is increased >10; see pp. 396–403). Absence of increased gap is evidence against elevated blood level of ethanol, methanol, or ethylene glycol.

Laboratory findings due to other drugs of abuse may be present.

Results of alcohol ingestion

- Hypoglycemia
- Hypochloremic alkalosis
- Low magnesium level
- Increased lactic acid (see pp. 397–398)
- Metabolic acidosis with increased anion gap (see pp. 42–43)
- Alcoholic ketoacidosis is preponderantly due to beta-hydroxybutyrate, and therefore increased levels in blood and urine are often negative or only weakly positive because nitroprusside test detects acetoacetic but not beta-hydroxybutyric acid. As the patient improves, the ketone test may become more strongly positive (although total ketone level declines) because the improved liver function slows the conversion of acetoacetate to beta-hydroxybutyrate.
- Thrombocytopenia
- Anemia most often due to folic acid deficiency; less frequently due to iron deficiency, hemorrhage, etc. (see appropriate separate sections)
- Alcohol is the most common cause of ring sideroblasts
- Three types of hemolytic syndromes may occur (spur cell anemia, acquired stomatocytosis, Zieve syndrome).

Increase in these blood values with no other known cause that should arouse suspicion of alcoholism

- Mean corpuscular volume (MCV) (e.g., >97) (26% of cases) with round macrocytosis
- Serum gamma-glutamyl transferase (GGT)
- Uric acid (10% of cases)
- SGPT, SGOT (48% of cases)
- Alkaline phosphatase (16% of cases)
- Bilirubin (13% of cases)
- Triglycerides

After 4 weeks of abstention, alcohol challenge in "moderate drinkers" causes increased SGOT and GGT in 24 hours with slow decline thereafter. SGPT, lactic dehydrogenase (LDH), alkaline phosphatase show little or no change.

Declining serum potassium level to hypokalemia during alcohol withdrawal is said to be a reliable predictor of delirium tremens.

Laboratory findings due to major alcohol-associated illnesses (see these appropriate separate sections)

- Fatty liver, alcoholic hepatitis (see p. 193), cirrhosis, esophageal varices, peptic ulcer, chronic gastritis, pancreatitis, malabsorption, vitamin deficiencies
- Head trauma, Korsakoff's syndrome, delirium tremens, peripheral neuropathy, myopathy

Table 18-1. Drugs of Abuse

Drug	Street Name	Route	Usual Dose	Toxic Dose	Half-Life (hr)	Duration Effect (hr)	% Not Changed in Urine
Stimulants							
Cocaine[a]	Coke Crack Snow	Nasal Smoke IV Oral	1.5 mg/kg	>1.2 gm	2–5	1–2	<10
Amphetamine[b] (Benzedrine, Dexedrine)	Bennies Dexies Uppers	Oral IV	10 mg	30–500 mg	4–24	2–4	~30
Metamphetamine (Desoxyn, Methedrine)	Speed Meth Crystal	Oral IV	5–10 mg	>1 gm	9–24	2–4	10–20
Methylphenidate (Ritalin)		Oral IV	5–20 mg	>2 gm	2–3	2–4	<1
Phenmetrazine (Preludin)		Oral IV	75 mg		8	12	15–20
Cannabis							
Marijuana,[c] Hashish	Grass Mary Jane Pot THC Hash	Smoke Oral IV		50–200 μg/kg	14–38	2–4	<1
Narcotics							
Heroin[d]	Horse Smack White Lady Scag	IV Smoke Nasal	5–10 mg	100–250 mg	1.0–1.5	3–6	<1

Codeine[e] (e.g., with Empirin)		Oral IV IM	15–60 mg	500–1000 mg	2–4	3–6	5–20
Morphine[f] (Morphine SO_4, Duramorph)	M Junk Morpho White Stuff	IV IM Oral Smoke	5–10 mg	50–100 μg/kg	2–4	3–6	<10
Methadone[g] (Dolophine, Amidone)	Methadose	Oral IV IM	40–100 mg	100–200 mg	15–60	12–24	5–50
Meperidine (Demerol, Mepergan, Pethidine)		IV IM Oral	25–100 mg	500–2000 mg	2–5	3–6	5
Propoxyphene[h] (Darvon, Darvocet, Dolene)	Yellow footballs	Oral	65–400 mg	500 mg	8–24	1–6	<1
Barbiturates[i]							
Pentobarbital (Nembutal)	Yellow jackets Yellows	Oral IV IM	50–200 mg	2–10 gm	15–48	3–6	1
Amobarbital (Amytal, Tuinal)	Blues Bluebirds Rainbows	Oral IV IM	30–200 mg	1.5–10 gm	12–60	3–24	<1
Secobarbital (Seconal, Tuinal)	Reds Red devils M & Ms	Oral IV IM	100–200 mg	2–5 gm	15–40	3–6	5
Butabarbital (Butisol)		Oral	15–100 mg	>2 gm	30–40	3–6	5–10
Butalbital (Fiorinal)		Oral	50–100 mg	>1 gm	30–40	3–6	5
Phenobarbital (Luminal)	Downers	Oral IV IM	50–200 mg	6–20 gm	48–120	10–20	20–35

Table 18-1 (continued)

Drug	Street Name	Route	Usual Dose	Toxic Dose	Half-Life (hr)	Duration Effect (hr)	% Not Changed in Urine
Benzodiazepines[j]							
Alprazolam (Xanax)		Oral	0.25–1.0 mg		7–13	4–8	20
Chlordiazepoxide (Librium)		Oral IM	5–100 mg	>500 μg	6–27	4–8	<1
Diazepam (Valium)		Oral IV IM	5–30 mg	>250 mg	20–50	4–8	<1
Flurazepam (Dalmane)		Oral	15–30 mg	>500 mg	2–3	4–12	<1
Lorazepam (Ativan)		Oral IV IM	0.5–2.0 mg	25–100 mg	9–16	4–8	<1
Antidepressants							
Tricyclics, e.g., imipramine (Tofranil, Janimine)		Oral IM	100–500 mg	>1 gm	12–30		<1
Phenothiazines, e.g., chlorpromazine (Thorazine)		Oral IV IM Rectal	5–800 mg	>1 gm	7–120		<1
Sedatives/Depressants							
Ethanol		Oral		100 gm	2–14	2–6	2–10
Methaqualone[k] (Quaaludes)	Ludes Soapers	Oral	150–500 mg	2 gm	20–60	4–8	<1
Meprobamate (Equanil, Miltown, Pathibamate)		Oral	400–1000 mg	2–5 gm	6–16	4–8	5%

Glutethimide (Doricen)		Oral	150–500 mg	5 gm	5–22	4–8	<2
Chloral hydrate (Noctec)	Mickey Finn Joy Juice	Oral Rectal	300–1000 mg	3 gm	<1	5–8	<1
Hallucinogens							
Phencyclidine[l]	PCP Angel dust Killer weed	Oral Nasal Smoke IV	0.25 mg/kg	10–20 mg	7–16	2–4 (psychosis may last weeks)	30–50
LSD	Acid White lightning Microdots	Oral	1–2 μg/kg	100–200 μg	3–4	8–12	1
Amphetamine analogs	STP DOM	Oral IV	2 mg		4–8		20
Ketamine (Ketalar)		IV IM	1.0–4.5 mg/kg	>500 mg	3–4	0.5–2.0	2–5
Mescaline	Peyote Mesc Buttons	Oral		200–700 mg	6	8–12	50–60

Detection Times in Urine with EMIT Methods

[a]Cocaine — Up to 48 hours after a single dose.
[b]Amphetamines — Detectable within 24–48 hours after ingestion. "Cold" medicines that contain ephedrine, pseudoephedrine, or phenylpropanolamine may give positive reaction.
[c]Marijuana — ≤5 days after occasional use. 21–32 days after last dose in chronic users.
[d]Heroin — One dose of 10 mg detectable for up to 24 hours. 4–5 days in chronic users.
[e]Codeine — Excreted as morphine. 120-mg dose detectable for up to 48 hours.
[f]Morphine — Single 10-mg dose detectable for 24–48 hours.
[g]Methadone — ~3 days. Interference from high levels of chlorpromazine, promethazine, and dextromethorpan may occur.
[h]Propoxyphene — Up to 48 hours.
[i]Barbiturates — Up to 9 days after one 250-mg dose of phenobarbital. Other common barbiturates can be detected for 1–2 days.
[j]Benzodiazepine — Not usually positive after one dose with normal renal function. Up to 5–7 days in chronic users.
[k]Methaqualone — ≥5 days after a typical dose.
[l]Phencyclidine — 1 week after a single dose. Up to 2 weeks after last dose in chronic users.

Source: Data from J Wilson, *Clinical Chemistry News Laboratory Guide to Abused Drugs (for Roche Diagnostic Systems)*. Washington: AACC Press, 1990.

Table 18-2. Stages of Acute Alcoholic Intoxication

Ethanol Concentration (% weight/volume)		Stage of Alcohol Influence	Effects
Blood	Urine		
0.01–0.05	0.01–0.07	Sobriety	Little effect on most persons
0.04–0.12	0.03–0.16	Euphoria	Decreased inhibitions Decreased judgment Loss of fine control Increased reaction time (≤20%)
0.09–0.20	0.07–0.30	Excitement	Uncoordinated Loss of critical judgment Memory loss Increased reaction time (≤100%)
0.15–0.30	0.12–0.40	Confusion	Disoriented Emotional Balance impaired Speech slurred Sensation disturbed
0.25–0.40	0.20–0.50	Stupor	Paralyzed Incontinent
0.30–0.50	0.25–0.60	Coma	Reflexes depressed Respiration decreased Possible death

Cardiac myopathy
Various pneumonias, lung abscess, tuberculosis
Associated addictions

METHYL ALCOHOL POISONING

Onset is 12–24 hours after ingestion.

Severe metabolic acidosis with increased anion gap and increased osmolar gap similar to ethanol intoxication (see Alcoholism, preceding section) and ethylene glycol poisoning

Frequent concomitant acute pancreatitis

SALICYLATE INTOXICATION

(due to aspirin, sodium salicylate, oil of wintergreen, methylsalicylate)

Increased serum salicylate
>10 mg/dl when symptoms are present
>40 mg/dl when hyperventilation is present
At ~50 mg/dl, severe toxicity with acid-base imbalance and ketosis
At 45–70 mg/dl, death

15–30 mg/dl for optimal anti-inflammatory effect
5–27 mg/dl in patients with rheumatoid arthritis on dose of 65 mg/kg/day
19–45 mg/dl when tinnitus is first noted

Peak serum level is reached 2 hours after therapeutic and at least 6 hours after toxic dose. Serum levels drawn <6 hours after ingestion cannot be used to predict severity of toxic reaction using Done's nomogram, although they will confirm salicylate overdose. Done's nomogram cannot be used for enteric-coated aspirin.

When awaiting laboratory measurement, can estimate peak salicylate levels:

$$\text{mg/dl of salicylate} = \frac{\text{mg of salicylate ingested}}{70\% \text{ of body weight (in gm)*}} \times 100$$

In older children and adults, serum salicylate level corresponds well with severity; in younger children, correlation is more variable.

Gastric lavage may increase salicylate level ≤10 mg/dl.

Early, serum electrolytes and CO_2 are normal.

Later, progressive decrease in serum sodium and PCO_2 occurs. There is combined respiratory alkalosis and metabolic acidosis; change in blood pH reflects the net result. (*Infants may show immediate metabolic acidosis with the usual initial respiratory alkalosis. In older children and adults, the typical picture is respiratory alkalosis.*)

Hypokalemia accompanies the respiratory alkalosis.

Dehydration occurs.

Urine shows paradoxic acid pH despite the increased serum bicarbonate.

- Ferric chloride test is positive on boiled as well as unboiled urine (thus differentiating salicylate from ketone bodies); it may have a false positive result because of phenacetin.
- Tests for glucose (e.g., Clinistix), reducing substances (e.g., Clinitest), or ketone bodies (e.g., Ketostix) are positive. All positive urine screening tests should be confirmed by serum sample.
- RBCs may be present.
- Number of renal tubular cells is increased because of renal irritation.
- Hypoglycemia occurs, especially in infants on restricted diet and in diabetics.
- Serum SGOT and SGPT may be increased.
- Hypoprothrombinemia after some days of intensive salicylate therapy is temporary and occasional; rarely causes hemorrhage.
- Hydroxyproline is decreased in serum and urine.
- Monitor patient by following blood glucose, potassium, pH.

PHENACETIN—CHRONIC EXCESSIVE INGESTION

Laboratory findings due to increased incidence of peptic ulceration, especially of stomach, often with bleeding, may be present.

Laboratory findings associated with increased incidence of papillary necrosis and interstitial nephritis may be present.

- Proteinuria is slight or absent.
- Hematuria is often present in active papillary necrosis.
- WBC is increased in urine in absence of infection.
- Papillae are passed in urine.
- Creatinine clearance is decreased.
- Renal failure may occur.

Anemia is common and frequently precedes azotemia.

ACETAMINOPHEN POISONING

Blood levels

- 200 μg/ml within 4 hours after ingestion or >50 μg/ml at 12 hours forecasts severe liver damage, and treatment with acetylcysteine should begin.
- <150 μg/ml at 4 hours or <30–35 μg/ml at 12 hours indicates no liver damage will occur.
- *Liver toxicity cannot be predicted from blood levels earlier than 4 hours.*
- *Exact time of ingestion is often difficult to ascertain.*

* = Total body water.

Patients taking other drugs or with concomitant cirrhosis may develop liver toxicity at different blood levels.

Toxicity is less common in children <5 years old, and changes in liver function tests may be mild when serum drug levels are in toxic range.

With hepatotoxicity

During first 12–24 hours, no other laboratory test abnormalities are found, and serum drug levels are the chief guide to therapy; this is the only stage when treatment can prevent liver damage.

During next 24–48 hours, SGOT, SGPT, serum bilirubin, prothrombin time are increased.

Third to fourth day, liver function abnormalities peak; hypoglycemia, secondary renal failure may occur.

BROMISM

(should always be ruled out in the presence of mental symptoms or psychosis)

Serum and urine bromide levels are increased.

CSF protein is increased in acute bromide psychosis.

False increase of serum "chloride" when measured by AutoAnalyzer. *If result of chloride determination with AutoAnalyzer is increased out of proportion to result with Cotlove coulimetric titrator, bromism should be ruled out.*

Anion gap may be low or negative due to increased serum chloride.

SIDE EFFECTS OF STEROID THERAPY THAT CAUSE LABORATORY CHANGES

Endocrine effects (e.g., adrenal insufficiency after prolonged use, suppression of pituitary or thyroid function, development of diabetes mellitus)

Increased susceptibility to infections

Gastrointestinal effects (e.g., peptic ulcer, perforation of bowel, infarction of bowel, pancreatitis)

Musculoskeletal effects (e.g., osteoporosis, pathologic fractures, arthropathy, myopathy)

Decreased serum potassium, increased WBC, glycosuria, ecchymoses, etc.

PROCAINAMIDE THERAPY

Procainamide therapy may induce the findings of SLE.

Positive serologic tests for SLE are very frequent, especially in dosage of ≥1.25 gm/day, and may precede clinical manifestations.

Lupus erythematosus (LE) cell tests become positive in 50% of patients.

Anti-DNP tests become positive in 65% of patients.

Anti-DNA tests become positive in 35% of patients.

One of these tests becomes positive in 75% of patients.

Perform serologic tests for systemic lupus erythematosus (SLE) on all patients receiving procainamide.

APRESOLINE REACTION

(in hypertension therapy)

Anemia and pancytopenia occur infrequently.

Prolonged use causes a syndrome resembling SLE (microscopic hematuria, leukopenia, increased erythrocyte sedimentation rate [ESR], presence of LE cells, altered serum proteins with increased gamma globulin). After cessation of drug, remission is aided by administration of adrenocorticotropic hormone (ACTH).

ENTERIC-COATED POTASSIUM CHLORIDE

Laboratory findings due to small-intestine ulceration, obstruction, or perforation.

COMPLICATIONS OF PHENYTOIN SODIUM (DILANTIN) THERAPY

Megaloblastic anemia may occur. It is completely responsive to folic acid (even when Dilantin therapy is continued) but not always to vitamin B_{12}. This is the most common hematologic complication.

Rarely pancytopenia, thrombocytopenia alone, or leukopenia including agranulocytosis may occur.

Laboratory findings of hepatitis may be present.

Laboratory findings resembling those of malignant lymphomas may be present.

Laboratory findings resembling those of infectious mononucleosis may occur, but heterophil agglutination is not increased.

Increased T-3 uptake, but RAIU, serum cholesterol, etc., are normal (because of competition for binding sites of thyroxin-binding globulin).

Dilantin therapy may induce a lupuslike syndrome.

LABORATORY CHANGES AND SIDE EFFECTS FROM LIPID-LOWERING DRUGS

Nicotinic acid may cause
- Dramatic lowering (often) of blood triglyceride in hyperlipidemia, Types II and IV and probably also Types III and V
- Increased blood sugar
- Increased blood uric acid
- Abnormal liver function tests
- Jaundice (rarely)

Cholestyramine in the form of a chloride salt may cause
- Lowering of cholesterol in familial Type II hyperlipidemia
- Mild hyperchloremic acidosis

HYPERVITAMINOSIS A

Acute intoxication after ingestion of 150–600 mg (500,000–2,000,000 IU).

Chronic hypervitaminosis after ingestion of 7.5–90 mg/day (25,000–300,000 IU) for minimum of 1 month up to 2 years

Plasma vitamin A, 300–1000 μg/dl.

May also show
- Increased ESR
- Increased serum alkaline phosphatase
- Decreased serum albumin
- Increased serum bilirubin
- Decreased hemoglobin
- Slight proteinuria
- Slightly increased serum carotene
- Increased prothrombin time (PT)

VITAMIN D INTOXICATION

Serum calcium may be increased.

Serum phosphorus is usually also increased but sometimes is decreased, with increased urinary phosphorus.

ARSENIC POISONING

From insecticides, rodenticides, herbicides, or therapeutic arsenic, e.g., Fowler's solution.

Chronic

Increased arsenic appears in urine (usually >0.1 mg/L; in acute cases may be >1.0 mg/L). Can be present for up to 10 days after a single exposure. With high industrial exposure, urine level may reach 1600 μg/L. After large seafood meal, level may reach 400 μg/L in 4 hours.

Increased arsenic appears in hair (normal = 0.05 mg/100 gm of hair; chronic toxicity = 0.1–0.5 mg/100 gm of hair; acute toxicity = 1–3 mg/100 gm of hair); may take several weeks to appear.

Increased arsenic appears in nails 6–9 months after exposure.

Moderate anemia is present; commonly normocytic, normochromic, basophilic stippling.

Moderate leukopenia occurs (2000–5000/cu mm), with mild eosinophilia.

Liver function tests show mild abnormalities.

Abnormal renal function is frequent (oliguria, proteinuria, hematuria, casts).

CSF is normal.

Acute

E.g., arsine gas (hydrogen arsenide) causes hemolysis with hemoglobinuria; may cause oliguric renal failure. Cleared from blood in 10 hours; 40% is excreted in 48 hours and 70% within 1 week of ingestion; thus toxic blood levels may be missed. Urine levels are most useful to detect current (1–3 days previously) poisoning.

Laboratory findings due to
- Vomiting
- Profuse watery or bloody diarrhea
- Circulatory collapse
- Renal damage (oliguria, proteinuria, hematuria)

LEAD POISONING (PLUMBISM)

Rapid micromethods for measurement of zinc protoporphyrin (ZPP) (hematofluorometer) and free erythrocyte protoporphyrin (FEP) are recommended as more sensitive indicators of lead poisoning than delta-aminolevulinic acid (delta-ALA) in urine. Especially useful for screening children. ZPP appears only in new RBCs and remains for life of RBC; therefore ZPP does not increase until several weeks after onset of lead exposure and remains high long after lead exposure has ended; therefore is good indicator of total body burden of lead. After therapy or removal of exposure, blood lead becomes normal weeks to months before RBCs.

Delta-ALA is increased in urine. Since it is increased in 75% of asymptomatic lead workers who have normal coproporphyrin in urine, it can be used to detect early excess lead absorption.

Increased coproporphyrin in urine is a reliable sign of intoxication and is often demonstrable before basophilic stippling (but one should rule out a false positive reaction due to drugs such as barbiturates and salicylates). This is a useful rapid screening test.

Confirm diagnosis with determination of
- Blood lead—a single determination cannot distinguish chronic from acute exposure.
  - <20 μg/dl is considered normal.
  - 25–40 μg/dl is evidence of increased lead exposure.
  - >50 μg/dl is a treatable level.
  - 80 μg/dl in children is an indication for emergency treatment.
- Urine lead—must be collected in special lead-free containers.
  - <150 μg/L is normal for adults.
  - <80 μg/L is normal for children.
  - >500 μg/24 hours in children indicates excess mobile total body lead burden and suggests chelation therapy.

Lead mobilization test—administer 500 mg/m^2 (up to 1000 mg) of $CaNa_2EDTA$ followed by measurement of 8-hour urine excretion of lead. Children who excrete >1.0 μg of lead/1 mg of $CaNA_2EDTA$ are defined as having plumbism, and some authors suggest trial of chelation therapy.

Anemia is common, is usually mild (rarely <9 gm/dl). Is usually normochromic and normocytic but may be hypochromic and microcytic, especially in children. Mean corpuscular hemoglobin concentration (MCHC) is reduced only moderately. Is often the first manifestation of chronic lead poisoning; due to decreased hemoglobin production and increased hemolysis. In acute lead poisoning, hemolytic crisis may occur. Anemia may be seen at blood lead levels of 50–80 μg/dl in adults and 40–70 μg/dl in children.

Anisocytosis and poikilocytosis may be found, and a few nucleated RBCs may be seen. Some polychromasia is usual.

Stippled RBCs occur later. Basophilic stippling is not pathognomonic of lead poisoning.

Bone marrow shows erythroid hyperplasia, and 65% of erythroid cells show stippling, some of which are ringed sideroblasts (thus this may be considered a secondary sideroblastic anemia).

Osmotic fragility is decreased, but mechanical fragility is increased.

Hematologic changes of lead poisoning are more marked in patients with iron deficiency.

Urine urobilinogen and uroporphyrin are increased.

Porphobilinogen is normal or slightly increased in urine.

Renal tubular damage occurs, with Fanconi's syndrome (hypophosphatemia, aminoaciduria, and glycosuria), usually in very severe or very chronic cases. Albuminuria, increased WBC, and transient rising serum urea nitrogen (BUN) may occur. Increased serum uric acid is most frequent renal finding; causes saturnine gout.

CSF protein is increased, and frequently up to 100 mononuclear cells/cu mm are present in encephalopathy.

In children, acute encephalopathy may be seen with blood lead ≥ 80 μg/dl; abdominal and GI symptoms may occur with levels of 50 μg/dl but usually indicate levels ≥ 70 μg/dl.

Laboratory changes due to drug therapy

- Dimercaprol (BAL)
  - Daily check for hematuria, proteinuria, cast formation
  - Check every other day for hypokalemia and hypercalcemia
  - Rule out glucose-6-PD deficiency and liver disease before starting therapy.

In adults, usually due to occupational exposure

In children, usually due to pica

In adolescents, may be due to gasoline sniffing

In all groups, epidemics may be due to contamination of water supply, using contaminated pottery, etc.

All blood and urine specimens for lead must be collected in special containers.

ALUMINUM TOXICITY

May occur in chronic renal failure patients on long-term dialysis treatment. Serum aluminum should always be <200 μg/L (7.4 μmol/L); frequent monitoring and close observation for toxicity if serum >100 μg/L. Can be prevented by treatment of dialysate water (e.g., reverse osmosis) so that final aluminum concentration in dialysate is <15 μg/L.

Microcytic hypochromic anemia (non-iron-deficient type)

Osteomalacic osteodystrophy is progressive, associated with a myopathy, resists treatment with vitamin D or its metabolites; may be associated with hypercalcemia. Metastatic calcification is common. Bone biopsy (special techniques) is most reliable test.

Dialysis encephalopathy

Chelation treatment with deferoxamine increases serum level with decrease in protein-bound fraction.

MERCURY POISONING

Levels of mercury in serum, urine, and CSF are increased.

95% of asymptomatic normal people (not exposed to mercury) have a urine value

Table 18-3. Screening for Lead Poisoning in High-Risk Children

	FEP (μg/dl)[a]			
Lead (μg/dl)	≤34	35–109	110–249	≥250
≤24	Retest in 1 year.	Rule out other causes of ↑ FEP.[b] Retest in 3 mos.	Rule out iron deficiency. Retest in 3 mos.	Rule out erythropoietic protoporphyria. Retest in 3 mos.
25–49	Retest next visit.	Retest in 1–3 mos, then every 3–6 mos.[c]	Rule out iron deficiency. Retest in 2–4 weeks.[c]	
50–69	Usual pattern. Retest to confirm.	Retest in 2 weeks, then every 1–3 mos.[d]	Retest stat. Rule out iron deficiency.[d]	Retest stat. Mobilization test or treat.
≥70	Unusual pattern. Retest to rule out contaminated specimen.	Retest stat and treat.	Retest stat and treat.	Hospitalize stat.

[a]Other causes of increased FEP are iron deficiency, anemia of chronic disease, sickle cell disease, erythropoietic protoporphyria.
[b]Iron deficiency and thalassemia should be ruled out even if lead level is increased, since iron deficiency and lead poisoning can occur together. Use blood lead and ZPP together for possible lead poisoning, blood ZPP with serum iron and ferritin for iron deficiency.
[c]Consider mobilization test if lead ≥35 μg/dl.
[d]Consider mobilization test if lead = 35–55 μg/dl. Treat if lead = 56–69 μg/dl.
Source: Westchester County (N.Y.) Dept. of Health (Rev. 8.85).

<20 μg/L and blood level <3 μg/L. Urine and blood levels are nondiagnostic, in that they vary among patients with symptoms, and daily urine levels vary in the same patient. Thus in one epidemic, urine levels ≤1000 μg/L occurred in asymptomatic patients, whereas other patients had symptoms at levels of 200 μg/L. The above values apply to mercury vapor and inorganic mercury salts.

Organic mercury (e.g., ethyl and methyl mercury) is more toxic; accumulates in RBCs and CNS. Most is slowly excreted in feces with half-life of 70 days. Only 10% is excreted in urine; urine levels may be normal even with significant exposure. Phenyl and methoxyethyl mercuries are less toxic and show higher urine levels.

Clinical correlation with organic mercury

	Whole Blood Total Mercury (μg/L or ng/ml or ppm)
Safe level	<100
Probably no symptoms	100–200
Symptoms occasionally present	>650
Symptoms usually present	>1000

ACUTE IRON POISONING

(occurs in children who have ingested medicinal iron preparations)

Increased serum iron. Peak usually occurs 2–4 hours after ingestion.
Levels begin to fall after 6 hours. If the first sample was taken 1–2 hours

after ingestion, a second sample should be obtained several hours later. Serum should be obtained after absorption is complete and before peak serum level falls due to protein-binding and tissue distribution.

- <350 μg/dl is rarely significant clinically; may have mild symptoms.
- 350–500 μg/dl frequently have symptoms but risk of serious abnormality is mild; usually do not require prolonged chelation. 10% develop coma or shock.
- >500 μg/dl within 6 hours of ingestion with severe intoxication; need urgent chelation treatment in hospital. 25% develop coma or shock.
- >1000 μg/dl may be lethal; may require hemodialysis or exchange transfusion. 70% may develop coma or shock.

Increased total iron-binding capacity (TIBC) itself is not useful. Poor prognostic sign when serum iron greatly exceeds TIBC.

Serum glucose >150 mg/dl or WBC >15,000/cu mm and radiopaque material on flat plate of abdomen correlate with increased serum iron level.

Deferoxamine challenge (50 mg/kg up to 1 gm IM) chelates free iron in circulation (100 mg binds 9 mg of iron, chiefly ferric); later appears in urine bound to iron, causing light orange to dark red-brown ("vin rose") color. Parenteral chelation should continue until serum iron <100 μg/dl or urine loses vin rose color.

Renal changes may occur (e.g., acute renal failure, nephrotic syndrome, specific tubular defects).

ORGANIC PHOSPHATE (INSECTICIDES—PARATHION, MALATHION, ETC.) POISONING

Decreased RBC and serum cholinesterase by ≥50% due to inhibition of cholinesterase by organic phosphate pesticides (e.g., diazinon, malathion) and carbamates (e.g., carbaryl).

- Decrease in serum of 40% when first symptoms of acute ingestion appear
- Decrease in serum of 80% when neuromuscular effects occur
- Chronic low-level exposure may be asymptomatic even with decreased levels.

RBC assay is a better reflection of cholinesterase activity in nerve tissue than is serum assay.

In industrial exposure, worker should not return to work until these values rise to 75% of normal. RBC cholinesterase regenerates at rate of 1%/day and returns to baseline in 5–7 weeks. Serum cholinesterase regenerates at rate of 25% in 7–10 days and returns to baseline in 4–6 weeks.

Because of wide normal range, patient may lose 50% of their cholinesterase activity and still be within normal range. Therefore baseline levels should be determined for all workers at risk with organophosphates or carbamates. A decrease of 30–50% from baseline indicates toxicity even if still within normal range.

Without baseline levels, retrospective diagnosis by serial measurements that increase after exposure

Normal variation of ±20% in serum activity and ±10% in RBC activity prevents assessment of mild toxicity and recovery by only one or two assays.

Serum cholinesterase may also be decreased in

- Liver diseases
  - Especially hepatitis (30–50% decrease). Lowest level corresponds to peak of disease and becomes normal with recovery.
  - Cirrhosis with ascites or jaundice (50–70% decrease). Persistent decrease may indicate a poor prognosis.
  - Some patients with metastatic carcinoma (50–70% decrease), obstructive jaundice, congestive heart failure

Congenital inherited recessive decrease. Such patients are *particularly sensitive to administration of succinylcholine during anesthesia.*
Some conditions that may have decreased serum albumin (e.g., malnutrition, anemias, infections, dermatomyositis, acute myocardial infarction, pregnancy, recent surgery, liver diseases—see above)
Other drugs (e.g., prostigmine, quinine, fluoride, neostigmine, tetramethylammonium chloride, carbamate insecticides)

MOTHBALLS (CAMPHOR, PARADICHLOROBENZENE, NAPHTHALENE) POISONING

Paradichlorobenzene inhalation may cause liver damage.
Naphthalene ingestion may cause hemolytic anemia in patients with RBCs deficient in glucose 6-phosphate dehydrogenase (see pp. 315–316).

YELLOW PHOSPHORUS POISONING

(rat poison ingestion)

Acute yellow atrophy of liver occurs.
Vomitus may glow in the dark.

PHENOL AND LYSOL POISONING

Severe acidosis often occurs.
Acute tubular necrosis may develop.

OXALATE POISONING

(due to ingestion of stain remover or ink eradicator containing oxalic acid)

Hypocalcemic tetany (due to formation of insoluble calcium oxalate)

MILK SICKNESS ("TREMBLES")

(poisoning from goldrenrod, snakeroot, richweed, etc., or from eating poisoned animals)

Acidosis
Hypoglycemia
Increased nonprotein nitrogen (particularly guanidine)
Acetonuria

HEAT STROKE

Uniformly increased SGOT (mean is 20 times normal), SGPT (mean is 10 times normal), and LDH (mean is 5 times normal) reach peak on third day and return to normal by 2 weeks. Increased creatine kinase (CK), MM type. Very high levels are often associated with lethal outcome. Consecutive normal values rule out diagnosis of heat stroke.
CSF GOT, GPT, and LDH are normal.
Serum potassium is almost always decreased.
Serum sodium is often decreased but may be high, especially in exertional heat stroke.
Respiratory alkalosis may be mixed with lactic acidosis.
Evidence of kidney damage may vary from mild proteinuria and slight abnormalities of urine sediment and azotemia to acute oliguric renal insufficiency.
Increased WBC count is usual.
Disseminated intravascular coagulation (DIC) is common in severe cases.
Rhabdomyolysis, DIC, and acute renal failure are relatively uncommon in elderly because exertional heat stroke is less common than classic type.

MALIGNANT HYPERTHERMIA

Rare, familial disease triggered by inhalational anesthetics (e.g., halothane, succinylcholine) and other drugs, which cause hyperthermia, muscle rigidity, and 70% fatality, usually during anesthesia.
Marked elevation of serum CK (may be >10,000 IU/L), LDH, and SGOT with peak at 24–48 hours.

Myoglobinemia and myoglobinuria
Serum potassium >7 mEq/l
Combined metabolic and respiratory acidosis
  pH < 7.2
  Base excess > −10
  $PaCO_2$ = 70–120 mmHg
Diagnosis confirmed by in vitro exposure of biopsied skeletal muscle to incremental doses of caffeine and halothane is done in very few laboratories.
Resting serum CK levels may be elevated in relatives. However, serum CK has sensitivity and specificity too low to warrant use for diagnosis or screening and should not be used to diagnose susceptibility to malignant hyperthermia.

ACCIDENTAL HYPOTHERMIA

Acid-base disturbances are very common.
  Initial hyperventilation causes respiratory alkalosis followed by respiratory acidosis due to CO_2 retention.
  Metabolic acidosis due to lactate accumulation. During rewarming, metabolic acidosis may become worse as lactic acid is mobilized from poorly perfused tissues.
Hemoconcentration is common.
WBC frequently falls, but differential is usually normal.
DIC may occur during rewarming.
"Cold diuresis," glycosuria, and natriuresis may occur; oliguria suggests complicating hypovolemia, acute tubular necrosis, rhabdomyolysis, or drug overdose.
Pancreatitis is a frequent complication.
Marked abnormalities in liver function tests are unusual.
Extreme hyperkalemia (>6.8 mEq/L) is a good indicator of death during acute hypothermia.

DROWNING AND NEAR-DROWNING

Hypoxemia (decreased PO_2)
Metabolic acidosis (decreased blood pH)
In severe freshwater aspiration
  Decreased serum sodium and chloride
  Increased serum potassium
  Increased plasma hemoglobin
In severe seawater aspiration
  Hypovolemia
  Increased serum sodium and chloride
  Normal plasma hemoglobin

Aforementioned changes follow aspiration of very large amounts of water. Electrolytes return toward normal within 1 hour following survival, even without therapy.

In near-drowning in fresh water, often
  Normal serum sodium and chloride
  Variable serum potassium
  Increased free plasma hemoglobin; hemoglobinuria may occur.
  Oliguria with transient azotemia and proteinuria may develop.
  Fall in RBC, hemoglobin, and hematocrit in 24 hours
In near-drowning in seawater, often
  Moderate increase in serum sodium and chloride
  Normal or decreased serum potassium
  Normal hemoglobin, hematocrit, and plasma hemoglobin

Blood count may appear normal even when considerable hemolysis is present because usual methodology does not distinguish between hemoglobin within

RBC and free hemoglobin in serum. Fall in hemoglobin and hematocrit may be delayed 1–2 days.

ACUTE CARBON MONOXIDE POISONING

Arterial PO_2 is normal, although O_2 is significantly decreased.
Arterial PCO_2 may be normal or slightly decreased.
Blood pH is markedly decreased (metabolic acidosis due to tissue hypoxia).
Symptoms are correlated with the percentage of carbon monoxide in hemoglobin:

% CO Hb	Symptoms
0–2%	Asymptomatic
2–5%	Found in moderate cigarette smokers; usually asymptomatic but may be slight impairment of intellect
5–10%	Found in heavy cigarette smokers; slight dyspnea with severe exertion
10–20%	Dyspnea with moderate exertion; mild headache
20–30%	Marked headache, irritability, disturbed judgment and memory, easy fatigability
30–40%	Severe headache, dimness of vision, confusion, weakness, nausea
40–50%	Headache, confusion, fainting, ataxia, collapse, hyperventilation
50–60%	Coma, intermittent convulsions
>60%	Respiratory failure and death if exposure is long continued
80%	Rapidly fatal

INJURY DUE TO ELECTRIC CURRENT (INCLUDING LIGHTNING)

Increased WBC with large immature granulocytes
Albuminuria; hemoglobinuria in presence of severe burns
CSF sometimes bloody
Myoglobinuria and increased SGOT, serum CK, etc., indicate severe tissue damage.

BURNS

Decreased plasma volume and blood volume. This decrease follows (and therefore is not due to) marked drop in cardiac output. Greatest fall in plasma volume occurs in the first 12 hours and continues at a much slower rate for only 6–12 hours more. In a 40% burn, plasma volume falls to 25% below preburn levels.

Infection

Burn sepsis: Gram-positive organisms predominate until the third day, when gram-negative organisms become dominant. By fifth day, untreated infection is active. *Fatal burn-wound sepsis shows no noteworthy spread of bacteria beyond wound in half the cases. Before antibiotic therapy, this caused 75% of deaths due to burns; it now causes 10–15% of deaths.*

Laboratory findings due to pneumonia, which now causes most deaths that result from infection. Two-thirds of pneumonia cases are airborne infections. One-third are hematogenous infections and are often due to septic phlebitis at sites of old cutdowns.

Local and systemic infection due to *Candida* and *Phycomycetes*

Laboratory findings due to renal failure. Reported frequency varies—1.3% of total admissions to 15% of patients with burns involving >15% of body surface.

Laboratory findings due to Curling's ulcer—occurs in 11% of burn patients. *Gastric ulcer is more frequent in general, but duodenal ulcer occurs twice as often in children as in adults. Gastric lesions are seen throughout the first month with equal frequency in all age groups, but duodenal ulcers are most frequent in adults during the first week and in children during the third and fourth weeks after the burns.*

Blood viscosity rises acutely; remains elevated for 4–5 days although hematocrit has returned to normal.
Fibrin split products are increased for 3–5 days.
Other findings that may occur in all types of trauma
- Platelet count rises slowly, lasting for 3 weeks.
- Platelet adhesiveness is increased.
- Fibrinogen falls during first 36 hours, then rises steeply for up to 3 months.
- Factors V and VIII may be 4–8 times normal level for up to 3 months.

CONVULSIVE THERAPY

(e.g., electroshock therapy)

Increased CSF GOT and LDH peak (3 times normal) in 12 hours; return to normal by 48 hours.

SNAKEBITE

(mortality <1% in U.S.; 95% due to rattlesnakes)

Pit Vipers

(rattlesnake, copperhead, water moccasin; in U.S. all native snakes with elliptical pupils are poisonous)

Increased WBC (20,000–30,000/cu mm)
Platelets decreased to ~10,000/cu mm within an hour; return to normal in about 4 hours
Burrs on almost all RBCs
Clotting caused by some venoms; normal coagulation prevented by others, which destroy fibrinogen so that fibrin split products are detected, fibrinogen levels are very low or absent, and PT and partial thromboplastin time (PTT) are very high. As a screening test, blood drawn into a modified Lee-White clotting tube that fails to clot within a few minutes of constant agitation is a reliable indication of envenomization.
Albuminuria

Elapidae

(coral snakes, kraits, cobras)

Hemolytic manifestations

Monitor patients with CBC, platelet count, fibrinogen, PT, activated PTT (aPTT), BUN, bilirubin, electrolytes, bilirubin. Platelet count and fibrinogen are most sensitive.
80% of patients treated with antivenin will develop serum sickness reaction. Blood alcohol >0.1% in 40% of people bitten.

SPIDER BITE

Black Widow Spider

(*Latrodectus mactans*)

Moderately increased WBC
Findings of acute nephritis

Brown Spider

(*Loxosceles reclusa*)

Hemolytic anemia with hemoglobinuria and hemoglobinemia
Increased WBC
Thrombocytopenia
Proteinuria

INSECT BITE

(e.g., due to ticks, lice, fleas, bugs, beetles, ants, flies, bees, wasps)

No specific laboratory findings unless secondary infection occurs

SERUM SICKNESS

Decreased WBC due to decreased polymorphonuclear neutrophils; occasionally WBC is increased.

Eosinophils are usually normal.

ESR is normal.

Heterophil agglutination test is often positive and is decreased by guinea pig kidney absorption (see pp. 324–325).

ALLERGIC DISORDERS

Increased serum total IgE is not a sensitive test but extreme values may be helpful:

- Very low levels (<50 μg/L) help exclude atopic disease but not IgE sensitivity to special allergens such as penicillin or Hymenoptera venoms.
- If >900 μg/L, atopic disease is likely, but tests for specific allergens are needed.
- Very high levels (2000 to >60,000 μg/L) are found in asthma associated with severe atopic dermatitis, allergic bronchopulmonary aspergillosis, Buckley syndrome (staphylococcal infections with hyper-IgE), systemic parasitic infestations, IgE myeloma, immune deficiency,

RAST (radioallergosorbent test)—serum IgE antibodies specific for various allergens. Useful when skin testing cannot be done (e.g., children, risk of anaphylaxis) or when skin testing is unreliable (e.g., generalized dermatitis, severe dermographism). Less sensitive than skin and bronchial provocation tests.

Blood eosinophil count >450/cu mm in adults and >750/cu mm in children suggests allergic disorders. Significant number of false positive and false negative results occur.

Nasal cytology smears stained with Wright-Giemsa showing >5% eosinophils, >1% basophils, and/or >50% goblet/epithelial cells suggest allergic disease of respiratory tract. Does not correlate with blood eosinophilia. Large numbers of neutrophils suggest infection. Both eosinophils and neutrophils suggest chronic allergy with superimposed infection. Significant number of false positive and false negative results occur.

Measurement of serum complement is not useful.

IV

Drugs and Laboratory Test Values

Effects of Drugs on Laboratory Test Values

With the coincident ingestion of a large number of drugs and the performance of many laboratory tests (many of which are unsolicited because they are performed on a multitest analyzer), test abnormalities may be due to drugs as often as to disease. Correct interpretation of laboratory tests requires that the physician be aware of all drugs that the patient is taking. It is important to remember that patients often do not tell their physician about medications they are taking (prescribed by other doctors or by the patients themselves). In addition, there is environmental exposure to many drugs and chemicals.

The classes of drugs most often involved include the anticoagulants, anticonvulsants, antihypertensives, anti-infectives, oral hypoglycemics, hormones, and psychoactive agents.

The following lists of the more frequently performed laboratory test values that may be altered by commonly used drugs are only a general guide to the direction of increase or decrease, not an all-inclusive collection of such information.

The selection and arrangement of data by clinical groups provide the most useful, most rapid, and simplest summary of a very complex subject. Only generic names for drugs are used. The frequency of such modified laboratory test values is variable. A number of causative mechanisms may operate, sometimes simultaneously. Thus some changes are due to interference with the chemical reaction used in the testing procedure. Other changes reflect damage to a specific organ, such as the liver or kidney. In some cases, specific metabolic alterations are induced, such as accelerated or retarded formation or excretion of a specific chemical, competition for binding sites, stimulation or suppression of degradative enzymes, etc. Often the mechanism of these altered laboratory test values is not known.

This chapter is meant only as an illustration of various possible mechanisms of such alterations and as a list of some of the more common responsible drugs. It is not to be considered a complete or exhaustive list, nor should it be used to rule out drug-caused effect on a laboratory test by virtue of a drug's not appearing on the lists. For the most specific information, the reader should consult more detailed sources about an individual drug, such as the manufacturer's insert sheets and data, computer-file based data, and the most current literature available published since this and other compilations.

DRUGS THAT MAY CAUSE MARKED ELEVATION OF URINE SPECIFIC GRAVITY

Dextran
Radiopaque contrast media
Sucrose

DRUGS THAT MAY ALTER URINE COLOR

Urine coloration due to drugs may mask other abnormal colors (e.g., due to blood, bile, porphyrins) as well as interfere with various chemical determinations (fluorometric, colorimetric, photometric).

Drug	Resulting Color
Acetophenetidin	Hematuria or pink-red due to metabolite
Aminopyrine	Red or pink
Aminosalicylic acid (PAS)	Discoloration abnormal but not distinctive. May turn red on contact with hypochlorite bleach used as toilet bowl cleaner

Amitriptyline	Blue-green
Anisindione (indanedione)	Orange (alkaline urine), pink-red-brown (acid urine)
Anthraquinones laxatives	Pink to brown
Anticoagulants	Pink to red to brown (due to bleeding)
Antipyrine	Red or pink
Cascara	Brown (acid urine), yellow-pink (alkaline urine), black on standing
Chloroquine	Brown
Chlorzoxazone (metabolite)	Purple, red, pink, rust
Cinchophen	Red-brown
Dihydroxyanthraquinone	Pink to orange (alkaline urine)
Doxorubicin	Red or pink
Emodin	Pink to red to red-brown (alkaline urine)
Ethoxazene	Orange, red, pink, rust
Furazolidone	Brown
Ibuprofen	Red or pink
Indomethacin	Green (due to biliverdin)
Iron sorbitol	Brown
Levodopa	Red-brown
Methocarbamol	Dark brown, black, blue or green on standing
Methyldopa	Red darkens on standing, pink or brown
Methylene blue	Greenish-yellow to blue
Metronidazole (metabolite)	Dark brown
Nitrofurantoin and derivatives	Brown, yellow
Oxamniquine (antiparasitic agent)	Red-orange
Pamaquine	Brown
Phenacetin	Dark brown
Phenazopyridine	Orange to red
Phenindione	Red-orange in alkaline urine
Phenolphthalein	Pink to red to magenta (alkaline urine), orange, rust (acid)
Phenothiazines	Pink, red, purple, orange, rust
Phensuximide	Pink, red, purple, orange, rust
Phenytoin	Red or pink
Primaquine	Rust yellow to brown
Quinacrine (mepacrine)	Deep yellow on acidification
Quinine and derivatives	Brown to black
Rhubarb	Yellow-brown (acid), yellow-pink (alkaline), darkens
Riboflavin	Yellow
Rifampin	Red-orange
Salicylates	Pink to red to brown (due to bleeding)
Salicylazosulfapyridine	Pink, red, purple, orange, rust
Senna	Red (alkaline urine), yellow-brown (acid urine)
Sulfonamides	Rust, yellow, brown
Thiazolsulfone	Pink, red, purple, orange, rust
Tolonium	Blue, green
Triamterene	Green, blue with blue fluorescence

DRUGS THAT MAY CAUSE FALSE POSITIVE TEST FOR URINE PROTEIN

Drugs with nephrotoxic effect (e.g., gold, arsenicals, antimony compounds)

Drugs that may interfere with sulfosalicylic acid methods

- Cephalothin
- Sulfamethoxazole
- Tolbutamide

- Tolmetin sodium
- Other

Drugs that may cause false positive turbidity tests
- Chlorpromazine, promazine
- Penicillin (massive doses)
- Radiopaque contrast media (for up to 3 days)
- Sulfisoxazole
- Thymol
- Other

Drugs that react with Folin-Ciocalteu reagent of Lowry procedure
- Aminosalicylic acid (PAS)
- Dithiazanine
- Other

Drugs that cause false positive reaction with Labstix because of high pH
- Sodium bicarbonate
- Acetazolamide
- Other

DRUGS THAT MAY CAUSE POSITIVE TEST FOR URINE GLUCOSE

Drugs that may cause hyperglycemia with secondary glycosuria (e.g., corticosteroids, indomethacin, isoniazid)

Drugs that cause renal damage (e.g., degraded tetracycline)

Vaginal powders that contain glucose, causing artifactual false positive (e.g., furazolidone)

Drugs that cause false positive test by reducing action with Benedict's solution and Clinitest but not with Clinistix or Tes-Tape
- Acetylsalicylic acid
- Aminosalicylic acid (PAS)
- Cephaloridine (abnormal dark color)
- Cephalothin (brown-black color)
- Chloral hydrate
- Cinchophen
- Nitrofurantoin
- Streptomycin
- Sulfonamides
- Other

DRUGS THAT MAY CAUSE FALSE NEGATIVE TEST FOR URINE GLUCOSE

(glucose oxidase method, e.g., Clinistix, Tes-Tape)

Ascorbic acid
Levodopa (with Clinistix but not Tes-Tape)
Phenazopyridine

DRUGS THAT MAY CAUSE FALSE POSITIVE URINE ACETONE TEST

Ketostix or Acetest Methods	Labstix, Bili-Labstix, etc.
Phenolsulfonphthalein (PSP)	Levodopa
Inositol or methionine	
Metformin, phenformin	

DRUGS THAT MAY CAUSE FALSE POSITIVE URINE DIACETIC ACID TEST

(Gerhardt ferric chloride test; Phenistix)

Aminosalicylic acid (PAS)
Chlorpromazine
Levodopa
Phenothiazines
Salicylates

DRUGS THAT MAY CAUSE POSITIVE TEST FOR URINE AMINO ACIDS

ACTH and cortisone
Tetracyclines (degraded) and other nephrotoxic agents
Gentamicin, neomycin, and kanamycin cause spurious spots on thin-layer chromatograms (Ninhydrin reaction).

DRUGS THAT MAY ALTER URINE TESTS FOR OCCULT BLOOD

Guaiac

False positive
- Bromides
- Copper
- Iodides
- Oxidizing agents

False negative
- Ascorbic acid (high doses)

Benzidine

False positive
- Bromides
- Copper
- Iodides
- Permanganate

DRUGS THAT MAY CAUSE POSITIVE TESTS FOR HEMATURIA OR HEMOGLOBINURIA

Drugs that cause nephrotoxicity (e.g., amphotericin B, bacitracin)
Drugs that cause actual bleeding (e.g., phenylbutazone, indomethacin, coumarin)
Drugs that cause hemolysis (e.g., acetylsalicyclic acid, acetophenetidin, acetanilid)

DRUGS THAT MAY CAUSE POSITIVE TESTS FOR BILE IN URINE

Drugs that cause cholestasis
Drugs that are hepatotoxic
Drugs that interfere with testing methods
- Acriflavine (yellow color when urine is shaken)
- Chlorpromazine (interferes with Bili-Labstix)
- Ethoxazene (atypical red color with Bili-Labstix and Ictotest)
- Mefenamic acid
- Phenazopyridine (false positive with Bili-Labstix and Ictotest)
- Phenothiazines (may interfere with Bili-Labstix)
- Thymol (affects Hay's test for bile acids)

DRUGS THAT MAY CAUSE INCREASED OR DECREASED URINE UROBILINOGEN

Increased

Drugs that interfere with testing methods
- Aminosalicylic acid (PAS)
- Antipyrine
- Bromsulphalein (BSP)
- Cascara
- Chlorpromazine
- Phenazopyridine
- Phenothiazines
- Sulfonamides

Drugs that cause hemolysis

Decreased

Drugs that cause cholestasis

Drugs that reduce the bacterial flora in the GI tract (e.g., chloramphenicol)

DRUGS THAT MAY CAUSE POSITIVE TESTS FOR URINE PORPHYRINS (FLUOROMETRIC METHODS)

Drugs that produce fluorescence
- Acriflavine
- Ethoxazene
- Phenazopyridine

Sulfamethoxazole
Tetracycline

Drugs that may precipitate porphyria

Antipyretics
Barbiturates
Phenylhydrazine
Sulfonamides

DRUGS THAT MAY CAUSE INCREASED OR DECREASED URINE CREATINE

Increased	Decreased
Caffeine	Androgens, anabolic steroids
Methyltestosterone	Thiazides
PSP	

DRUGS THAT MAY CAUSE INCREASED OR DECREASED URINE CREATININE

Increased	Decreased
Ascorbic acid	Androgens, anabolic steroids
Corticosteroids	Thiazides
Levodopa	
Methyldopa	
Nitrofurans	
PSP	

DRUGS THAT MAY CAUSE INCREASED OR DECREASED URINE CALCIUM

Increased	Decreased
Androgens, anabolic steroids	Sodium phytate
Cholestyramine	Thiazides
Corticosteroids	
Dihydrotachysterol, vitamin D parathyroid injections	
Viomycin	

DRUGS THAT MAY CAUSE FALSE POSITIVE PSP TEST IN URINE

Kaolin
Magnesium
Methylene blue
Nicotinic acid
Quinacrine (mepacrine)
Quinidine
Quinine

DRUGS THAT MAY CAUSE INCREASED OR DECREASED URINE 17-KETOSTEROIDS

Increased	Decreased
Ampicillin	Chlordiazepoxide
Cephaloridine	Estrogens
Cephalothin	Meprobamate
Chloramphenicol	Metyrapone
Chlorpromazine	Probenecid
Cloxacillin	Promazine
Dexamethasone	Reserpine
Erythromycin	
Ethinamate	
Meprobamate	

Increased
Nalidixic acid
Oleandomycin
Penicillin
Phenaglycodol
Phenazopyridine
Phenothiazines
Quinidine
Secobarbital
Spironolactone

DRUGS THAT MAY CAUSE INCREASED OR DECREASED URINE 17-HYDROXYCORTICOSTEROIDS

Increased	Decreased
Acetazolamide	Estrogens, oral contraceptives
Chloral hydrate	Phenothiazines
Chlordiazepoxide	Reserpine
Chlorpromazine	
Colchicine	
Erythromycin	
Etryptamine	
Meprobamate	
Oleandomycin	
Paraldehyde	
Quinine and quinidine	
Spironolactone	

DRUGS THAT MAY CAUSE INCREASED URINE CATECHOLAMINES

Alpha$_1$ blockers
Ampicillin
Ascorbic acid
Aspirin
Bananas
Beta blockers
Chloral hydrate
Epinephrine
Erythromycin
Hydralazine
Isoproterenol
Labetalol
Methenamine
Methyldopa
Nicotinic acid (large doses)
Quinine and quinidine
Reserpine
Tetracycline and derivatives
Vitamin B complex
Nose drops, cough and sinus remedies, bronchodilators, appetite suppressants

DRUGS THAT MAY CAUSE DECREASED URINE CATECHOLAMINES

Alpha$_2$ agonists
Bromocriptine
Calcium channel blockers (chronic use)
Converting enzyme inhibitors
Chlorpromazine
Clonidine
Guanethidine
Methenamine mandelate (destroys catecholamines in bladder urine)
Reserpine

DRUGS THAT MAY CAUSE INCREASED OR DECREASED URINARY METANEPHRINES

Increased
Chlorpromazine
Imipramine
Monoamine oxidase (MAO) inhibitors
Phenacetin

Decreased
Levodopa
Propranolol
Radiographic contrast medium (methylglucamine)

DRUGS THAT MAY CAUSE INCREASED OR DECREASED URINE VANILLYLMANDELIC ACID (VMA)

Increased
Aminosalicylic acid (PAS)
Anileridine
Aspirin
Bromosulphalein (BSP)
Certain foods (bananas, caffeine, chocolate, vanilla)
Glyceryl guaiacolate
Isoproterenol
Mephenesin
Methocarbamol
Nalidixic acid
Oxytetracycline
Penicillin
Phenazopyridine
PSP
Sulfa drugs

Decreased
(Usually not depressed to normal in patients with pheochromocytoma)
Clofibrate
Chlorpromazine
Disulfiram
Imipramine
Monoamine oxidase (MAO) inhibitors
Levodopa
Reserpine

DRUGS THAT MAY CAUSE INCREASED OR DECREASED URINE 5-HYDROXYINDOLEACETIC ACID (5-HIAA)

Increased
Acetanilid
Acetophenetidin
Glyceryl guaiacolate
Mephenesin
Methocarbamol
Reserpine

Decreased
Chlorpromazine, promazine
Imipramine
Isoniazid
Monoamine oxidase (MAO) inhibitors
Methenamine
Methyldopa
Phenothiazines
Promethazine

DRUGS THAT MAY CAUSE A FALSE POSITIVE URINE PREGNANCY TEST

Chlorpromazine (frog, rabbit, immunologic)
Phenothiazines (frog, rabbit, immunologic)
Promethazine (Gravindex)

DRUG THAT MAY CAUSE A FALSE NEGATIVE URINE PREGNANCY TEST

Promethazine (DAP test)

DRUGS THAT MAY CAUSE INCREASED OR DECREASED ERYTHROCYTE SEDIMENTATION RATE (ESR)

Increased
Dextran
Methyldopa

Decreased
Quinine (therapeutic)
Salicylates (therapeutic)

Increased	Decreased
Methysergide	Drugs that cause a high glucose level
Penicillamine	
Theophylline	
Trifluperidol	
Vitamin A	

DRUGS THAT MAY CAUSE A POSITIVE DIRECT COOMBS' TEST

Acetophenetidin
Cephalosporins (most common with cephalothin; less frequent with cefazolin and cephapirin; reported in 3–50% of patients)
Chlorpromazine
Chlorpropamide
Dipyrone
Ethosuximide
Hydralazine
Isoniazid
Levodopa
Mefenamic acid
Melphalan
Oxyphenisatin
Penicillin (with daily IV dose of 20 million units/day for several weeks)
Phenacetin (low incidence)
Phenylbutazone
Phenytoin sodium
Procainamide
Quinidine, quinine
Rifampin (rare)
Streptomycin
Sulfonamides
Tetracyclines
Tolbutamide (rare)

Illustrative information: For methyldopa, a positive direct Coombs' test occurs in 10–20% of patients on continued therapy. Occurs rarely in first 6 months of treatment. If not found within 12 months, is unlikely to occur. Is dose-related, with lowest incidence in patients receiving ≤ 1 gm daily. Reversal may take weeks to months after the drug is discontinued.

DRUGS THAT MAY CAUSE POSITIVE TESTS FOR LUPUS ERYTHEMATOSUS CELLS AND/OR ANTINUCLEAR ANTIBODIES (lupus induction)

- Definite
  - High risk
    - Procainamide
    - Hydralazine
  - Low risk
    - Isoniazid
    - Lithium
    - Quinidine
    - Thiouracils
    - Hydantoins
    - Ethosuximide
    - Trimethadione
- Possible (rare)
  - D-Penicillamine
  - Chlorpromazine
  - Reserpine
- Unlikely
  - Allopurinol
  - Gold salts
  - Griseofulvin
  - Methysergide
  - Oral contraceptives
  - Penicillin
  - Streptomycin
  - Sulfonamides
  - Tetracycline

DRUGS THAT MAY CAUSE INCREASED BLEEDING TIME (WHEN PLATELET COUNT IS NORMAL)

Anticoagulants
- Dextran
- Heparin
- Prostacyclin
- Streptokinase-streptodornase

Anti-inflammatory drugs
- Acetylsalicyclic acid
- Indomethacin
- Naproxen

Antibiotics
- Penicillin
- Ampicillin
- Carbenicillin
- Nafcillin
- Piperacillin
- Ticarcillin
- Azlocillin
- Mithramycin
- Moxalactam
- Nitrofurantoin

Others
- Aminocaproic acid
- Ethanol
- Halothane
- Nitroglycerin
- Radiographic contrast agents

DRUGS THAT MAY CAUSE INCREASED OR DECREASED COAGULATION TIME

Increased	**Decreased**
Anticoagulants	Corticosteroids
Tetracyclines	Epinephrine

DRUGS THAT POTENTIATE COUMARIN ACTION
(increase prothrombin time [PT])

Anabolic steroids
Chloral hydrate
Chloramphenicol
Clofibrate
Glucagon
Indomethacin
Mefenamic acid
Neomycin
Oxyphenbutazone
Phenylbutazone
Phenyramidol
Phenytoin sodium
Quinidine
Salicylates
D-Thyroxine

DRUGS THAT *MAY* POTENTIATE COUMARIN ACTION
(increase PT)

Acetaminophen
Allopurinol
Dizzoxide
Disulfiram
Ethacrynic acid
Heparin
Mercaptopurine
Methyldopa
Methylphenidate
Monamine oxidase (MAO) inhibitors
Nalidixic acid
Nortriptyline
Sulfinpyrazone
Sulfonamides (long-acting)
Thyroid drugs
Tolbutamide

DRUGS THAT INHIBIT COUMARIN ACTION
(decrease PT)

Barbiturates
Ethchlorvynol
Glutethimide
Griseofulvin
Heptabarbital
Vitamin K

DRUGS THAT MAY INHIBIT COUMARIN ACTION
(decrease PT)

Adrenocortical steroids
Birth control pills
Cholestyramine
Colchicine
Meprobamate
Rifampin

Patients on long-term coumarin treatment should not take barbiturates, chloral hydrate, chloramphenicol, ethchlorvynol, glutethimide, phenylbutazone (or its congeners), phenyramidol, quinidine, or salicylates.

Patients on long-term coumarin treatment should not take any other drugs without consideration of possible drug interaction.

DRUGS THAT MAY INHIBIT HEPARIN

Antihistamines
Digitalis
Nicotine
Penicillin (intravenous)
Protamine
Tetracycline
Tranquilizers (phenothiazine)

DRUGS THAT MAY CAUSE THROMBOCYTOPENIA BY DEPRESSION OF BONE MARROW

Alkylating agents
Antipurines
Antipyrimidines
D-Asparaginase
Bleomycin
Doxorubicin hydrochloride (Adriamycin)

DRUGS THAT MAY CAUSE IDIOSYNCRATIC THROMBOCYTOPENIA

- Antibacterial agents
  - Isoniazid (INH)
  - Sulfonamides
- Antibiotics
  - Chloramphenicol
  - Streptomycin
- Anticonvulsant drugs
  - Ethosuximide (Zarontin)
  - Methylhydantoin
  - Paramethadione
  - Phenacemide
  - Trimethadione
- Antirheumatic drugs
  - Colchicine
  - Gold salts
  - Indomethacin
  - Phenylbutazone
- Hypoglycemic agents
  - Carbutamide
  - Chlorpropamide
  - Tolbutamide
- Tranquilizers
  - Chlordiazepoxide
  - Chlorpromazine
  - Meprobamate
  - Promazine
- Miscellaneous
  - Acetazolamide
  - Chlorthiazide
  - Hydralazine
  - Quinacrine
  - Tripelennamine
  - Quinidine
- Acetaminophen

DRUGS THAT MAY CAUSE ALLERGIC VASCULAR PURPURA WITH NORMAL PLATELET FUNCTION AND NUMBERS

Acetophenetidin
Aspirin
Camphenazine
Carbromal
Chloral hydrate
Chlorothiazide
Chlorpromazine
Colchicine
Coumarin congeners
Diphenhydramine (Benadryl)
Erythromycin
Griseofulvin
Iodides
Isoniazid
Meprobamate
Oxytetracycline
Phenothiazines
Procaine penicillin
Quinidine
Sulfonamides
Tetracycline
Trifluoperazine

DRUGS THAT MAY CAUSE COLOR CHANGES IN STOOL

Drug	Resulting Color
Alkaline antacids and aluminum salts	White discoloration or speckling
Anticoagulants (excess)	Due to bleeding
Anthraquinones	Brown staining
Bismuth salts	Black
Charcoal	Black
Dithiazanine	Green to blue
Indomethacin	Green (due to biliverdin)
Iron salts	Black
Mercurous chloride	Green
Phenazopyridine	Orange-red
Phenolphthalein	Red
Phenybutazone and oxyphenbutazone	Black (due to bleeding)
Pyrvinium pamoate	Red
Rhubarb	Yellow
Salicylates	Due to bleeding
Santonin	Yellow
Senna	Yellow to brown
Tetracyclines in syrup (due to glucosamine)	Red

DRUGS THAT MAY CAUSE FALSE NEGATIVE TEST FOR OCCULT BLOOD IN STOOL

Vitamin C (usually >500 mg/day)

DRUGS THAT MAY CAUSE INCREASED SERUM GLUCOSE AND/OR IMPAIRED GLUCOSE TOLERANCE

Hormones (e.g., oral contraceptives, thyroid hormone, glucocorticoids, progestins)
Anti-inflammatory agents (e.g., indomethacin)
Diuretic and antihypertensive drugs (e.g., thiazides, furosemide, clonidine)
Neuroactive drugs (e.g., phenothiazines, tricyclics, lithium carbonate, haloperidol, adrenergic agonists)
Others (e.g., isoniazid, heparin, cimetidine, nicotinic acid)

DRUGS THAT MAY CAUSE INCREASED SERUM UREA NITROGEN

Due To

Nephrotoxic effect (see Table 19-1, pp. 750, 752, 754)
Methodologic interference
- Nesslerization (chloral hydrate, chloramphenicol, ammonium salts)
- Berthelot (aminophenol, asparagine, ammonium salts)
- Fearon (acetohexamide, sulfonylureas)

DRUGS THAT MAY CAUSE DECREASED SERUM UREA NITROGEN

Due To

Methodologic interference—Berthelot (chloramphenicol, streptomycin)

DRUGS THAT MAY CAUSE INCREASED SERUM CREATININE

Due To

Interference with tubular secretion of creatinine
- Acetohexamide
- Cephalosporins
- Cimetidine
- Trimethoprim

Methodologic interference (e.g., ascorbic acid, PSP, para-aminohippurate, levodopa)

DRUGS THAT MAY CAUSE INCREASED SERUM URIC ACID

Due To

Cytotoxic effect causing increased turnover rate of nucleic acids (e.g., antimetabolite and chemotherapeutic agents in neoplastic diseases [e.g., methotrexate, busulfan, vincristine, azathioprine, prednisone])
Decreased renal clearance or tubular secretion (e.g., various diuretics [thiazides, furosemide, mercurials])
Nephrotoxic effect (e.g., mitomycin C)
Other effects (e.g., levodopa, phenytoin sodium)
Methodologic interference (e.g., ascorbic acid, levodopa, methyldopa)

DRUGS THAT MAY CAUSE DECREASED SERUM URIC ACID

Due To

Decreased production (allopurinol [xanthine oxidase inhibition])
Uricosuric effect (e.g., probenecid, high doses of salicylates, cinchophen, corticotropin, coumarins, thiazide diuretics, acetohexamide)
Other effects (e.g., corticosteroids, indomethacin)

DRUGS THAT MAY CAUSE INCREASED SERUM CALCIUM

Diuretics (thiazide and chlorthalidone rarely increase serum calcium >1.0 mg/dl)
Therapeutic agents (estrogens, androgens, progestins, tamoxifen, lithium)
Others (e.g., vitamin A, thyroid hormone)
Vitamin D intoxication
Milk-alkali (Burnett's) syndrome
Aluminum-associated osteomalacia

DRUGS THAT MAY CAUSE DECREASED SERUM CALCIUM

Chronic therapeutic use of anticonvulsant drugs (e.g., phenobarbital, phenytoin)

DRUGS THAT MAY CAUSE INCREASED SERUM PHOSPHORUS

Phosphate enemas or infusions
Massive blood transfusions
Excess Vitamin D

DRUGS THAT MAY CAUSE DECREASED SERUM PHOSPHORUS

Hyperalimentation
Nutritional recovery syndrome (rapid refeeding after prolonged starvation)
Administration of IV glucose (e.g., recovery after severe burns, hyperalimentation)
Administration of anabolic steroids, androgens, epinephrine, glucagon, insulin
Administration of diuretics
Administration of phosphate-binding antacids
Salicylate poisoning

DRUGS THAT MAY CAUSE INCREASED SERUM BILIRUBIN

Due To

Hepatotoxic effect
Cholestatic effect
Hemolysis and hemolytic anemia (e.g., antimalarials, streptomycin)
Hemolysis in glucose-6-PD deficiency (e.g., primaquine, sulfa drugs)
Methodologic interference
- Evelyn-Malloy (dextran, novobiocin)
- Diazo reaction (ethoxazene, histidine, indican, phenazopyridine, rifampin, theophylline, tyrosine)
- SMA 12/60 (aminophenol, ascorbic acid, epinephrine, isoproterenol, levodopa, methyldopa, phenelzine)

Spectrophotometric methods (drugs that cause lipemia)

FACTORS THAT MAY CAUSE DECREASED SERUM BILIRUBIN

Presence of hemoglobin
Exposure to sunlight or fluorescent light
Barbiturates (in newborns)

DRUGS THAT MAY CAUSE INCREASED SERUM CHOLESTEROL

Due To

Hepatotoxic effect (e.g., phenytoin sodium)
Cholestatic effect (e.g., androgens and anabolic steroids, thiazides, sulfonamides, promazines, chlorpropamide, cinchophen)
Hormonal effect (e.g., corticosteroids, birth control pills)
Methodologic interference (Zlatkis-Zak reaction) (e.g., bromides, iodides, chlorpromazine, corticosteroids, viomycin, vitamin C, vitamin A)
10% of patients on long-term levodopa therapy

DRUGS THAT MAY CAUSE DECREASED SERUM CHOLESTEROL

Due To

Hepatotoxic effect (e.g., allopurinol, tetracyclines, erythromycin, isoniazid, MAO inhibitors)
Synthesis inhibition (e.g., androgens, chlorpropamide, clomiphene, phenformin)
Diminished synthesis (probable mechanism) (e.g., clofibrate)
Other mechanisms (e.g., azathioprine, kanamycin, neomycin, estrogens, cholestyramine)
Methodologic interference (Zlatkis-Zak reaction) (e.g., thiouracil, nitrates, nitrites)

DRUGS THAT MAY CAUSE INCREASED SERUM TRIGLYCERIDES

Estrogens and birth control pills
Cholestyramine

Due To

Methodologic interference (enzyme reaction) (glyceraldehyde)

DRUGS THAT MAY CAUSE DECREASED SERUM TRIGLYCERIDES

Ascorbic acid	Clofibrate
Phenformin	Asparaginase
Metformin	Other

DRUGS THAT MAY CAUSE INCREASED SERUM SODIUM

Due To

Retention of salt and water (e.g., corticosteroids, guanethidine, phenylbutazone)
Alkalosis (e.g., bicarbonates)

Table 19-1. Effects of Various Drugs on Laboratory Test Values

Drugs	Hepatotoxic and/or cholestatic	Nephrotoxic	Intestinal malabsorption	Serum iron	Serum TIBC	Serum folate (inhibit *L. casei*)	Creatinine	BUN	Uric acid	Calcium	Bilirubin	SGOT/SGPT	Glucose
Antihistamines													
Antimony compounds	+	+											
Arsenicals	+	+											
Caffeine											D		I
Cholinergics											I	I	
Cinchophen	+								D				
Clofibrate	+								D				
Coumarins	+								D				
Cyclophosphamide	+												
Dextran				I				I	I		I		I
Phenytoin sodium	+		+			D							I
Heparin										[a]			
Levodopa									I				
Methotrexate	+					+			I[a]				
Procainamide	+												
Propylthiouracil	+								I[a]				
Quinacrine	+												
Quinine, Quinidine													
Radiopaque contrast media		+							D		+		
Theophylline									I		I		
Vitamins													
Ascorbic acid							I		I		I	I	I
Nicotinic acid (large doses)	+										I		
Vitamin A											I		
Vitamin D		[a]											
Vitamin K													
Hormones													
ACTH				D	D				D				I
Anabolic steroids and androgens	+												
Corticosteroids									D	D			I
Estrogens	+					D							I
Birth control pills (estrogens + progestin)	+			I	I	D							
D-Thyroxine													I

See footnotes on p. 755.

Glucose tolerance	Cholesterol	T-3 uptake	T-4	^{131}I uptake	Amylase/lipase	Sodium	Potassium	Chloride	Prothrombin time	Comments
									D	
I										
					I					Changes due to spasm of sphincter of Oddi
	D								I	D–triglycerides, total lipids, LDH
									I	
										I–protein
D		I	D							D–IgA
		I	D						I	[a]Alters turbidity tests and lipoprotein electrophoresis pattern. May interfere with calcium
			I							
										[a]In gout
		D	D	D					I	[a]SMA methodology
									I	
										I–protein. Serum protein electrophoresis pattern cannot be interpreted.
				D						I–ESR
										D–LDH
	I									
	I									[a]With hypervitaminosis D
									D	
D			D	D	I	I	D	D		
D		D	I							
	I					I	D	I		
D	D	D	I	I						
									D	
	D	I	I						I	

Table 19-1 (continued)

Drugs	Hepatotoxic and/or cholestatic	Nephrotoxic	Intestinal malabsorption	Serum iron	Serum TIBC	Serum folate (inhibit *L. casei*)	Creatinine	BUN	Uric acid	Calcium	Bilirubin	SGOT/SGPT	Glucose
Anti-inflammatory anti-gout, anti-arthritis													
Allopurinol	+								D				
Colchicine	+		+										
Gold	+	+											
Indomethacin	+												
Phenylbutazone	+												
Probenecid	+	+							D				
Salicylates	+	+							I[a]				
Psychoactive Agents													
Chloral hydrate								I[a]					
Chlordiazepoxide	+												
Imipramine	+												
Lithium		+											
Phenobarbital	+					D							
Phenothiazines													
Chlorpromazine	+								D				I
Chlorprothixene	+								D				
Fluphenazine													
Thiothixene	+												
Narcotics													
Codeine											I	I	
Meperidine (Demerol)											I	I	
Morphine (heroin)											I	I	
Marihuana								I	D				D
Antidiabetic (oral)													
Acetohexamide (sulfonylurea)	+							I					
Chlorpropamide	+												
Tolbutamide	+												I[a]
Antihypertensives													
Guanethidine analogs								I				I	D
Hydralazine									I	I		I	I
MAO inhibitors	+		+										
Methyldopa	+						I		I				
Reserpine													I

See footnotes on p. 755.

Glucose tolerance	Cholesterol	T-3 uptake	T-4	^{131}I uptake	Amylase/lipase	Sodium	Potassium	Chloride	Prothrombin time	Comments
									D[a]	[a]On coumarins
										[a]With some methods
									I	
		I		D					I	
		I	D							[a]High doses decrease uric acid
									D	[a]React with Neisler's reagent
		D		D						
										D–VMA and 5-HIAA
		D		D						I–TSH. Mild to moderate I in WBC
									D	
D										D–5-HIAA. May cause false positive pregnancy test
					I					I–LDH. Laboratory changes due to spasm of sphincter of Oddi
					I					
					I					
						I	I	I		
										[a]SMA methodology
I						I		I	I	D–VMA
										D–VMA and 5-HIAA
									I	D–5-HIAA
			D							I–5-HIAA

Table 19-1 (continued)

Drugs	Hepatotoxic and/or cholestatic	Nephrotoxic	Intestinal malabsorption	Serum iron	Serum TIBC	Serum folate (inhibit *L. casei*)	Creatinine	BUN	Uric acid	Calcium	Bilirubin	SGOT/SGPT	Glucose
Diuretics													
Acetazolamide									I				
Chlorthalidone		+											I
Ethacrynic acid	+								I				I
Furosemide								I	I				I
Thiazides	+								I	I			I
Antibiotics, etc.													
Aminosalicylic acid (PAS)	+					D							
Amphotericin B	+	+											
Ampicillin		+				D							
Cephaloridine		+											
Cephalothin													
Chloramphenicol	+			I	D	D		I or D[a]					
Colistin		+											
Erythromycin	+					D						I[a]	
Gentamicin	+	+											
Griseofulvin	+	+											
Isoniazid	+	+										I[a]	
Kanamycin	+	+	+										
Lincomycin	+					D							
Methicillin		+											
Nalidixic acid	+	a											I[b]
Neomycin		+	+										
Nitrofurantoin	+	+											
Novobiocin	+												
Oleandomycin	+												
Oxacillin	+	+											
Penicillin						D							
Polymyxin B		+											
Rifampin	+	+											
Streptomycin		+						D					
Sulfonamides	+	+						I		D			
Tetracyclines	+	+				D							

Table 19-1 (continued)

Glucose tolerance	Cholesterol	T-3 uptake	T-4	^{131}I uptake	Amylase/lipase	Sodium	Potassium	Chloride	Prothrombin time	Comments
D									I	
D						D	D	D	I	
D						D	D	D		
D					I	D	D	D		D–PSP and creatinine tolerance
										[a]Depends on method
										[a]Colorimetric method
			D							[a]SMA method. D–5-HIAA
										[a]Nitrogen retention [b]Copper reduction method
										With massive dosage D–PSP
			D							I–PAH clearance

+ = presence of laboratory test changes due to drug effect on organ; I = values may be increased, elevated, or falsely positive; D = values may be decreased, lowered, or falsely negative.

[a] and [b] See last column on right.

Hepatotoxic refers to liver damage that may alter one or more laboratory tests of liver function, including alkaline phosphatase, bilirubin, transaminase. When this column is marked with a + sign, the individual columns (e.g., bilirubin, SGOT) are not also marked with a + sign.

Nephrotoxic refers to renal damage that may cause changes in BUN, creatinine, urine protein, casts, or cells. When this column is marked with a + sign, the individual columns (e.g., BUN, creatinine) are not also marked with a + sign.

Mineralocorticoid effect (e.g., anabolic steroids, cortisone)
Effect on renal tubules (e.g., clonidine, methoxyflurane, tetracycline)

DRUGS THAT MAY CAUSE DECREASED SERUM SODIUM

Due To

Diuretic effect (e.g., ethacrynic acid, furosemide, thiazides, triamterene, mannitol, ammonium chloride, spironolactone)

DRUGS THAT MAY CAUSE INCREASED SERUM POTASSIUM

Due To

Effect on renal tubules (e.g., spironolactone)
Renal toxicity (e.g., amphotericin B, methicillin, tetracycline)
Antineoplastic agents due to rapid lysis of cells, especially in leukemia and lymphoma
Potassium content (e.g., 1 million units of penicillin G potassium contains 1.7 mEq of potassium)
Heparin sodium (especially in patients with renal insufficiency due to reduction of aldosterone synthesis)
Others (e.g., triamterene)

DRUGS THAT MAY CAUSE DECREASED SERUM POTASSIUM

Due To

Diuretic effect (e.g., ethacrynic acid, furosemide, thiazides)
Increased renal excretion (e.g., corticosteroids, IV EDTA)
Other loss (e.g., chronic laxative abuse, aldosterone, licorice)
Alkalosis (e.g., bicarbonates)
Potassium shift into cells (e.g., glucose, insulin)

DRUGS THAT MAY CAUSE INCREASED SERUM CHLORIDE

Due To

Hyperchloremic alkalosis during prolonged treatment
Chlorothiazide
Hydrochlorothiazide
Retention of salt and water (e.g., corticosteroids, guanethidine, phenylbutazone)
False (methodologic) elevation due to drugs that contain bromides or other halogens

DRUGS THAT MAY CAUSE DECREASED SERUM CHLORIDE

Due To

Alkalosis (e.g., bicarbonates, aldosterone, corticosteroids)
Diuretic effect (e.g., ethacrynic acid, furosemide, thiazides)
Other loss (e.g., chronic laxative abuse)

DRUGS THAT MAY CAUSE INCREASED SERUM CARBON DIOXIDE

Due To

Alkalosis (e.g., bicarbonates, aldosterone, hydrocortisone, thiazides, ethacrynic acid)
Diuretic effect (e.g., metolazone)

DRUGS THAT MAY CAUSE DECREASED SERUM CARBON DIOXIDE

Due To

Nephrotoxic effect (e.g., methicillin, nitrofurantoin, tetracycline, triamterene)
Acidosis (e.g., dimercaprol, paraldehyde, phenformin)

DRUGS THAT MAY CAUSE INCREASED SERUM LACTIC DEHYDROGENASE

Any agent that causes in vivo hemolysis or damage to liver, heart, or skeletal muscle

Alcohol	Levodopa
Anabolic steroids	Meperidine
Anesthetics	Methotrexate
Aspirin	Methyltestosterone
Bismuth salts (LDH_1 and LDH_2)	Mithramycin
Carbenicillin	Morphine
Clindamycin	Nitrofurantoin
Clofibrate	Norethandrolone
Codeine	Oxyphenisatin
Dicumarol	Propoxyphene
Floxuridine	Quinidine
Fluorides (LDH_4 and LDH_5)	Sulfamethoxazole
Halothane	Sulfisoxazole
Imipramine	Xylitol (LDH_5)

DRUGS THAT MAY CAUSE INCREASED SERUM AMYLASE

Due To

Spasm of sphincter of Oddi (e.g., codeine, morphine, meperidine, methacholine, cholinergics)
Liver damage (e.g., birth control pills)
Induced acute pancreatitis (e.g., aminosalicylic acid, azathioprine, corticosteroids, dexamethasone, ethacrynic acid, ethanol, furosemide, thiazides, mercaptopurine, phenformin, triamcinolone)
Methodologic inteference (e.g., pancreozymin [contains amylase], chloride and fluoride salts [enhance amylase activity], lipemic serum [turbidimetric methods])

DRUGS THAT MAY CAUSE DECREASED SERUM AMYLASE

Due To

Methodologic interference (e.g., citrate and oxalate—decrease activity by binding calcium ions)

DRUGS THAT MAY CAUSE INCREASED SERUM LIPASE

Due To

Spasm of sphincter of Oddi (e.g., codeine, morphine, meperidine, methacholine, cholinergics)
Induced acute pancreatitis (see preceding section on serum amylase)
Cholestatic effect (e.g., indomethacin)
Methodologic interference (e.g., pancreozymin [contains lipase], deoxycholate, glycocholate, taurocholate [prevent inactivation of enzyme], bilirubin [turbidimetric methods])

FACTORS THAT MAY CAUSE DECREASED SERUM LIPASE

Due To

Methodologic interference (e.g., presence of hemoglobin, calcium ions)

DRUGS THAT MAY CAUSE INCREASED OR DECREASED T-4

Increased

By increasing thyroxine-binding globulin (TBG)
- Clofibrate (Atromid-S)
- Heroin
- Methadone

Decreased

By decreasing TBG
- Anabolic steroids, androgens
- Aspirin (high doses >2 gm/day; TSH is normal and patient is euthyroid)

Increased	Decreased
Perphenazine (Trilafon)	Chlorpropamide
Phenothiazines	Corticotropin, cortisone, prednisone
Progestins, estrogens	Sulfonamides
Fluorouracil (Adrucil)	Asparaginase (Elspar)
By altering T-4 peripheral conversion	By decreasing T-4 synthesis
Amiodarone	Aminosalicylic acid
L-Thyroxine	Dopamine
Radiopaque agents	Iodides
Iopanoic acid (Telepaque)	Liothyronine
Ipodate (Oragrafin)	Lithium
Propranolol (Inderal) (25–50% increase at doses > 160 mg/day)	Methimazone
	Propylthiouracil
	Sulfonamides
	Sulfonylureas
By stimulating TSH secretion	By displacing T-4 from binding sites
Amphetamines (transient)	Aspirin
	Halofenate (Lipivas)
	Heparin (acute administration)
	Phenylbutazone (Butazolidin)
	Phenytoin
	Tolbutamide
By assay cross reaction	By increasing T-4 hepatic metabolism
Dextrothyroxine	Chlorpromazine
	Phenytoin
	Reserpine

DRUGS THAT MAY CAUSE INCREASED SERUM TSH

Aminoglutethimide	Phenylbutazone
Amphetamine abuse	Nitroprusside
Ethionamide	Resorcinol
Inorganic iodides	Sulfonamides
6-Mercaptopurine	Sulfonylureas

Domperidone and metoclopramide (mild transient effect)
Lithium (can cause hypothyroidism with increased TSH; antimicrosomal and antithyroglobulin antibodies may be present)

DRUGS THAT MAY CAUSE DECREASED SERUM TSH OR TSH RESPONSE TO TRH

Dopamine (prolonged use can cause secondary hypothyroidism with low/normal TSH)
L-Dopa
Glucocorticoids
Phenytoin
Thyroid hormones

DRUGS THAT MAY CAUSE INCREASED PLASMA RENIN ACTIVITY

Diazoxide	Minoxidil
Estrogens	Nitroprusside
Furosemide	Saralasin
Guanethidine	Spironolactone
Hydralazine	Thiazides

DRUGS THAT MAY CAUSE DECREASED PLASMA RENIN ACTIVITY

Clonidine	Propranolol
Methyldopa (slight)	Reserpine

DRUGS THAT MAY CAUSE INCREASED SERUM PROLACTIN

Estrogens and oral contraceptives
Neuroleptics (e.g., phenothiazines, thioxanthenes, butyrophenones)
Antipsychotics (e.g., Compazine, Thorazine, Stelazine, Mellaril, Haldol)
Opiates (morphine, methadone)
Amphetamines
Reserpine
Alpha-methyldopa (Aldomet)
Thyrotropin-releasing hormone
Isoniazid
Dopamine antagonists (e.g., metoclopramide, sulpiride)

DRUGS THAT MAY CAUSE DECREASED SERUM PROLACTIN

Dopamine agonists and ergot derivatives (e.g., bromocriptine, gergotrile mesylate, lisuride hydrogen maleate)
Levodopa, apomorphine, clonidine

DRUGS THAT MAY CAUSE INCREASED PLASMA CATECHOLAMINES

Alpha$_1$ blockers
Aminophylline
Ampicillin
Beta blockers
Caffeine
Chlorpromazine
Diazoxide
Drug withdrawal (alcohol, clonidine)
Epinephrine
Isoproterenol
Labetalol
MAO inhibitors
Methyldopa
Nicotine
Quinidine
Tetracycline
Theophylline

Vasodilator therapy (e.g., nitroglycerin, sodium nitroprusside; calcium channel blockers acutely)

DRUGS THAT MAY CAUSE DECREASED PLASMA CATECHOLAMINES

Alpha$_2$ agonists
Bromocriptine
Calcium channel blockers (chronic use)
Converting enzyme inhibitors
Reserpine

DRUGS THAT MAY CAUSE INCREASED SERUM NOREPINEPHRINE

(see also Urine Catecholamines, p. 742)

Marked
- Some vasodilators (minoxidil, hydralazine)
- Acute clonidine withdrawal
- Some beta blockers (atenolol, metoprolol, propranolol)

Moderate to slight
- Amphetamines
- Ephedrine
- Labetalol
- Methylxanthines
- Metoclopramide
- Naloxone
- Nifedipine
- Phenoxybenzamine
- Phentolamine
- Prazosin
- TRH
- Tricyclic antidepressants

DRUGS THAT MAY CAUSE DECREASED SERUM NOREPINEPHRINE

Alpha-methyltyrosine
Bromocriptine
Chlorpromazine
Cimetidine
Clonidine
Guanabenz
Guanethine
Haloperidol
Methyldopa
Reserpine
Thyroxine

DRUGS THAT HAVE BEEN REPORTED TO CAUSE INCREASED OR DECREASED SERUM NOREPINEPHRINE

Atenolol
Metoprolol
Nadolol
Propranolol
Timolol

DRUGS THAT HAVE BEEN REPORTED TO CAUSE INCREASED SERUM VMA

Anileridine
Nalidixic acid

DRUGS THAT HAVE BEEN REPORTED TO CAUSE DECREASED SERUM VMA

Clofibrate
MAO inhibitors
Methyldopa

DRUGS THAT ALTER CATECHOLAMINE METABOLISM AND MAY PRODUCE VARIABLE CHANGE IN ANY TEST FOR PHEOCHROMOCYTOMA

Levodopa
Phenothiazines
Tricyclic antidepressants

Therapeutic Drug Monitoring and Toxicology

The determination of toxic and effective therapeutic levels of drugs has become one of the most important and widely used functions of the laboratory. In the past, drugs were measured by their effects (e.g., coumadins prolonged prothrombin time, antimicrobials inhibited growth of microorganisms). Newer methodologies now permit determinations of drug levels in the blood that were previously impossible or not available to local laboratories and physicians.

The clinician must be aware of the various influences on pharmacokinetics, factors such as half-life, time to peak and to steady state, protein binding, and excretion, which are not within the province of this book but are useful for the physician in prescribing these drugs appropriately.

The route of administration and sampling time after last dose of drug must be known for proper interpretation. For some drugs, different assay methods produce different values (e.g., quinidine), and the clinician must know the normal range for the test method used on his or her patient.

In general, peak levels alone are useful when testing for toxicity, and trough levels alone are useful for demonstrating a satisfactory therapeutic level. Trough levels can usually be drawn at the time the next dose is administered (*this does not apply to digoxin*). IV and IM administration should usually be sampled 1/2 to 1 hour after administration is ended to determine peak levels.

Levels are meant only as a general guide; the laboratory performing the tests should supply its own values.

Blood should be drawn at a time specified by that laboratory, e.g., 1 hour before the next dose is due to be administered. This trough level should ideally be greater than the minimum effective serum level.

If a drug is administered by IV infusion, blood should be drawn from the opposite arm.

The drug should have been administered at a constant rate for at least 3–5 half-lives before blood levels are drawn.

INDICATIONS FOR THERAPEUTIC DRUG MONITORING

Symptoms or signs of toxicity occur.

Therapeutic effect is not obtained.

Noncompliance is suspected.

Drug has a narrow therapeutic range.

Provide or confirm an optimal dosing schedule

Confirm cause of organ toxicity (e.g., abnormal liver or kidney function tests)

Presence of other diseases or conditions that affect drug utilization

Suspect drug interactions have altered desired or previously achieved therapeutic levels

Drug shows large variations in utilization or metabolism between individuals.

Need medicolegal verification of treatment, cause of death, or injury (e.g., suicide, homicide, accident investigation); detect use of forbidden drugs (e.g., steroids in athletes, narcotics)

Differential diagnosis of coma

CRITERIA FOR THERAPEUTIC DRUG MONITORING

An available methodology that is specific and reliable

Correlation of blood levels with therapeutic and toxic effects

Narrow therapeutic window with danger of toxicity on therapeutic doses

Poor correlation between blood level and dose

Clinical effect of drug not easily determined

DRUGS FOR WHICH THERAPEUTIC DRUG MONITORING MAY BE USEFUL

Antiepileptic drugs
- Phenytoin (Dilantin)
- Phenobarbital

Theophylline
Antimicrobials
- Aminoglycoside
- Chloramphenicol
- Vancomycin
- Flucytosine (5-fluorocytosine)

Antipsychotic drugs
Cyclic antidepressants
Lithium
Cardiac glycosides (digoxin)
Cardiac antiarrhythmics and antianginal drugs
Antihypertensive drugs
Antineoplastic drugs
Cannabinoids
Other drugs of abuse (e.g., cocaine)
Androgenic anabolic steroids
Immunosuppressant drugs
Cyclosporine
Anti-inflammatory drugs
Nonsteroidal drugs
- Salicylates
- Propionic acids
- Oxicams
- Indoleacetic acids

Steroids
Total parenteral nutrition

At present, four drugs (digoxin, phenytoin, phenobarbital, theophylline) account for about 50% of drug monitoring.

LITHIUM

Use: treatment of mania, maintenance for prevention of manic and depressive episodes in bipolar disorders

Therapeutic level = 0.8–1.2 mEq/L based on serum trough level drawn 12 ± 1/2 hours after evening dose; significant time differences can be misleading. Blood should be drawn after steady state (3–10 days) has been achieved. About 25% of manic patients do not respond, and they can be tried at levels of 1.5–2.0 mEq/L if closely monitored. Patient compliance is a major problem in these patients.

Toxic levels >1.5 mEq/L. >3.0 mEq/L can be lethal.

Thyroid and renal function tests should be monitored along with lithium levels and clinical progress.

Peak levels occur 1–2 hours after lithium carbonate or citrate, 4 hours after slow-release preparations.

Recommended blood screening tests before beginning lithium therapy: sodium, potassium, calcium, phosphate, BUN, creatinine, TSH, T-4, CBC, urinalysis with specific gravity and osmolality

Drugs that may cause increased serum lithium levels
- Indomethacin
- Hydrochlorothiazide
- Diclofenac

Drugs that may cause decreased serum lithium levels
- Theophylline
- Aminophylline
- Acetazolamide
- Sodium bicarbonate
- Spironolactone
- Urea

Drug interactions may cause lithium toxicity at low lithium levels, e.g., methyldopa, tetracycline.

Effect of lithium on other laboratory test values
- Increased TSH in 30% of patients (clinically euthyroid)
- Increased parathormone with resultant increased serum calcium and decreased phosphorus
- Decreased serum testosterone
- May affect TRH, growth hormone, ADH

Serum lithium values may be increased by
- Decreased glomerular filtration rate (GFR) (e.g., aging)
- Sodium deprivation and dehydration

Serum lithium values may be decreased by
- Increased GFR (e.g., pregnancy, hemodialysis)
- Burn patients

DIGOXIN

Draw blood 6–8 hours (or 8–24 hours) after last oral dose after steady state has been achieved in 1–2 weeks.

Therapeutic range = 0.5–2.0 ng/ml

Toxic range >3.0 ng/ml, but 10% of patients may show toxicity at <2 ng/ml. Pediatric toxic levels may be higher. Therapeutic index is very low, i.e., small difference between therapeutic and toxic blood levels. But ~10% of patients have serum levels 2–4 ng/ml without evidence of toxicity. On dose of 0.25 mg/day, mean serum level = 1.2 ± 0.4 ng/ml; on dose of 0.5 mg/day, mean serum level = 1.5 ± 0.4 ng/ml; on dose of 0.1 mg/day, mean serum level = 17 ± 6 ng/ml. Digitalis leaf dose of 0.1 gm/day produces same serum level as 0.1 mg/day of crystalline digitoxin. ECG evidence of toxicity in one-third to two-thirds of patients with no symptoms or signs.

Toxicity may occur at lower blood levels in presence of hypokalemia, hypercalcemia, hypomagnesemia, hypoxia, chronic heart disease.

Drugs that may cause increased digoxin blood levels
- Quinidine
- Verapamil
- Amiodarone
- Indomethacin
- Cyclosporine A

Endogenous digoxinlike substances may give a positive test in persons who have not received the drug, especially in
- Uremia
- Postmortem

Increased levels due to endogenous digoxin-like substances may also occur in severe agonal states and postmortem. Thus a high postmortem level may not have been high before death and a normal postmortem level suggests that the antemortem level was not toxic. Thus only high-pressure liquid chromatography (HPLC) or mass spectrometry can definitely identify digoxin as a possible cause of death.

Because most methods measure both endogenous digoxinlike substances and inactive metabolites of digoxin, therapeutic monitoring should mostly be used to assess patient compliance and to confirm drug toxicity.

DIGITOXIN

Draw blood just before next dose or > 6 hours after last dose.
Therapeutic range = 15–30 ng/ml
Toxicity is common with levels > 30 ng/ml.

LIDOCAINE (XYLOCAINE)

(for prevention and treatment of ventricular arrhythmias)

Draw blood 12 hours after beginning therapy.
Indications for monitoring
- Repeat every 12 hours when drug clearance is altered by liver disease, heart failure, acute myocardial infarction.
- Toxicity is suspected.
- Ventricular arrhythmias occur despite therapy.

Therapeutic range = 2–5 μg/ml
Toxic level >6 μg/ml
Levels may be falsely low if blood is collected in some rubber-stoppered tubes.

OTHER ANTIARRHYTHMIC AGENTS

Amiodarone (Cordarone)/Desethylamiodarone

Used for supraventricular and some ventricular arrhythmias
Therapeutic range = 1.5–2.5 μg/ml
Toxic level >3.5 μg/ml
Effect on other laboratory test values
- Abnormal TSH and T-4 values are common and should be monitored during therapy.
- Laboratory changes due to pulmonary fibrosis, which occurs in >2% of patients

Drug interactions: may increase the plasma levels of
- Digoxin
- Diltiazem
- Phenytoin
- Procainamide
- Quinidine

Levels may be increased by severe liver disease (amiodarone) or decreased renal function (desethylamiodarone).

Flecainide (Tambocor)

Used for ventricular arrhythmias
Therapeutic range: trough plasma levels of 0.2–1.0 μg/ml
Toxic level >1.0 μg/ml

Mexiletine (Mexitil)

Used for ventricular arrhythmias
Therapeutic range: plasma trough levels of 0.75–2.0 μg/ml
Toxic level >2.0 μg/ml
Drugs that may cause decreased plasma mexiletine levels
- Phenobarbital
- Phenytoin
- Rifampin

Tocainide (Tonocard)

For long-term use of lidocaine-responsive ventricular arrhythmias
Therapeutic range: plasma level of 5–12 μg/ml
Toxic level >12 μg/ml (peak)
Effect on other laboratory test values
- ANA antibodies or lupus syndrome is rare (unlike procainamide).
- Agranulocytosis—rare
- Hepatitis

Verapamil (Calan)

Calcium channel blocker used for supraventricular dysrhythmias, angina pectoris, hypertension

Therapeutic range: serum levels 50–200 ng/ml (peak)

Toxic levels >400 ng/ml

Drug levels that may be increased by verapamil

- Carbamazepine
- Digoxin

Rifampin may decrease verapamil serum levels.

Nifedipine

Calcium channel blocker used for angina pectoris and hypertension

Therapeutic range: serum levels 25–100 ng/ml

Effect on other laboratory tests

- Decreased glucose tolerance in normal and diabetic patients
- Digoxin levels may be increased by nifedipine.

Diltiazem

Calcium channel blocker used for angina pectoris and hypertension

Therapeutic range: plasma levels 40–200 ng/ml

Effect of diltiazem on other laboratory tests

- Increased bleeding time due to platelet dysfunction

ANTIHYPERTENSIVE DRUGS

There is little correlation between plasma levels and clinical effect.

ETHANOL

For treatment of methanol or ethylene glycol poisoning, desirable blood level = 100 mg/dl.

Criterion for driving an automobile while intoxicated = 100 mg/dl (= 0.1%; 1000 μg/ml).

For diagnosis of alcoholism

- Major criterion
  - Blood level >150 mg/dl without gross evidence of intoxication
- Minor criteria
  - Blood level >300 mg/dl at any time
  - Blood level >100 mg/dl in routine examination

ANTINEOPLASTIC DRUG MONITORING

Despite the large number of classes and drugs available, is clinically useful only in the following instances and the clinical result is improved only with methotrexate.

5-Fluorouracil

To monitor systemic levels with intrahepatic or intraperitoneal use

Melphalan

To monitor absorbance of oral drug

Doxorubicin

To determine kinetics in patients with liver dysfunction

Methotrexate

Therapeutic level $\leq 1.0 \times 10^{-7}$ mol/L

CANNABINOIDS

(marijuana, hashish)

Testing is done to detect drug abuse rather than for therapeutic monitoring.

Plasma levels >1 ng/ml may be found up to 6 days after smoking one marijuana cigarette.

In chronic marijuana users, cannabinoid metabolites have been detected in the urine up to 46 days after last use.
Urines adulterated with bleach, detergent, blood, salt, vinegar may produce negative tests with EMIT (enzyme immunoassay) methods.
Screening tests positive with one method (e.g., EMIT, RAI) should be confirmed with another method (e.g., chromatography, mass spectrometry).

PHENOBARBITAL

(Luminaal)

For treatment of seizure disorders
Draw blood just before next oral dose, after steady state has occurred (11–25 days in adults; 8–15 days in children).
Therapeutic range: 20–40 μg/ml in adults; 15–30 μg/ml in children
Toxic level >55 μg/ml
Monitoring is indicated when patients are poorly controlled, have toxic symptoms, or 2–3 weeks after change in dose or drug (e.g., primidone and mephobarbital, which are metabolized to phenobarbital).
Valproic acid may cause increased serum levels.

PHENYTOIN

(Dilantin)

For monitoring therapeutic oral maintenance, patient should be on stable dose for at least 1 week; draw blood just before next dose. Draw trough level 1 week after beginning treatment and again in 3–5 weeks. After IV administration, draw blood 2–4 hours after loading dose.
Therapeutic drug monitoring is indicated if
- Medication or dosage has changed (allow 1 week to reach steady state)
- Seizures are poorly controlled
- Toxic symptoms occur
- Children (10–13 years old) every 3–4 months until stable level occurs.

Effect on other laboratory tests
- Decreased serum free testosterone
- Increased total testosterone

May be artifactually increased in uremia by various methods (e.g., immunoassay) compared to HPLC
Therapeutic or toxic effects may occur at a lower blood level in presence of decreased serum albumin, increased bilirubin, increased BUN; not altered by dialysis.
Drugs that may cause increased phenytoin blood levels
- Isoniazid
- Phenylbutazone
- Bishydroxycoumarin
- Diazepam
- Chlorpromazine
- Others

Some drugs that may cause decreased phenytoin blood levels
- Ethanol
- Valproic acid
- Carbamazepine

Therapeutic range
- Total = 10–20 μg/ml
- Free = 1–2 μg/ml.

Toxic level
- Total ≥25 μg/ml
- Free ≥2.5 μg/ml

CYCLOSPORINE

(Sandimmune)

Use: Immunosuppressant to prevent rejection of kidney, heart, liver, marrow, pancreas transplants. Possible use in graft-versus-host disease and treatment of autoimmune diseases. Acts by selective inhibition of certain T-lymphocytes; does not affect granulocytes. Often used in combination with corticosteroids. Initial oral dose 4–12 hours prior to transplantation surgery. Oral dose needs to be decreased. (e.g., 5%) during the following weeks or months to maintain constant blood levels. Half-life = 4–6 hours. Peak level 2–6 hours after oral dose. Trough levels 12–18 hours after maintenance oral dose but longer after initial oral dose. Trough level about 12 hours after one IV dose.

Therapeutic range: No immunosuppression with trough whole blood <100 ng/ml. 100–300 ng/ml (trough) in whole blood for kidney transplants. For first weeks after transplantation, rejection occurs with trough values <170 ng/ml; quiescence is usually maintained at ≥200 ng/ml; requirements diminish to 50–75 ng/ml by about 3 months and are maintained for rest of patient's life.

Monitoring: Draw blood just before next dose (trough level). Periodic monitoring (e.g., daily for liver transplant, 3 times/week for kidney transplant) should be performed, but this is not recommended as an emergency procedure.

Threshold for renal toxicity ≥400 ng/ml in whole blood.

- Nephrotoxicity occurs in up to one-half of renal transplant cases and about one-third of heart and liver transplant cases.
- Urine sediment unchanged.
- Nephrotoxicity includes 4 discrete syndromes:
  - Delayed graft function in 10% of cases without cyclosporine and 35% of cases with cyclosporine therapy; resolves when cyclosporine is withdrawn.
  - Acute reversible functional impairment begins to occur at levels of 200 ng/ml and is universal >400 ng/ml. Serum creatinine begins to rise 3–7 days after rise in cyclosporine and falls 2–14 days after cyclosporine is reduced. Decreased GFR, hyperkalemia, acidosis.
  - Hemolytic-uremic syndrome (see Hematology, p. 590).
  - Chronic nephropathy with interstitial fibrosis causes irreversible loss of renal function.

Hepatotoxicity in 4–7% of cases is mild, transient, dose-related; is monitored by increased serum total bilirubin, SGOT, SGPT, alkaline phosphatase, liver biopsy showing hepatocyte damage.

Lymphoma and epithelial malignancy are uncommon (0.1–0.4%); increase with combined immunosuppression.

Acute graft rejection occurs in 50% of patients after renal, heart, liver transplants. May be difficult to differentiate from renal graft rejection, and renal biopsy may be indicated. Monitoring T-cell subsets is reported not useful by some, while others have used rise in T4 and decline in T8 counts to reflect graft rejection. To distinguish nephrotoxicity from renal graft rejection, tests of complement-dependent cytotoxicity, antibody-dependent cell-mediated cytotoxicity, and lymphocyte-mediated cytotoxicity to donor spleen cells obtained at time of donor nephrectomy. Also in bacterial or viral infection, all target cells are destroyed, but with graft rejection, only donor cells are destroyed.

RIA measures parent compound and certain metabolite; high-performance liquid chromatography (HPLC) measures only parent compound. Serum levels are ~60% lower than whole blood.

Drugs that may cause increased serum cyclosporine levels

- Amphotericin B
- Cimetidine
- Corticosteroids

- Diltiazem
- Erythromycin
- Furosemide
- Ketoconazole
- Nicardipine

Drugs that may cause decreased serum cyclosporine levels

- Carbamazepine
- Glutethimide
- Phenobarbital
- Phenytoin
- Rifampin with isoniazid
- Sulfadimidine
- Trimethoprim/sulfamethoxazole (TMP/SMX)

Since cyclosporine contains ethanol, drug interactions may occur with

- Disulfiram (Antabuse)
- Cefamandole
- Cefoperazone
- Chlorpropamide (Diabinase)
- Metronidazole (Flagyl)
- Moxalactam

FLUCYTOSINE (5-FLUOROCYTOSINE)

Antimycotic agent (e.g., *Cryptococcus neoformans, Candida*)

Therapeutic range: serum level of 50–100 mg/L.

Most susceptible organisms are killed at 0.5–12.5 mg/L concentrations. Serum and CSF fungistatic levels of 10–40 mg/L. Bone marrow toxicity becomes prominent at serum levels >125 mg/L or in presence of renal dysfunction.

In addition to drug monitoring, patients should be monitored for liver, kidney, and bone marrow toxicity.

CYCLIC ANTIDEPRESSANTS

Utility of plasma levels is decreased by the lack of objective monitoring criteria, poor correlation of plasma levels with clinical response, and the presence of active metabolites.

Drug levels are usually requested because of lack of clinical response.

Some conditions that may increase tricyclic antidepressant plasma levels

- Aging
- Alcoholic liver disease
- Chloramphenicol
- Cimetidine
- Haloperidol
- Methylphenidate
- Renal failure

Some conditions that may decrease tricyclic antidepressant plasma levels

- Barbiturates
- Chloral hydrate
- Smoking

Should maintain uniformity of collection, e.g., time related to last dose, serum versus plasma, type of container

NONSTEROIDAL ANTI-INFLAMMATORY DRUGS

Salicylates

- Aspirin
- Diflunisal

Propionic acids

- Ibuprofen
- Diclofenac

- Naproxen
- Oxicams
  - Piroxicam
- Indoleacetic acids
  - Indomethacin
  - Sulindac

Except for salicylates, serum levels do not correlate with drug effects, therapeutic ranges have not been established, and routine drug monitoring is not clinically useful.

Therapeutic drug monitoring of salicylates is indicated because of
- Unreliability of clinical symptoms (e.g., tinnitus) as an indication of toxicity
- Narrow anti-inflammatory
- Therapeutic range = 2–20 mg/dl
- Toxic level >50 mg/dl
- Intraindividual variation of up to 300%
- Drug interaction may significantly lower serum salicylate levels (e.g., antacids, ACTH, prednisone).
- After 4 weeks of therapy, serum salicylate levels decline to 65–80% of 1-week levels.

THEOPHYLLINE

Therapeutic range = 10–15 μg/ml; <5 μg/ml is usually ineffective.

Toxic level >25 μg/ml is toxic in 75% of persons.

Levels are usually measured at peak rather than trough. Peak occurs 2 hours after oral standard form and about 5 hours after sustained-release form.

Table 20-1. Reported Reference Ranges of Some Common Therapeutic Drugs

Drug	Therapeutic	Toxic
Acetaminophen (e.g., Anacin, Dristan, Excedrin, Nyquil, Sinutab, Tylenol)	<50 μg/ml	>120 μg/ml
Amitriptyline + nortriptyline	75–225 ng/ml	>500 ng/ml
Nortriptyline (only)	50–150 ng/ml	>500 ng/ml
Bromide	1000–2000 μg/ml	>3000 μg/ml
Butabarbital	1–5 μg/ml	≥10 μg/ml
Butalbital	10–20 μg/ml	>40 μg/ml
Caffeine	5–15 μg/ml	>30 μg/ml
Carbamazepine (P) (Tegretol for seizures)	2–10 μg/ml	>12 μg/ml
Carotene (S)	48–200 μg/dl	
Chlordiazepoxide (S) (Librium)	5–10 μg/ml	>15 μg/ml
Chlorpromazene (S) (Thorazine)	>50 ng/ml	>1500 ng/ml
Clonazepam (seizures)	10–50 ng/ml	>100 ng/ml
Cyclosporine (B)	100–300 mg/ml	>400 ng/ml
Diazepam	0.2–0.8 μg/ml	
Nordiazepam	0.2–1.0 μg/ml	
Total for both	0.4–1.8 μg/ml	>5.0 μg/ml
Dicumarol (P) (Warfarin)	2–5 μg/ml	>10 μg/ml
Digitoxin	15–30 mg/ml	>30 ng/ml
Digoxin	0.5–2.0 ng/ml	≥3.0 ng/ml
Disopyramide (P)	2.0–4.5 μg/ml	≥8.0 μg/ml
Doxepin (combined with metabolite desmethyldoxepin)	100–275 ng/ml	>500 ng/ml
Ethchlorvynol (S)	5–10 μg/ml	>20 μg/ml
Ethosuximide (P)	40–75 μg/ml	>100 μg/ml
Fluoride (P)		>15 μmol/L
Folate, RBC (B)		
≥12 years old	150–800 ng/ml	
1–11 years old	96–362 ng/ml	
<1 year old	74–995 ng/ml	
Glutethimide (S)	0.2–7.0 μg/ml	>10 μg/ml
Gold (S)	1.0–2.0 μg/ml	>5.0 μg/ml
(urine in 24-hr specimen)	<1.0 μg/specimen	>5000 μg/specimen
Imipramine plus desipramine (P)	125–225 ng/ml	>500 ng/ml
Lidocaine (P) (Xylocaine)	2.0–5.0 μg/ml	>6.0 μg/ml
Lithium (S)	0.8–1.2 mEq/L	>1.5 mEq/L
Mephobarbital (P) (phenobarbital should be determined on same specimen)	1–7 μg/ml	>15 μg/ml
Meprobamate (S)	<10 μg/ml	>100 μg/ml
Methaqualone (S)	1–5 μg/ml	>10 μg/ml
Methotrexate (S)	<0.1 μmol/L after 48 hr	
Methsuximide (S)	<1.0 μg/ml	
Methyprylon (S)	<10 μg/ml	>30 μg/ml
Mexiletine (S or P)	0.75–2.0 μg/ml (trough)	>2.0 μg/ml (trough)

Table 20-1 (continued)

Drug	Therapeutic	Toxic
Normethsuximide (should be performed with methsuximide)	20–40 μg/ml	>55 μg/ml
Pentobarbital (S)	1–5 μg/ml	>10 μg/ml
Phenobarbital (P)		
Adults	20–40 μg/ml	>55 μg/ml
Infants & children	15–30 μg/ml	
For reducing intracranial pressure	30–40 μg/ml	
Phenytoin		
Total (P)	10–20 μg/ml	>25 μg/ml
Free (P)	1–2 μg/ml	≥2.5 μg/ml
Primidone (P) (should be performed with phenobarbital determination)		
Adults	9–12.5 μg/ml	≥15 μg/ml
Children <5 years	7–10 μg/ml	
Procainamide (P)	4–8 μg/ml	>16 μg/ml
(should be performed with NAPA determination)	<46 μg/ml (both)	>46 μg/ml (both)
N-Acetylprocainamide (P) (NAPA)	≤30 μg/ml	>30 μg/ml
Propoxyphene (S)	0.2–0.5 μg/ml	>5 μg/ml
Propranolol (P)	50–100 ng/ml	>1000 ng/ml
Quinidine (P)	2.0–5.0 μg/ml	>7.0 μg/ml
Salicylates (S)	2–20 mg/dl (adults)	>50 mg/dl
Secobarbital (S)	1.0–5.0 μg/ml	>7.0 μg/ml
Theophylline (P)		
Adults	10–20 μg/ml	>30 μg/ml
Children	5–20 μg/ml	
Thiocyanate (S)	4–20 μg/ml	>60 μg/ml
Thioridazine (S)	>50 ng/ml	>1500 ng/ml
Tocainide (S)	5–12 μg/ml	>15 μg/ml
Trifluoperazine (S)	<10 ng/ml	>50 ng/ml
Lower limit for detection is 20 ng/ml. Only useful to detect toxic levels.		
Valproic acid (P)	40 μg/ml (trough) 100 μg/ml (peak)	>120 μg/ml
Vitamin A (S)		
Retinol	360–1200 μg/L	
Retinyl esters	≤10 μg/L	
Vitamin B_{12} (S)		
Females >20 years	190–765 ng/L	
Males		
0–29 years	281–1079 ng/L	
30–39 years	248–965 ng/L	
40–49 years	218–863 ng/L	
50–59 years	191–770 ng/L	
60–69 years	168–687 ng/L	
70–79 years	152–630 ng/L	
Folate (S)	2.0–20 μg/L	
Low	<2.0 μg/L	
Increased	>20 μg/L	

Table 20-1 (continued)

Drug	Therapeutic	Toxic
Vitamin C (P) (ascorbic acid)	0.6–2.0 mg/dl	
Vitamin D (S)		
25-hydroxy	14–42 ng/ml (winter) 15–80 ng/ml (summer)	
1,25-dihydroxy	15–60 pg/ml	
Vitamin E (S)		
Alpha-tocopherol	5.5–17.0 mg/L	
Deficiency	<3.0 mg/L	
Excess	>40 mg/L	
Beta/gamma-tocopherol	≤5.5 mg/L	
Antimicrobials		
Amikacin		
Peak	20–25 μg/ml	30 μg/ml
Trough	5–10 μg/ml	10 μg/ml
Chloramphenicol		
Peak	15–25 μg/ml	30 μg/ml
Trough	8–10 μg/ml	15 μg/ml
Flucytosine		
Peak	100 μg/ml	125 μg/ml
Trough	50 μg/ml	125 μg/ml
Gentamicin		
Peak	4–8 μg/ml	8 μg/ml
Trough	1–2 μg/ml	2 μg/ml
Netilmicin		
Peak	4–8 μg/ml	8 μg/ml
Trough	1–2 μg/ml	2 μg/ml
Streptomycin		
Peak	5–20 μg/ml	40 μg/ml
Trough	<5 μg/ml	40 μg/ml
Tobramycin		
Peak	4–8 μg/ml	8 μg/ml
Trough	1–2 μg/ml	>2 μg/ml
Sulfadiazine (S)	100–120 μg/ml	>300 μg/ml
Sulfamethoxazole (S)	90–100 μg/ml	>300 μg/ml
Sulfisoxazole (S)	90–100 μg/ml	>300 μg/ml
Trimethoprim/sulfamethoxazole (TMP/SMX)		
Trimethoprim (peak)	≥5 μg/ml	
Sulfamethoxazole (peak)	≥100 μg/ml	
Vancomycin		
Peak	20–40 μg/ml	40 μg/ml
Trough	5–10 μg/ml	15 μg/ml

P = plasma; S = serum; B = blood.
Source: Data from (1) JB Henry (ed), *Clin Lab Med* Sept 1981; (2) B Gerson (ed), *Clin Lab Med* Sept 1987; (3) S Bakerman, *ABC's of Interpretive Laboratory Data*. Greenville, NC: Interpretive Laboratory Data, Inc., 1984; (4) DE Leavelle (ed), *Mayo Medical Laboratories' Interpretive Handbook*. Rochester, MN: Mayo Medical Laboratories, 1990.

Table 20-2. Reported Reference Ranges of Some Common Toxic Substances

Chemical	Specimen	Normal Range	Toxic Level
Arsenic	Hair or nails	<1.0 μg/gm hair or nails	
	S	<0.07 μg/ml	
	U (24 hr)	<25 μg/specimen	>150 μg/specimen
Cadmium	B	<5.0 ng/ml	
	U (24 hr)	<3 μg/24 hr	
Carbon monoxide	B	<7% <15% in heavy smokers	>20%
Chromium	S	0.3–0.9 μg/L	
	U (24 hr)	<8.0 μg/specimen	
Copper	S	0.75–1.45 μg/ml	
	U (24 hr)	15–60 μg/specimen	
	Liver tissue	10–35 μg/gm dry weight	
Ethanol	B		Toxic >2000 μg/ml
Ethylene glycol	S		Toxic >2 mmol/L Lethal >20 mmol/L
Lead	B	<0.2 μg/ml	
	S	0.8–2.5 ng/ml	
	U (24 hr)	<80 μg/specimen Abnormal >400 μg/specimen Inconclusive 80–400 μg/specimen	
	Hair or nails	<25 μg/gm	
Manganese	S	0.4–0.85 ng/ml	
	U (24 hr)	<0.3 μg/specimen	
Mercury	B	<0.005 μg/ml	>0.05 μg/ml
	U (24 hr)	<20 μg/specimen	>50 μg/specimen
	Hair or nails	<1.0 μg/gm	
Selenium	S	95–165 ng/ml	
	U (24 hr)	<35 μg/specimen	
Silver	S	<0.2 μg/ml	
	U (24 hr)	<1.0 μg/specimen	
Thallium	S	<10 ng/ml	
	U (24 hr)	<10 μg/specimen	
Zinc	S	0.66–1.1 μg/ml	
	U (24 hr)	300–600 μg/specimen	

B = blood; S = serum; U = urine.
Urine level = reported as per 7-ml aliquot of 24-hour urine collection.

Table 20-3. Lower Detectability Limits for Screening Urine for Drugs of Abuse

Drug abuse screen (urine)	Lower limit of detectability (EMIT confirmed by GC/MS)
Alcohol	300 μg/ml
Amphetamines	500 ng/ml
Barbiturates	1000 ng/ml
Benzodiazepines	300 ng/ml
Benzoylecgonine	150 ng/ml
Cocaine	150 ng/ml
Opiates	300 ng/ml
Phencyclidine	25 ng/ml
Tetrahydrocannabinol carboxylic acid	15 ng/ml

EMIT = enzyme multiplied immunoassay technique; GC/MS = gas chromatography/mass sphincterometry.

Source: Adapted from DE Leavelle (ed), *Mayo Medical Laboratories' Interpretive Handbook*. Rochester, MN: Mayo Medical Laboratories, 1990.

Bibliography

Baron EJ and Finegold SM. *Bailey & Scott's Diagnostic Microbiology* (8th ed.). St. Louis: Mosby, 1990.

Baum GL and Wolinsky E (Eds). *Textbook of Pulmonary Diseases* (4th ed.). Boston: Little, Brown, 1989.

DeGroot LJ, et al. (Eds). *Endocrinology*. Philadelphia: Saunders, 1989.

Hurst JW (Ed). *Criteria for Diagnosis*. Boston: Butterworth, 1989.

Jandl JH. *Blood: Textbook of Hematology*. Boston: Little Brown, 1987.

Nyhan WL and Sakati NA. *Diagnostic Recognition of Genetic Disease*. Philadelphia: Lea & Febiger, 1987.

Schrier RW and Gottschalk CW (Eds). *Diseases of the Kidney* (4th ed.). Boston: Little, Brown, 1988.

Scriver CR, Beaudet AL, Sly WS, et al. (Eds). *The Metabolic Basis of Inherited Disease*. New York: McGraw-Hill, 1989.

Stein JH (Ed). *Internal Medicine* (3rd ed.). Boston: Little, Brown, 1990.

Tietz NW, et al. (Eds). *Clinical Guide to Laboratory Tests* (2nd ed.). Philadelphia: Saunders, 1990.

Wallach J. *Interpretation of Pediatric Tests*. Boston: Little, Brown, 1983.

Appendices

Abbreviations and Acronyms

AA	atomic absorption
Ab	antibody
ABG	arterial blood gas
ACh	acetylcholine
ACTH	adrenocorticotropic hormone
ADH	antidiuretic hormone
AF	amniotic fluid
AFB	acid-fast bacillus
AFP	alpha-fetoprotein
Ag	antigen
AG	anion gap
A/G	albumin-globulin ratio
AHF	antihemophilic factor
AIDS	acquired immune deficiency syndrome
ALA	aminolevulinic acid
ALL	acute lymphoblastic leukemia
ALP	alkaline phosphatase
ALT	alanine aminotransferase (SGPT)
AMI	acute myocardial infarction
AML	acute myeloblastic leukemia acute myelocytic leukemia acute myelogenous leukemia
ANA	antinuclear antibody
aPTT	activated partial thromboplastin time
ARC	AIDS-related complex
ARDS	acute respiratory distress syndrome
ASOT	antistreptolysin-O titer
AST	aspartate aminotransferase (SGOT)
BAL	bronchial alveolar lavage
BCG	bacillus Calmette-Guerin
BFP	biologically false positive
BJ protein	Bence-Jones protein
BT	bleeding time
BUN	blood urea nitrogen
C125	C125 tumor antigen
CAH	chronic active hepatitis congenital adrenal hyperplasia
CEA	carcinoembryonic antigen
CF	complement fixation
ChE	cholinesterase
CIE	counterimmunoelectrophoresis
CK	creatine kinase
CLL	chronic lymphocytic leukemia
CMV	cytomegalovirus
CNS	central nervous system
COPD	chronic obstructive pulmonary disease
CRP	C-reactive protein
CSF	cerebrospinal fluid
d	day
D	decreased
DFA	direct fluorescent antibody

DHEA-S	dehydroepiandrosterone sulfate
DIC	disseminated intravascular coagulation
DKA	diabetic ketoacidosis
DNA	deoxyribonucleic acid
DOC	deoxycorticosterone
EBV	Epstein-Barr virus
EIA	enzyme immunoassay
ELISA	enzyme-linked immunosorbent assay
EM	electron microscopy
EMIT	enzyme multiplied immunoassay technique
ENA	extractable nuclear antigen
ERCP	endoscopic retrograde cholangiopancreatography
ESR	erythrocyte sedimentation rate
Fab	antigen-binding fragment of immunoglobulin FAB
FAB	French-American-British classification for acute leukemias
FBS	fasting blood sugar
Fc	crystallizable fragment of immunoglobulin
fl	femtoliter
FNA	fine-needle aspiration
FSH	follicle-stimulating hormone
FTA	fluorescent treponemal antibody
FTA-ABS	fluorescent treponemal antibody absorption test
FTI	free thyroxine index
FT-4	free thyroxine
GFR	glomerular filtration rate
GGT	gamma-glutamyl transferase
GI	gastrointestinal
GOT	glutamic-oxaloacetic transaminase (aspartate aminotransferase [AST])
G-6-PD	glucose 6-phosphate dehydrogenase
GPT	glutamic-pyruvic transaminase (alanine aminotransferase [ALT])
GTT	glucose tolerance test
GU	genitourinary
h	hour
HA	hemagglutination
HAA	hepatitis-associated antigen
Hb A_{1c}	glycosylated hemoglobin, hemoglobin A_{1c}
HAI	hemagglutination inhibition
HAV	hepatitis A virus
Hb	hemoglobin
HB_cAb	hepatitis B core antibody
HB_cAg	hepatitis B core antigen
HB_eAb	hepatitis B e antibody
HB_eAg	hepatitis B e antigen
HBIG	hepatitis B immune globulin
HB_sAb	hepatitis B surface antibody
HB_sAg	hepatitis B surface antigen
HBV	hepatitis B virus
HCG	human chorionic gonadotropin
Hct	hematocrit
HCV	hepatitis C virus
HDL	high-density lipoprotein
HDN	hemolytic disease of the newborn
HDV	hepatitis delta virus
hGH	human growth hormone

HI	hemagglutination inhibition
HIAA	hydroxyindoleacetic acid
HIV	human immunodeficiency virus
HLA	human leukocyte antigen histocompatibility antigen
hpf	high-power field
HPLC	high-pressure liquid chromatography
HSV	herpes simplex virus
HTLV	human T-cell leukemia virus, human T-cell lymphotropic virus
HVA	homovanillic acid
I	increased
ICDH	isocitric dehydrogenase
IEP	immunoelectrophoresis
IF	immunofluorescence
IFA	immunofluorescent assay
Ig	immunoglobulin
IgA	immunoglobulin A
IgD	immunoglobulin D
IgE	immunoglobulin E
IgG	immunoglobulin G
IgM	immunoglobulin M
IHA	indirect hemagglutination
IM	infectious mononucleosis
INH	isoniazid
IRMA	immunoradiometric assay
ITP	idiopathic thrombocytopenic purpura
IV	intravenous
17-KGS	17-ketogenic steroids
17-KS	17-ketosteroids
L	liter
LA	latex agglutination
LAP	leucine aminopeptidase
	leukocyte alkaline phosphatase
LD or LDH	lactate dehydrogenase
LDL	low-density lipoprotein
LE	lupus erythematosus
LH	luteinizing hormone
MAO	monoamine oxidase
MCH	mean corpuscular hemoglobin
MCHC	mean corpuscular hemoglobin concentration
MCV	mean corpuscular volume
MEA, MEN	multiple endocrine neoplasia (syndrome)
mEq	milliequivalent
mg	milligram
MHA-TP	microhemagglutination test (for *Treponema pallidum*)
min	minute
mmHg	millimeters of mercury
mmol	millimole
mol	mole
MoM	multiple of the median (replaces mean of SD from mean when results are skewed rather than Gaussian distribution; e.g., see alpha-fetoprotein)
N	normal
NANB	non-A, non-B hepatitis (hepatitis C)

NBT	nitroblue tetrazolium
NIDDM	non-insulin-dependent diabetes mellitus
5′-NT	5′-nucleotidase
OGTT	oral glucose tolerance test
17-OHKS	17-hydroxyketosteroids
O & P	ova and parasites
PA	pernicious anemia
PAP	Papanicolaou smear prostatic acid phosphatase
PAS	*p*-aminosalicylic acid
PCO_2	partial pressure of carbon dioxide
PCV	packed cell volume
PDW	platelet distribution width
pH	hydrogen ion concentration
PKU	phenylketonuria
PMN	polymorphonuclear neutrophil
PNH	paroxysmal nocturnal hemoglobinuria
PO_2	partial pressure of oxygen
PRA	plasma renin activity
PSA	prostate-specific antigen
PSP	phenolsulfonphthalein
PT	prothrombin time
PTH	parathyroid hormone
PTT	partial thromboplastin time
RA	rheumatoid arthritis
RAIU	thyroid uptake of radioactive iodine
RAST	radioallergosorbent test
RBC	red blood cells
RDW	red cell distribution width
RE	reticuloendothelial
RF	rheumatoid factor
Rh	rhesus factor
RIA	radioimmunoassay
RNA	ribonucleic acid
ROC	receiver-operating characteristic
RSV	respiratory syncytial virus
rT-3	reverse T-3
s	second
SBE	subacute bacterial endocarditis
SGOT	serum glutamic-oxaloacetic transaminase (aspartate aminotransferase [AST])
SGPT	serum glutamic-pyruvic transaminase (alanine aminotransferase [ALT])
SI	Système International d'Unités
SIADH	syndrome of inappropriate antidiuretic hormone secretion
SLE	systemic lupus erythematosus
STD	sexually transmitted disease
T-3	triiodothyronine
T-4	thyroxine
TB	tuberculosis
TBG	thyroxine-binding globulin
TDM	therapeutic drug monitoring
TGT	thromboplastin generation time

THC	marijuana (delta-9-tetrahydrocannabinol)
TIBC	total iron-binding capacity
TLC	thin-layer chromatography
TORCH	toxoplasma, others, rubella, cytomegalovirus, herpes simplex
TP	total protein
TPN	total parenteral nutrition
TRH	thyrotropin-releasing hormone
TSH	thyroid-stimulating hormone
TSI	thyroid-stimulating immunoglobulin
TTP	thrombotic thrombocytopenic purpura
ULN	upper limit of normal
URI	upper respiratory infection
UTI	urinary tract infection
UV	ultraviolet
V	variable
VCA	viral capsid antigen
VDRL	Venereal Disease Research Laboratory (test for syphilis)
VIP	vasoactive intestinal polypeptide
VLDL	very-low-density lipoprotein
VMA	vanillylmandelic acid
vWF	von Willebrand factor
VZV	varicella-zoster virus
WBC	white blood cell, white blood cell count
X	times; e.g., 4 X increase = fourfold increase
Z-E	Zollinger-Ellison (syndrome)

Conversion Factors Between Conventional and Système International Units (SIU)

This list is included to assist the reader to convert values between conventional units and the newer SI units (Système International d'Unités) that have been mandated by many journals. Only common analytes are included.

Table A-1. Hematology

Analyte	Conventional Units	SI Units	Conversion Factors: Conventional to SI Units	Conversion Factors: SI to Conventional Units
WBC count (leukocytes) (B)	/μl or /cu mm or /mm^3	cells × 10^9/L	0.001	1000
(CSF)	/cu mm or	10^6/L	1	1
	/cu μl	10^6/L	10^6	10^{-6}
(SF)	#/μl	#/L	10^6	10^{-6}
Platelet count	10^3/cu mm	10^9/L	1	1
Reticulocytes	/cu mm	10^9/L	0.001	1000
RBC count (erythrocytes) (B)	10^6/μl or /cu mm or /mm^3	10^{12}/L	1	1
(CSF)	/cu mm	10^6/L	1	1
Hematocrit (packed cell volume [PCV])	%	Volume fraction	0.01	100
Mean corpuscular volume (MCV) (volume index)	μ^3 (cubic microns)	fl	1	1
Mean corpuscular hemoglobin (MCH) (color	pg (or μμg)	pg	1	1
index)	pg	fmol	0.06206	16.11
Mean corpuscular hemoglobin concentration	gm/dl	gm/L	10	0.1
(MCHC) (saturation index)	gm/dl	mmol/L	0.6206	1.611
Hemoglobin	gm/dl	gm/L	10	0.1
(whole blood)	gm/dl	mmol/L	0.155	6.45
(plasma)	mg/dl	μmol/L	0.155	6.45
Fetal hemoglobin	%	mol/mol (may omit symbol)	0.01	100
Haptoglobin	mg/dl	mg/L	10	0.1
Fibrinogen	mg/dl	gm/L	0.01	100

For abbreviations, see Table A-2 footnotes, p. 793.

Table A-2. Chemistry

Analyte	Conventional Units	SI Units	Conversion Factors: Conventional to SI Units	Conversion Factors: SI to Conventional Units
Adrenocorticotropic hormone (ACTH)	pg/ml	ng/L	1	1
	pg/ml	pmol/L	0.2202	4.541
Aldosterone				
(S)	ng/dl	nmol/L	0.0277	36.1
(U)	mEq/24 hr	mmol/d	1	1
(U)	µg/24 hr	nmol/d	2.77	0.36
Angiotensin	ng/dl	ng/L	10	0.1
	pg/ml	ng/L	1	1
Angiotensin-converting enzyme (ACE)	nmol/min/ml	U/L	1	1
Antidiuretic hormone (ADH) (vasopressin)	pg/ml	ng/L	1	1
Albumin				
(S)	gm/dl	gm/L	10	0.1
(CSF, AF)	mg/dl	mg/L	10	0.1
Alpha antitrypsin	mg/dl	gm/L	0.01	100
Alpha-fetoprotein (AFP)	ng/ml	µg/L	1	1
(S)	ng/dl	ng/L	10	0.1
	mg/dl	gm/L	0.01	100
	mg/dl	mg/L	10	0.1
	µg/dl	µg/L	10	0.1
Ammonia	µg/dl	µmol/L	0.714	1.4
(P)	µg/dl	µmol/L	0.5872	1.703
Anion gap	mEq/L	mmol/L	1	1
Base excess	mEq/L	mmol/L	1	1
Bicarbonate	mEq/L	mmol/L	1	1
Bilirubin	mg/dl	µmol/L	17.1	0.0584

Table A-2 (continued)

Analyte	Conventional Units	SI Units	Conversion Factors: Conventional to SI Units	Conversion Factors: SI to Conventional Units
Calcitonin	pg/ml	ng/L	1	1
Catecholamines (U)				
Norepinephrine	µg/24 hr	nmol/d	5.91	0.169
	µg/mg creatinine	µmol/mol creatinine	669	0.00149
	pg/ml	pmol/L	5.91	0.169
	ng/ml	nmol/L	5.91	0.169
Epinephrine	µg/24 hr	nmol/d	5.46	0.183
	µg/mg creatinine	µmol/mol creatinine	617	0.00162
	pg/ml	pmol/L	5.46	0.183
	ng/ml	nmol/L	5.46	0.183
Normetanephrine	ng/ml	nmol/L	5.46	0.183
Dopamine	µg/24 hr	nmol/d	6.53	0.153
	µg/mg creatinine	µmol/mol creatinine	738.	0.00136
	pg/ml	pmol/L	6.53	0.153
	ng/ml	nmol/L	6.53	0.153
Chorionic gonadotropin (HCG), beta-subunit	mU/ml	IU/L	1	1
	U/24 hr	IU/d	1	1
Calcium				
(S)	mg/dl	mmol/L	0.25	4.0
	mEq/L	mmol/L	0.5	2.0
(U)	mg/24 hr	mmol/d	0.025	40
Carbon dioxide total (content; CO_2 + bicarbonate)	mEq/L	mmol/L	1	1
CO_2 partial pressure, tension (PCO_2)	mmHg	kPa	0.133	7.52
Standard bicarbonate (hydrogen carbonate)	mEq/L	mmol/L	1	1
Chloride	mEq/L or mg/dl	mmol/L	1	1

CEA	ng/ml	µg/L	1	1
	µg/ml	mg/L	1	1
Ceruloplasmin	mg/dl	mg/L	10	0.1
Cholesterol	mg/dl	mmol/L	0.0259	38.61
HDL-cholesterol	mg/dl	mmol/L	0.0259	38.61
LDL-cholesterol	mg/dl	mmol/L	0.0259	38.61
Copper				
(S)	µg/dl	µmol/L	0.157	6.37
(U)	µg/24 hr	µmol/d	0.0157	63.69
Coproporphyrins (I and III)	µg/dl	nmol/L	15	0.067
(U)	µg/24 hr	nmol/d	1.5	0.67
(F)	µg/gm	nmol/gm	1.5	0.67
Porphobilinogen (PBG)				
(U)	mg/24 hr	µmol/d	4.42	0.226
Cortisol				
(S)	µg/dl	µmol/L	0.028	35.7
	ng/ml	nmol/L	2.76	0.362
17-OHKS (cortisol)	mg/24 hr	µmol/d	2.759	0.3625
(U)	µg/24 hr	nmol/d	2.759	0.3625
Creatine	mg/dl	µmol/L	76.3	0.0131
(S)				
Creatinine				
(S,AF)	mg/dl	µmol/L	88.4	0.0113
(U)	gm/24 hr	mmol/d	8.84	0.1131
(U)	mg/24 hr	mmol/d	0.00884	113.1
(U)	mg/kg/24 hr	µmol/kg/d	8.84	0.113
(C)	ml/min/1.73 m^2	ml/sec/m^2	0.00963	104
cAMP (cyclic adenosine monophosphate)				
(S)	µg/L	nmol/L	3.04	0.329
(B)	ng/ml	nmol/L	3.04	0.329
(U)	mg/24 hr	µmol/d	3.04	0.329
(U)	mg/gm creatinine	µmol/mol creatinine	344	0.00291

Table A-2 (continued)

Analyte	Conventional Units	SI Units	Conversion Factors: Conventional to SI Units	Conversion Factors: SI to Conventional Units
Dehydroepiandrosterone sulfate (DHEA-S)				
(S)	μg/ml	μmol/L	2.6	0.38
(AF)	ng/ml	nmol/L	2.6	0.38
17-Ketosteroids (as DHEA)				
(U)	mg/24 hr	μmol/d	3.467	0.2904
17-Ketogenic steroids (as DHEA)				
(U)	mg/24 hr	μmol/d	3.467	0.2904
17-Hydroxycorticosteroids (17-OHCS)				
(U)	mg/d of creatinine	mg/mol of creatinine	113.1	0.00884
11-Deoxy corticosterone (DOC)				
(S)	pg/ml	pmol/L	3.03	0.33
Glucose	mg/dl	mmol/L	0.0555	18.02
Ferritin	ng/ml	μg/L	1	1
Gastrin	pg/ml	ng/L	1	1
Growth hormone	ng/ml	μg/L	1	1
Homovanillic acid (HVA)				
(U)	mg/24 hr	μmol/d	5.49	0.182
	μg/24 hr	μmol/d	0.00549	182
	μg/mg of creatinine	mmol/mol of creatinine	0.621	1.61
5-Hydroxyindoleacetic acid (5-HIAA)				
(U)	mg/24 hr	μmol/d	5.2	0.19
Hormone receptors (T)				
Progesterone receptor assay (PRA)	fmol/mg of protein	nmol/kg of protein	1	1
Estrogen receptor assay (ERA)	fmol/mg of protein	nmol/kg of protein	1	1
Iron	μg/dl	μmol/L	0.179	5.587
Iron-binding capacity	μg/dl	μmol/L	0.179	5.587

Iron saturation	%	fraction saturation	0.01	100
Lactate	mg/dl	mmol/L	0.111	9.01
Lead				
(S)	μg/dl	μmol/L	0.0483	20.72
(S)	mg/dl	μmol/L	48.26	
(U)	μg/24 hr	μmol/d	0.00483	
Lipids (total)	mg/dl	gm/L	0.01	100
Magnesium	mEq/L	mmol/L	0.5	2
	mg/dl	mmol/L	0.411	2.433
Osmolality	mOsml/kg	same		
O_2 partial pressure (PaO_2)	mm Hg	kPa	0.133	7.5
Parathyroid hormone	pg/ml	ng/L	1	1
	μlEq/ml	mlEq/L	1	1
Phosphate (inorganic phosphorus)				
(S)	mg/dl	mmol/L	0.323	3.10
(U)	gm/24 hr	mmol/d	32.3	0.031
pH	nEq/L	nmol/L	1	1
Porphobilinogen	μg/d	μmol/d	4.42	0.226
Potassium				
(S)	mEq/L	mmol/L	1	1
(U)	mEq/24 hr	mmol/L	1	1
(U)	mg/24 hr	mmol/d	0.02558	39.1
Protein, total				
(S)	gm/dl	gm/L	10	0.1
(U)	mg/24 hr	gm/d	0.001	1000
(CSF)	mg/dl	mg/L	10	0.1
Renin (plasma renin activity [PRA])	ng/ml/hr	μg/L/hr	1	1
Sodium				
(S)	mEq/L	mmol/L	1	1
(U)	mEq/24 hr	mmol/L	1	1
(U)	mg/24 hr	mmol/d	0.0435	22.99

Table A-2 (continued)

Analyte	Conventional Units	SI Units	Conversion Factors	
			Conventional to SI Units	SI to Conventional Units
Serotonin				
(S)	ng/ml	μmol/L	0.00568	176
Testosterone (total)				
(S)	ng/dl	nmol/L	0.0347	28.8
Thyroid-binding globulin (TBG)	mg/dl	mg/L	10	0.1
	μg/dl	μg/L	10	0.1
Thyroglobulin	ng/ml	μg/L	1	1
TSH (thyroid-stimulating hormone)	μU/ml	mIU/L	1	1
Thyrotropin-releasing hormone (TRH)	pg/ml	ng/L	1	1
Triiodothyronine, total (T-3)	ng/dl	nmol/L	0.0154	65.1
Reverse T-3 (rT-3)	ng/dl	nmol/L	0.0154	65.1
Thyroxine, total (T-4)	μg/dl	nmol/L	12.9	0.0775
Transferrin (TIBC)	mg/dl	gm/L	0.01	100
Triglycerides	mg/dl	mmol/L	0.0113	88.5

Urea nitrogen				
(S)	mg/dl	mmol/L	0.357	2.8
(U)	gm/24 hr	mol/d	0.0357	28
Uric acid				
(S)	mg/dl	mmol/L	0.05948	16.9
(U)	mg/24 hr	mmol/d	0.0059	169
Vanillylmandelic acid (VMA)				
(U)	mg/24 hr	μmol/d	5.05	0.198
	μg/mg of creatinine	mmol/mol of creatinine	0.571	1.75
Viscosity (S)	centipoise	same		
Vitamin B_{12} (cyanocobalamin)	pg/ml	pmol/L	0.738	1.355
Unsaturated B_{12} binding capacity				
(S)	pg/ml	pmol/L	0.738	1.355
Vitamin C (ascorbic acid)	mg/dl	μmol/L	56.78	0.176
Vitamin A	μg/dl	μmol/L	0.0349	28.65
Vitamin D (calcitriol; 1,25-dihydroxy)	pg/ml	pmol/L	2.4	0.417
Xylose (U)	mg/dl	mmol/L	0.0666	15.01
	gm/5 hr	mmol/5 hr	6.66	0.15

μ = microns; μmol = micromoles; mmol = millimoles; nmol = nanomoles; fmol = fentamoles; mg = milligrams; gm = grams; pg = picograms; ng = nanograms; L = liter; ml = milliliter; mEq = milliequivalent; ml/sec = milliliter/second; ml/min = milliliter/minute; U = units; mU = milliunits; IU = international units; d = day; 24 hr = 24 hours; S = serum; U = urine; B = blood; C = clearance; F = feces; AF = amniotic fluid; SF = synovial fluid; T = tissue. All references are to serum unless otherwise indicated.

Table A-3. Enzymes

Conventional Unit	IU/L Equivalent	
Acid phosphatase (prostatic)		
Bodansky	5.37	
Shinowara-Jones-Reinhart	5.37	
King-Armstrong	1.77	
Bessey-Lowry-Brock	16.67	
Alkaline phosphatase		
Bodansky	5.37	
Shinowara-Jones-Reinhart	5.37	
King-Armstrong	7.1	0.14
Bessey-Lowry-Brock	16.67	
Babson	1.0	
Aldolase		
Sibley-Lehninger	0.74	
Amylase		
Somogyi (saccharogenic)	1.85	0.541
Somogyi	20.6	
Creatine kinase (CK)	1.0	
Hydroxybutyric dehydrogenase (α-HBD)		
Rosalki-Wilkinson	0.482	
Isocitrate dehydrogenase (ICD)		
Wolfson-Williams-Ashman	0.0167	
Taylor-Friedman	0.0167	
Lactate dehydrogenase (LDH)		
Wroblewski	0.482	
Lipase		
Cherry-Crandal	278	
Malic dehydrogenase (MD)		
Wacker-Ulmer-Valee	0.482	
Transaminases		
Reitman-Frankel	0.482	
Karmen	0.482	

Table A-4. Therapeutic and Toxic Drugs

Analyte	Conventional Units	SI Units	Conversion Factors	
			Conventional to SI Units	SI to Conventional Units
Acetaminophen	μg/ml	μmol/L	6.62	0.151
Amikacin	μg/ml	μmol/L	1.71	0.585
Amitriptyline	ng/ml	nmol/L	3.61	0.277
Amobarbital	μg/ml	μmol/L	4.42	0.226
Amphetamine	ng/ml	nmol/L	7.4	0.135
	μg/ml	μmol/L	7.4	0.135
Bromide	μg/ml	mmol/L	0.0125	79.9
Caffeine	μg/ml	μmol/L	5.15	0.194
Carbamazepine (Tegretol)	μg/ml	μmol/L	4.23	0.236
Carbenicillin	μg/ml	μmol/L	2.64	0.378
Chloral hydrate	μg/ml	μmol/L	6.69	0.149
Chloramphenicol	μg/ml	μmol/L	3.09	0.323
Chlordiazepoxide (Librium)	ng/ml	μmol/L	0.00334	300
Chlorpromazine (Thorazine)	ng/ml	nmol/L	3.14	0.319
Chlorpropamide (Diabinese)	μg/ml	μmol/L	3.61	0.227
Cimetidine (Tagamet)	μg/ml	μmol/L	3.96	0.252
Clonazepam (Clonopin)	ng/ml	nmol/L	3.17	0.316
Clonidine (Catapres)	ng/ml	nmol/L	4.35	0.230

Table A-4 (continued)

Analyte	Conventional Units	SI Units	Conversion Factors: Conventional to SI Units	Conversion Factors: SI to Conventional Units
Cocaine	ng/ml	nmol/L	3.3	0.303
Codeine	ng/ml	nmol/L	3.34	0.299
Demerol (Meperidine)	ng/ml	nmol/L	4.04	0.247
Desipramine (Norpramin)	ng/ml	nmol/L	3.75	0.267
Diazepam (Valium)	ng/ml	μmol/L	0.0035	285
Digitoxin	ng/ml	nmol/L	1.31	0.765
Digoxin	ng/ml	nmol/L	1.28	0.781
Dilaudid	ng/ml	nmol/L	4.85	0.206
Disulfiram	μg/ml	μmol/L	12.12	0.0761
Doxepin (Sinequan)	ng/ml	nmol/L	3.58	0.279
Ethanol	mg/dl	mmol/L	0.217	4.61
Ethchlorvynol (Placidyl)	μg/ml	μmol/L	6.92	0.145
Ethosuximide (Zarontin)	μg/ml	μmol/L	7.08	0.141
Gentamicin	μg/ml	μmol/L	2.09	0.478
Glutethimide (Doriden)	μg/ml	μmol/L	4.60	0.217
Haloperidol (Haldol)	ng/ml	nmol/L	2.66	0.376

Ibuprofen	μg/ml	μmol/L	4.85	0.206
Imipramine (Tofranil)	ng/ml	nmol/L	3.57	0.28
Isoniazid	μg/ml	μmol/L	7.29	0.137
Kanamycin (Kantrex)	μg/ml	μmol/L	2.06	0.485
Lidocaine (Xylocaine)	μg/ml	μmol/L	4.27	0.234
Lithium	mEq/L	mmol/L	1	1
Lorazepam	ng/ml	nmol/L	3.11	0.321
LSD (lysergic acid diethylamide)	μg/ml	μmol/L	3.09	0.323
Meprobamate	mg/L	μmol/L	4.58	0.218
Methadone	ng/ml	μmol/L	0.00323	309
Methaqualone (Quaalude)	μg/ml	μmol/L	4.0	0.250
Methotrexate	ng/ml	nmol/L	2.2	0.454
Methsuximide	μg/ml	μmol/L	5.29	0.189
Methyldopa (Aldomet)	μg/ml	μmol/L	4.73	0.211
Morphine	ng/ml	nmol/L	3.5	0.285
	ng/ml	μmol/L	0.0035	285
Nortriptyline	ng/ml	nmol/L	3.8	0.263
Oxazepam	μg/ml	μmol/L	3.49	0.287
Paraldehyde	μg/ml	μmol/L	7.57	0.132
Pentobarbital (Nembutal)	μg/ml	μmol/L	4.42	0.179
Percodan	ng/ml	nmol/L	3.17	0.315
Phenacetin	μg/ml	μmol/L	5.58	0.179
Phenobarbital (Luminal)	μg/ml	μmol/L	4.31	0.232

Table A-4 (continued)

Analyte	Conventional Units	SI Units	Conversion Factors	
			Conventional to SI Units	SI to Conventional Units
Phenylbutazone (Butazolidin)	μg/ml	μmol/L	3.08	0.324
Phenytoin (Dilantin)	μg/ml	μmol/L	3.96	0.253
Primidone	μg/ml	μmol/L	4.58	0.218
Procainamide (Pronestyl), procaine (Novocain)	μg/ml	μmol/L	4.23	0.236
Propoxyphene (Darvon)	μg/ml	μmol/L	3.07	0.326
Propranolol	ng/ml	nmol/L	3.86	0.259
Quinidine	μg/ml	μmol/L	3.08	0.324
Quinine	μg/ml	μmol/L	3.08	0.324
Salicylic acid	μg/ml	μmol/L	7.24	0.138
Secobarbital (Seconal)	μg/ml	μmol/L	4.2	0.238
Theophylline (aminophylline)	μg/ml	μmol/L	5.55	0.180
Tobramycin	μg/ml	μmol/L	2.14	0.467
Valproic acid	μg/ml	μmol/L	6.93	0.144
Vancomycin	μg/ml	mg/L	1	1
Warfarin (Coumadin)	μg/ml	μmol/L	3.24	0.308

Table A-5. Multiples of SI Units

Prefix	Factor	Prefix	Factor
kilo	10^3	milli	10^{-3}
mega	10^6	micro	10^{-6}
giga	10^9	nano	10^{-9}
tetra	10^{12}	pico	10^{-12}
		femto	10^{-15}
		atto	10^{-18}

BIBLIOGRAPHY

McQueen MJ. *SI Unit Pocket Guide.* Chicago: ASCP Press, 1990.

Système International Conversion Factors for Frequently Used Laboratory Components. *JAMA* 260:74, 1988.

Tietz NW and Finley PR. *Clinical Guide to Laboratory Tests.* Philadelphia: Saunders, 1983.

Tietz NW, et al. *Textbook of Clinical Chemistry.* Philadelphia: Saunders, 1986.

Young DS. Implementation of SI Units for clinical laboratory data: Style specification and conversion tables. *Ann Intern Med* 106:114, 1987.

Index